# THE BIG SKINNY

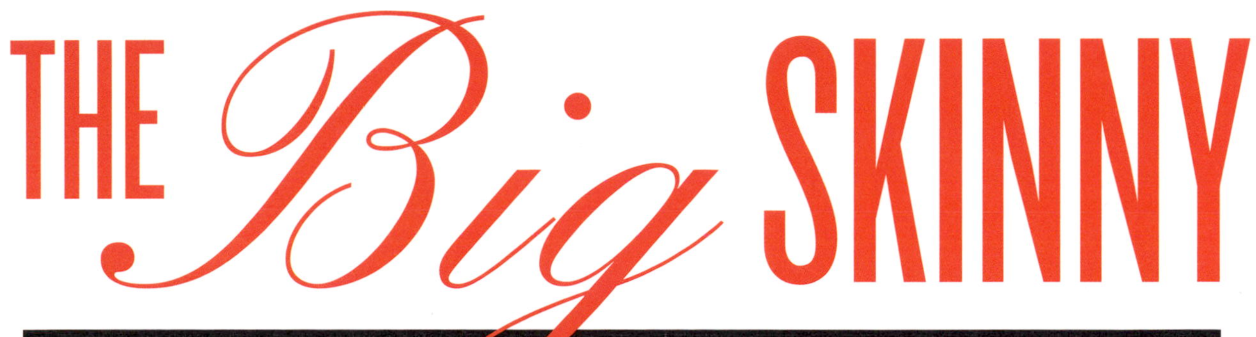

# THE Big SKINNY

## HOW I CHANGED MY FATTITUDE

*a memoir*

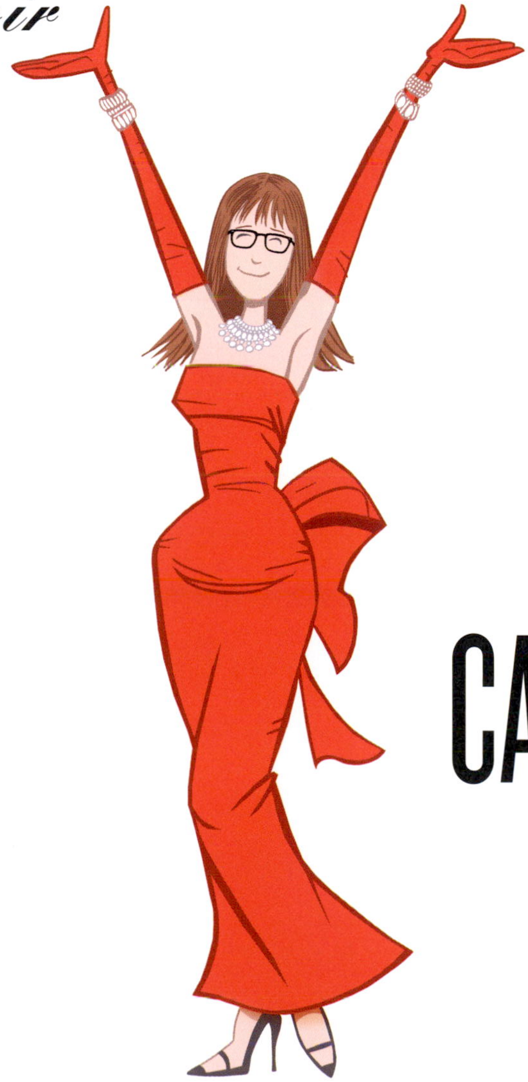

CAROL LAY

VILLARD BOOKS NEW YORK

This book includes detailed information about the diet and exercise choices I have made and found helpful. Obviously, I'm not a physician, and you should consult a qualified medical professional (and, if you are pregnant, your ob-gyn) before starting any serious weight control or fitness program.

A Villard Books Trade Paperback Original



Published in the United States by Villard Books, an imprint of The Random House Publishing Group, a division of Random House, Inc., New York.

VILLARD and "V" CIRCLED Design are registered trademarks of Random House, Inc.

ISBN 978-0-345-50404-3

Printed in the United States of America

www.villard.com

2 4 6 8 9 7 5 3 1

# CONTENTS

# THE BIG SKINNY

# What's It All About?

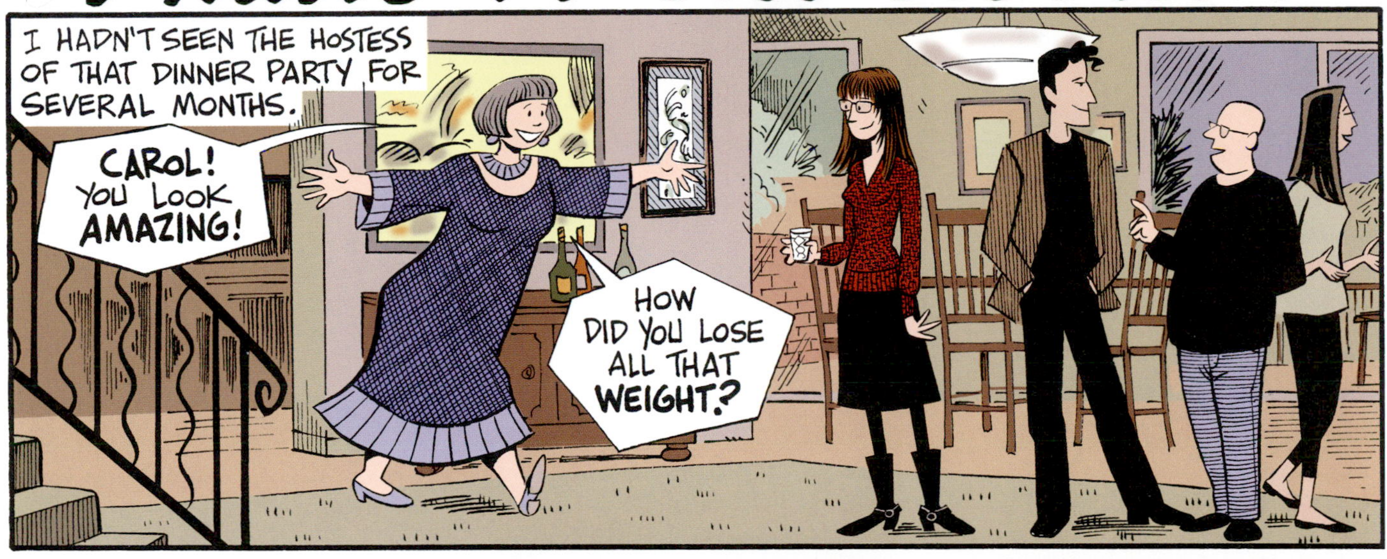
I HADN'T SEEN THE HOSTESS OF THAT DINNER PARTY FOR SEVERAL MONTHS.
CAROL! YOU LOOK AMAZING!
HOW DID YOU LOSE ALL THAT WEIGHT?

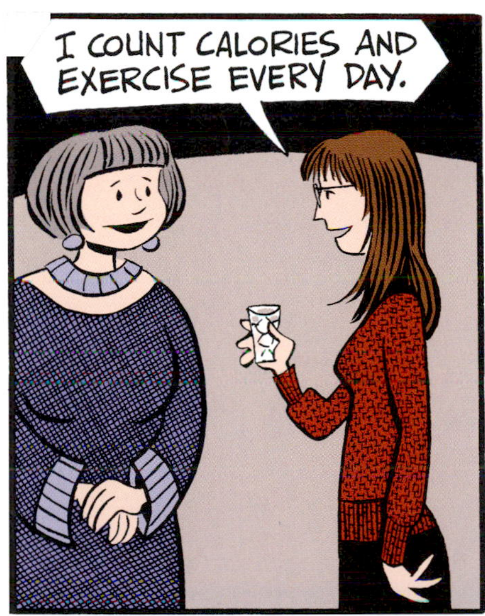
I COUNT CALORIES AND EXERCISE EVERY DAY.

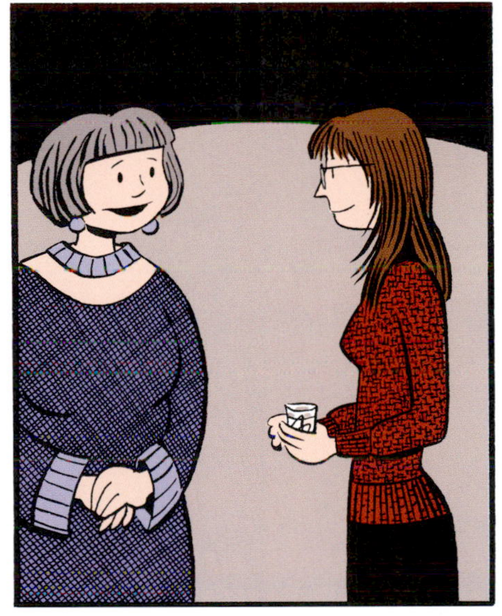

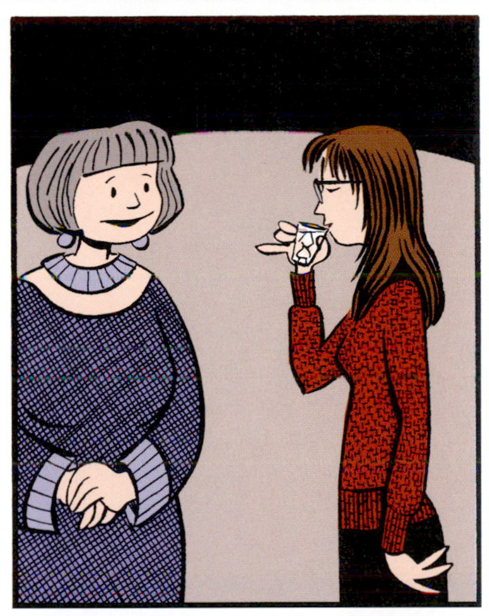

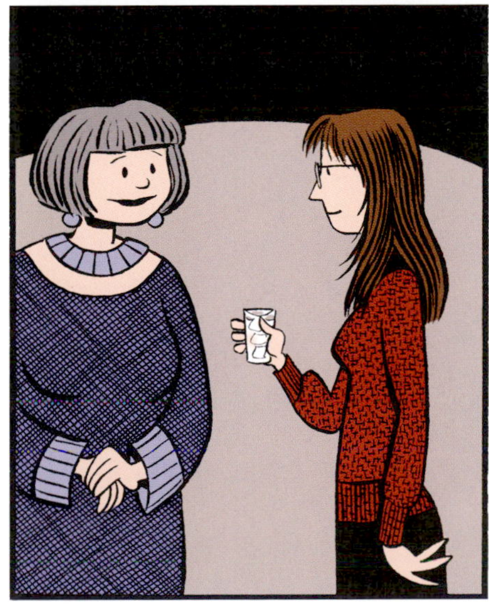

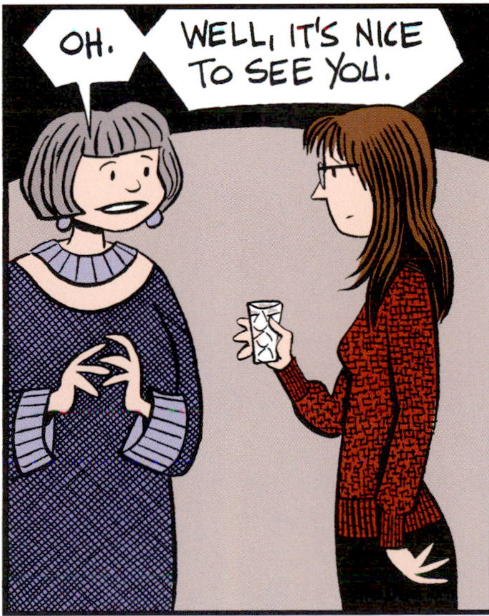
OH.
WELL, IT'S NICE TO SEE YOU.

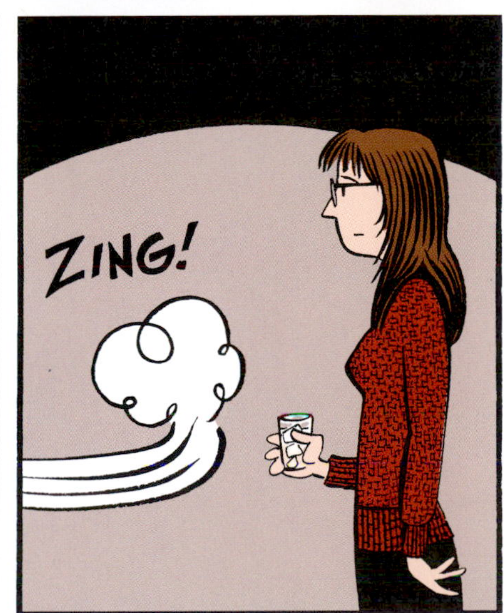
ZING!

I COULD IMAGINE WHAT SHE **WANTED** TO HEAR.

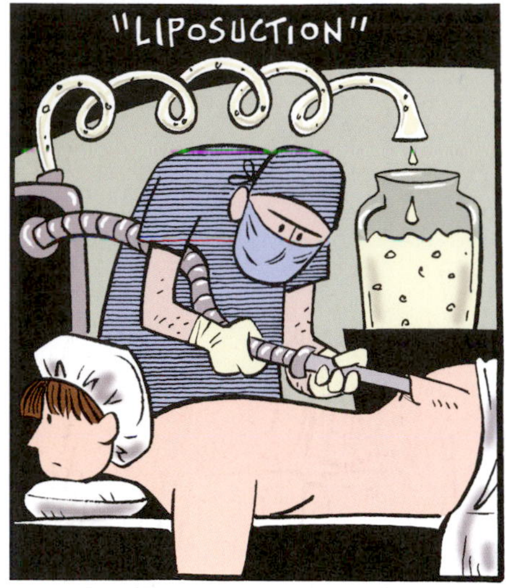


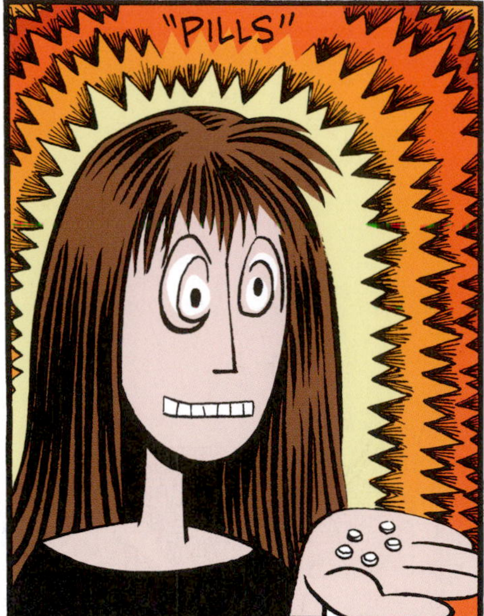


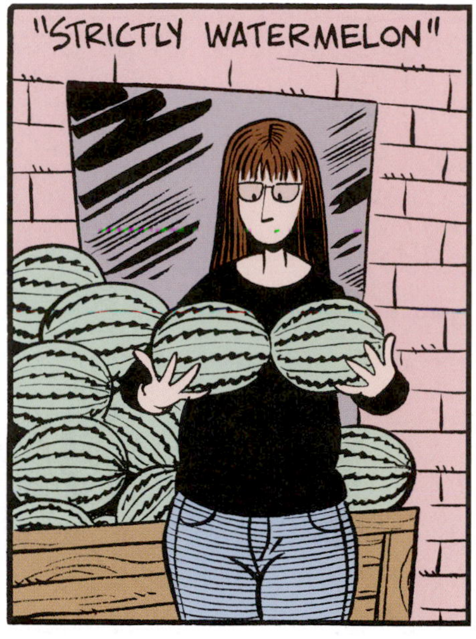


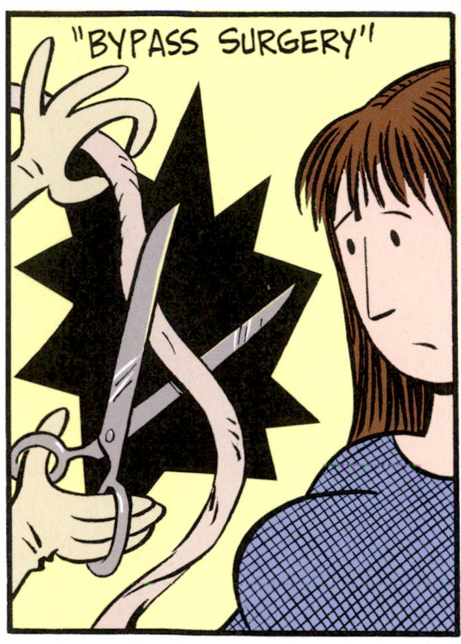


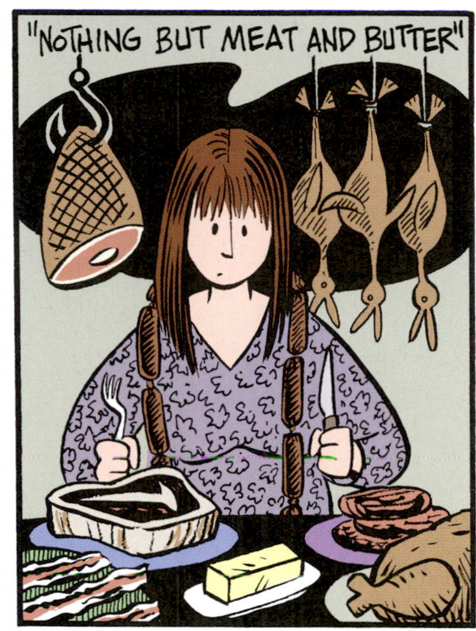


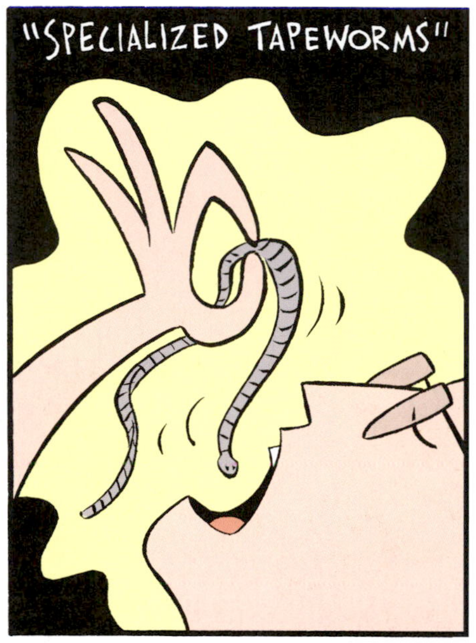


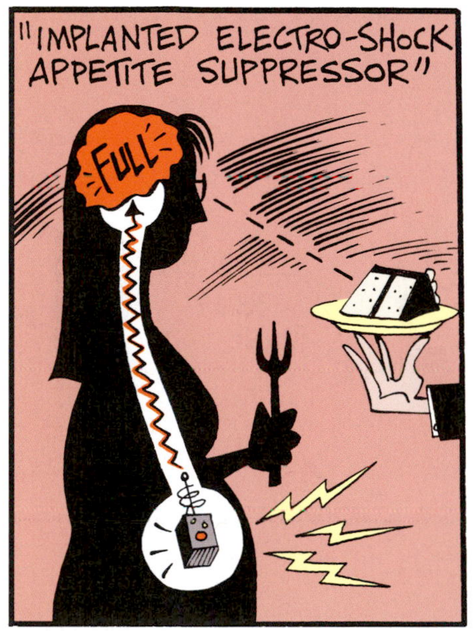


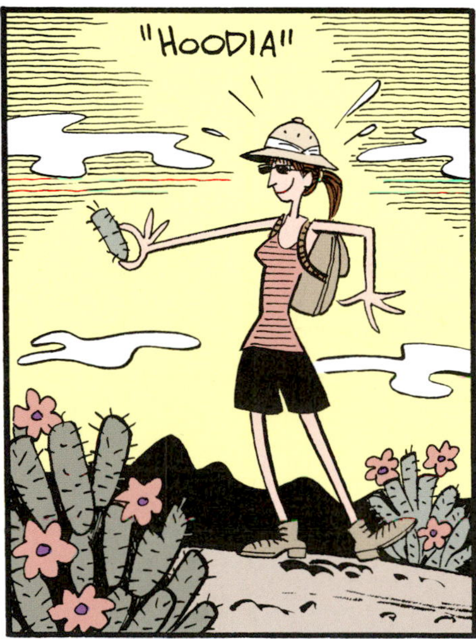


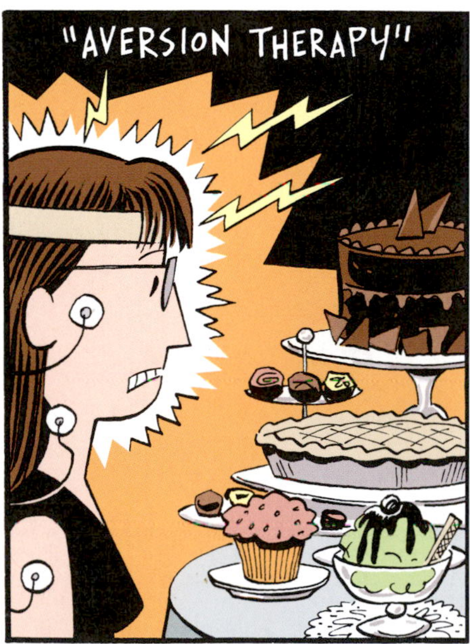

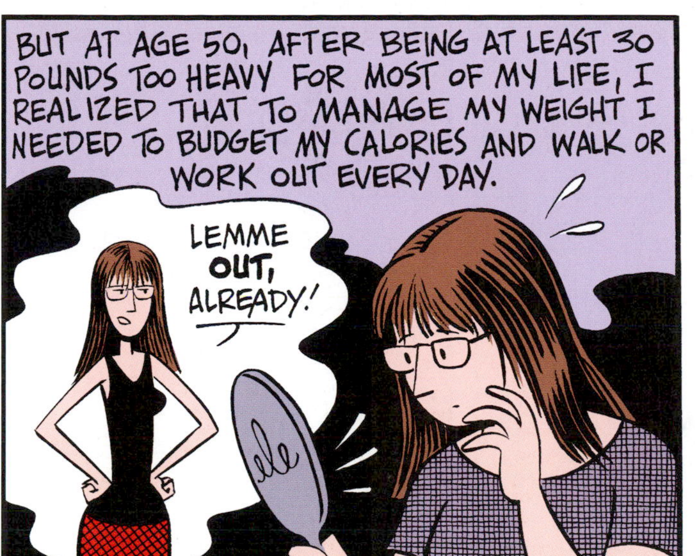
BUT AT AGE 50, AFTER BEING AT LEAST 30 POUNDS TOO HEAVY FOR MOST OF MY LIFE, I REALIZED THAT TO MANAGE MY WEIGHT I NEEDED TO BUDGET MY CALORIES AND WALK OR WORK OUT EVERY DAY.
LEMME OUT, ALREADY!

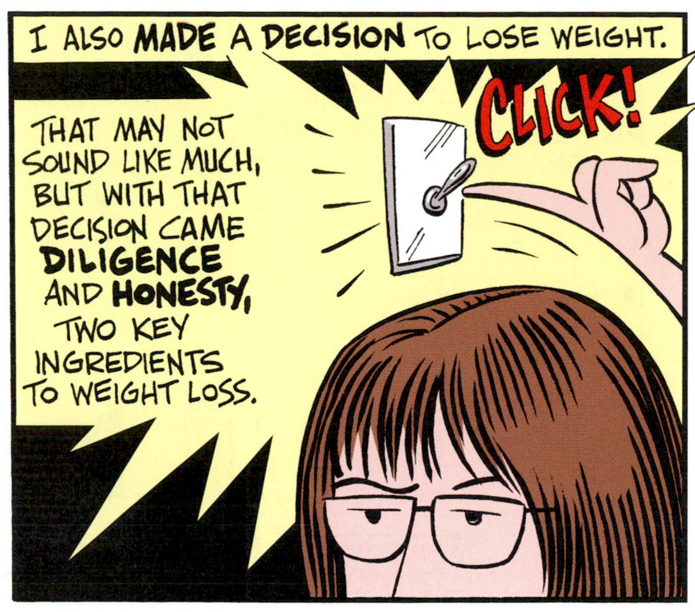
I ALSO MADE A DECISION TO LOSE WEIGHT.
CLICK!
THAT MAY NOT SOUND LIKE MUCH, BUT WITH THAT DECISION CAME DILIGENCE AND HONESTY, TWO KEY INGREDIENTS TO WEIGHT LOSS.

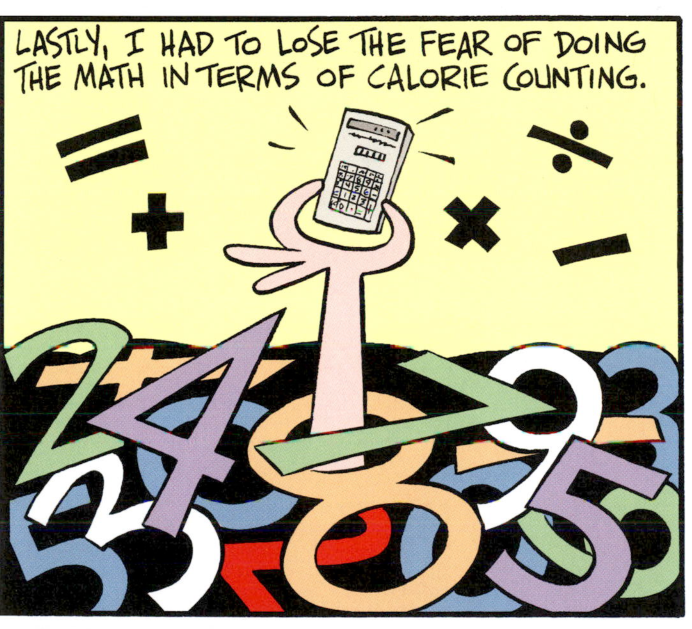
LASTLY, I HAD TO LOSE THE FEAR OF DOING THE MATH IN TERMS OF CALORIE COUNTING.

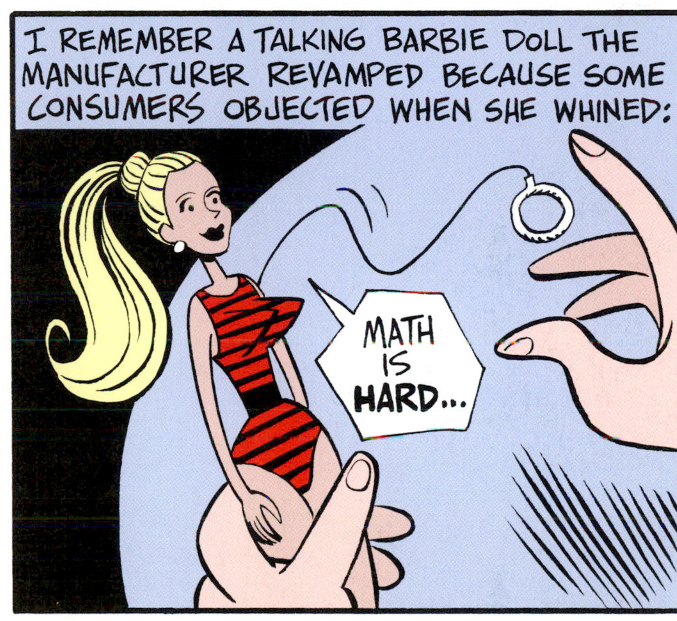
I REMEMBER A TALKING BARBIE DOLL THE MANUFACTURER REVAMPED BECAUSE SOME CONSUMERS OBJECTED WHEN SHE WHINED:
MATH IS HARD...

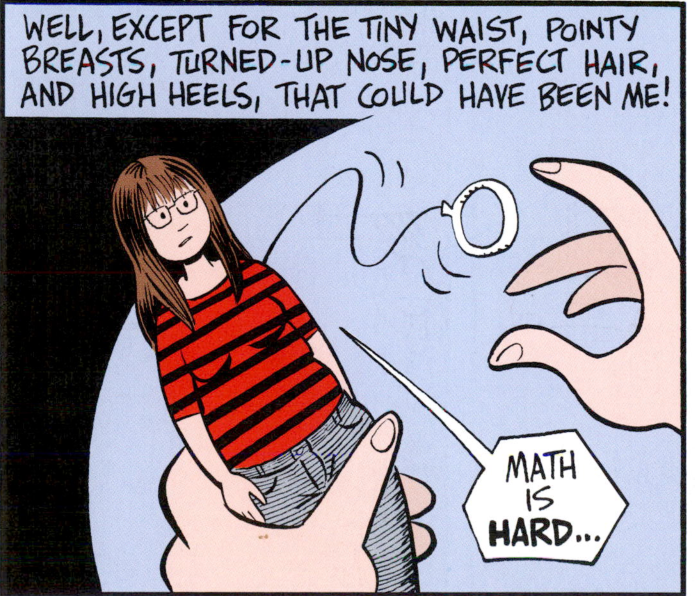
WELL, EXCEPT FOR THE TINY WAIST, POINTY BREASTS, TURNED-UP NOSE, PERFECT HAIR, AND HIGH HEELS, THAT COULD HAVE BEEN ME!
MATH IS HARD...

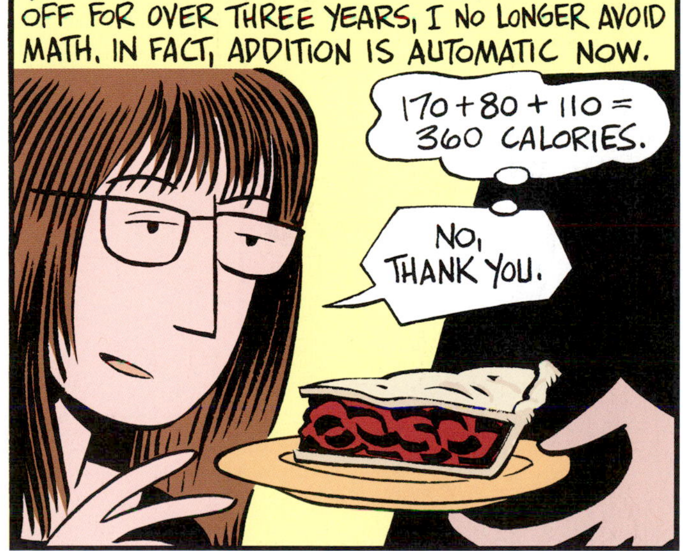
BUT AFTER LOSING 35 POUNDS AND KEEPING IT OFF FOR OVER THREE YEARS, I NO LONGER AVOID MATH. IN FACT, ADDITION IS AUTOMATIC NOW.
170 + 80 + 110 = 360 CALORIES.
NO, THANK YOU.

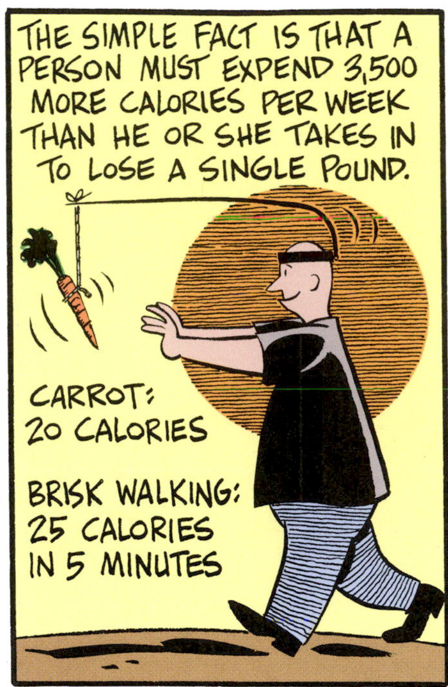
THE SIMPLE FACT IS THAT A PERSON MUST EXPEND 3,500 MORE CALORIES PER WEEK THAN HE OR SHE TAKES IN TO LOSE A SINGLE POUND.
CARROT: 20 CALORIES
BRISK WALKING: 25 CALORIES IN 5 MINUTES

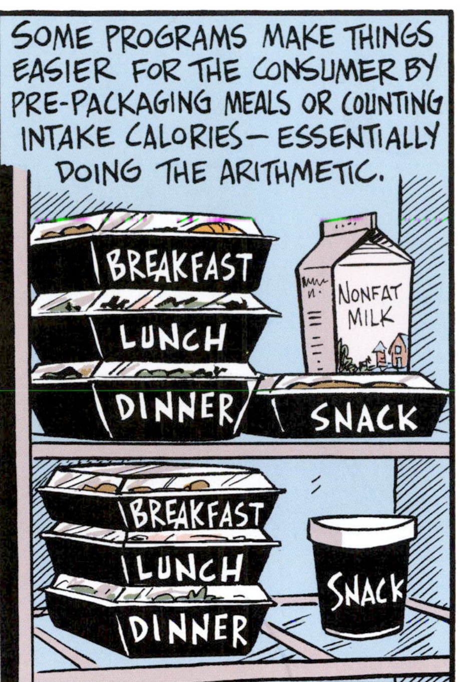
SOME PROGRAMS MAKE THINGS EASIER FOR THE CONSUMER BY PRE-PACKAGING MEALS OR COUNTING INTAKE CALORIES—ESSENTIALLY DOING THE ARITHMETIC.
BREAKFAST
LUNCH
DINNER
NONFAT MILK
SNACK
BREAKFAST
LUNCH
DINNER
SNACK

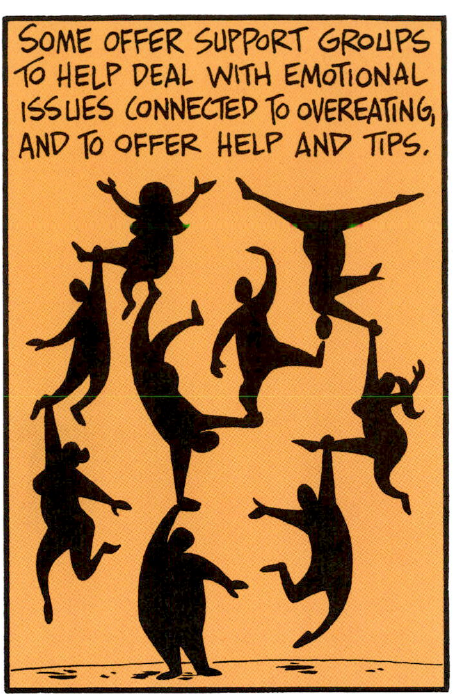
SOME OFFER SUPPORT GROUPS TO HELP DEAL WITH EMOTIONAL ISSUES CONNECTED TO OVEREATING, AND TO OFFER HELP AND TIPS.

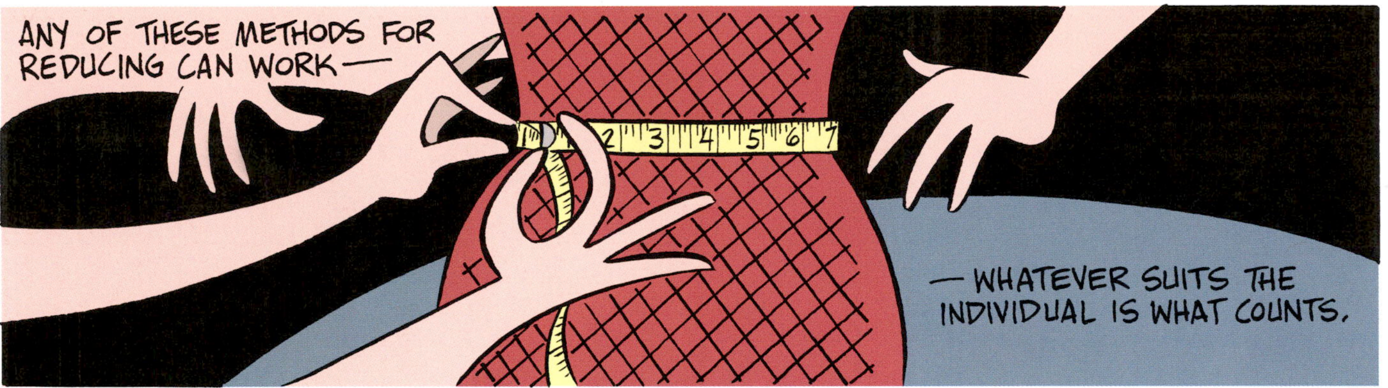
ANY OF THESE METHODS FOR REDUCING CAN WORK—
—WHATEVER SUITS THE INDIVIDUAL IS WHAT COUNTS.

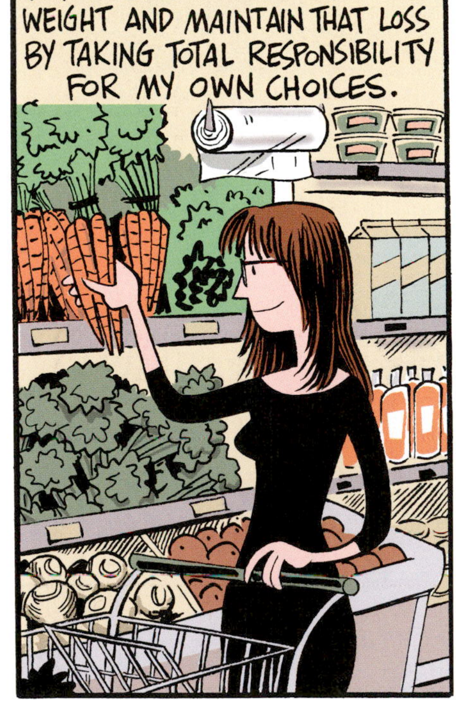
IN THIS BOOK I TELL HOW I LOST WEIGHT AND MAINTAIN THAT LOSS BY TAKING TOTAL RESPONSIBILITY FOR MY OWN CHOICES.

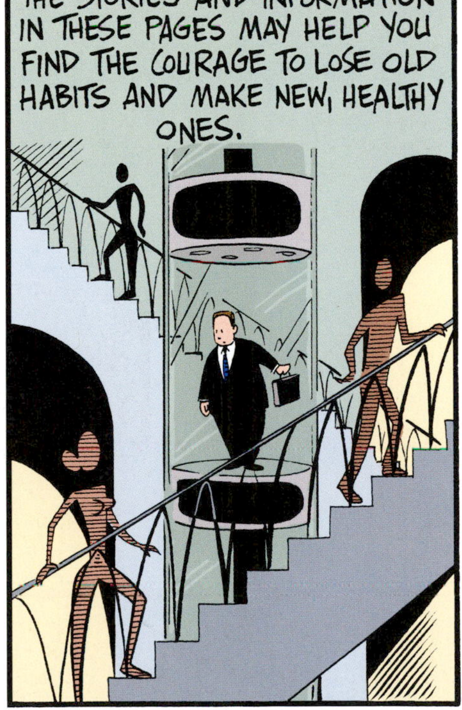
THE STORIES AND INFORMATION IN THESE PAGES MAY HELP YOU FIND THE COURAGE TO LOSE OLD HABITS AND MAKE NEW, HEALTHY ONES.

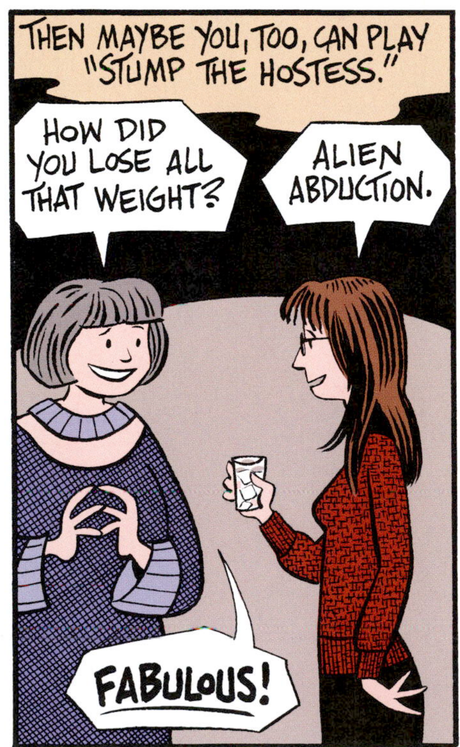
THEN MAYBE YOU, TOO, CAN PLAY "STUMP THE HOSTESS."
HOW DID YOU LOSE ALL THAT WEIGHT?
ALIEN ABDUCTION.
FABULOUS!

# MY BIG FAT LIFE

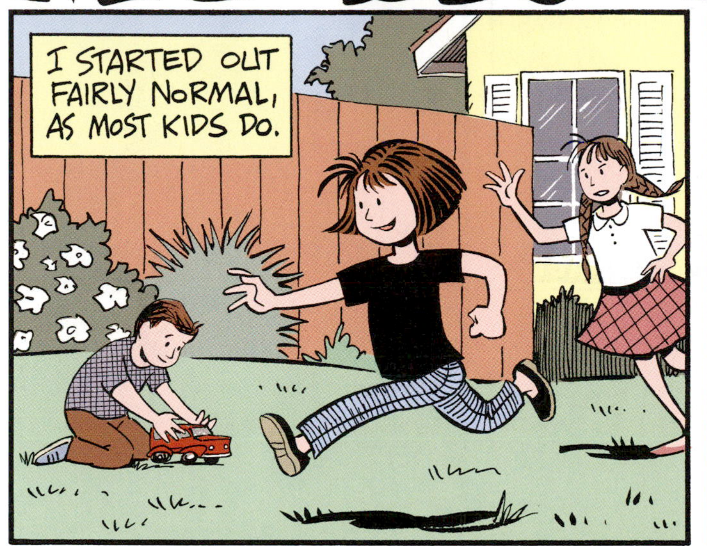

I STARTED OUT FAIRLY NORMAL, AS MOST KIDS DO.

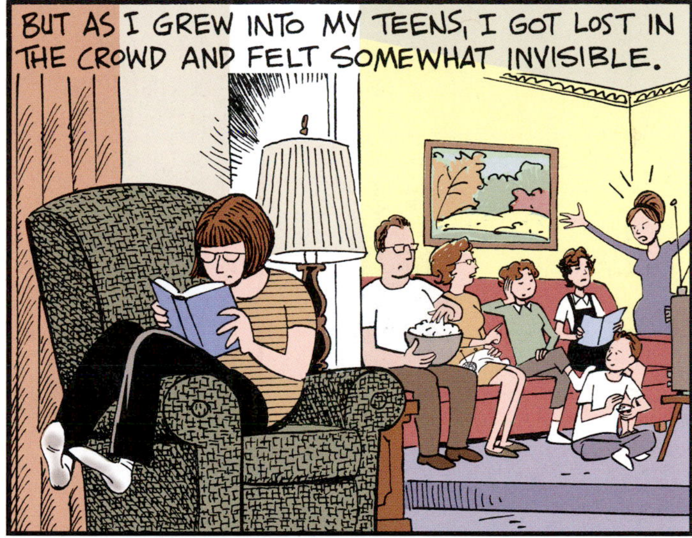

BUT AS I GREW INTO MY TEENS, I GOT LOST IN THE CROWD AND FELT SOMEWHAT INVISIBLE.

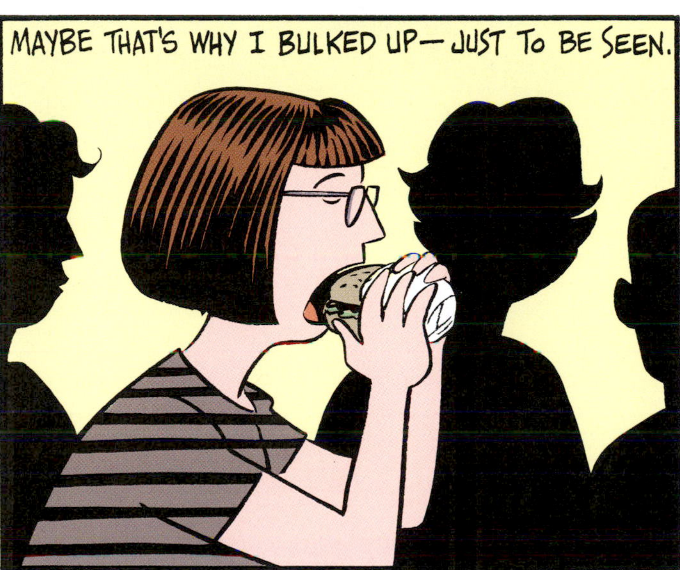

MAYBE THAT'S WHY I BULKED UP— JUST TO BE SEEN.

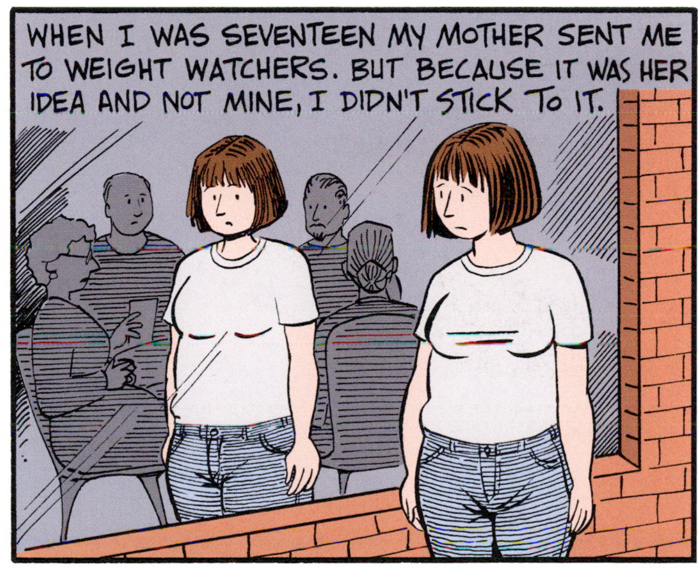

WHEN I WAS SEVENTEEN MY MOTHER SENT ME TO WEIGHT WATCHERS. BUT BECAUSE IT WAS HER IDEA AND NOT MINE, I DIDN'T STICK TO IT.

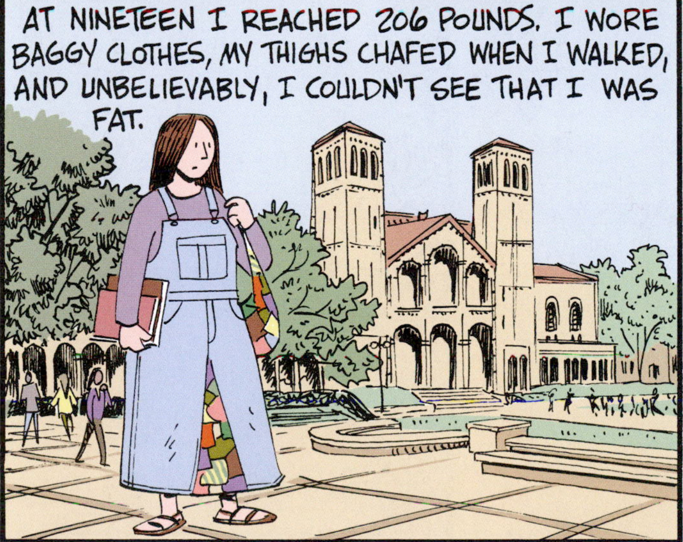

AT NINETEEN I REACHED 206 POUNDS. I WORE BAGGY CLOTHES, MY THIGHS CHAFED WHEN I WALKED, AND UNBELIEVABLY, I COULDN'T SEE THAT I WAS FAT.

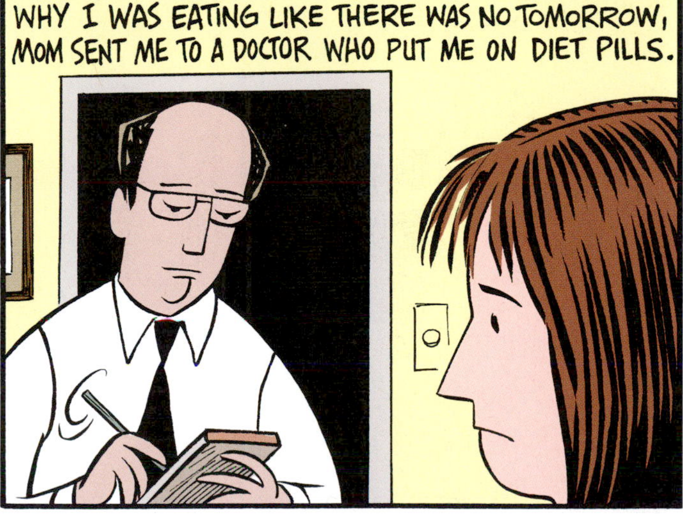

INSTEAD OF SENDING ME TO A SHRINK TO FIND OUT WHY I WAS EATING LIKE THERE WAS NO TOMORROW, MOM SENT ME TO A DOCTOR WHO PUT ME ON DIET PILLS.

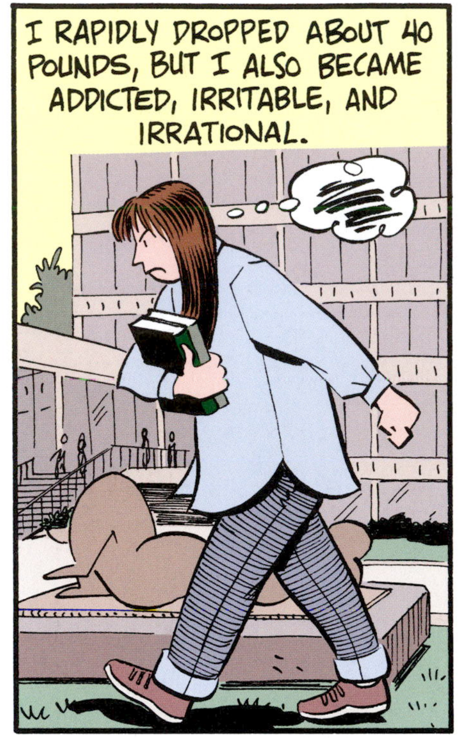
I RAPIDLY DROPPED ABOUT 40 POUNDS, BUT I ALSO BECAME ADDICTED, IRRITABLE, AND IRRATIONAL.

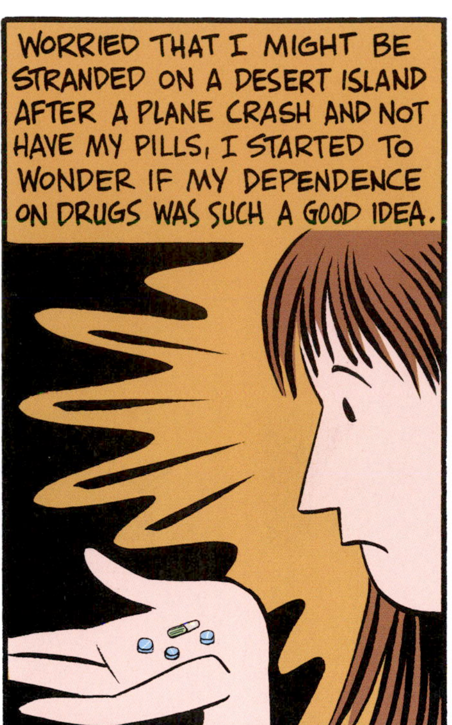
WORRIED THAT I MIGHT BE STRANDED ON A DESERT ISLAND AFTER A PLANE CRASH AND NOT HAVE MY PILLS, I STARTED TO WONDER IF MY DEPENDENCE ON DRUGS WAS SUCH A GOOD IDEA.

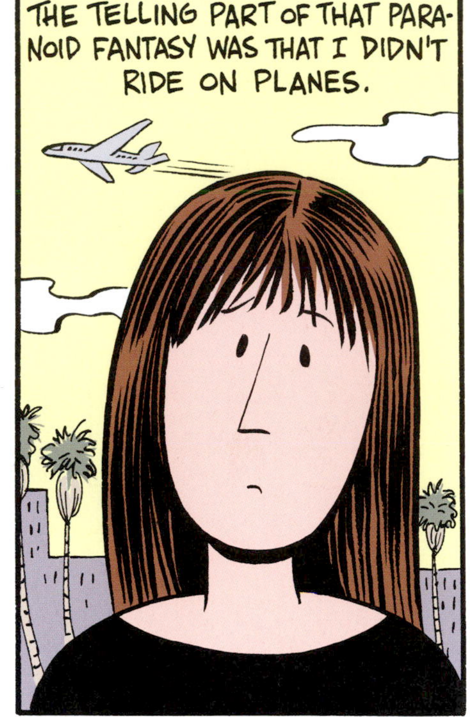
THE TELLING PART OF THAT PARANOID FANTASY WAS THAT I DIDN'T RIDE ON PLANES.

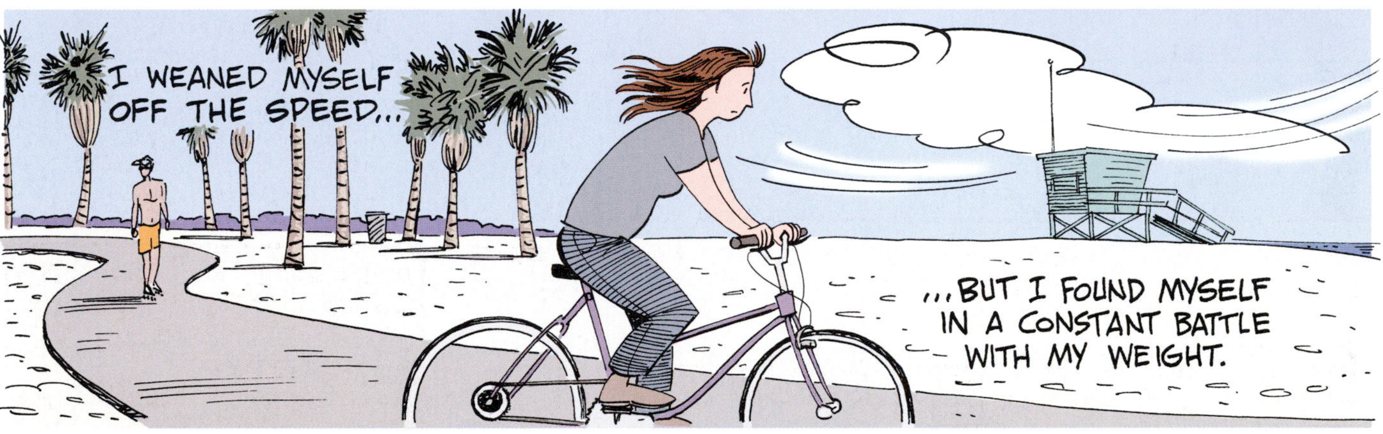
I WEANED MYSELF OFF THE SPEED...
...BUT I FOUND MYSELF IN A CONSTANT BATTLE WITH MY WEIGHT.

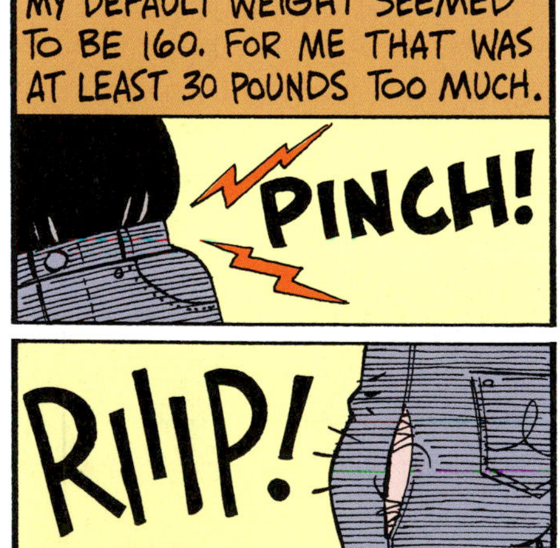
MY DEFAULT WEIGHT SEEMED TO BE 160. FOR ME THAT WAS AT LEAST 30 POUNDS TOO MUCH.
PINCH!
RIIIP!

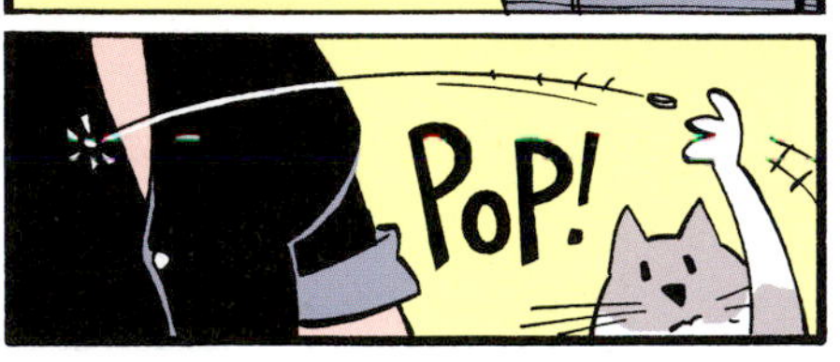
POP!

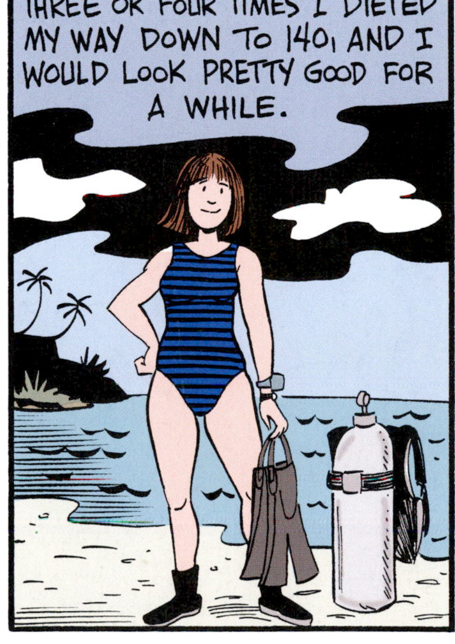
THREE OR FOUR TIMES I DIETED MY WAY DOWN TO 140, AND I WOULD LOOK PRETTY GOOD FOR A WHILE.

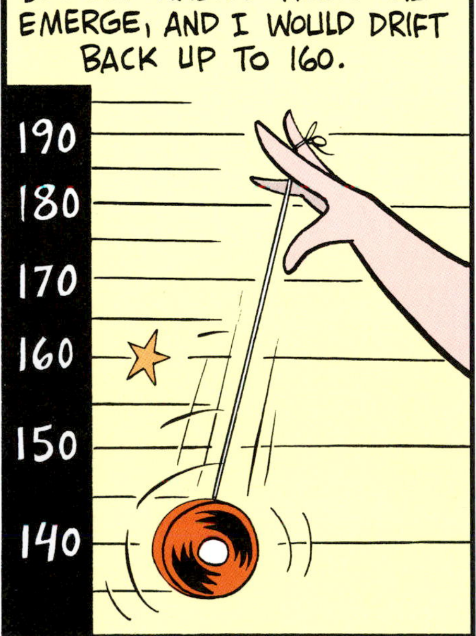
BUT OLD HABITS WOULD RE-EMERGE, AND I WOULD DRIFT BACK UP TO 160.
190
180
170
160
150
140

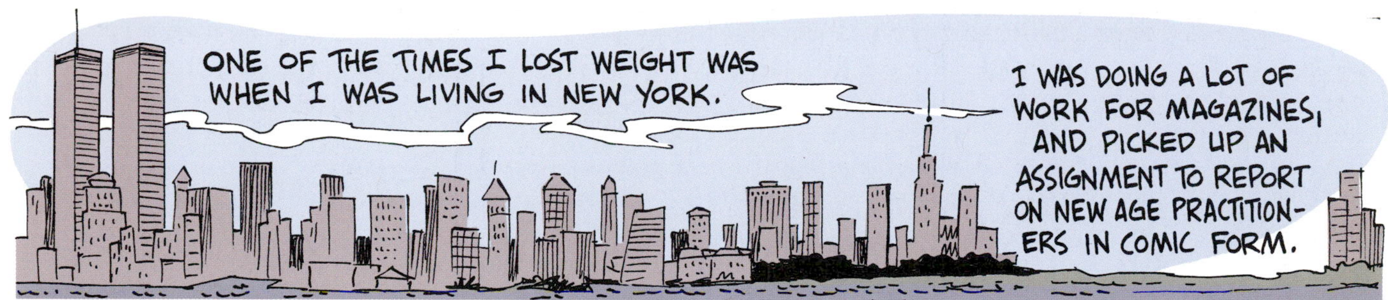

ONE OF THE TIMES I LOST WEIGHT WAS WHEN I WAS LIVING IN NEW YORK.
I WAS DOING A LOT OF WORK FOR MAGAZINES, AND PICKED UP AN ASSIGNMENT TO REPORT ON NEW AGE PRACTITIONERS IN COMIC FORM.

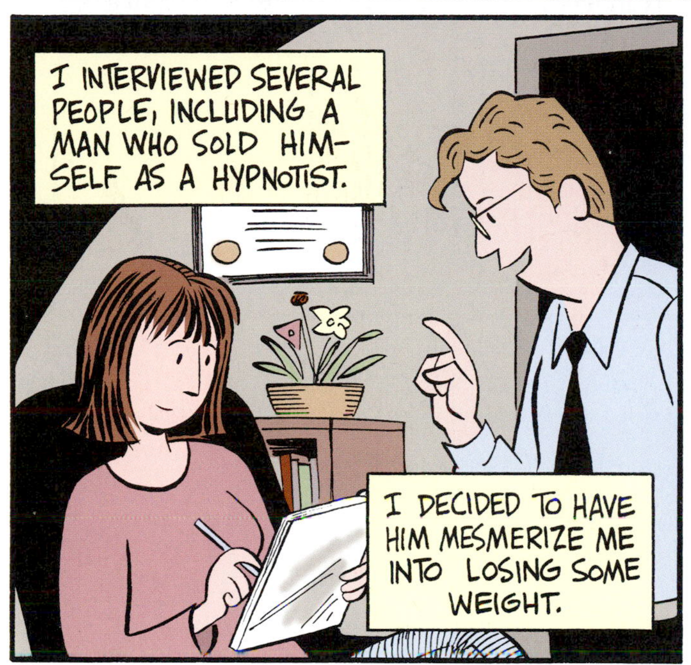

I INTERVIEWED SEVERAL PEOPLE, INCLUDING A MAN WHO SOLD HIMSELF AS A HYPNOTIST.
I DECIDED TO HAVE HIM MESMERIZE ME INTO LOSING SOME WEIGHT.

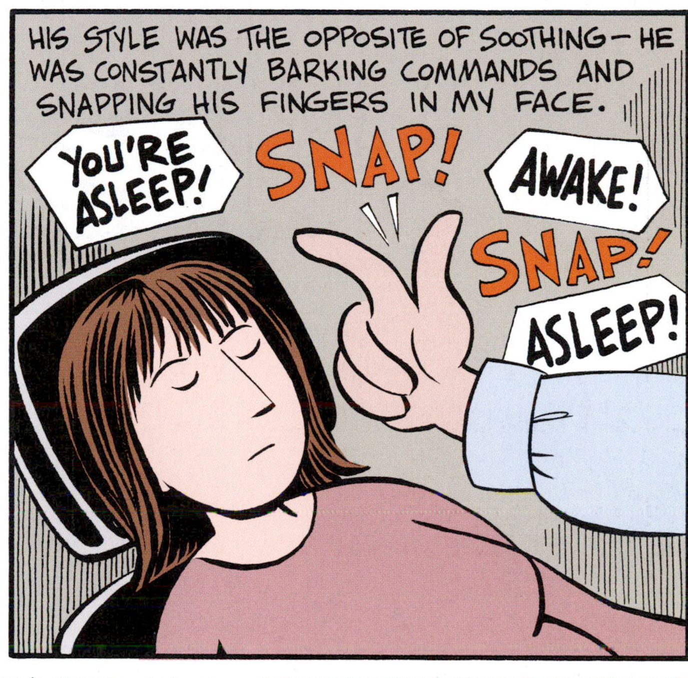

HIS STYLE WAS THE OPPOSITE OF SOOTHING—HE WAS CONSTANTLY BARKING COMMANDS AND SNAPPING HIS FINGERS IN MY FACE.
YOU'RE ASLEEP!
SNAP!
AWAKE!
SNAP!
ASLEEP!

WORSE, I HAD TO PEE, AND THAT WAS PRETTY MUCH ALL I COULD THINK ABOUT EVEN AS THE MAN KEPT TELLING ME WHAT A DEEP SLEEP I WAS IN.

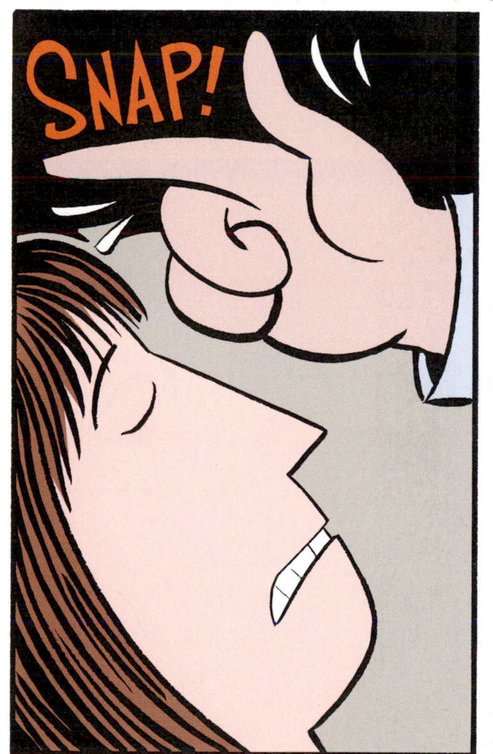


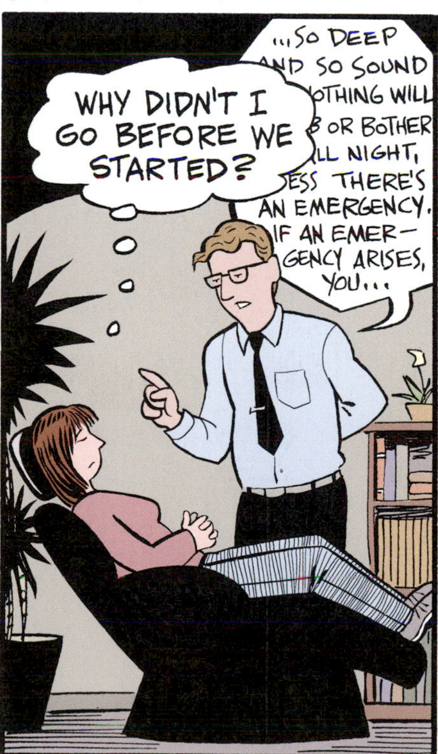


ND SO SOUND

B OR BOTHER

ESS THERE'S
AN EMERGENCY. IF AN EMERGENCY ARISES, YOU...
WHY DIDN'T I GO BEFORE WE STARTED?

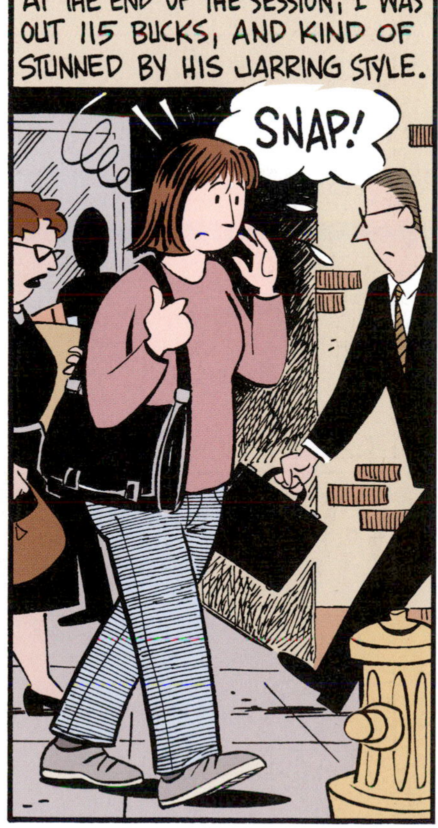

AT THE END OF THE SESSION, I WAS OUT 115 BUCKS, AND KIND OF STUNNED BY HIS JARRING STYLE.

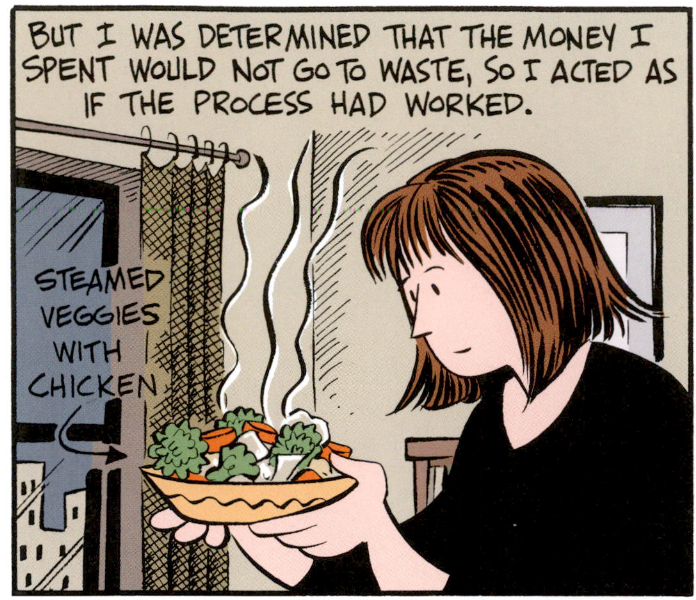
BUT I WAS DETERMINED THAT THE MONEY I SPENT WOULD NOT GO TO WASTE, SO I ACTED AS IF THE PROCESS HAD WORKED.
STEAMED VEGGIES WITH CHICKEN

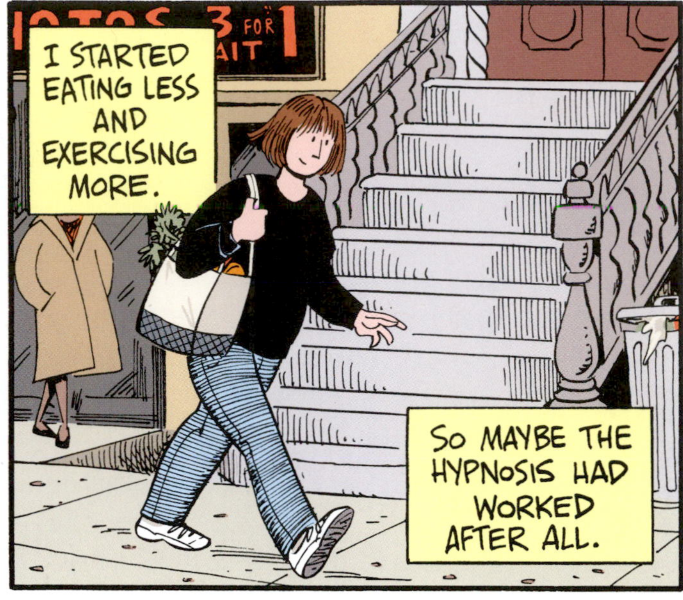
I STARTED EATING LESS AND EXERCISING MORE.
SO MAYBE THE HYPNOSIS HAD WORKED AFTER ALL.

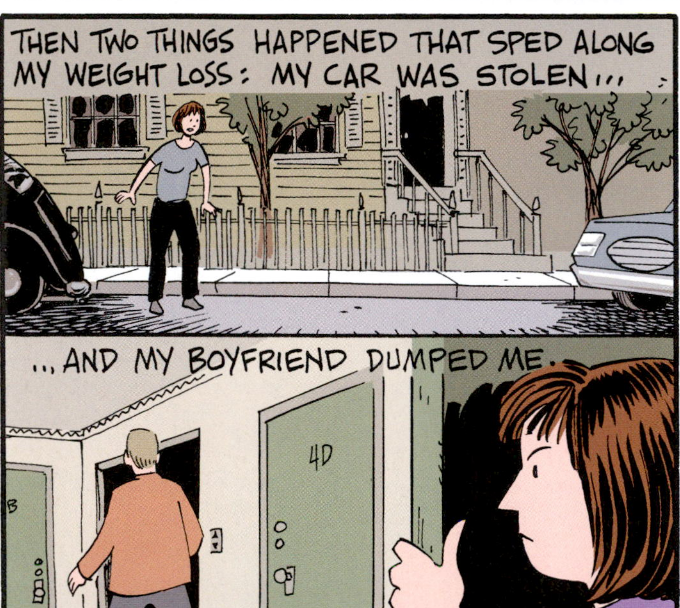
THEN TWO THINGS HAPPENED THAT SPED ALONG MY WEIGHT LOSS: MY CAR WAS STOLEN...
...AND MY BOYFRIEND DUMPED ME.
4D

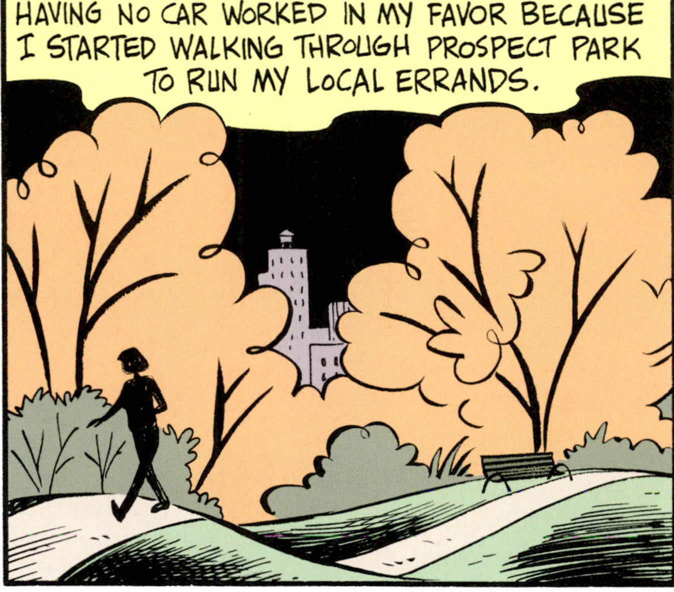
HAVING NO CAR WORKED IN MY FAVOR BECAUSE I STARTED WALKING THROUGH PROSPECT PARK TO RUN MY LOCAL ERRANDS.

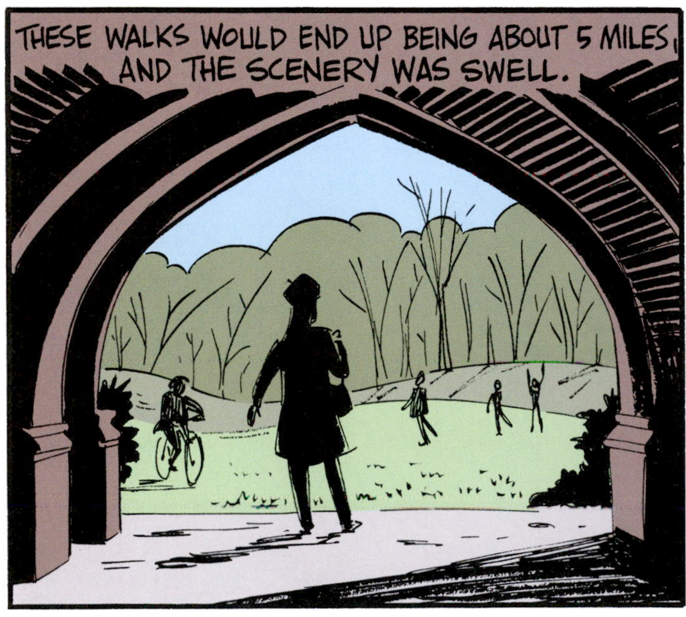
THESE WALKS WOULD END UP BEING ABOUT 5 MILES, AND THE SCENERY WAS SWELL.

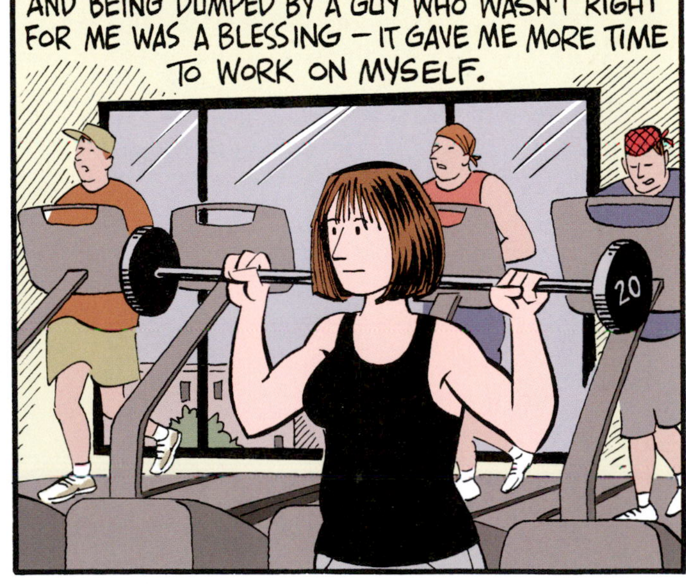
AND BEING DUMPED BY A GUY WHO WASN'T RIGHT FOR ME WAS A BLESSING — IT GAVE ME MORE TIME TO WORK ON MYSELF.
20

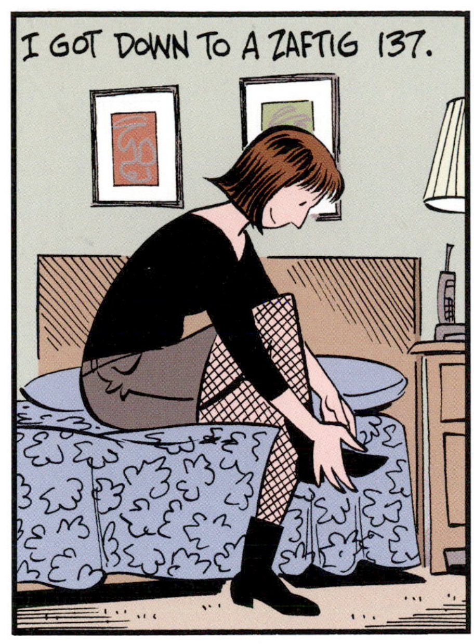
I GOT DOWN TO A ZAFTIG 137.

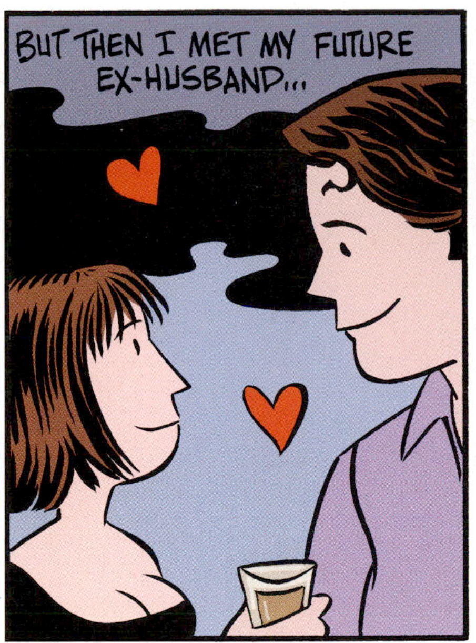
BUT THEN I MET MY FUTURE EX-HUSBAND...

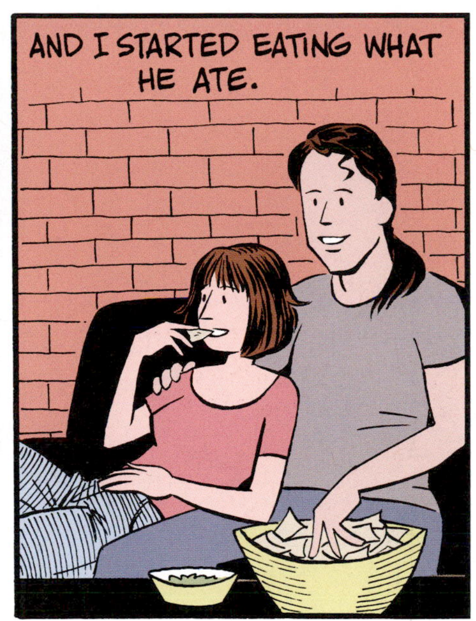
AND I STARTED EATING WHAT HE ATE.

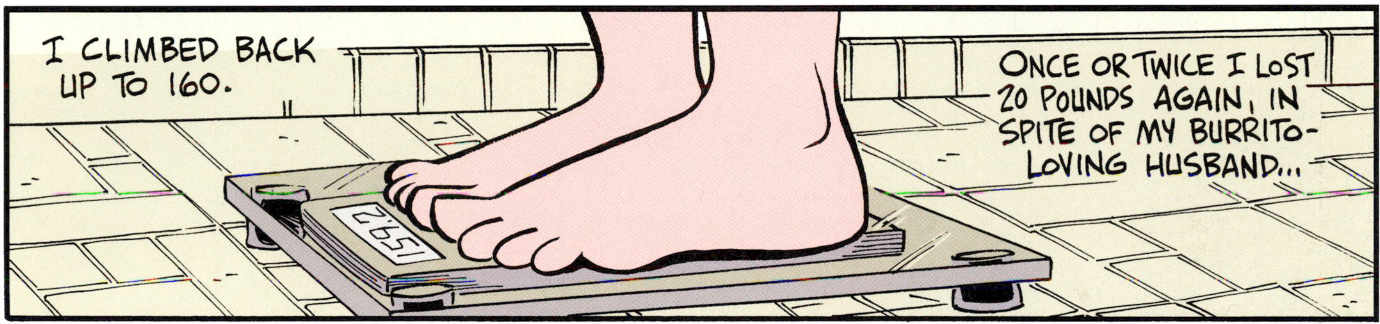
I CLIMBED BACK UP TO 160.
ONCE OR TWICE I LOST 20 POUNDS AGAIN, IN SPITE OF MY BURRITO-LOVING HUSBAND...
159.2

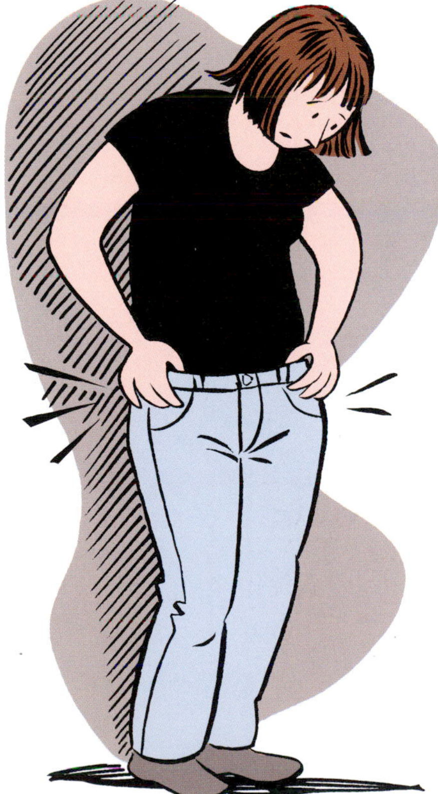
BUT I COULDN'T KEEP IT OFF.

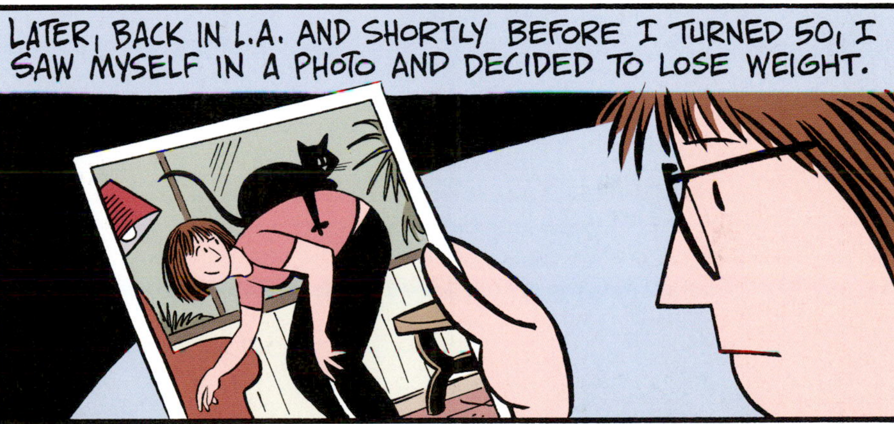
LATER, BACK IN L.A. AND SHORTLY BEFORE I TURNED 50, I SAW MYSELF IN A PHOTO AND DECIDED TO LOSE WEIGHT.

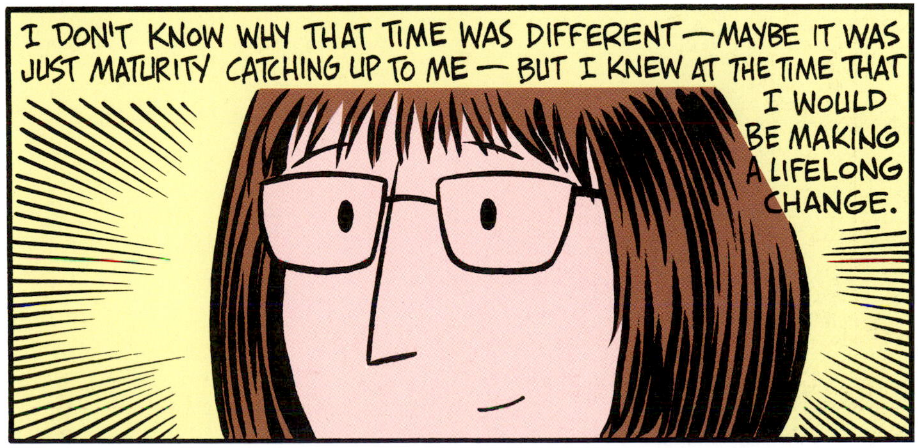
I DON'T KNOW WHY THAT TIME WAS DIFFERENT—MAYBE IT WAS JUST MATURITY CATCHING UP TO ME—BUT I KNEW AT THE TIME THAT I WOULD BE MAKING A LIFELONG CHANGE.

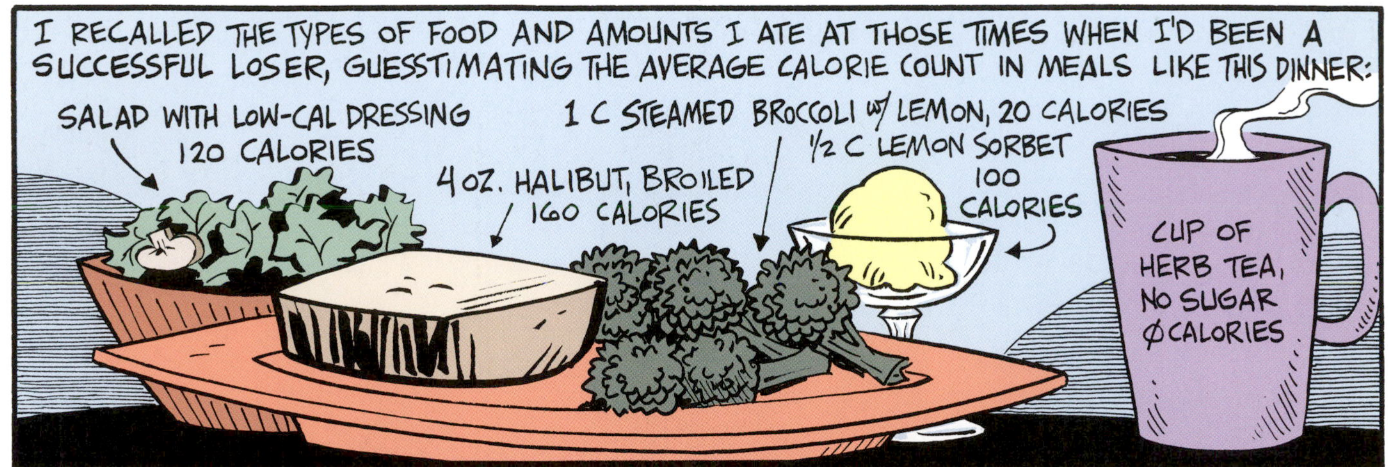
I RECALLED THE TYPES OF FOOD AND AMOUNTS I ATE AT THOSE TIMES WHEN I'D BEEN A SUCCESSFUL LOSER, GUESSTIMATING THE AVERAGE CALORIE COUNT IN MEALS LIKE THIS DINNER:
SALAD WITH LOW-CAL DRESSING 120 CALORIES
4 OZ. HALIBUT, BROILED 160 CALORIES
1 C STEAMED BROCCOLI W/ LEMON, 20 CALORIES
1/2 C LEMON SORBET 100 CALORIES
CUP OF HERB TEA, NO SUGAR Ø CALORIES

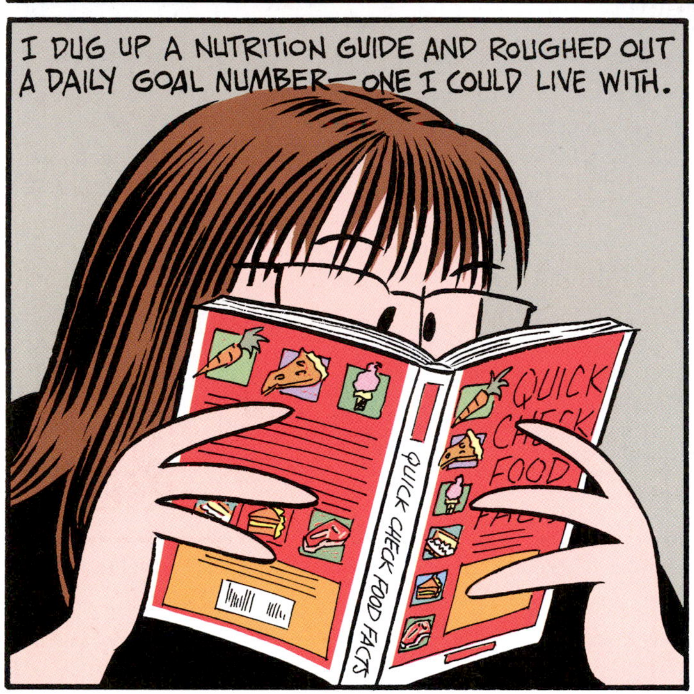
I DUG UP A NUTRITION GUIDE AND ROUGHED OUT A DAILY GOAL NUMBER—ONE I COULD LIVE WITH.
QUICK CHECK FOOD FACTS

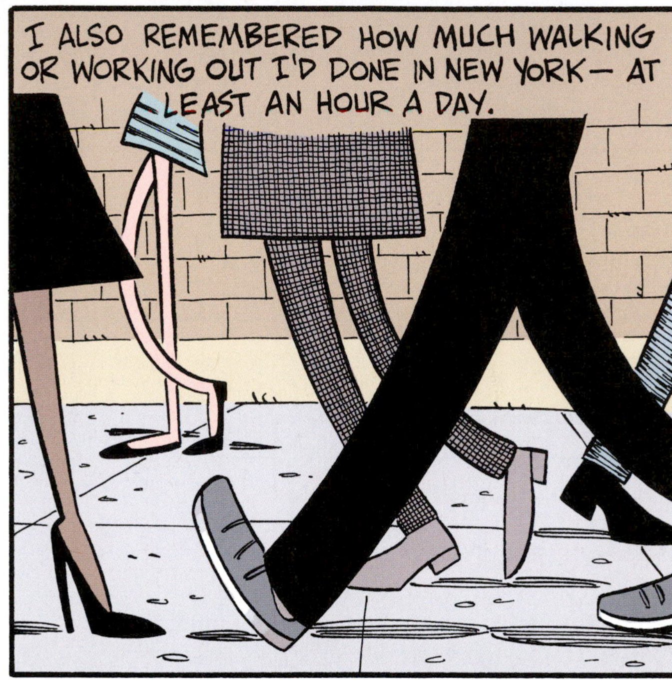
I ALSO REMEMBERED HOW MUCH WALKING OR WORKING OUT I'D DONE IN NEW YORK— AT LEAST AN HOUR A DAY.

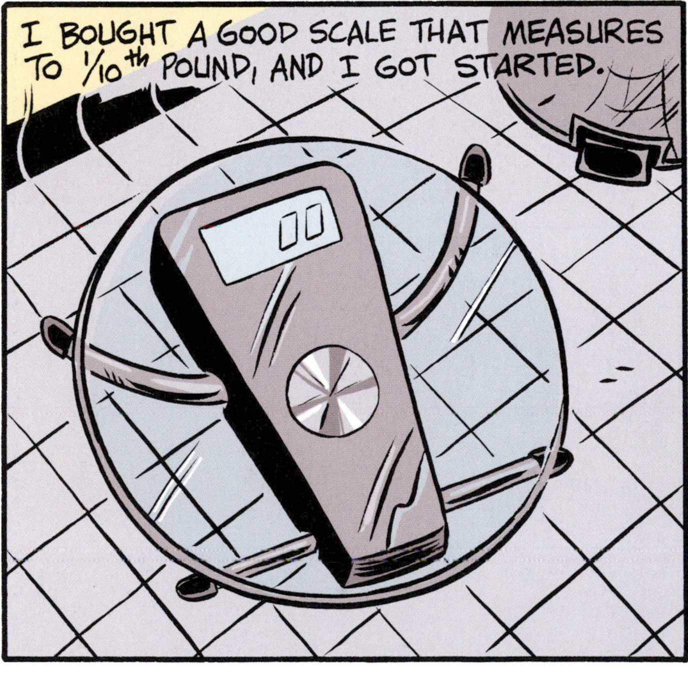
I BOUGHT A GOOD SCALE THAT MEASURES TO 1/10th POUND, AND I GOT STARTED.
00

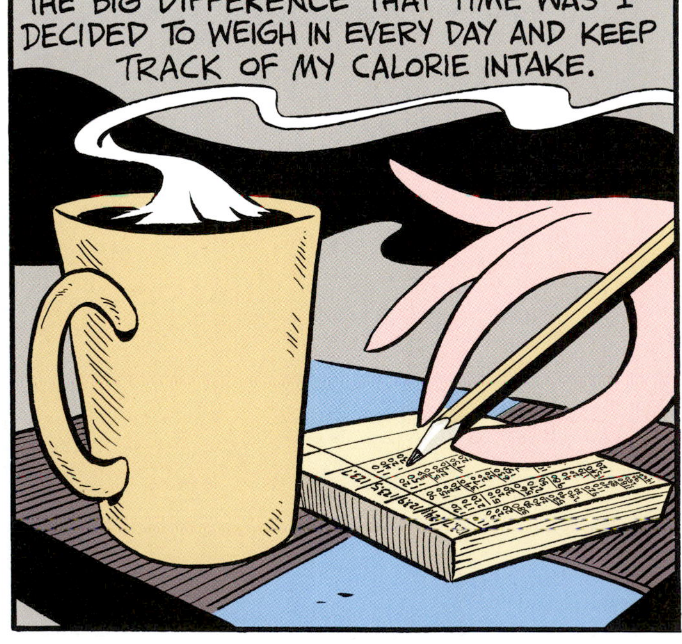
THE BIG DIFFERENCE THAT TIME WAS I DECIDED TO WEIGH IN EVERY DAY AND KEEP TRACK OF MY CALORIE INTAKE.

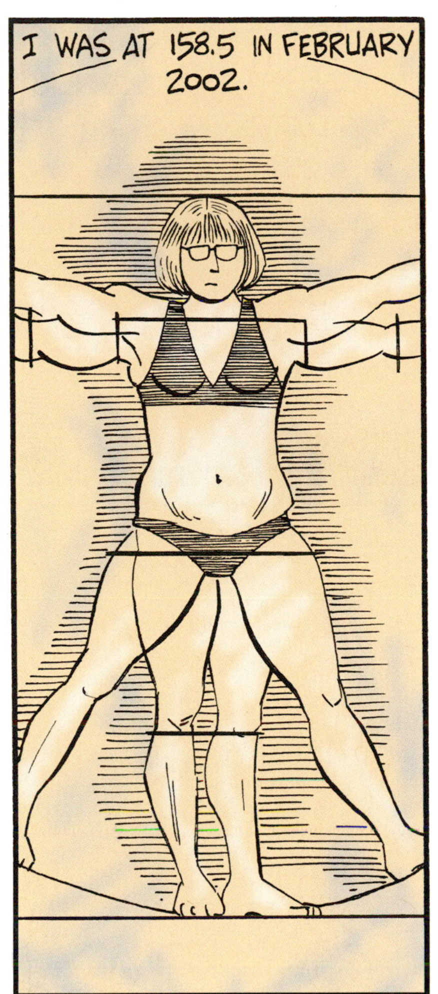
I WAS AT 158.5 IN FEBRUARY 2002.

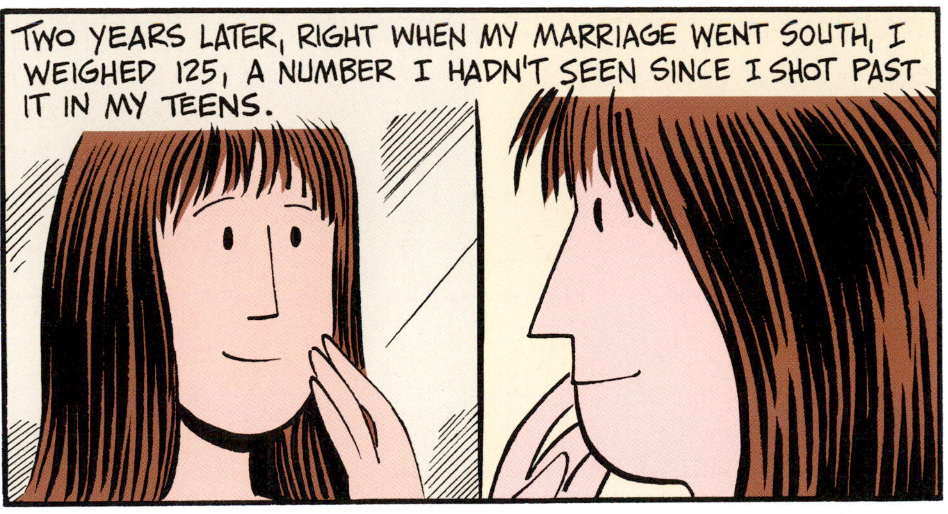
TWO YEARS LATER, RIGHT WHEN MY MARRIAGE WENT SOUTH, I WEIGHED 125, A NUMBER I HADN'T SEEN SINCE I SHOT PAST IT IN MY TEENS.

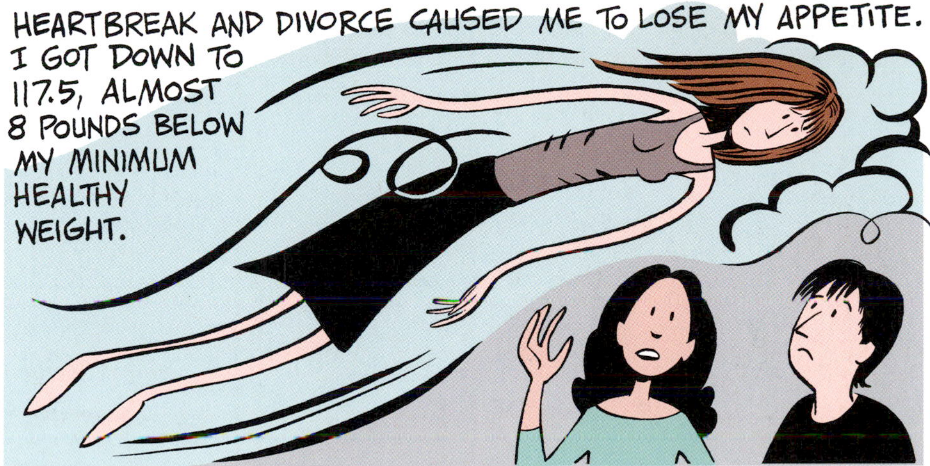
HEARTBREAK AND DIVORCE CAUSED ME TO LOSE MY APPETITE. I GOT DOWN TO 117.5, ALMOST 8 POUNDS BELOW MY MINIMUM HEALTHY WEIGHT.

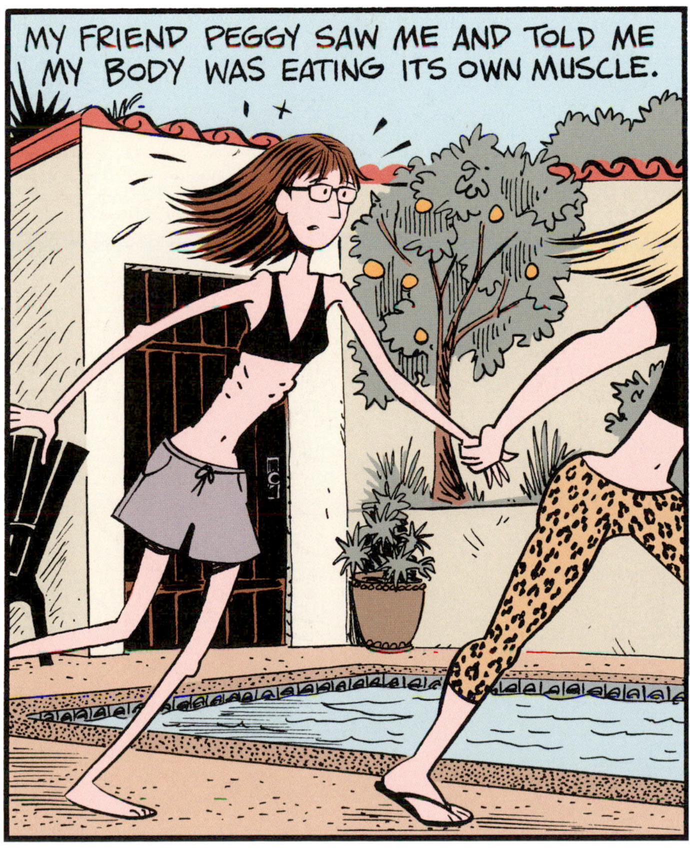
MY FRIEND PEGGY SAW ME AND TOLD ME MY BODY WAS EATING ITS OWN MUSCLE.

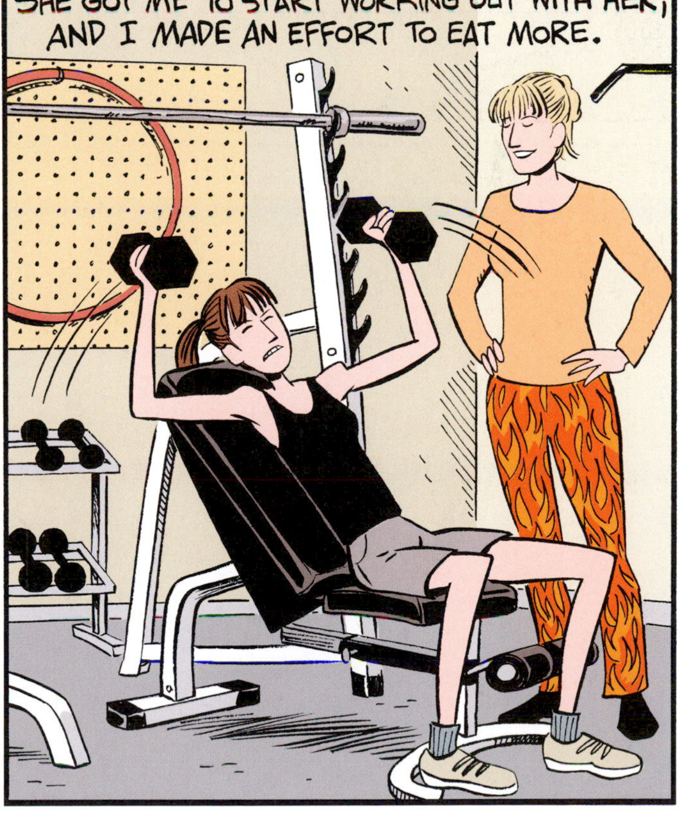
SHE GOT ME TO START WORKING OUT WITH HER, AND I MADE AN EFFORT TO EAT MORE.

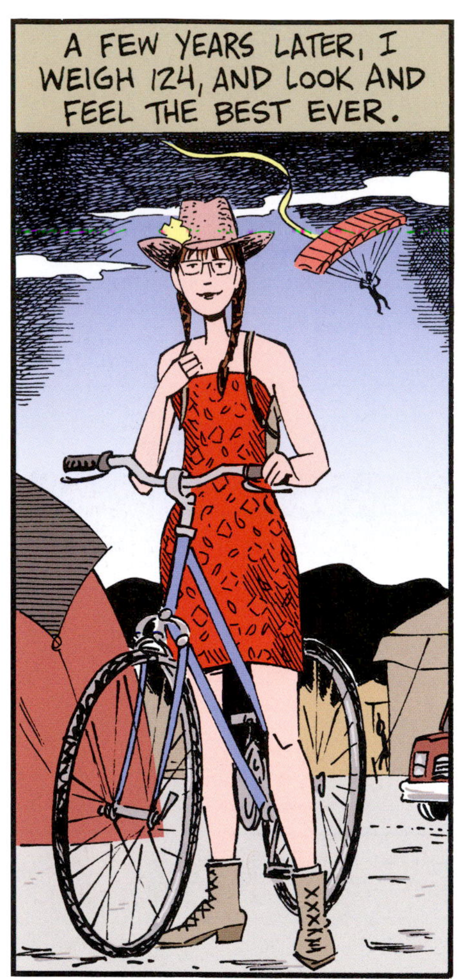
A FEW YEARS LATER, I WEIGH 124, AND LOOK AND FEEL THE BEST EVER.

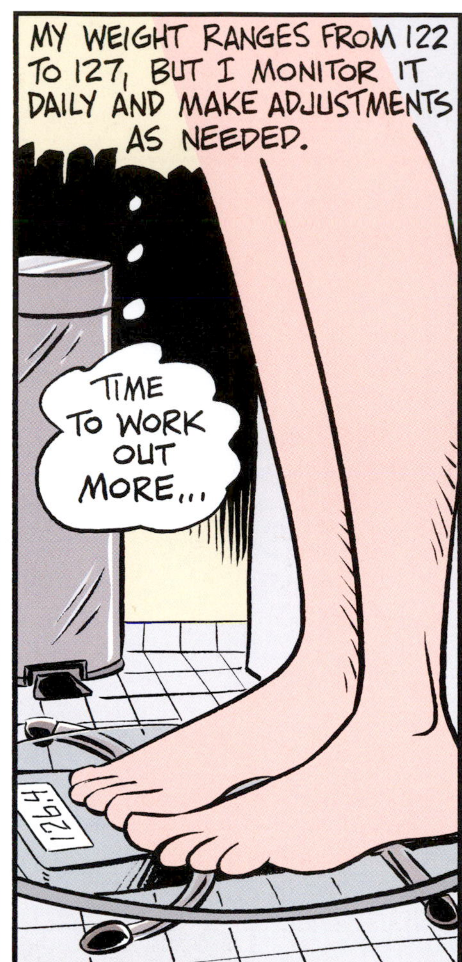
MY WEIGHT RANGES FROM 122 TO 127, BUT I MONITOR IT DAILY AND MAKE ADJUSTMENTS AS NEEDED.
TIME TO WORK OUT MORE...
126.4

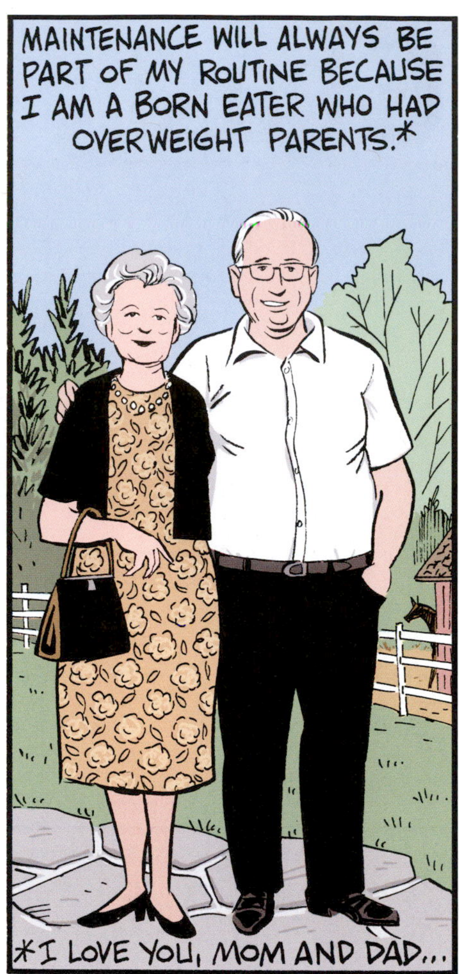
MAINTENANCE WILL ALWAYS BE PART OF MY ROUTINE BECAUSE I AM A BORN EATER WHO HAD OVERWEIGHT PARENTS.*
*I LOVE YOU, MOM AND DAD...

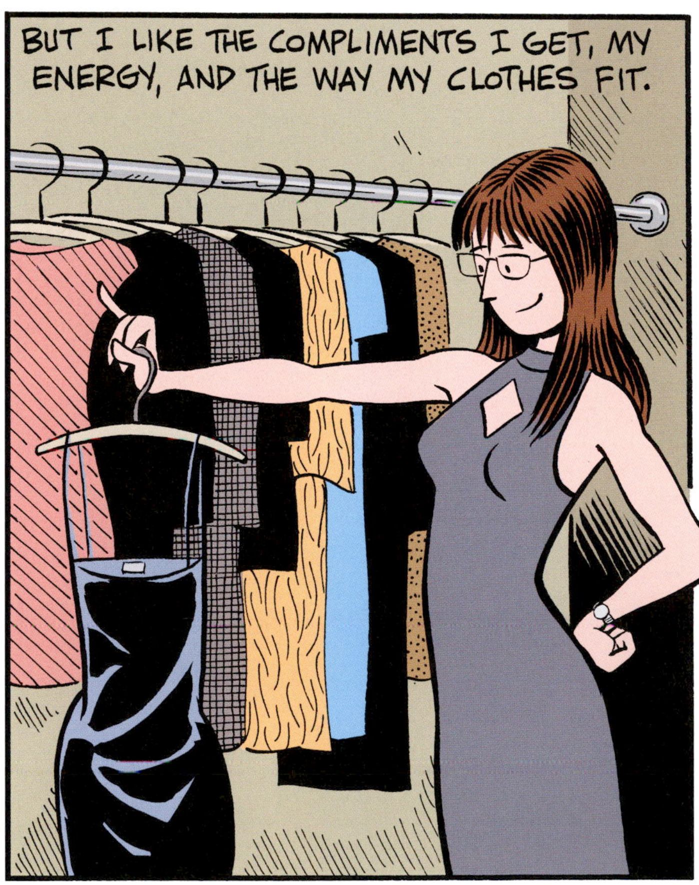
BUT I LIKE THE COMPLIMENTS I GET, MY ENERGY, AND THE WAY MY CLOTHES FIT.

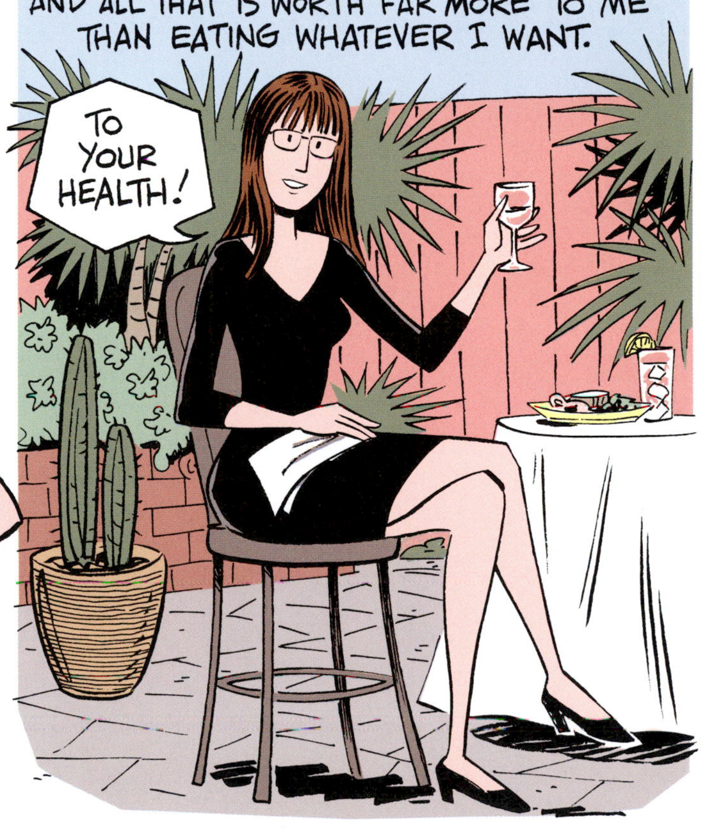
AND ALL THAT IS WORTH FAR MORE TO ME THAN EATING WHATEVER I WANT.
TO YOUR HEALTH!

# Ghosts in the Graveyard

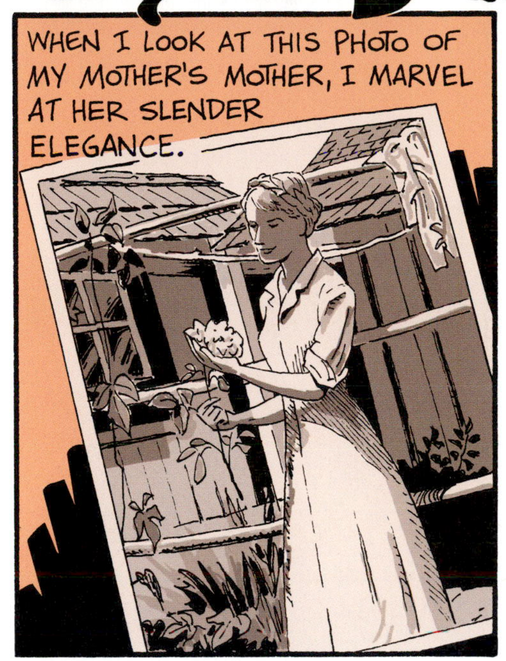

WHEN I LOOK AT THIS PHOTO OF MY MOTHER'S MOTHER, I MARVEL AT HER SLENDER ELEGANCE.

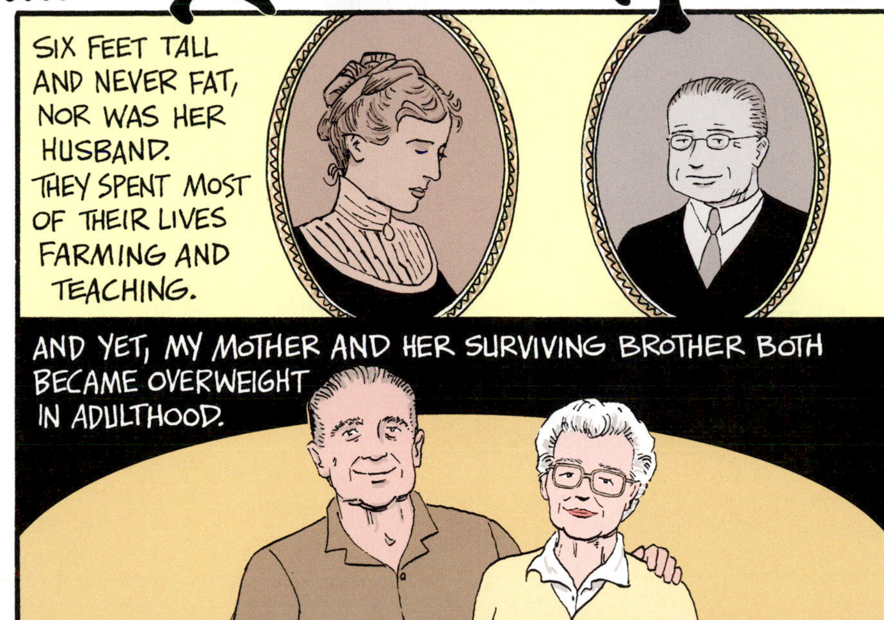

SIX FEET TALL AND NEVER FAT, NOR WAS HER HUSBAND. THEY SPENT MOST OF THEIR LIVES FARMING AND TEACHING.
AND YET, MY MOTHER AND HER SURVIVING BROTHER BOTH BECAME OVERWEIGHT IN ADULTHOOD.

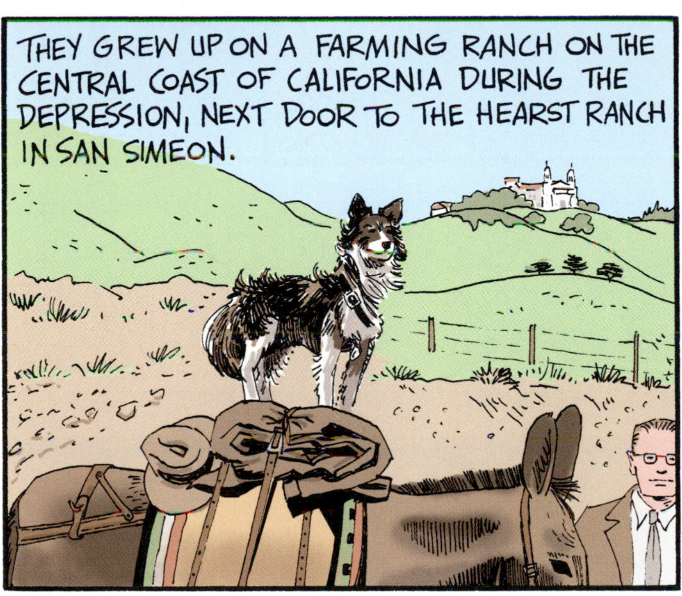

THEY GREW UP ON A FARMING RANCH ON THE CENTRAL COAST OF CALIFORNIA DURING THE DEPRESSION, NEXT DOOR TO THE HEARST RANCH IN SAN SIMEON.

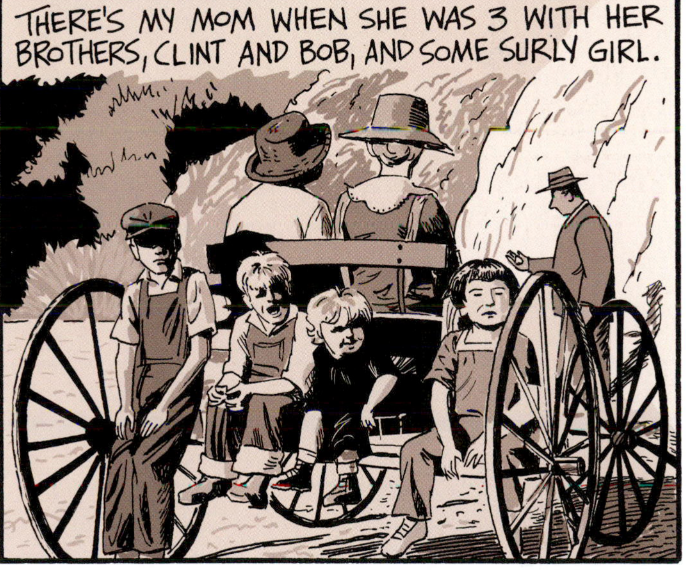

THERE'S MY MOM WHEN SHE WAS 3 WITH HER BROTHERS, CLINT AND BOB, AND SOME SURLY GIRL.

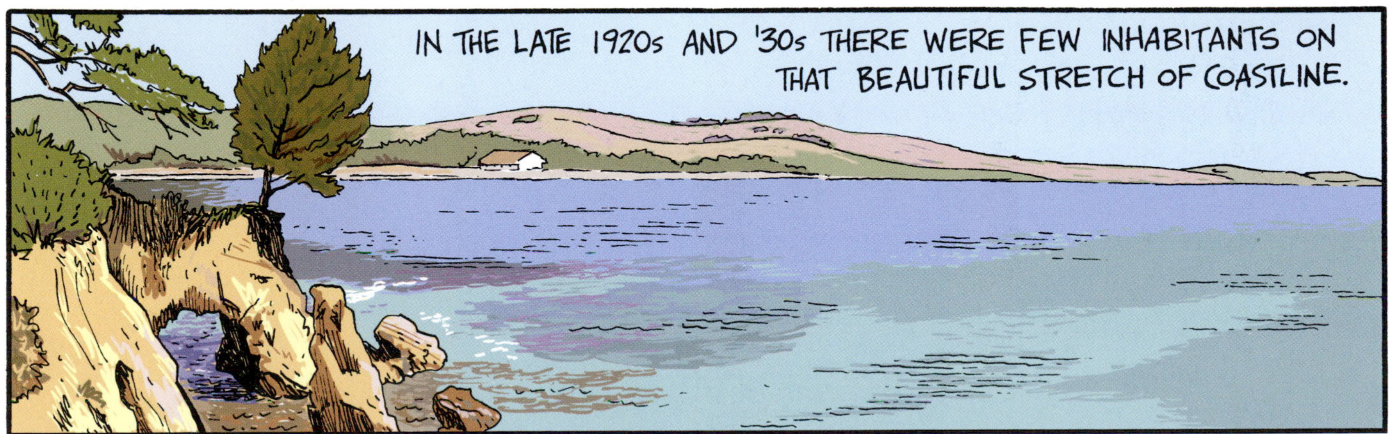

IN THE LATE 1920s AND '30s THERE WERE FEW INHABITANTS ON THAT BEAUTIFUL STRETCH OF COASTLINE.

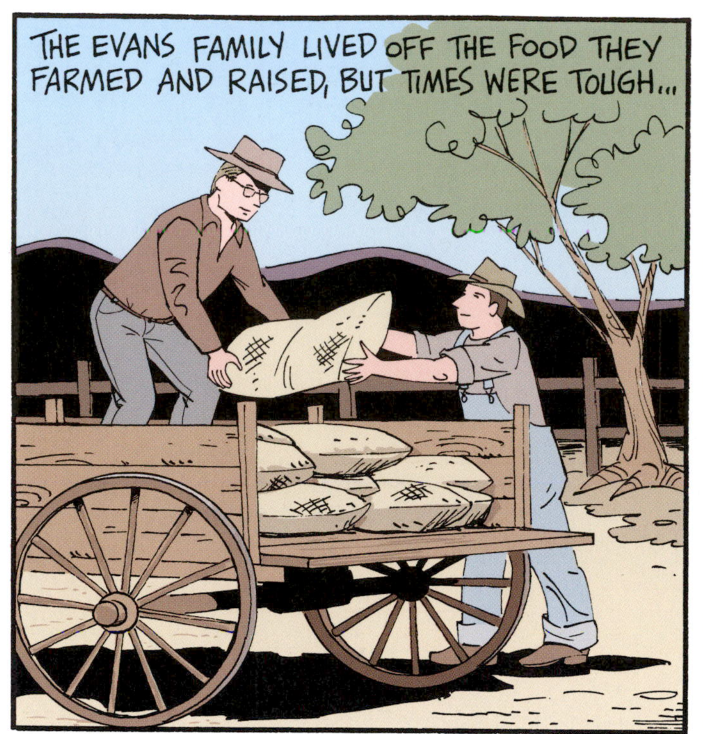
THE EVANS FAMILY LIVED OFF THE FOOD THEY FARMED AND RAISED, BUT TIMES WERE TOUGH...

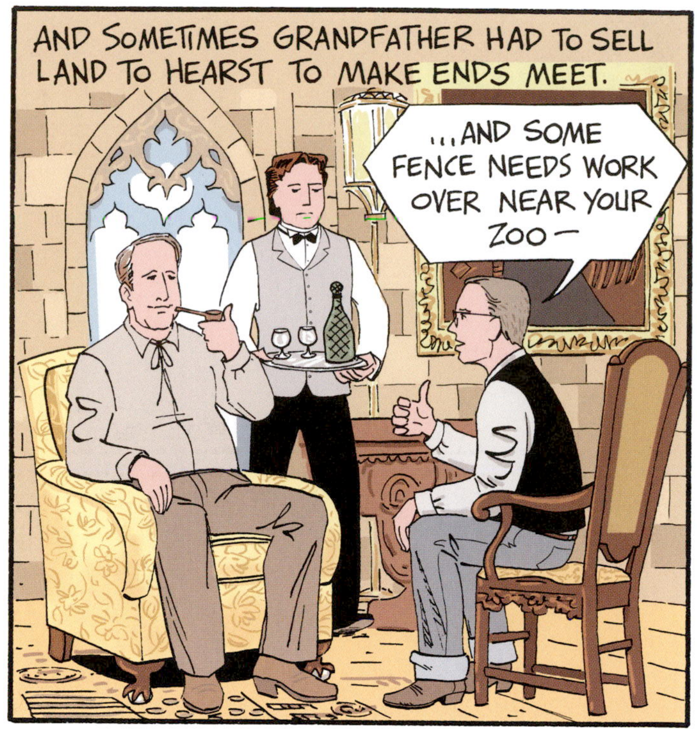
AND SOMETIMES GRANDFATHER HAD TO SELL LAND TO HEARST TO MAKE ENDS MEET.
...AND SOME FENCE NEEDS WORK OVER NEAR YOUR ZOO—

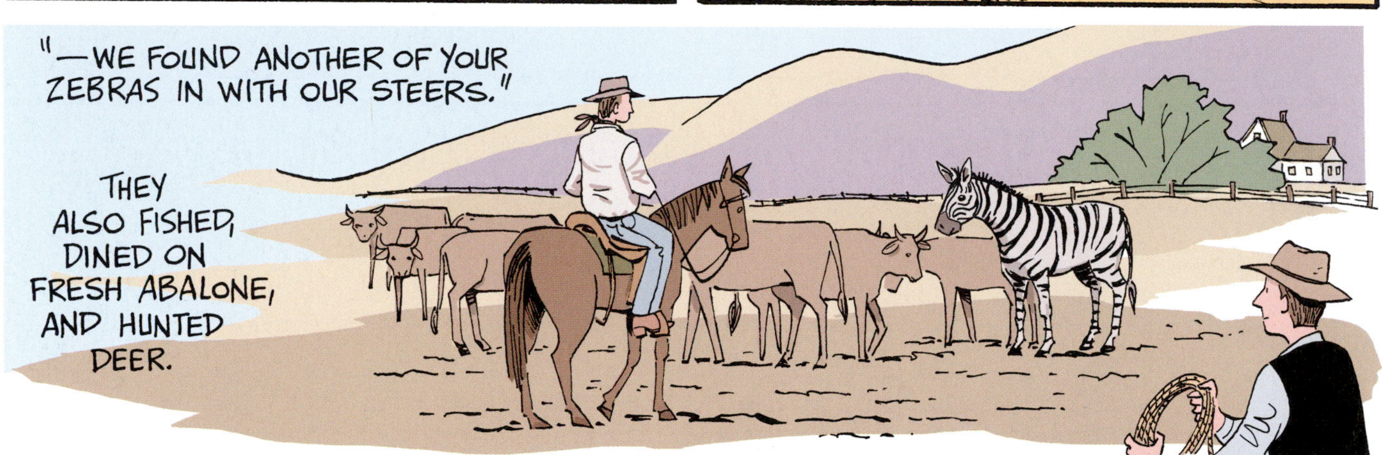
"—WE FOUND ANOTHER OF YOUR ZEBRAS IN WITH OUR STEERS."
THEY ALSO FISHED, DINED ON FRESH ABALONE, AND HUNTED DEER.

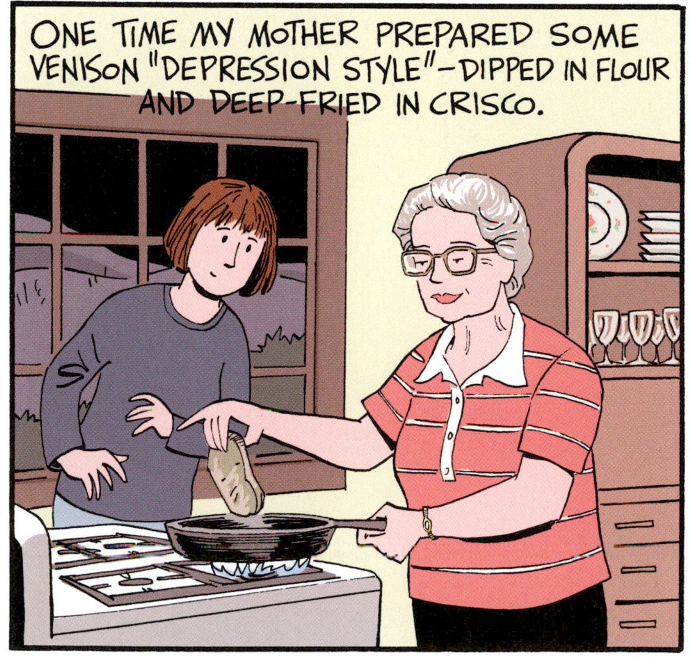
ONE TIME MY MOTHER PREPARED SOME VENISON "DEPRESSION STYLE"—DIPPED IN FLOUR AND DEEP-FRIED IN CRISCO.

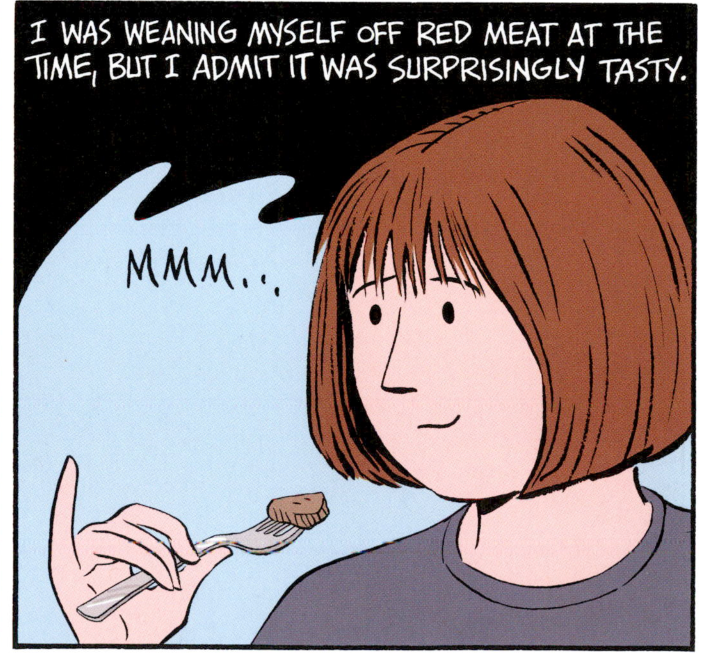
I WAS WEANING MYSELF OFF RED MEAT AT THE TIME, BUT I ADMIT IT WAS SURPRISINGLY TASTY.
MMM...

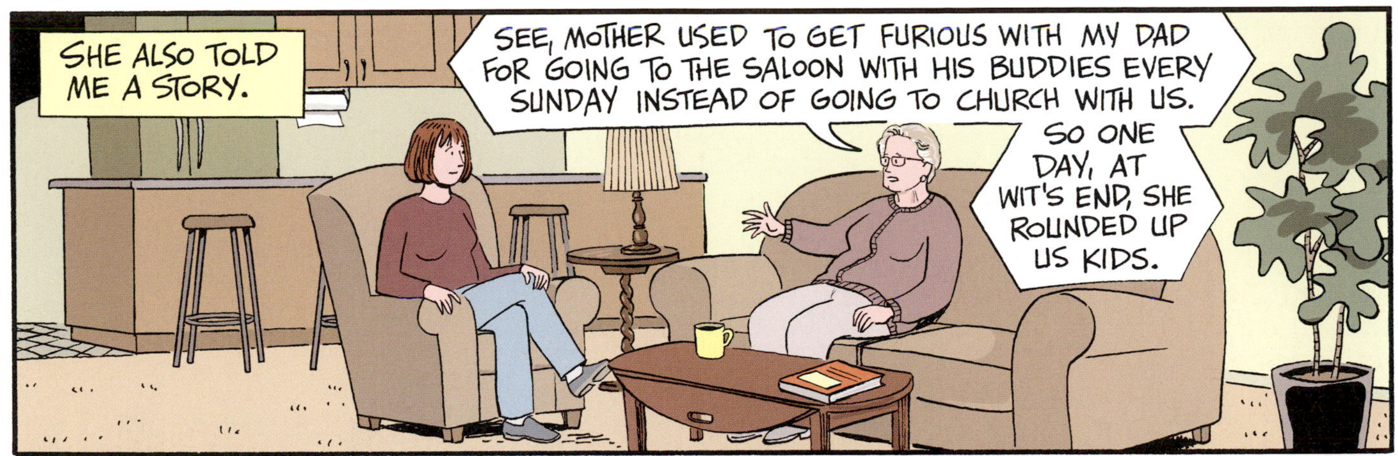
SHE ALSO TOLD ME A STORY.
SEE, MOTHER USED TO GET FURIOUS WITH MY DAD FOR GOING TO THE SALOON WITH HIS BUDDIES EVERY SUNDAY INSTEAD OF GOING TO CHURCH WITH US.
SO ONE DAY, AT WIT'S END, SHE ROUNDED UP US KIDS.

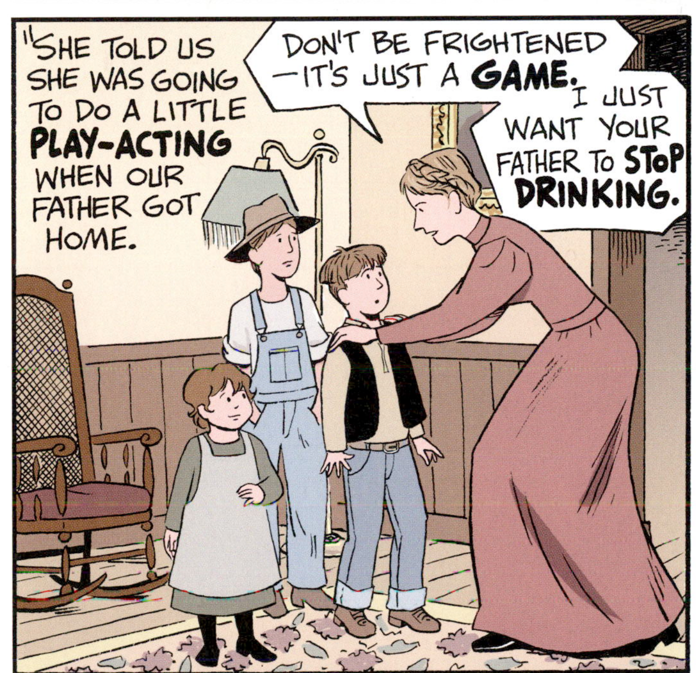
"SHE TOLD US SHE WAS GOING TO DO A LITTLE **PLAY-ACTING** WHEN OUR FATHER GOT HOME.
DON'T BE FRIGHTENED —IT'S JUST A **GAME.**
I JUST WANT YOUR FATHER TO **STOP DRINKING.**

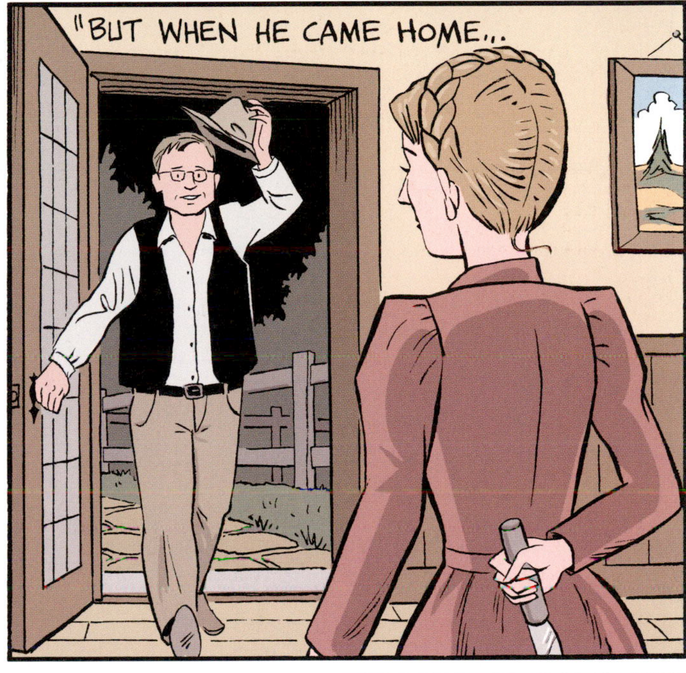
"BUT WHEN HE CAME HOME...

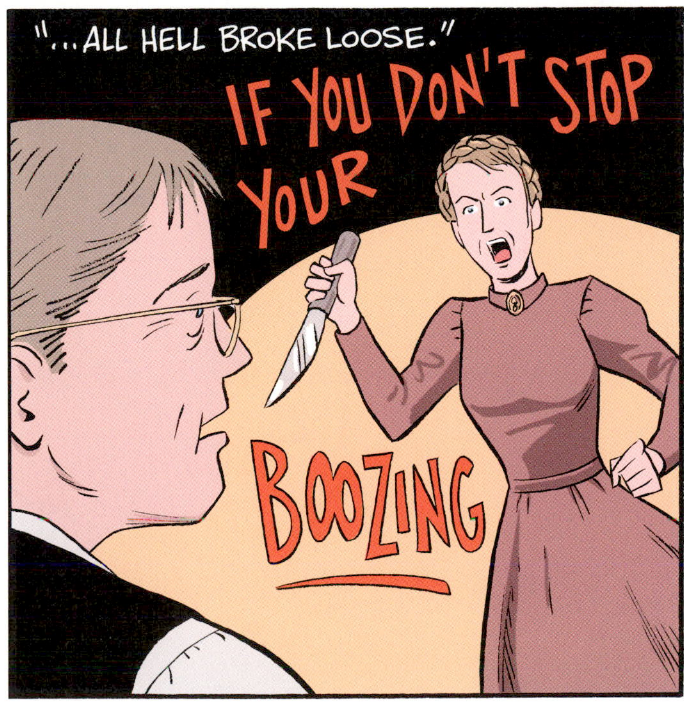
"...ALL HELL BROKE LOOSE."
IF YOU DON'T STOP YOUR
BOOZING

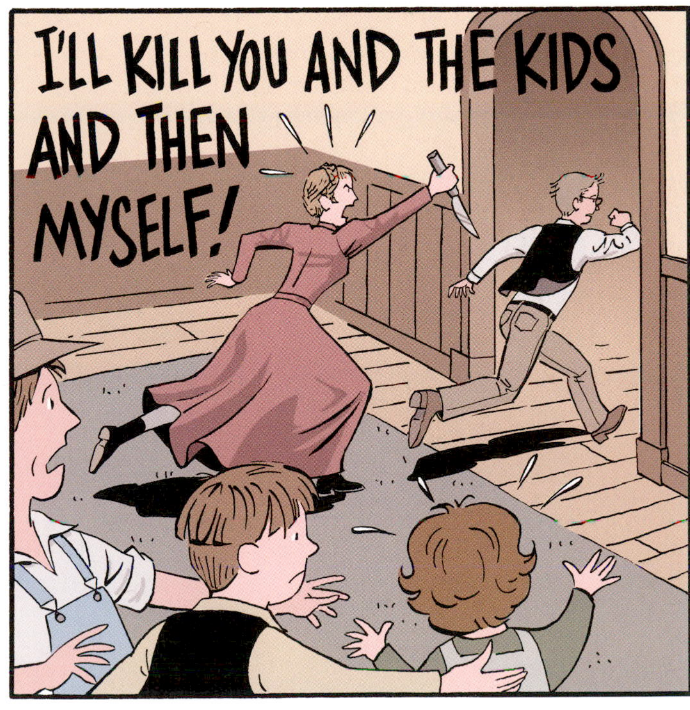
I'LL KILL YOU AND THE KIDS AND THEN MYSELF!

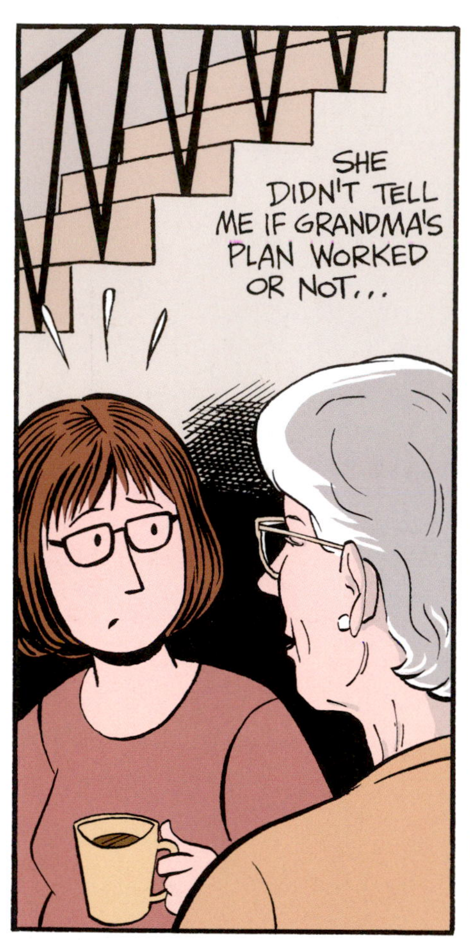
SHE DIDN'T TELL ME IF GRANDMA'S PLAN WORKED OR NOT...

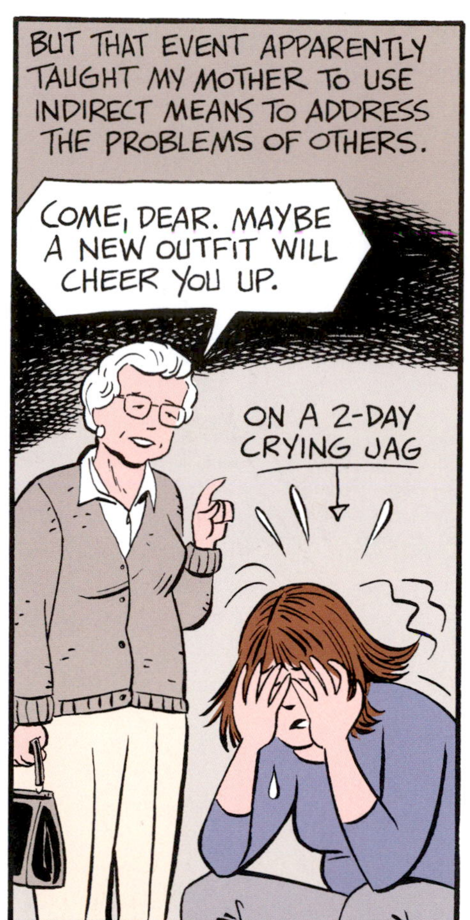
BUT THAT EVENT APPARENTLY TAUGHT MY MOTHER TO USE INDIRECT MEANS TO ADDRESS THE PROBLEMS OF OTHERS.
COME, DEAR. MAYBE A NEW OUTFIT WILL CHEER YOU UP.
ON A 2-DAY CRYING JAG

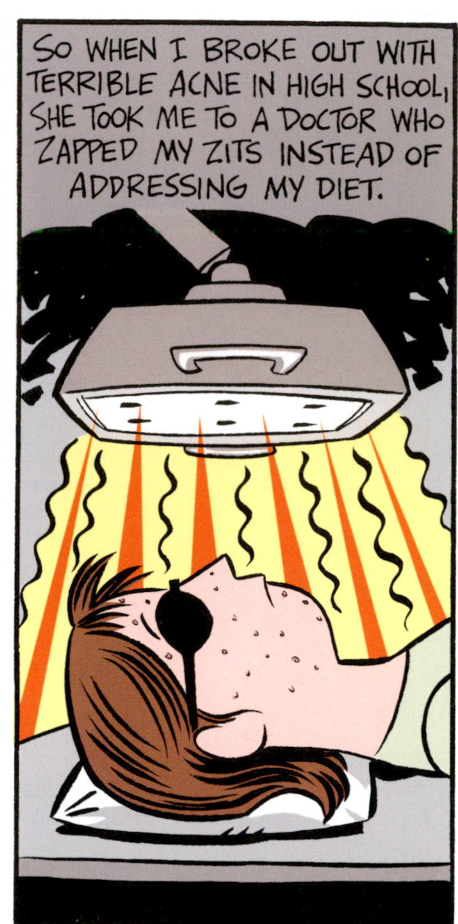
SO WHEN I BROKE OUT WITH TERRIBLE ACNE IN HIGH SCHOOL, SHE TOOK ME TO A DOCTOR WHO ZAPPED MY ZITS INSTEAD OF ADDRESSING MY DIET.

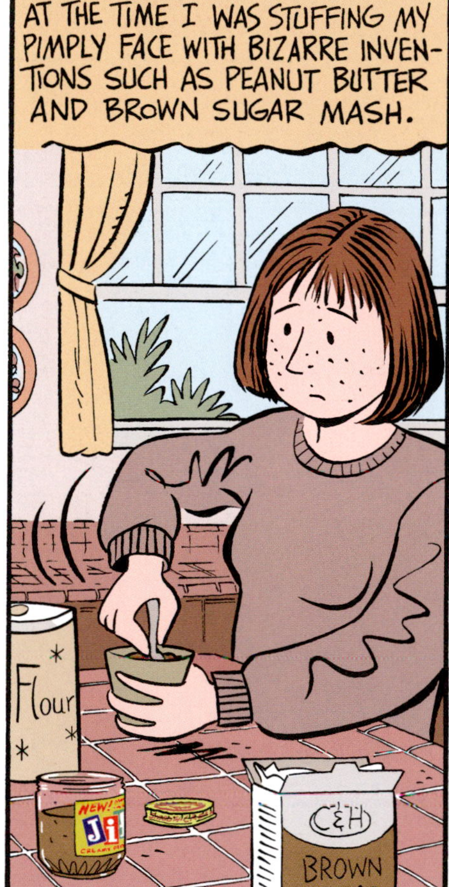
AT THE TIME I WAS STUFFING MY PIMPLY FACE WITH BIZARRE INVENTIONS SUCH AS PEANUT BUTTER AND BROWN SUGAR MASH.
Flour
Jif
C&H
BROWN

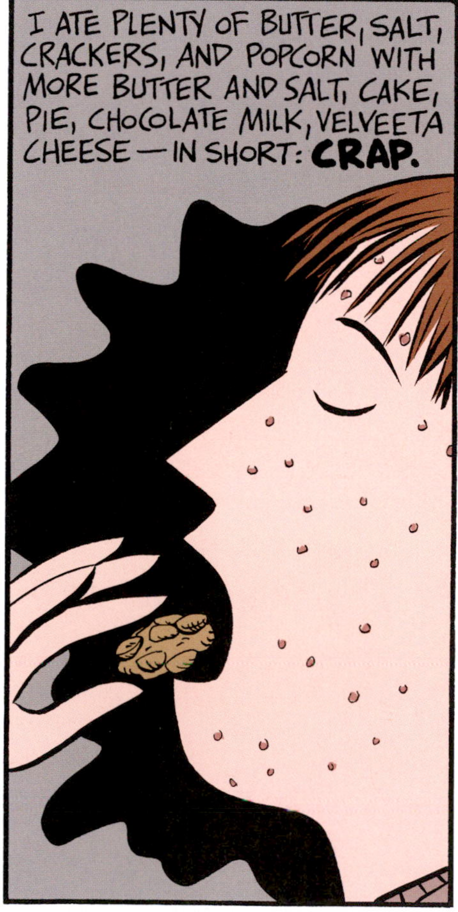
I ATE PLENTY OF BUTTER, SALT, CRACKERS, AND POPCORN WITH MORE BUTTER AND SALT, CAKE, PIE, CHOCOLATE MILK, VELVEETA CHEESE — IN SHORT: **CRAP.**

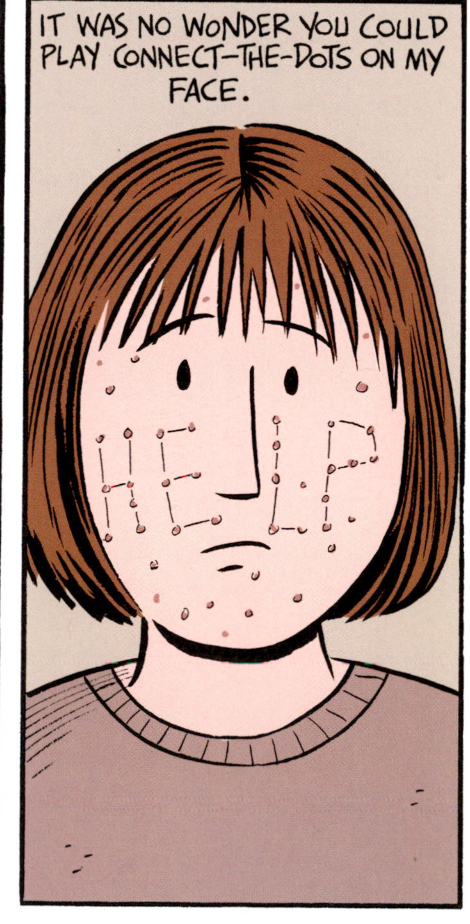
IT WAS NO WONDER YOU COULD PLAY CONNECT-THE-DOTS ON MY FACE.
HELP

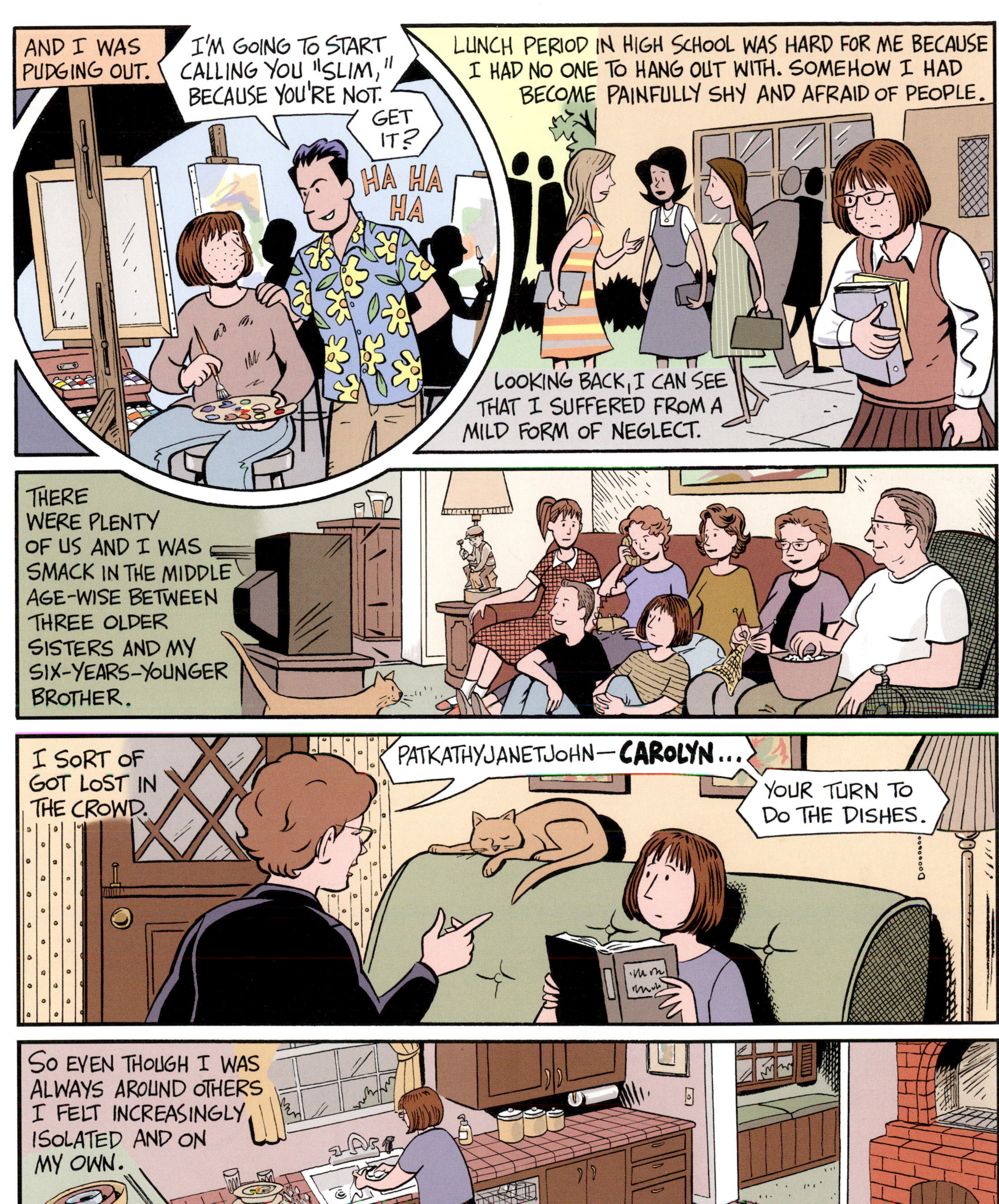

AND I WAS PUDGING OUT.
I'M GOING TO START CALLING YOU "SLIM," BECAUSE YOU'RE NOT.
GET IT?
HA HA HA
LUNCH PERIOD IN HIGH SCHOOL WAS HARD FOR ME BECAUSE I HAD NO ONE TO HANG OUT WITH. SOMEHOW I HAD BECOME PAINFULLY SHY AND AFRAID OF PEOPLE.
LOOKING BACK, I CAN SEE THAT I SUFFERED FROM A MILD FORM OF NEGLECT.
THERE WERE PLENTY OF US AND I WAS SMACK IN THE MIDDLE AGE-WISE BETWEEN THREE OLDER SISTERS AND MY SIX-YEARS-YOUNGER BROTHER.
I SORT OF GOT LOST IN THE CROWD.
PATKATHYJANETJOHN—**CAROLYN**...
YOUR TURN TO DO THE DISHES.
SO EVEN THOUGH I WAS ALWAYS AROUND OTHERS I FELT INCREASINGLY ISOLATED AND ON MY OWN.
AND HOW DID I REACT? I ATE LOTS OF **SNACKS**.

AND THAT WAS ON TOP OF THE NUTRITIONALLY DUBIOUS FOODS WE ATE AT MEALTIMES:

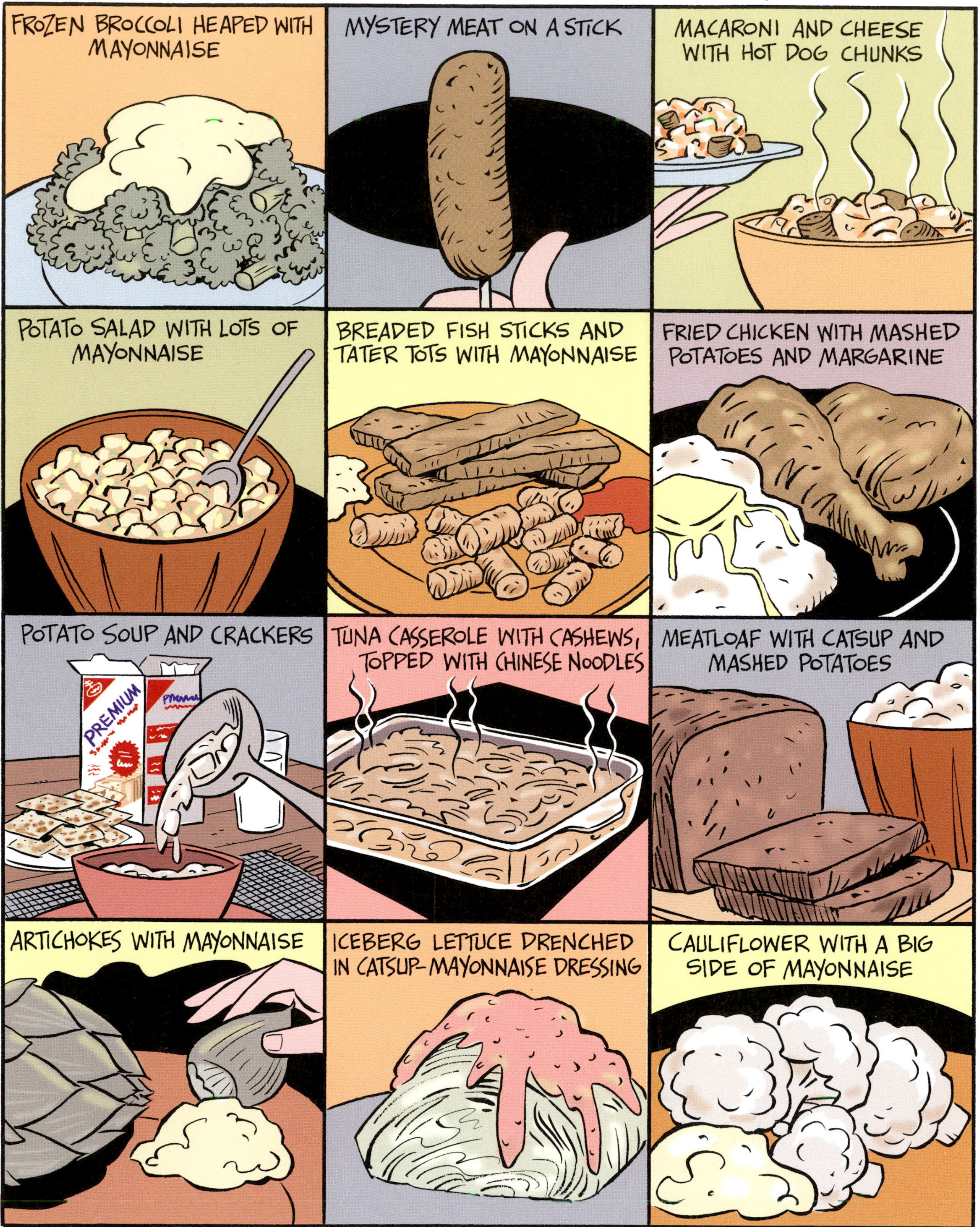
FROZEN BROCCOLI HEAPED WITH MAYONNAISE
MYSTERY MEAT ON A STICK
MACARONI AND CHEESE WITH HOT DOG CHUNKS
POTATO SALAD WITH LOTS OF MAYONNAISE
BREADED FISH STICKS AND TATER TOTS WITH MAYONNAISE
FRIED CHICKEN WITH MASHED POTATOES AND MARGARINE
POTATO SOUP AND CRACKERS
PREMIUM
TUNA CASSEROLE WITH CASHEWS, TOPPED WITH CHINESE NOODLES
MEATLOAF WITH CATSUP AND MASHED POTATOES
ARTICHOKES WITH MAYONNAISE
ICEBERG LETTUCE DRENCHED IN CATSUP-MAYONNAISE DRESSING
CAULIFLOWER WITH A BIG SIDE OF MAYONNAISE

AND THIS WAS BEFORE THERE WERE ANY LOW-FAT OR "LIGHT" MAYONNAISE OPTIONS.

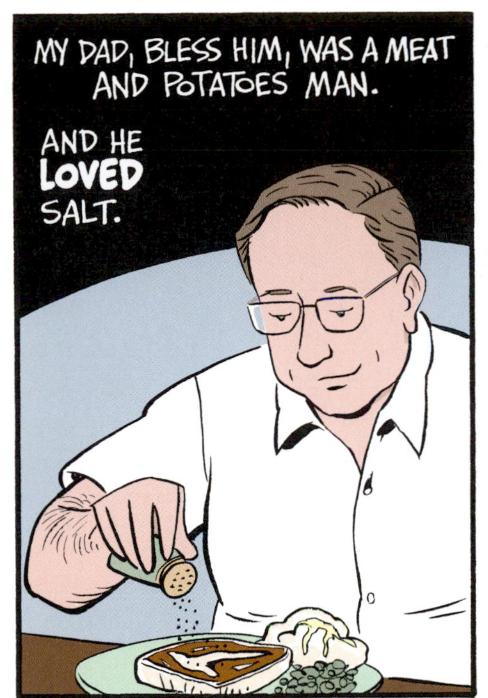
MY DAD, BLESS HIM, WAS A MEAT AND POTATOES MAN.
AND HE **LOVED** SALT.

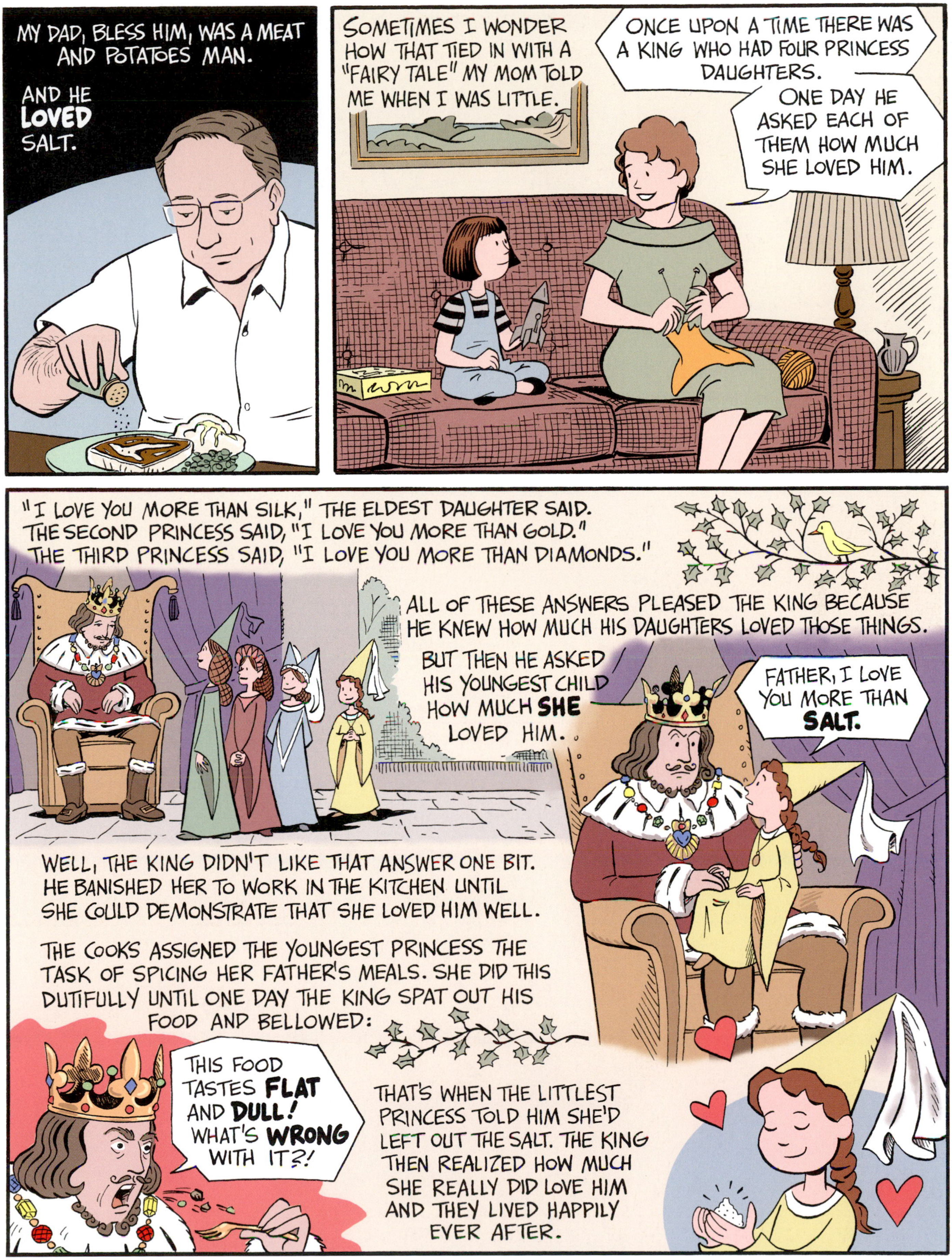

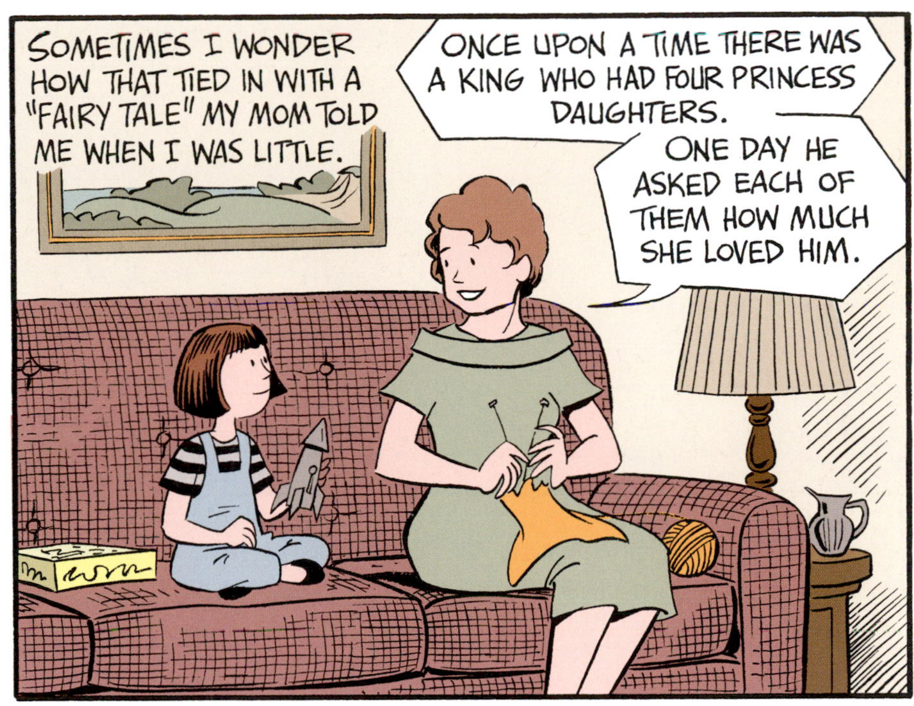
SOMETIMES I WONDER HOW THAT TIED IN WITH A "FAIRY TALE" MY MOM TOLD ME WHEN I WAS LITTLE.
ONCE UPON A TIME THERE WAS A KING WHO HAD FOUR PRINCESS DAUGHTERS.
ONE DAY HE ASKED EACH OF THEM HOW MUCH SHE LOVED HIM.

"I LOVE YOU MORE THAN SILK," THE ELDEST DAUGHTER SAID. THE SECOND PRINCESS SAID, "I LOVE YOU MORE THAN GOLD." THE THIRD PRINCESS SAID, "I LOVE YOU MORE THAN DIAMONDS."

ALL OF THESE ANSWERS PLEASED THE KING BECAUSE HE KNEW HOW MUCH HIS DAUGHTERS LOVED THOSE THINGS.

BUT THEN HE ASKED HIS YOUNGEST CHILD HOW MUCH **SHE** LOVED HIM.

FATHER, I LOVE YOU MORE THAN **SALT.**

WELL, THE KING DIDN'T LIKE THAT ANSWER ONE BIT. HE BANISHED HER TO WORK IN THE KITCHEN UNTIL SHE COULD DEMONSTRATE THAT SHE LOVED HIM WELL.

THE COOKS ASSIGNED THE YOUNGEST PRINCESS THE TASK OF SPICING HER FATHER'S MEALS. SHE DID THIS DUTIFULLY UNTIL ONE DAY THE KING SPAT OUT HIS FOOD AND BELLOWED:

THIS FOOD TASTES **FLAT** AND **DULL!** WHAT'S **WRONG** WITH IT?!

THAT'S WHEN THE LITTLEST PRINCESS TOLD HIM SHE'D LEFT OUT THE SALT. THE KING THEN REALIZED HOW MUCH SHE REALLY DID LOVE HIM AND THEY LIVED HAPPILY EVER AFTER.

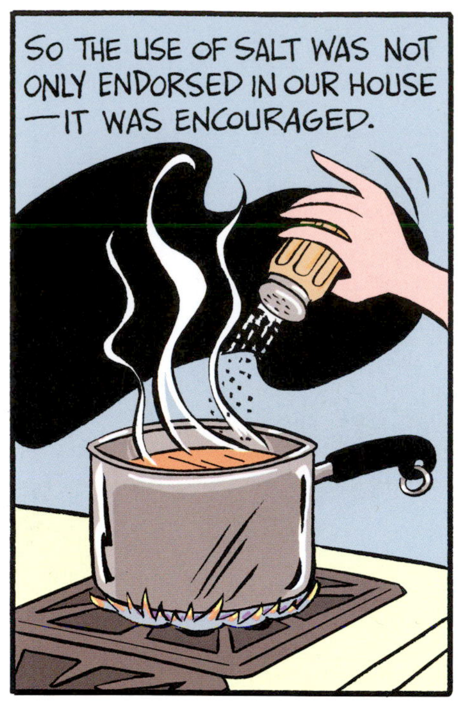
SO THE USE OF SALT WAS NOT ONLY ENDORSED IN OUR HOUSE —IT WAS ENCOURAGED.

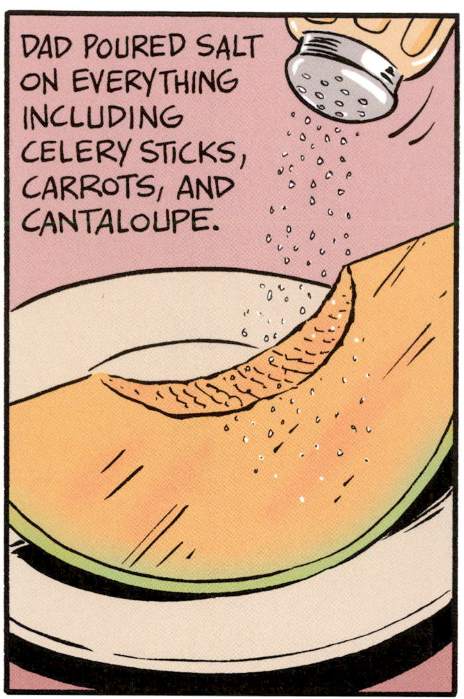
DAD POURED SALT ON EVERYTHING INCLUDING CELERY STICKS, CARROTS, AND CANTALOUPE.

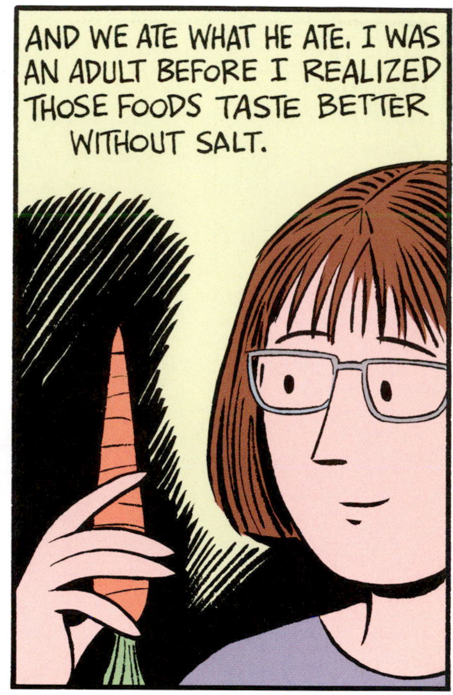
AND WE ATE WHAT HE ATE. I WAS AN ADULT BEFORE I REALIZED THOSE FOODS TASTE BETTER WITHOUT SALT.

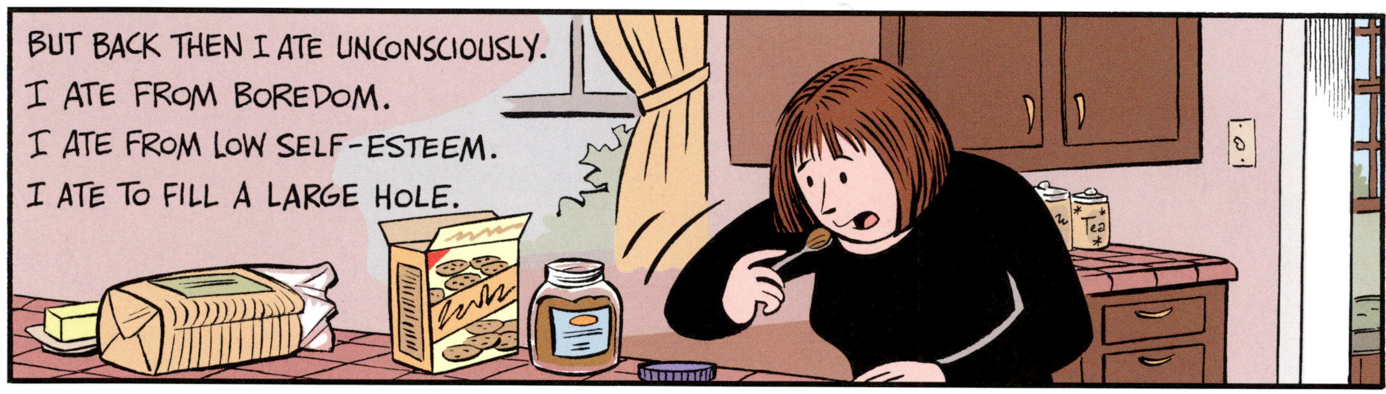
BUT BACK THEN I ATE UNCONSCIOUSLY.
I ATE FROM BOREDOM.
I ATE FROM LOW SELF-ESTEEM.
I ATE TO FILL A LARGE HOLE.
Tea

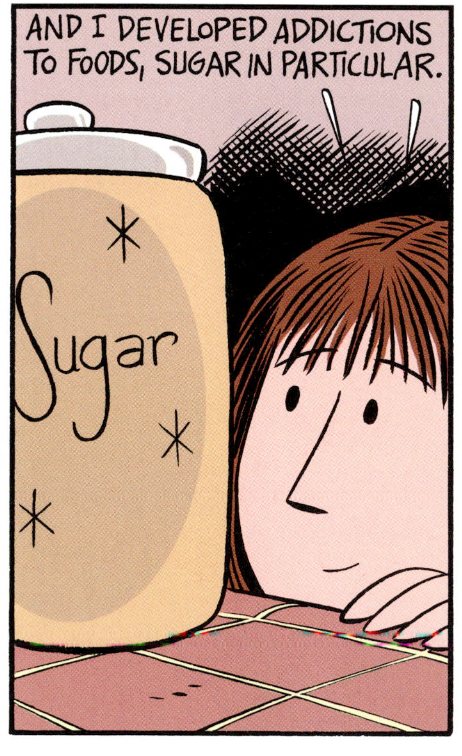
AND I DEVELOPED ADDICTIONS TO FOODS, SUGAR IN PARTICULAR.
Sugar

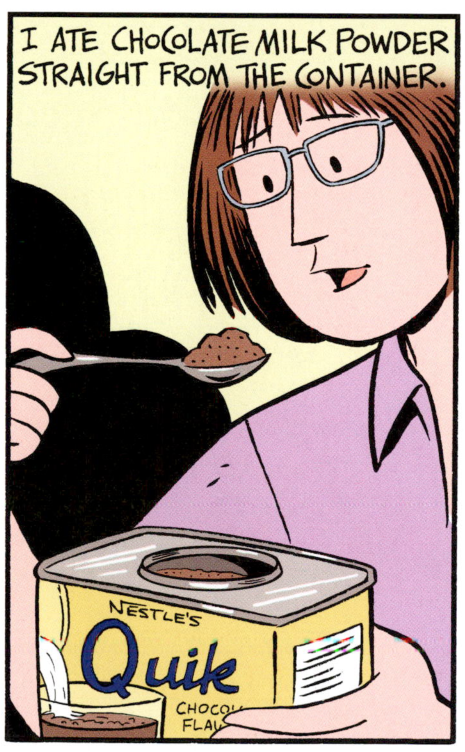
I ATE CHOCOLATE MILK POWDER STRAIGHT FROM THE CONTAINER.
NESTLE'S
Quik

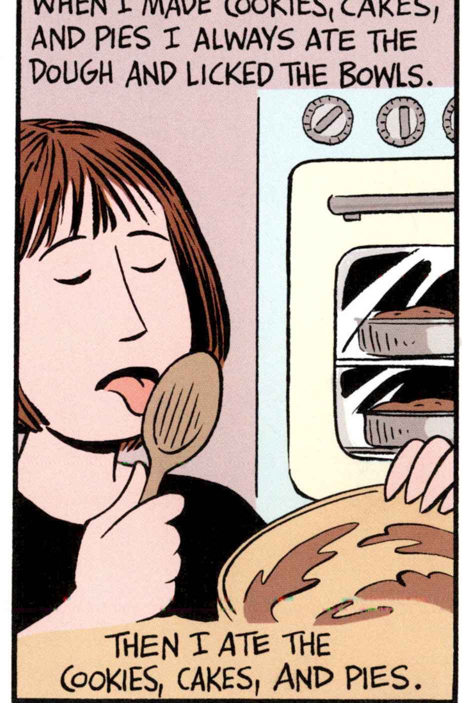
WHEN I MADE COOKIES, CAKES, AND PIES I ALWAYS ATE THE DOUGH AND LICKED THE BOWLS.
THEN I ATE THE COOKIES, CAKES, AND PIES.

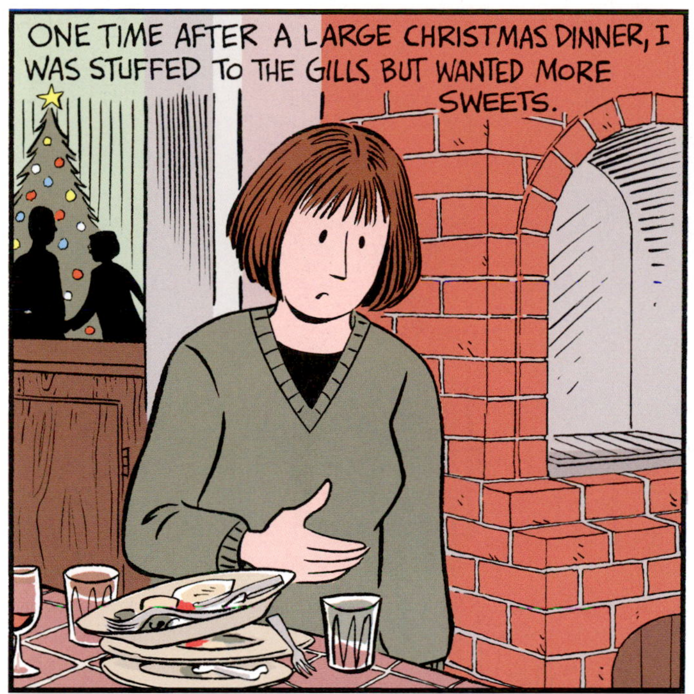
ONE TIME AFTER A LARGE CHRISTMAS DINNER, I WAS STUFFED TO THE GILLS BUT WANTED MORE SWEETS.

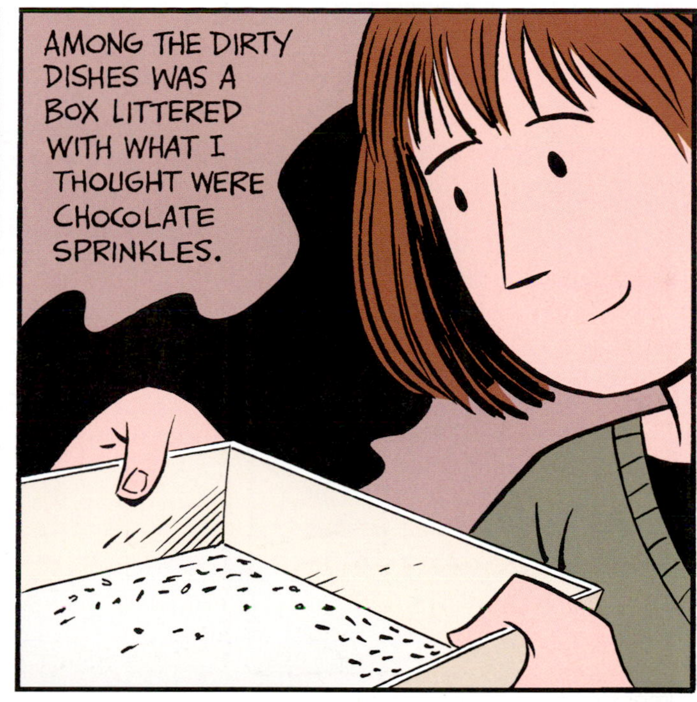
AMONG THE DIRTY DISHES WAS A BOX LITTERED WITH WHAT I THOUGHT WERE CHOCOLATE SPRINKLES.

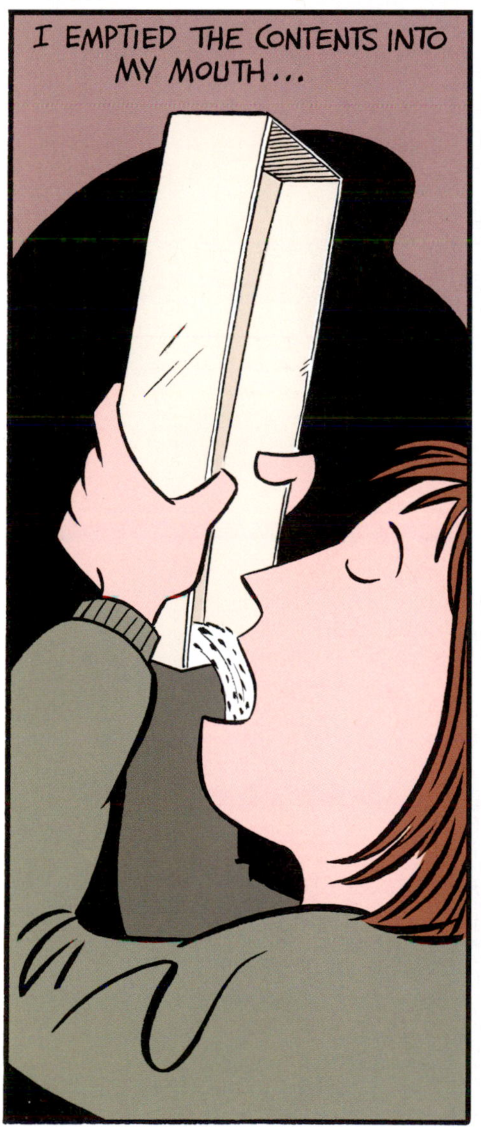
I EMPTIED THE CONTENTS INTO MY MOUTH...

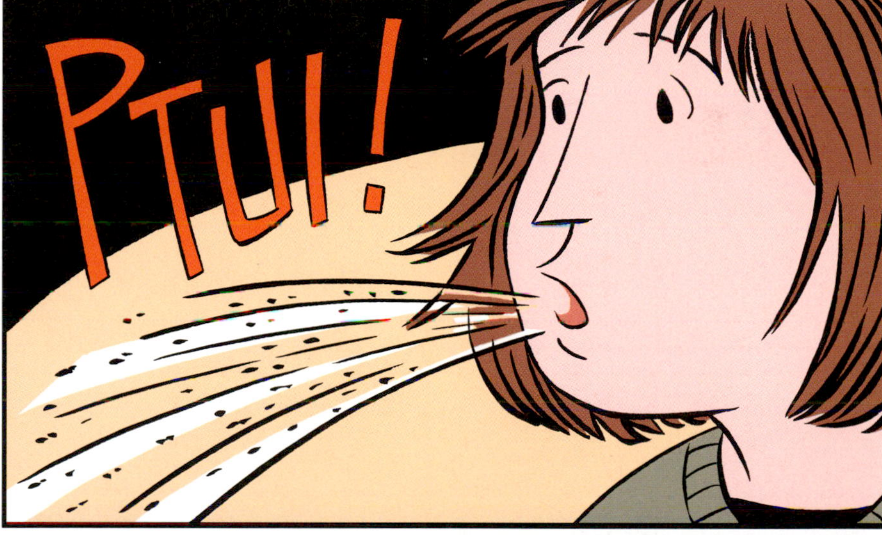
PTUI!

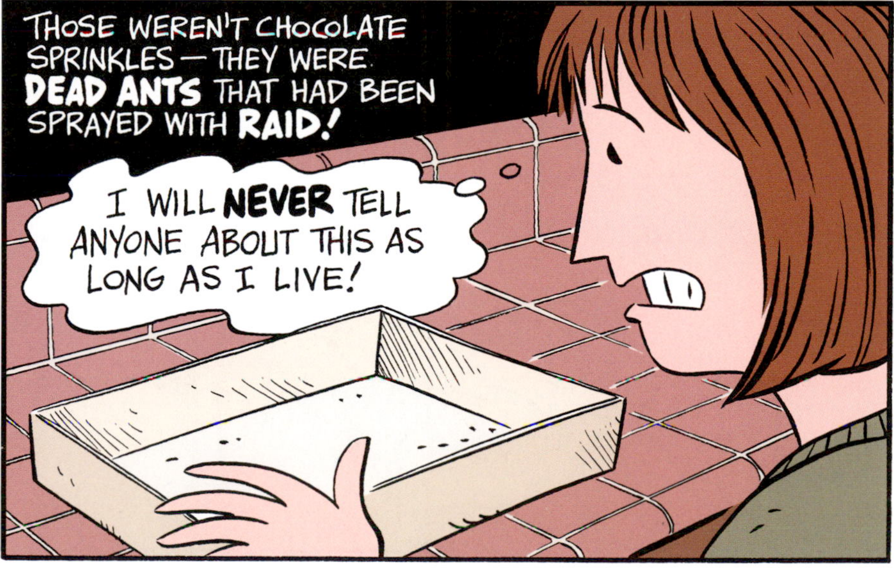
THOSE WEREN'T CHOCOLATE SPRINKLES—THEY WERE **DEAD ANTS** THAT HAD BEEN SPRAYED WITH **RAID!**
I WILL **NEVER** TELL ANYONE ABOUT THIS AS LONG AS I LIVE!

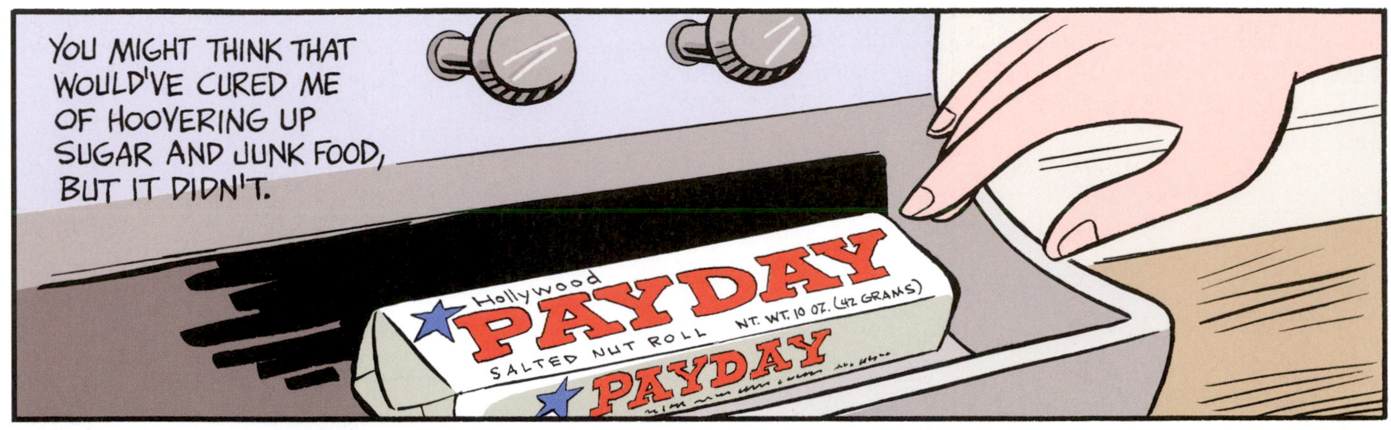
YOU MIGHT THINK THAT WOULD'VE CURED ME OF HOOVERING UP SUGAR AND JUNK FOOD, BUT IT DIDN'T.
Hollywood
PAYDAY
SALTED NUT ROLL
NT. WT. 1.0 OZ. (42 GRAMS)
PAYDAY

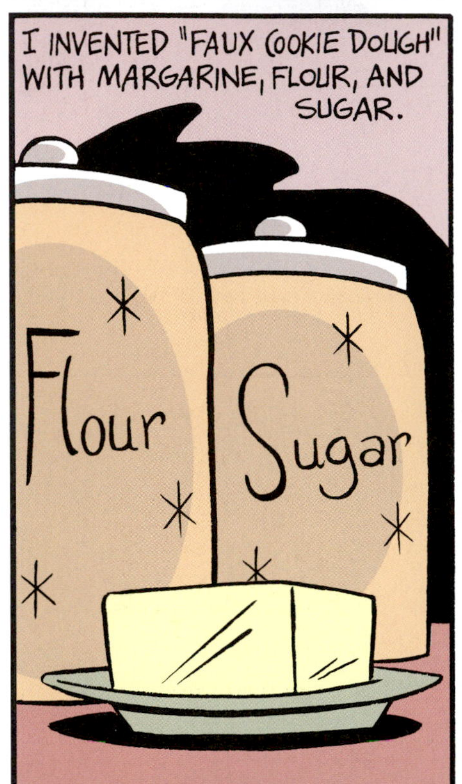
I INVENTED "FAUX COOKIE DOUGH" WITH MARGARINE, FLOUR, AND SUGAR.
Flour
Sugar

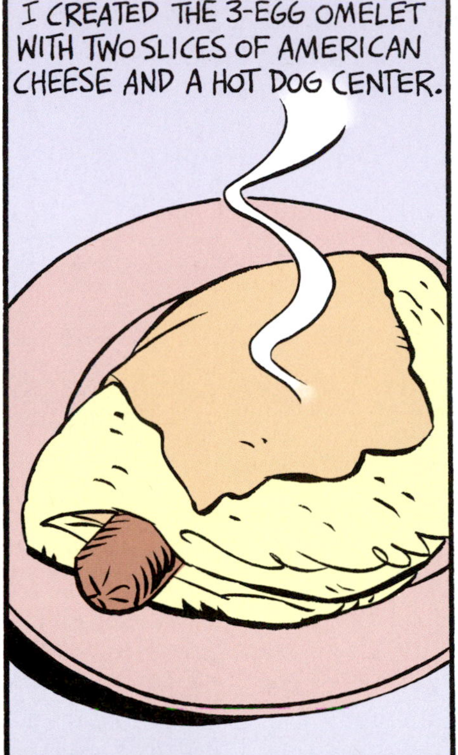
I CREATED THE 3-EGG OMELET WITH TWO SLICES OF AMERICAN CHEESE AND A HOT DOG CENTER.

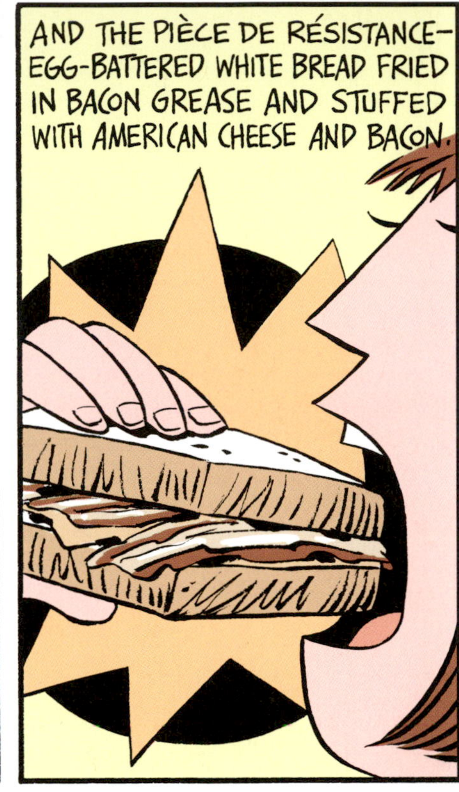
AND THE PIÈCE DE RÉSISTANCE—EGG-BATTERED WHITE BREAD FRIED IN BACON GREASE AND STUFFED WITH AMERICAN CHEESE AND BACON.

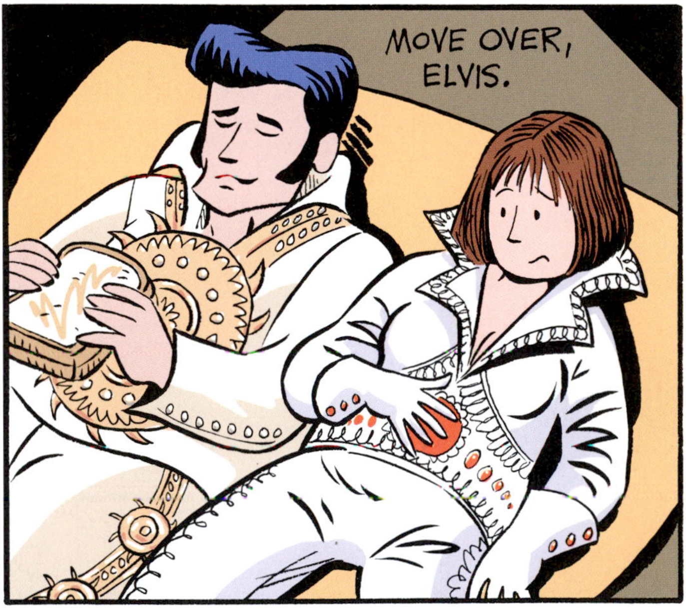
MOVE OVER, ELVIS.

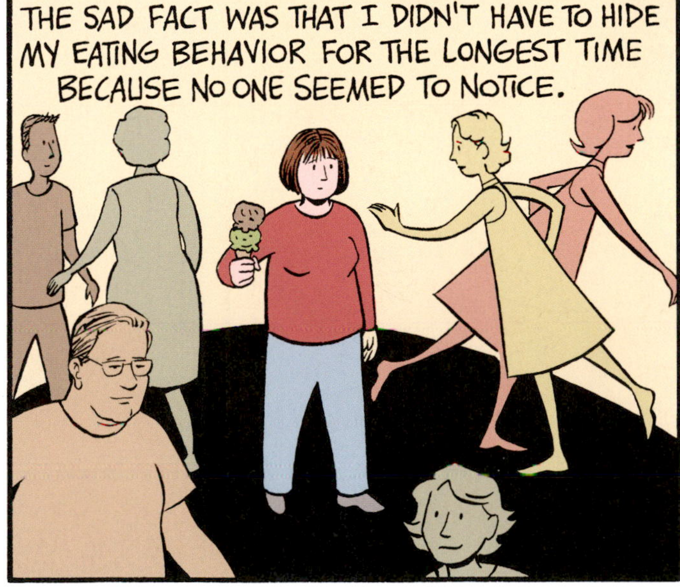
THE SAD FACT WAS THAT I DIDN'T HAVE TO HIDE MY EATING BEHAVIOR FOR THE LONGEST TIME BECAUSE NO ONE SEEMED TO NOTICE.

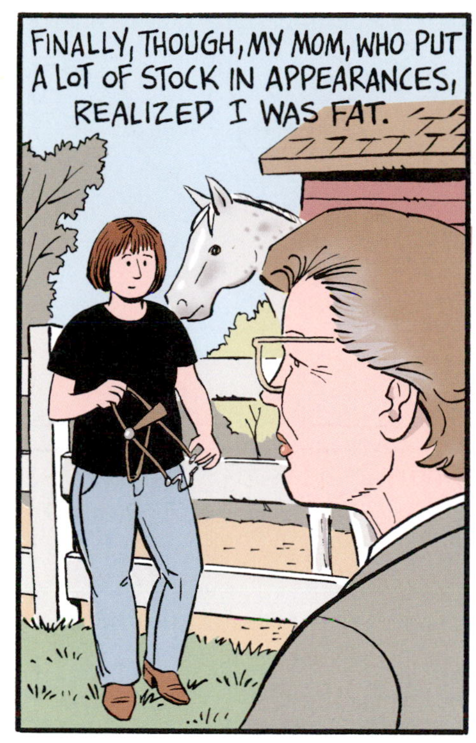
FINALLY, THOUGH, MY MOM, WHO PUT A LOT OF STOCK IN APPEARANCES, REALIZED I WAS FAT.

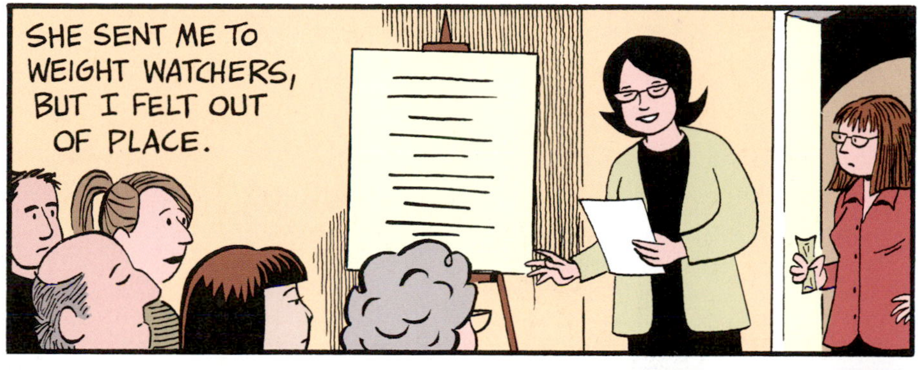
SHE SENT ME TO WEIGHT WATCHERS, BUT I FELT OUT OF PLACE.

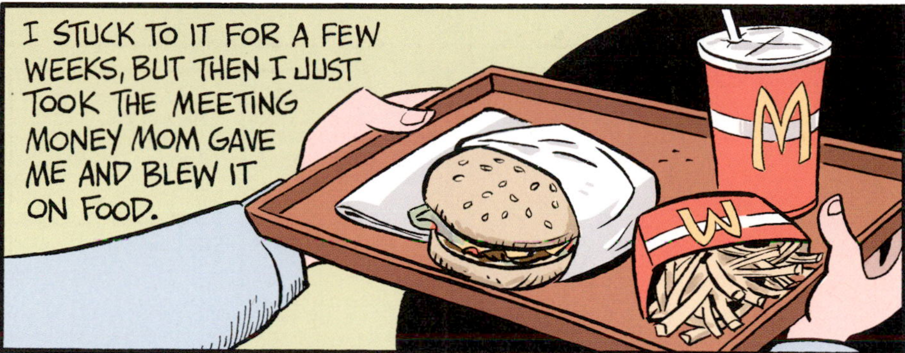
I STUCK TO IT FOR A FEW WEEKS, BUT THEN I JUST TOOK THE MEETING MONEY MOM GAVE ME AND BLEW IT ON FOOD.

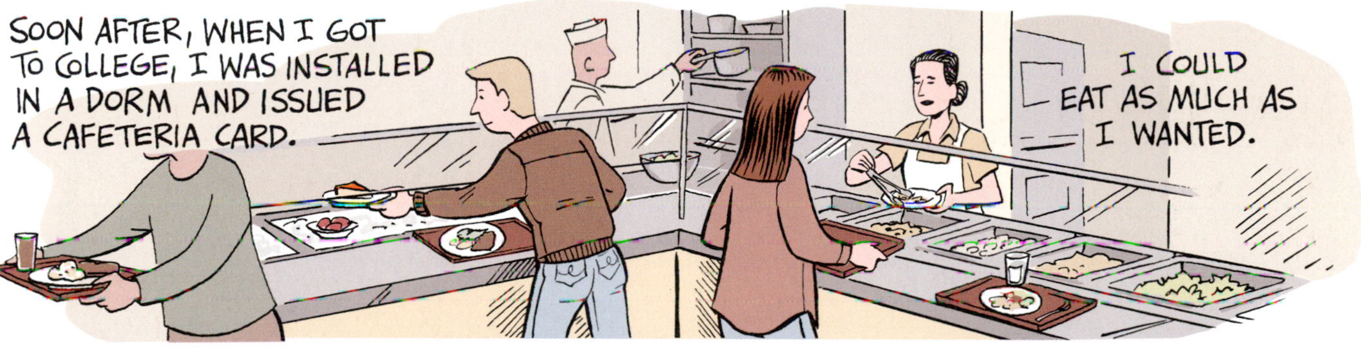
SOON AFTER, WHEN I GOT TO COLLEGE, I WAS INSTALLED IN A DORM AND ISSUED A CAFETERIA CARD.
I COULD EAT AS MUCH AS I WANTED.

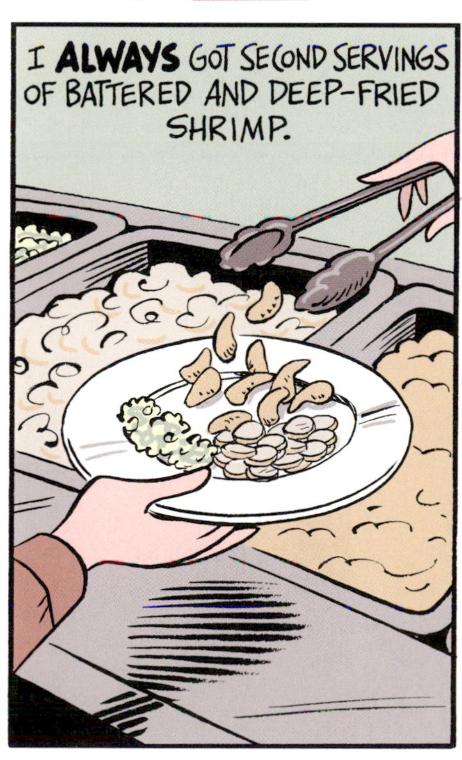
I **ALWAYS** GOT SECOND SERVINGS OF BATTERED AND DEEP-FRIED SHRIMP.

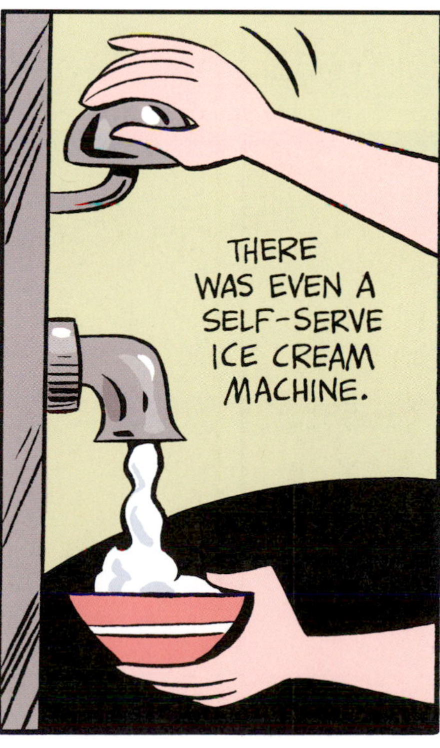
THERE WAS EVEN A SELF-SERVE ICE CREAM MACHINE.

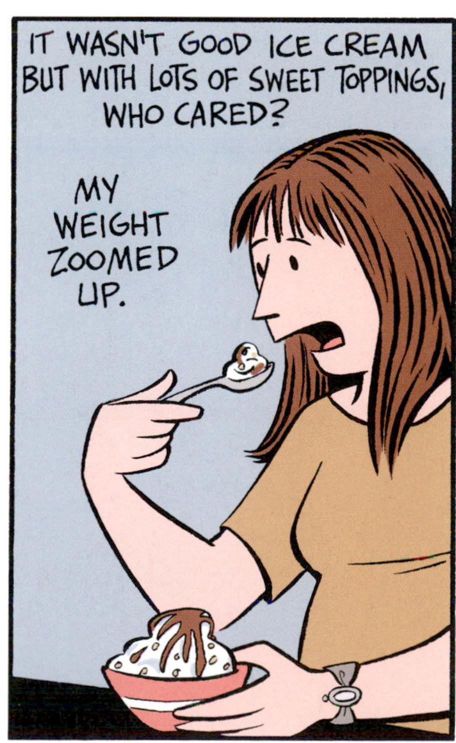
IT WASN'T GOOD ICE CREAM BUT WITH LOTS OF SWEET TOPPINGS, WHO CARED?
MY WEIGHT ZOOMED UP.

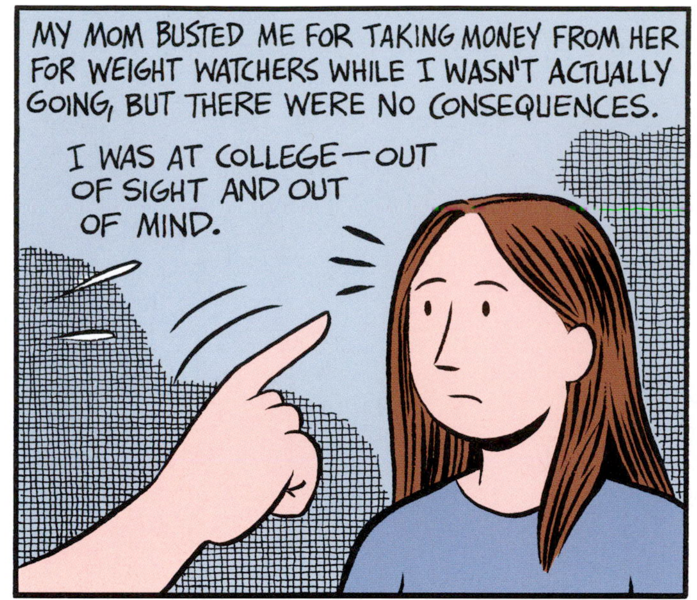
MY MOM BUSTED ME FOR TAKING MONEY FROM HER FOR WEIGHT WATCHERS WHILE I WASN'T ACTUALLY GOING, BUT THERE WERE NO CONSEQUENCES.
I WAS AT COLLEGE—OUT OF SIGHT AND OUT OF MIND.

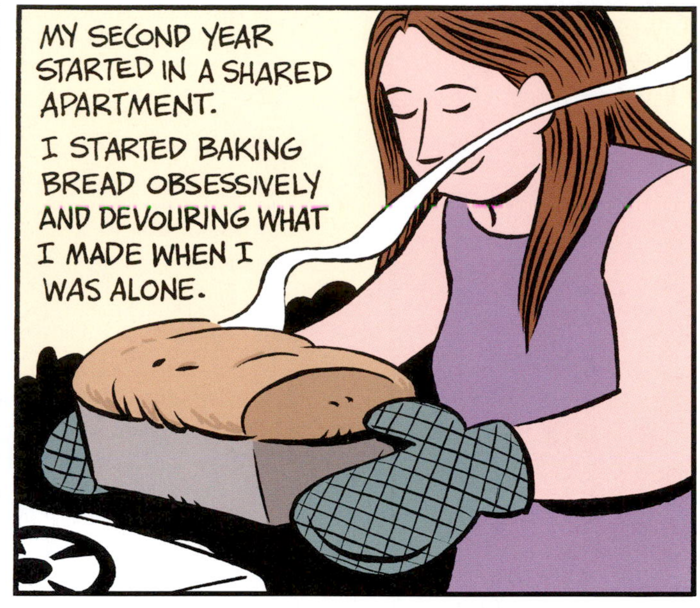
MY SECOND YEAR STARTED IN A SHARED APARTMENT.
I STARTED BAKING BREAD OBSESSIVELY AND DEVOURING WHAT I MADE WHEN I WAS ALONE.

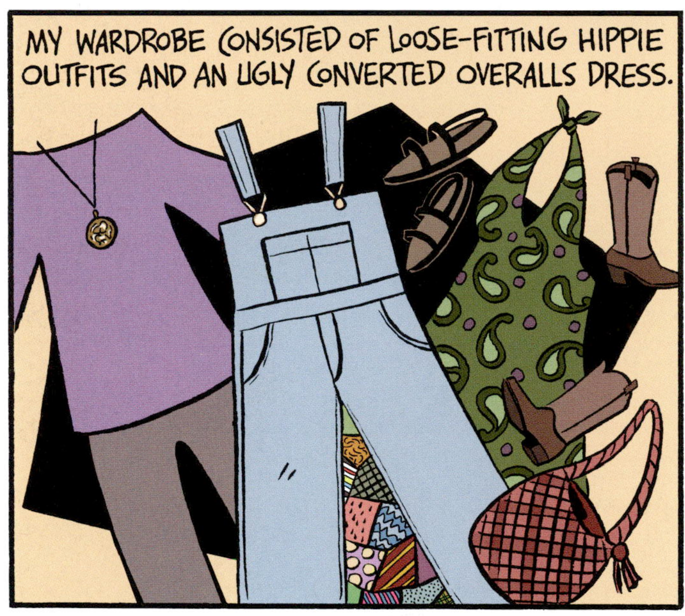
MY WARDROBE CONSISTED OF LOOSE-FITTING HIPPIE OUTFITS AND AN UGLY CONVERTED OVERALLS DRESS.

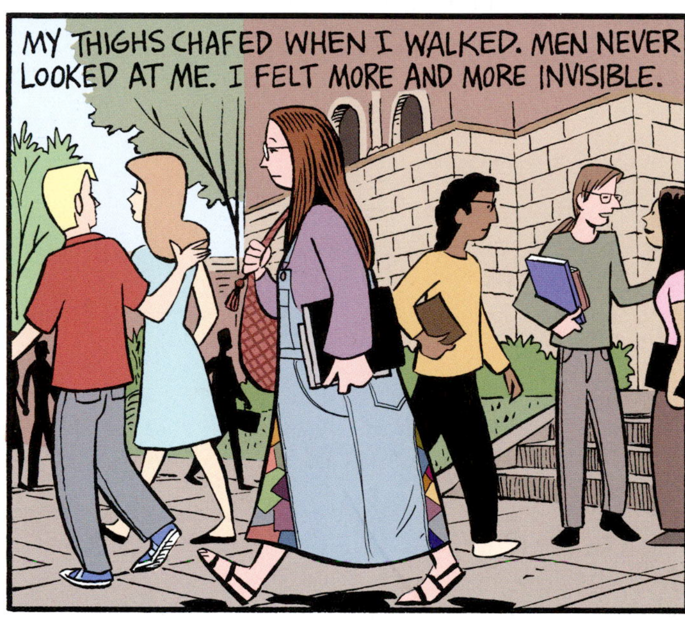
MY THIGHS CHAFED WHEN I WALKED. MEN NEVER LOOKED AT ME. I FELT MORE AND MORE INVISIBLE.

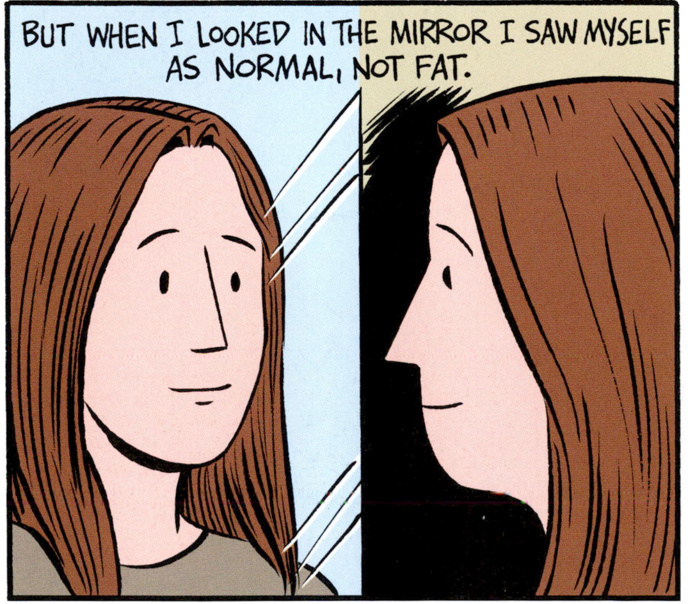
BUT WHEN I LOOKED IN THE MIRROR I SAW MYSELF AS NORMAL, NOT FAT.

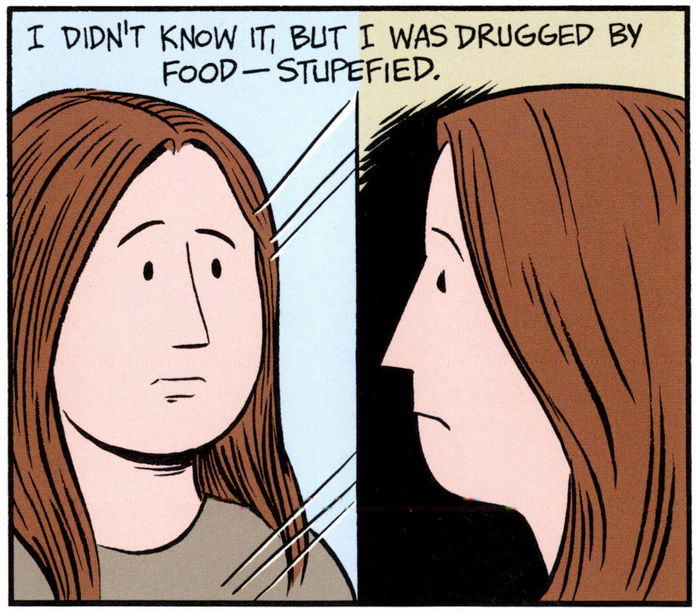
I DIDN'T KNOW IT, BUT I WAS DRUGGED BY FOOD—STUPEFIED.

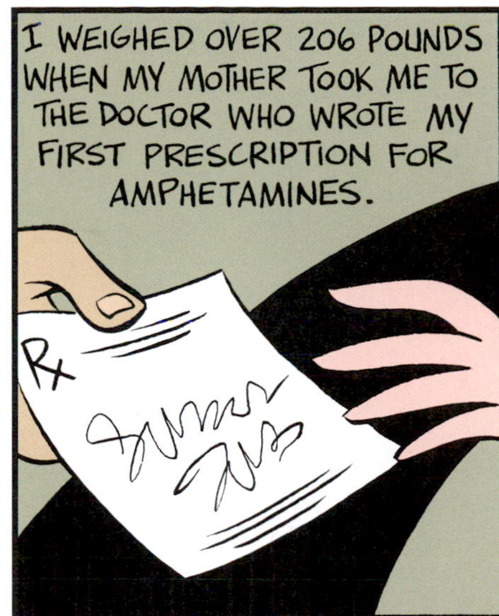
I WEIGHED OVER 206 POUNDS WHEN MY MOTHER TOOK ME TO THE DOCTOR WHO WROTE MY FIRST PRESCRIPTION FOR AMPHETAMINES.
Rx

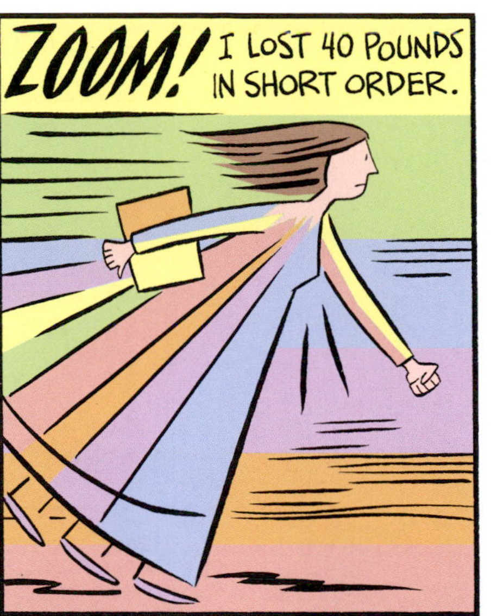
ZOOM!
I LOST 40 POUNDS IN SHORT ORDER.

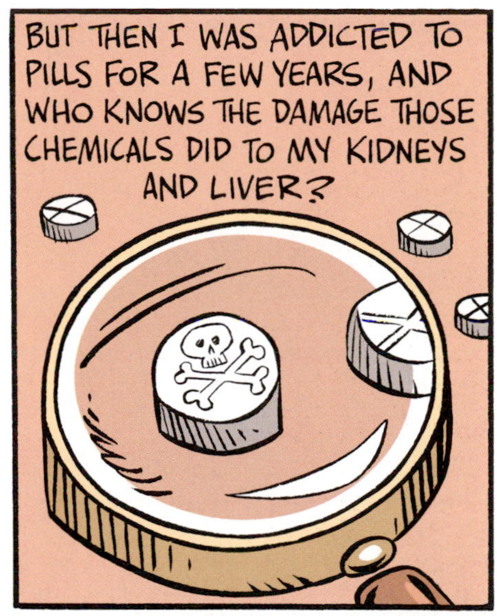
BUT THEN I WAS ADDICTED TO PILLS FOR A FEW YEARS, AND WHO KNOWS THE DAMAGE THOSE CHEMICALS DID TO MY KIDNEYS AND LIVER?

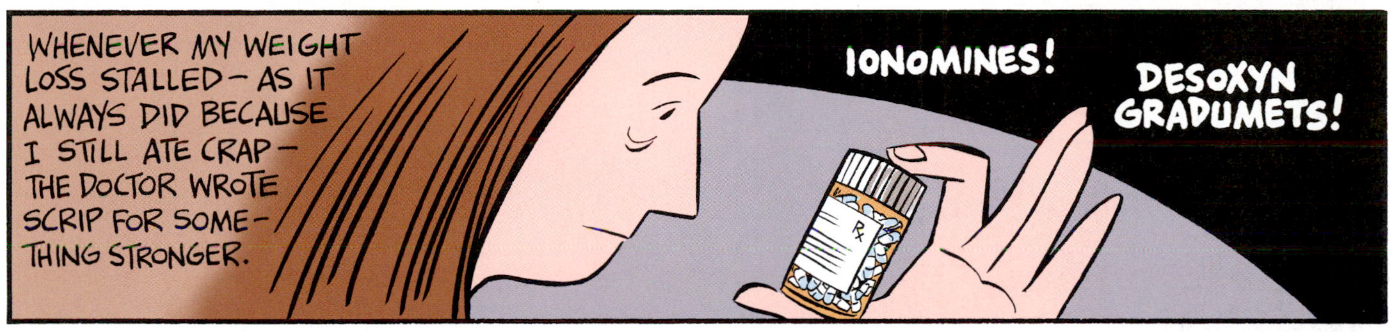
WHENEVER MY WEIGHT LOSS STALLED—AS IT ALWAYS DID BECAUSE I STILL ATE CRAP—THE DOCTOR WROTE SCRIP FOR SOMETHING STRONGER.
IONOMINES!
DESOXYN GRADUMETS!

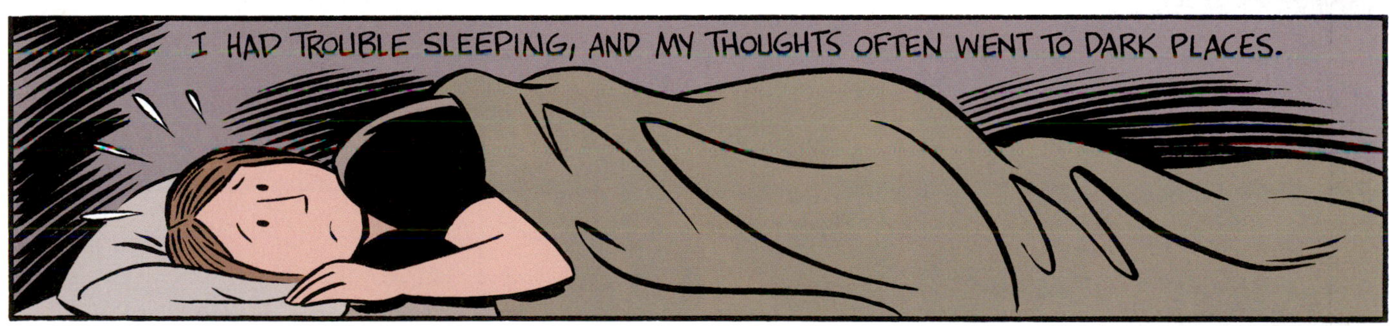
I HAD TROUBLE SLEEPING, AND MY THOUGHTS OFTEN WENT TO DARK PLACES.

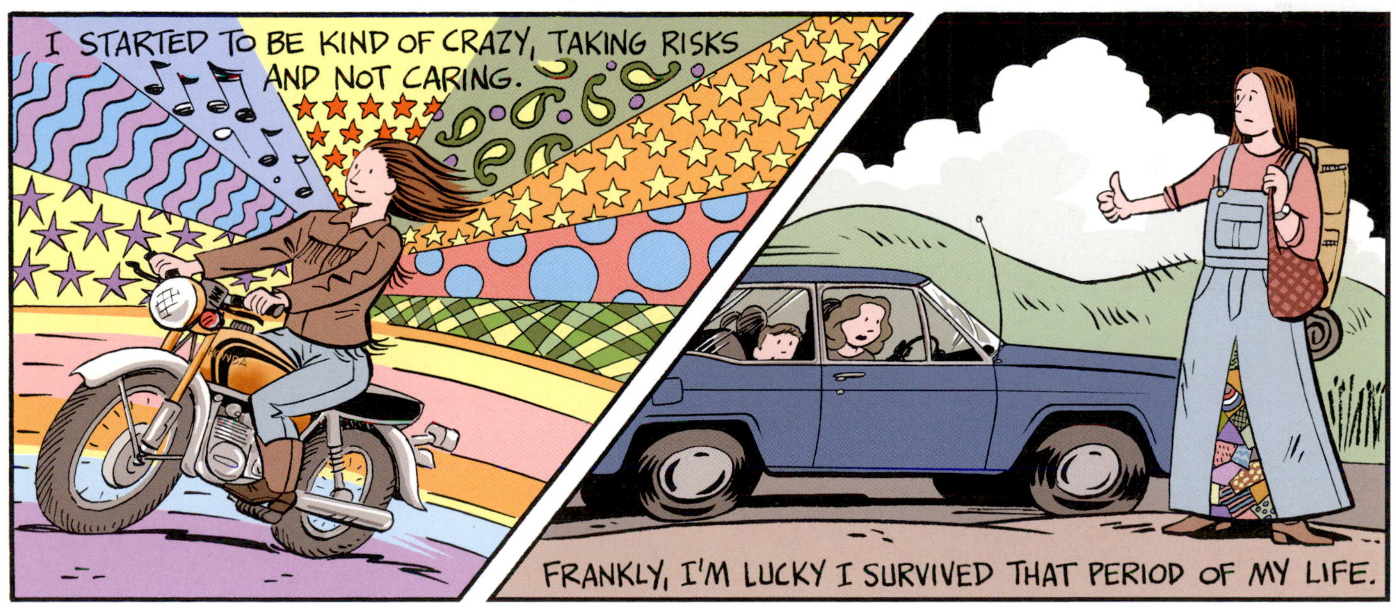
I STARTED TO BE KIND OF CRAZY, TAKING RISKS AND NOT CARING.
FRANKLY, I'M LUCKY I SURVIVED THAT PERIOD OF MY LIFE.

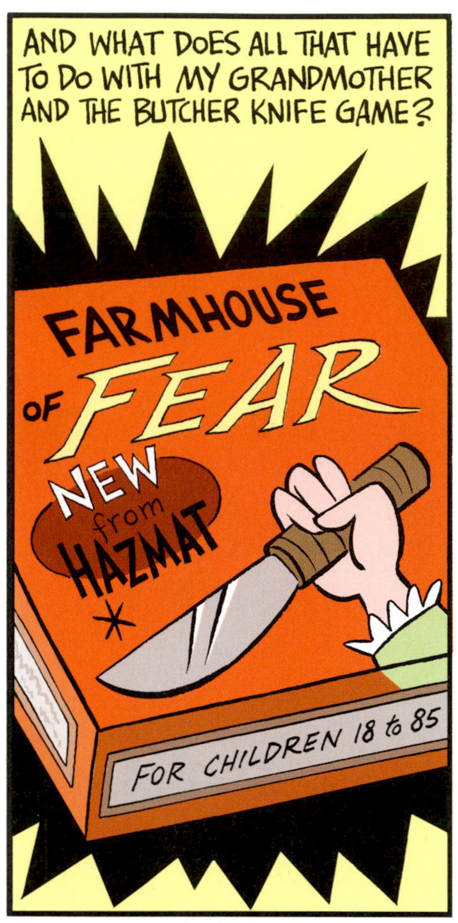
AND WHAT DOES ALL THAT HAVE TO DO WITH MY GRANDMOTHER AND THE BUTCHER KNIFE GAME?
FARMHOUSE OF FEAR
NEW from HAZMAT
FOR CHILDREN 18 to 85

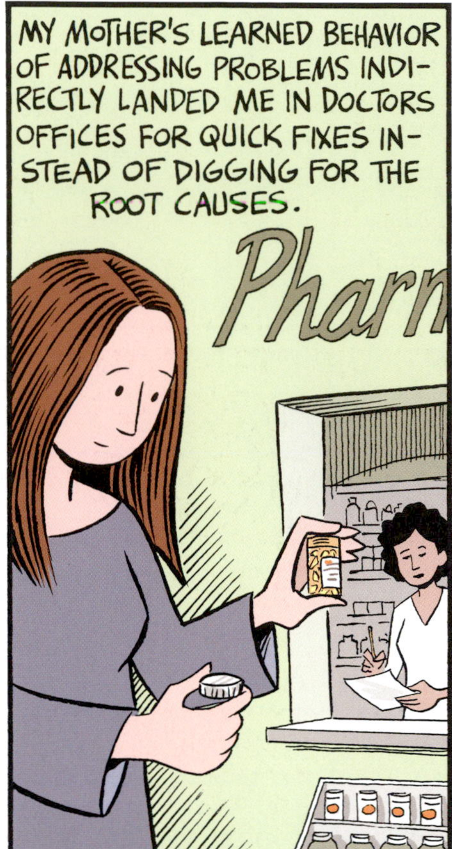
MY MOTHER'S LEARNED BEHAVIOR OF ADDRESSING PROBLEMS INDIRECTLY LANDED ME IN DOCTORS OFFICES FOR QUICK FIXES INSTEAD OF DIGGING FOR THE ROOT CAUSES.
Pharm

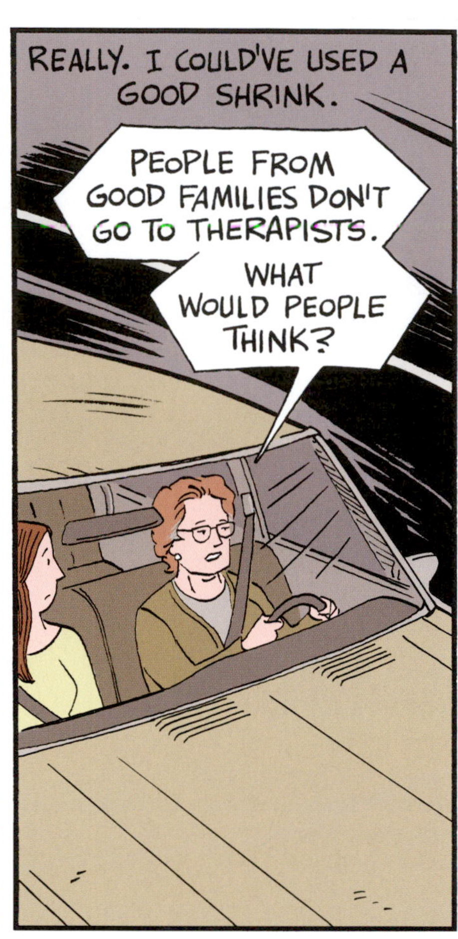
REALLY. I COULD'VE USED A GOOD SHRINK.
PEOPLE FROM GOOD FAMILIES DON'T GO TO THERAPISTS.
WHAT WOULD PEOPLE THINK?

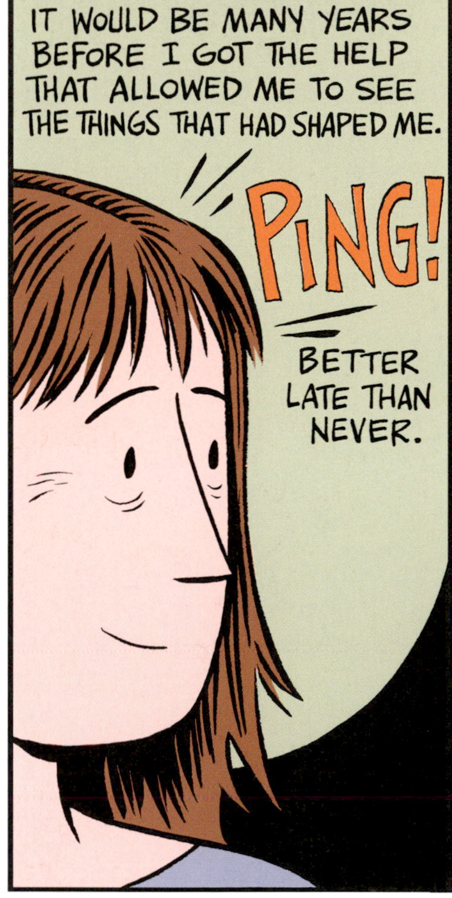
IT WOULD BE MANY YEARS BEFORE I GOT THE HELP THAT ALLOWED ME TO SEE THE THINGS THAT HAD SHAPED ME.
PING!
BETTER LATE THAN NEVER.

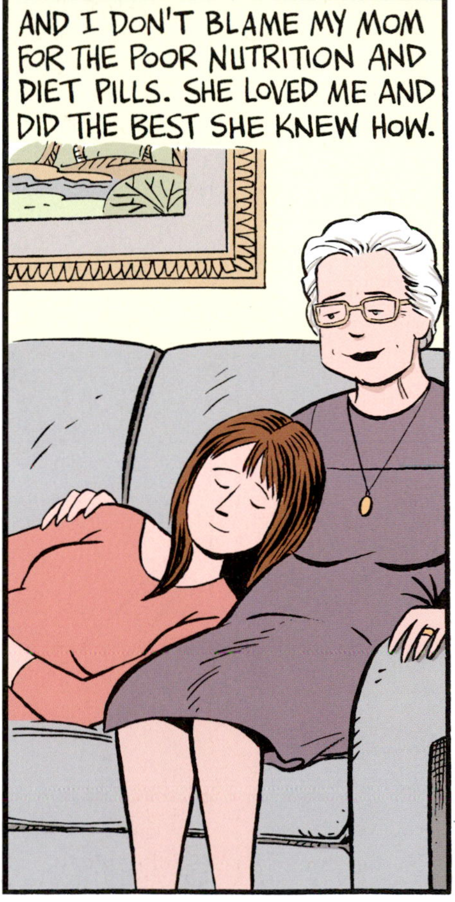
AND I DON'T BLAME MY MOM FOR THE POOR NUTRITION AND DIET PILLS. SHE LOVED ME AND DID THE BEST SHE KNEW HOW.

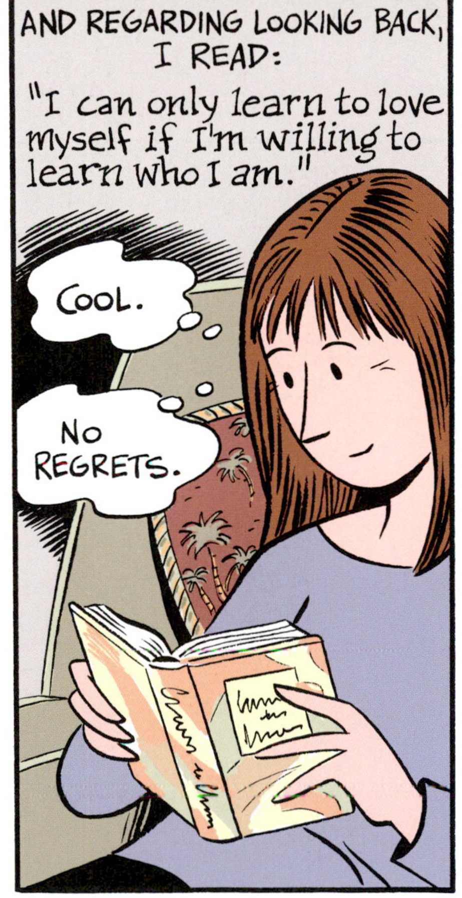
AND REGARDING LOOKING BACK, I READ:
"I can only learn to love myself if I'm willing to learn who I am."
COOL.
NO REGRETS.

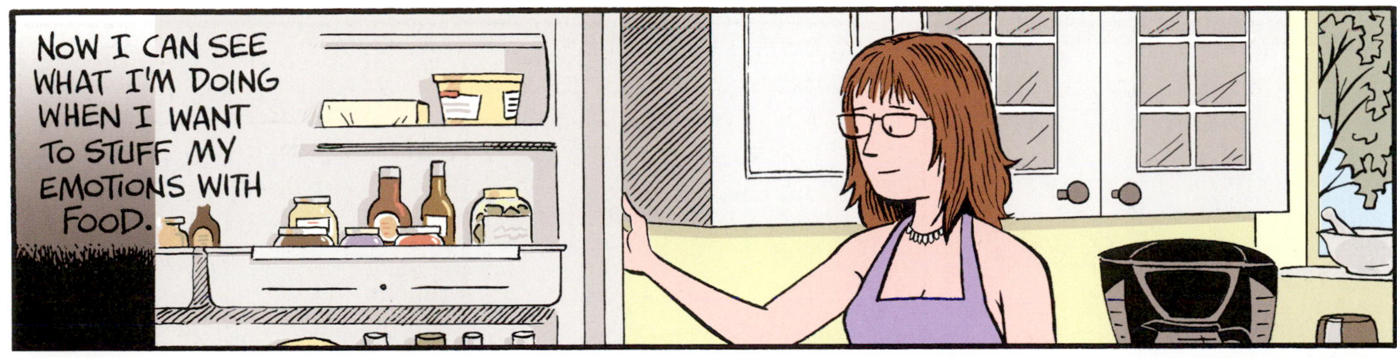
NOW I CAN SEE WHAT I'M DOING WHEN I WANT TO STUFF MY EMOTIONS WITH FOOD.

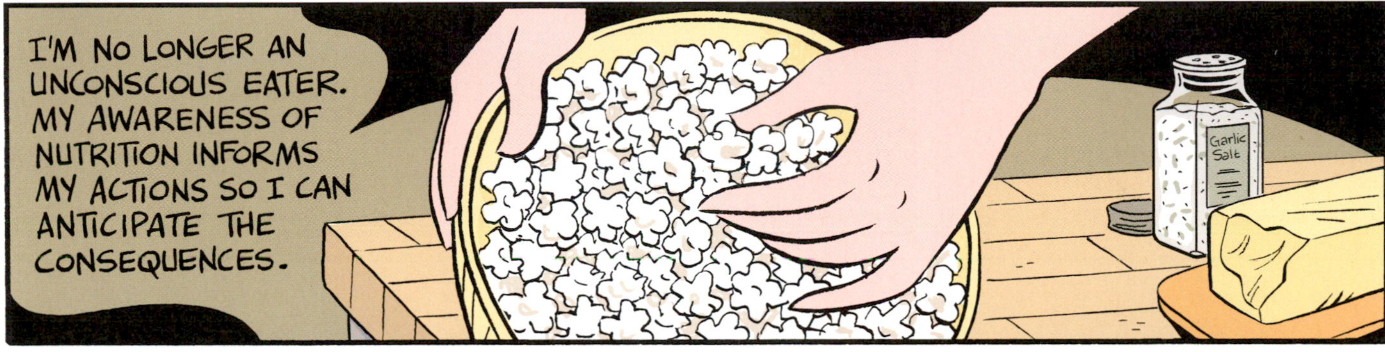
I'M NO LONGER AN UNCONSCIOUS EATER. MY AWARENESS OF NUTRITION INFORMS MY ACTIONS SO I CAN ANTICIPATE THE CONSEQUENCES.
Garlic Salt

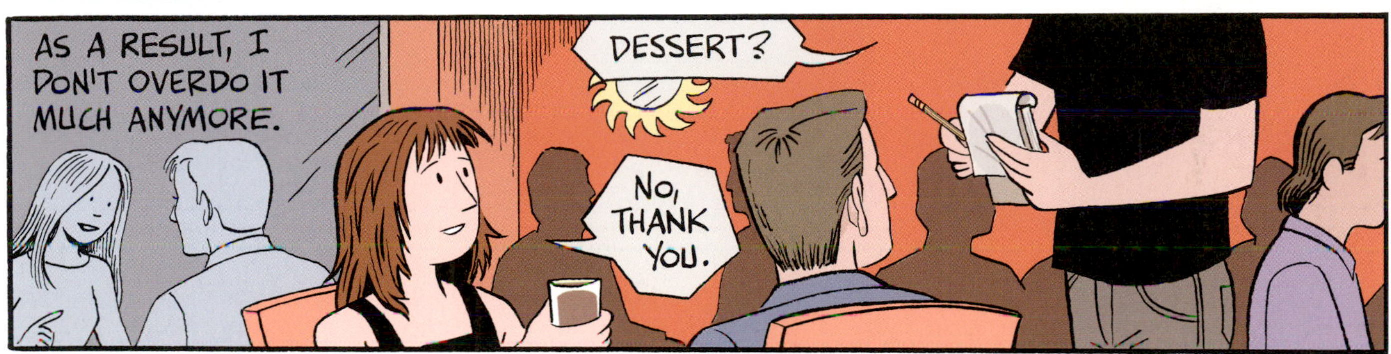
AS A RESULT, I DON'T OVERDO IT MUCH ANYMORE.
DESSERT?
NO, THANK YOU.

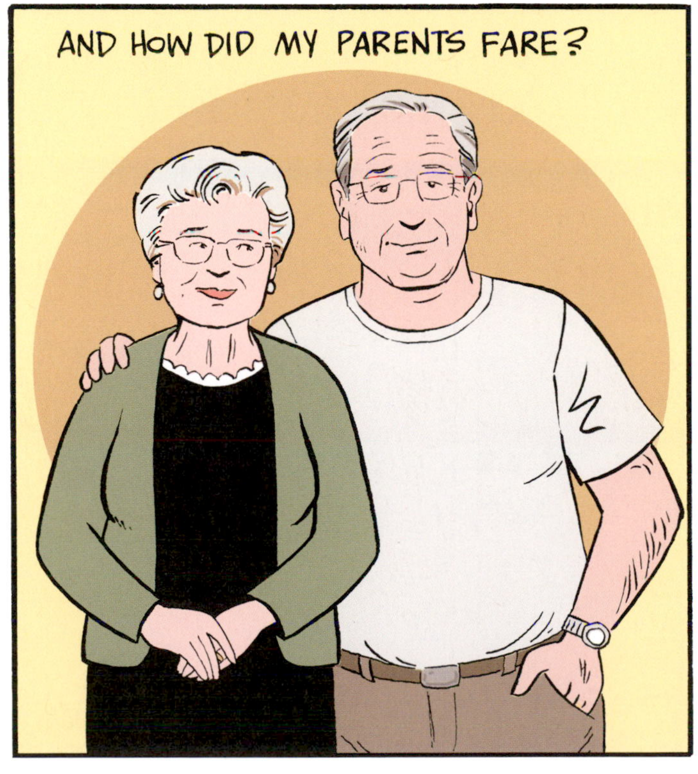
AND HOW DID MY PARENTS FARE?

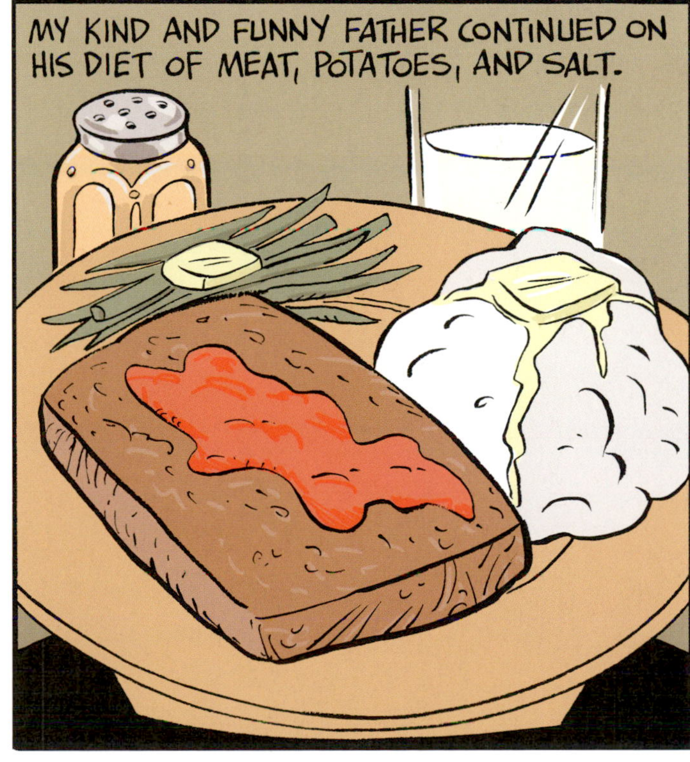
MY KIND AND FUNNY FATHER CONTINUED ON HIS DIET OF MEAT, POTATOES, AND SALT.

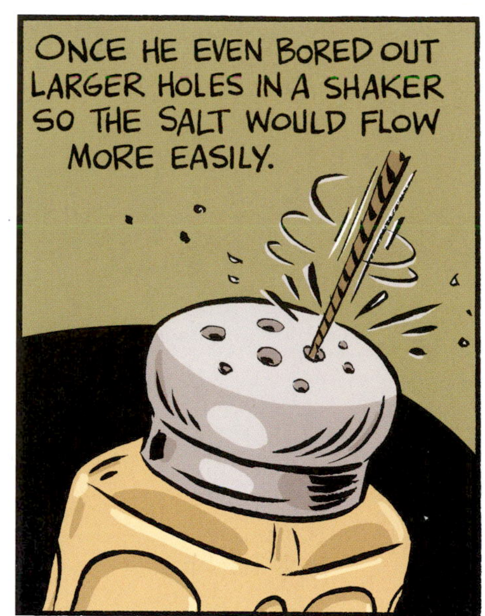
ONCE HE EVEN BORED OUT LARGER HOLES IN A SHAKER SO THE SALT WOULD FLOW MORE EASILY.

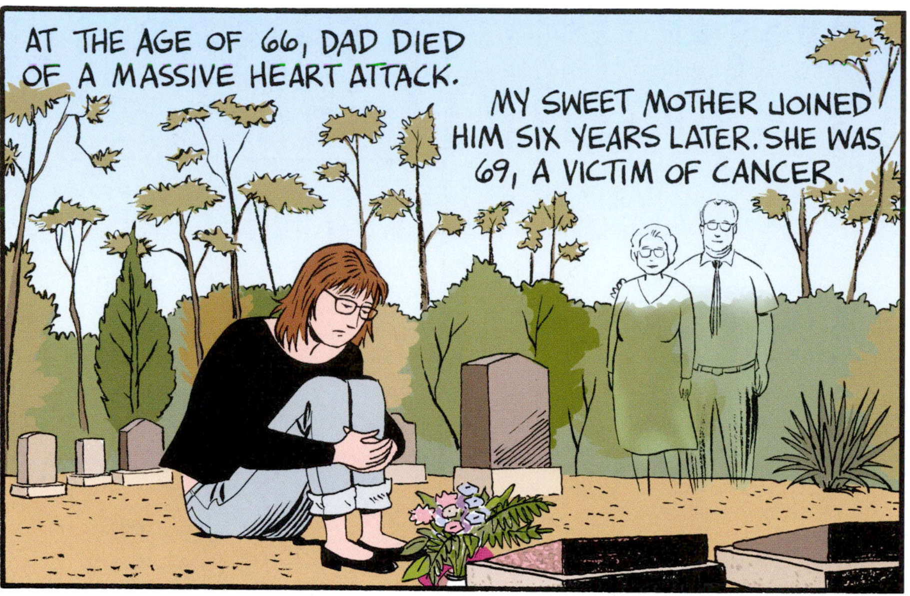
AT THE AGE OF 66, DAD DIED OF A MASSIVE HEART ATTACK.
MY SWEET MOTHER JOINED HIM SIX YEARS LATER. SHE WAS 69, A VICTIM OF CANCER.

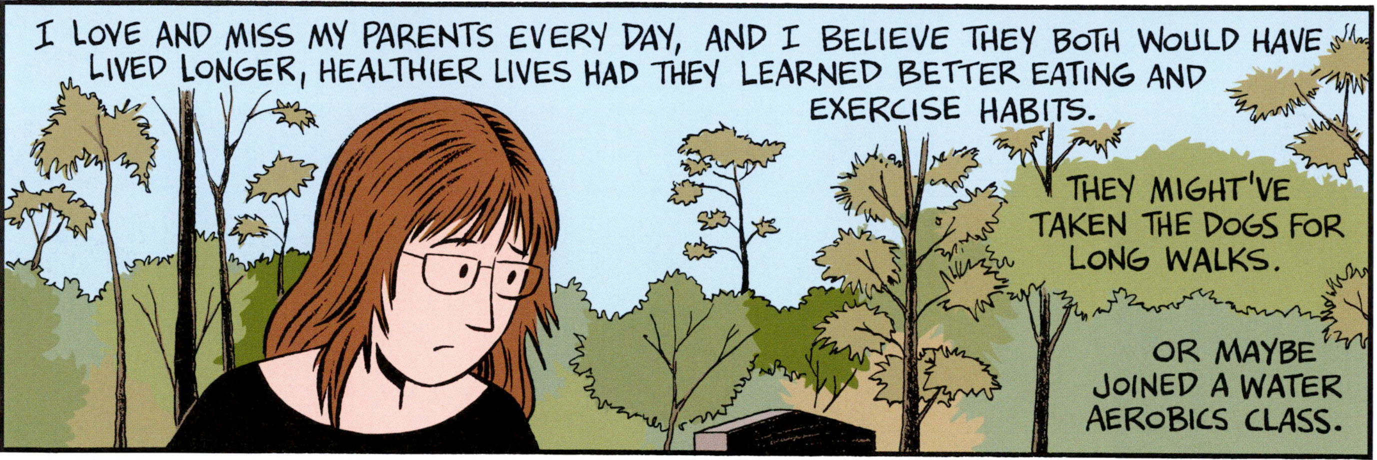
I LOVE AND MISS MY PARENTS EVERY DAY, AND I BELIEVE THEY BOTH WOULD HAVE LIVED LONGER, HEALTHIER LIVES HAD THEY LEARNED BETTER EATING AND EXERCISE HABITS.
THEY MIGHT'VE TAKEN THE DOGS FOR LONG WALKS.
OR MAYBE JOINED A WATER AEROBICS CLASS.

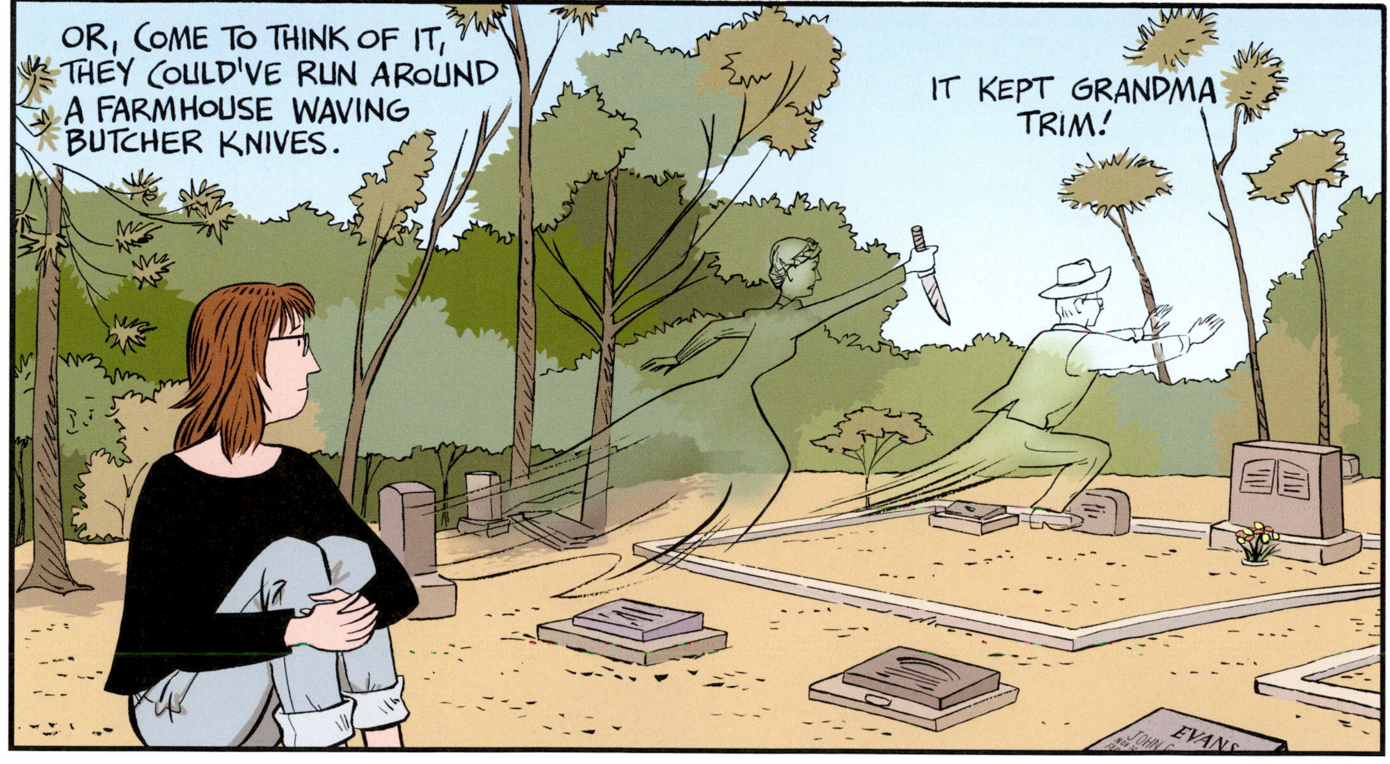
OR, COME TO THINK OF IT, THEY COULD'VE RUN AROUND A FARMHOUSE WAVING BUTCHER KNIVES.
IT KEPT GRANDMA TRIM!
EVANS

# HOW WHAT WHEN WHY HUH?

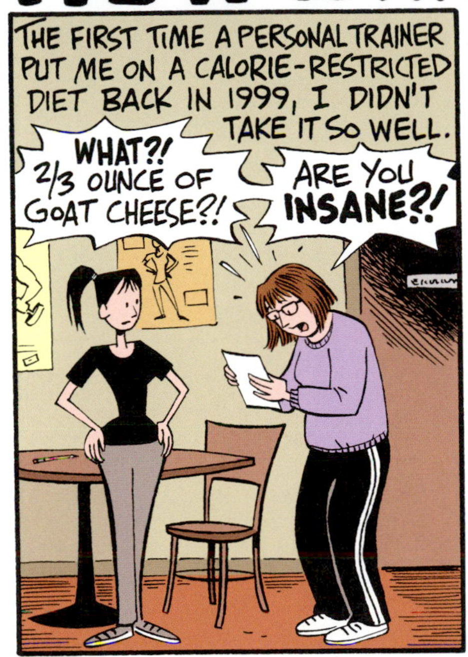
THE FIRST TIME A PERSONAL TRAINER PUT ME ON A CALORIE-RESTRICTED DIET BACK IN 1999, I DIDN'T TAKE IT SO WELL.
WHAT?! 2/3 OUNCE OF GOAT CHEESE?!
ARE YOU INSANE?!

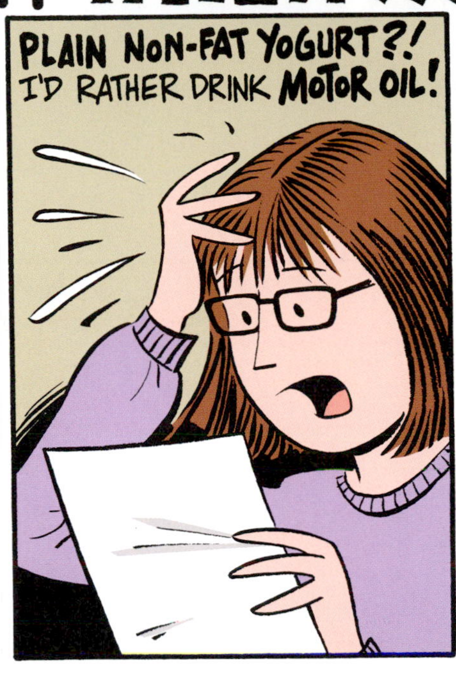
PLAIN NON-FAT YOGURT?! I'D RATHER DRINK MOTOR OIL!

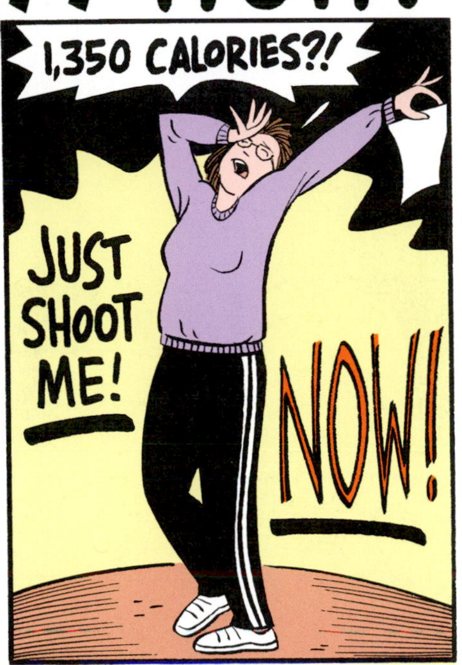
1,350 CALORIES?!
JUST SHOOT ME!
NOW!

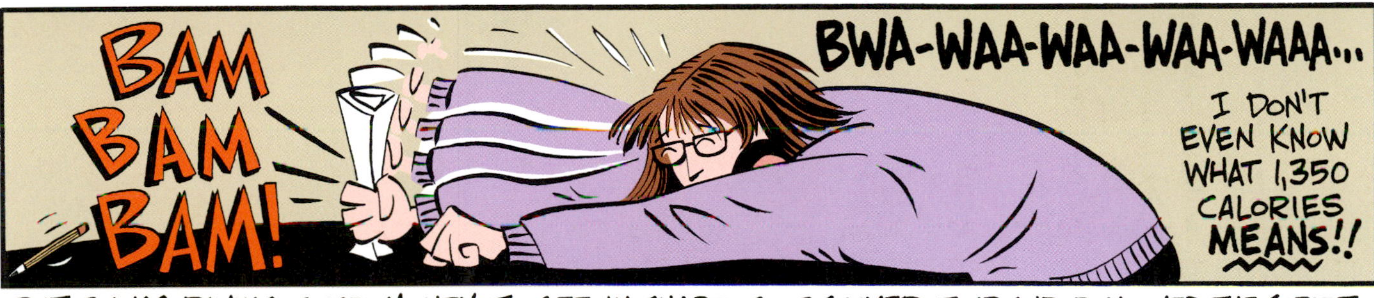
BAM BAM BAM!
BWA-WAA-WAA-WAA-WAAA...
I DON'T EVEN KNOW WHAT 1,350 CALORIES MEANS!!

BUT I WAS PAYING GOOD MONEY TO GET IN SHAPE, SO I SUCKED IT UP AND FOLLOWED THE SCRIPT.

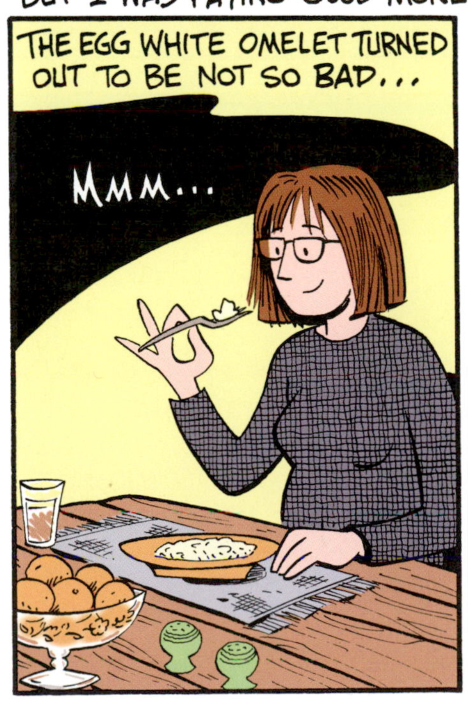
THE EGG WHITE OMELET TURNED OUT TO BE NOT SO BAD...
MMM...

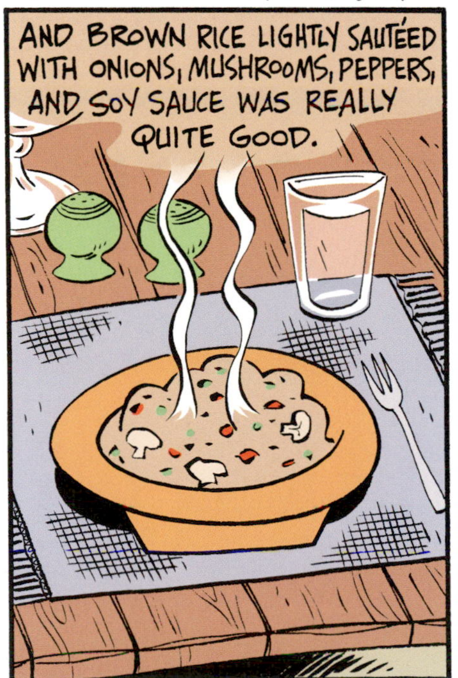
AND BROWN RICE LIGHTLY SAUTÉED WITH ONIONS, MUSHROOMS, PEPPERS, AND SOY SAUCE WAS REALLY QUITE GOOD.

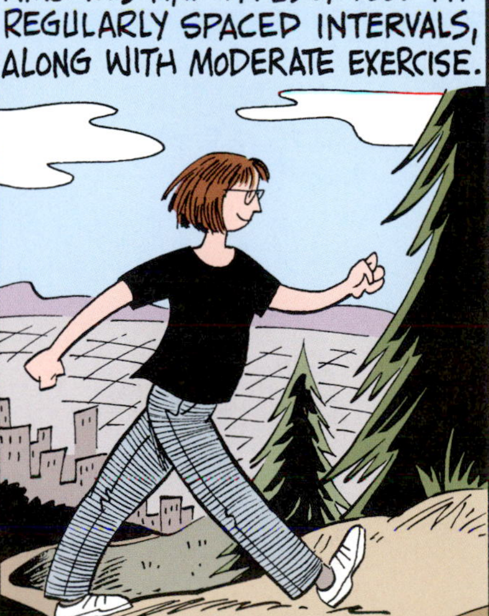
THE PLAN SUGGESTED SPECIFIC AMOUNTS AND TYPES OF FOOD AT REGULARLY SPACED INTERVALS, ALONG WITH MODERATE EXERCISE.

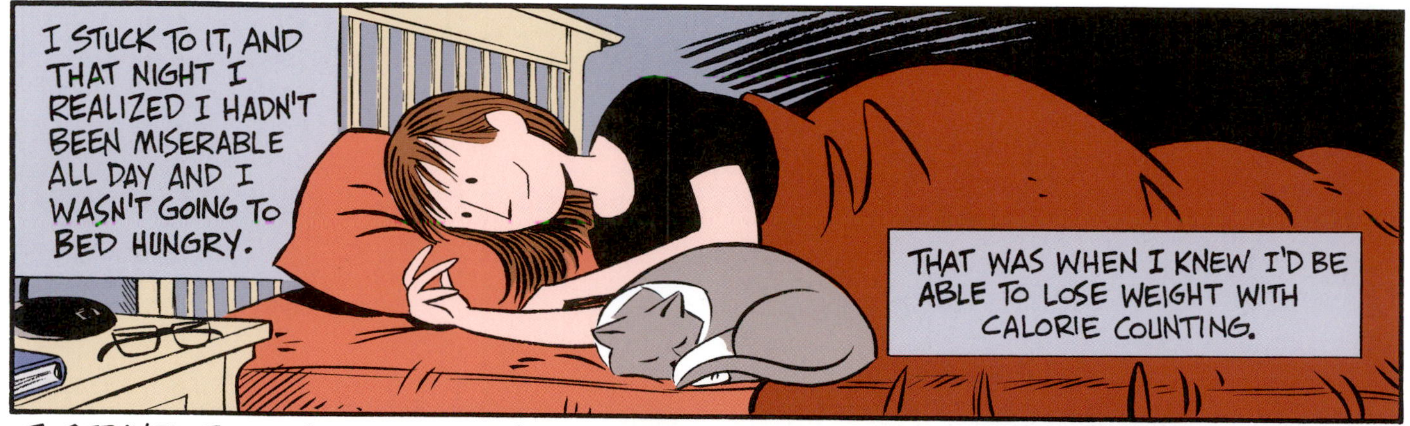
I STUCK TO IT, AND THAT NIGHT I REALIZED I HADN'T BEEN MISERABLE ALL DAY AND I WASN'T GOING TO BED HUNGRY.
THAT WAS WHEN I KNEW I'D BE ABLE TO LOSE WEIGHT WITH CALORIE COUNTING.

I STRAYED FROM THAT DIET WHEN I STOPPED WORKING WITH THE GYM COACH, BUT WHEN I FINALLY DECIDED TO PERMANENTLY CHANGE MY EATING HABITS, I KNEW WHAT TO DO.

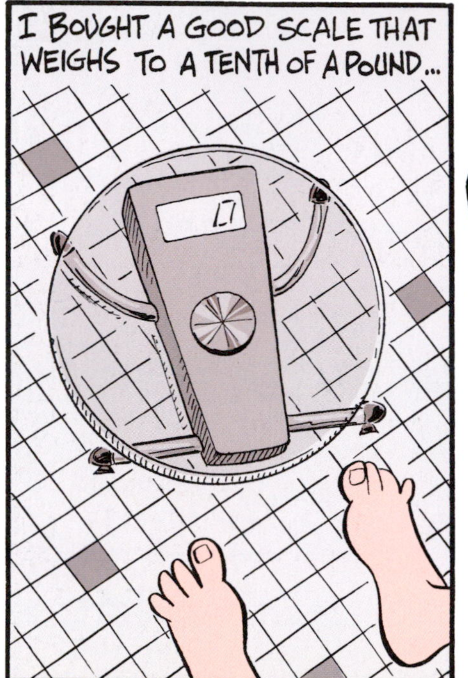


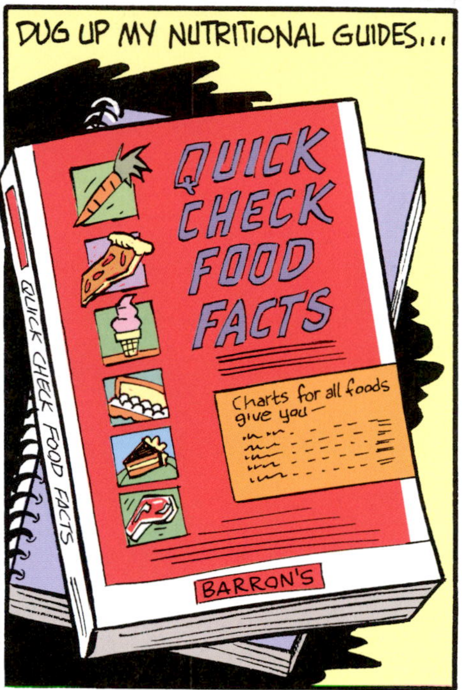
DUG UP MY NUTRITIONAL GUIDES...
QUICK CHECK FOOD FACTS
Charts for all foods give you—
QUICK CHECK FOOD FACTS
BARRON'S

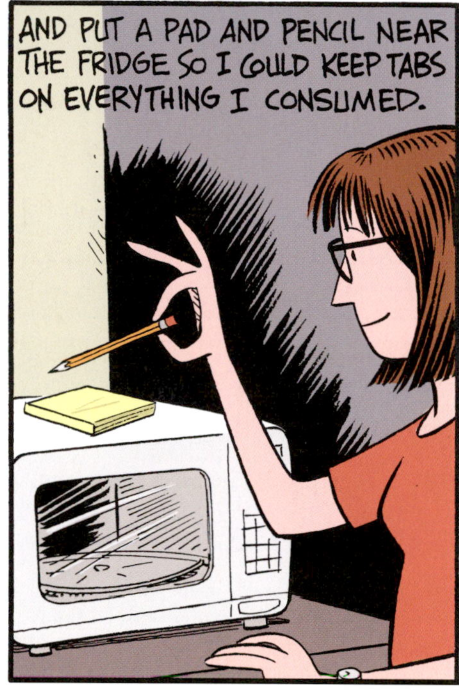
AND PUT A PAD AND PENCIL NEAR THE FRIDGE SO I COULD KEEP TABS ON EVERYTHING I CONSUMED.

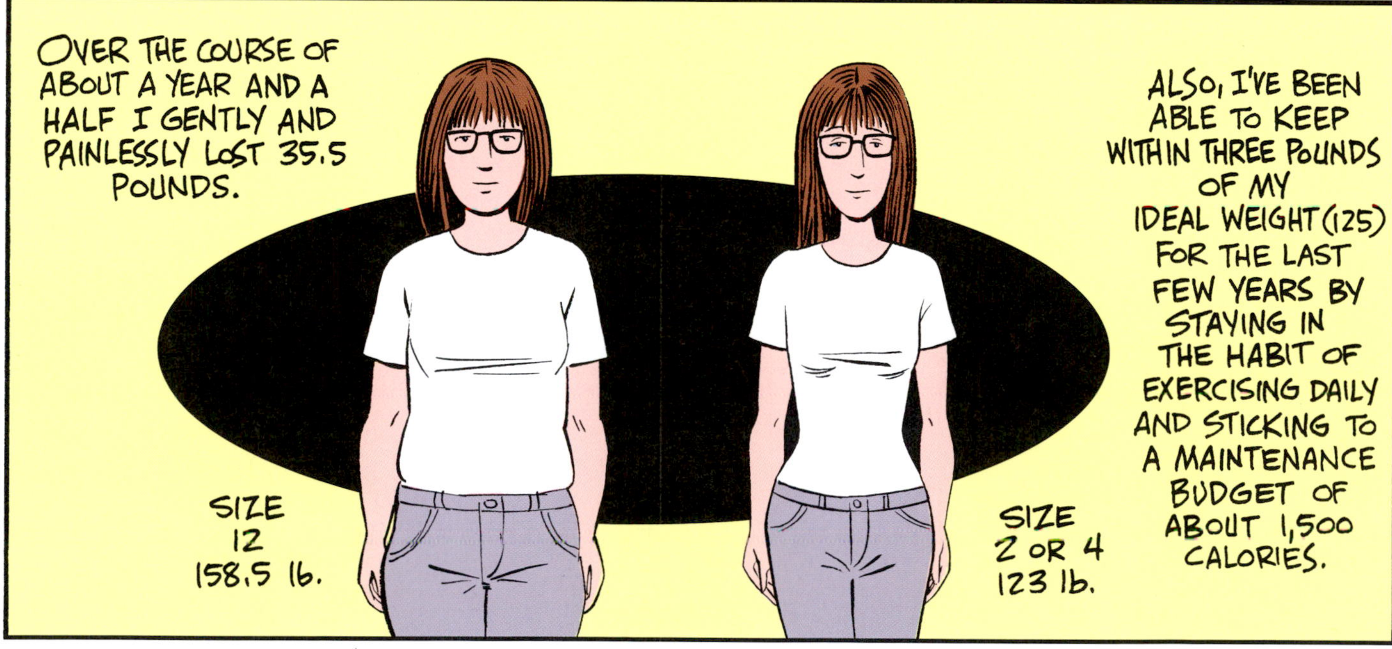
OVER THE COURSE OF ABOUT A YEAR AND A HALF I GENTLY AND PAINLESSLY LOST 35.5 POUNDS.
SIZE 12 158.5 lb.
SIZE 2 OR 4 123 lb.
ALSO, I'VE BEEN ABLE TO KEEP WITHIN THREE POUNDS OF MY IDEAL WEIGHT (125) FOR THE LAST FEW YEARS BY STAYING IN THE HABIT OF EXERCISING DAILY AND STICKING TO A MAINTENANCE BUDGET OF ABOUT 1,500 CALORIES.

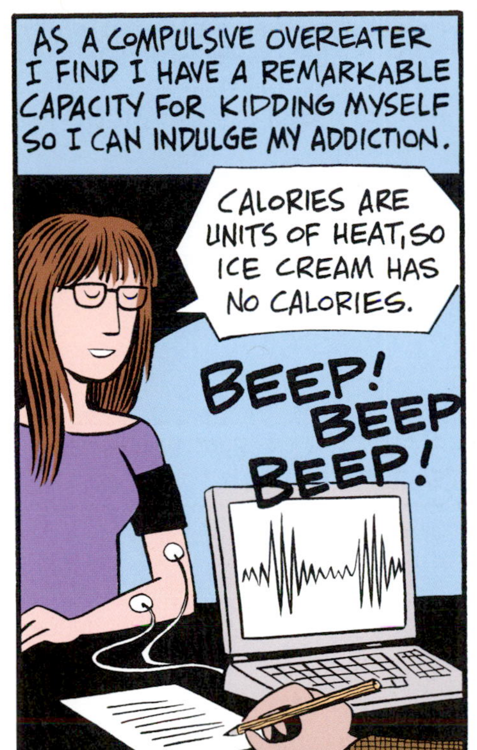

AS A COMPULSIVE OVEREATER I FIND I HAVE A REMARKABLE CAPACITY FOR KIDDING MYSELF SO I CAN INDULGE MY ADDICTION.
CALORIES ARE UNITS OF HEAT, SO ICE CREAM HAS NO CALORIES.
BEEP! BEEP BEEP!

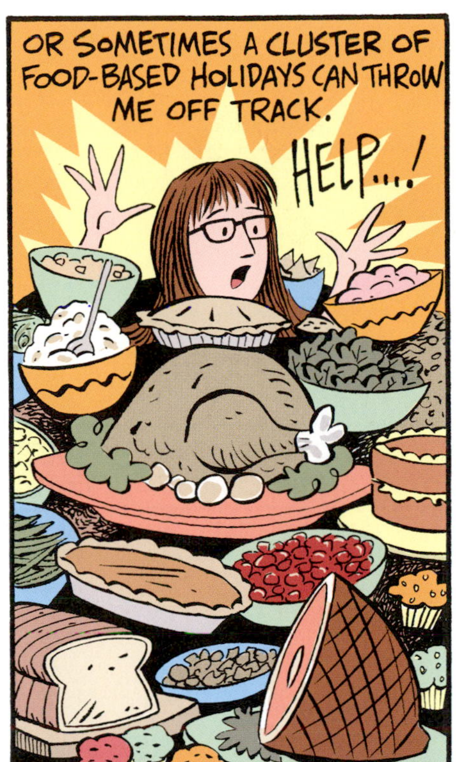

OR SOMETIMES A CLUSTER OF FOOD-BASED HOLIDAYS CAN THROW ME OFF TRACK.
HELP...!

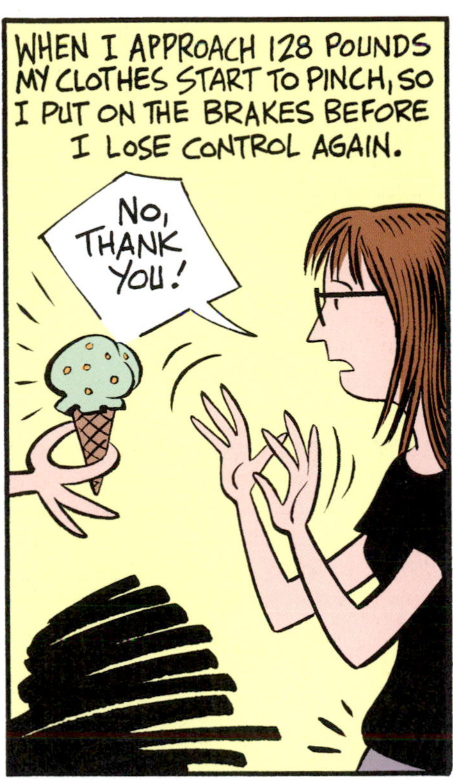

WHEN I APPROACH 128 POUNDS MY CLOTHES START TO PINCH, SO I PUT ON THE BRAKES BEFORE I LOSE CONTROL AGAIN.
NO, THANK YOU!

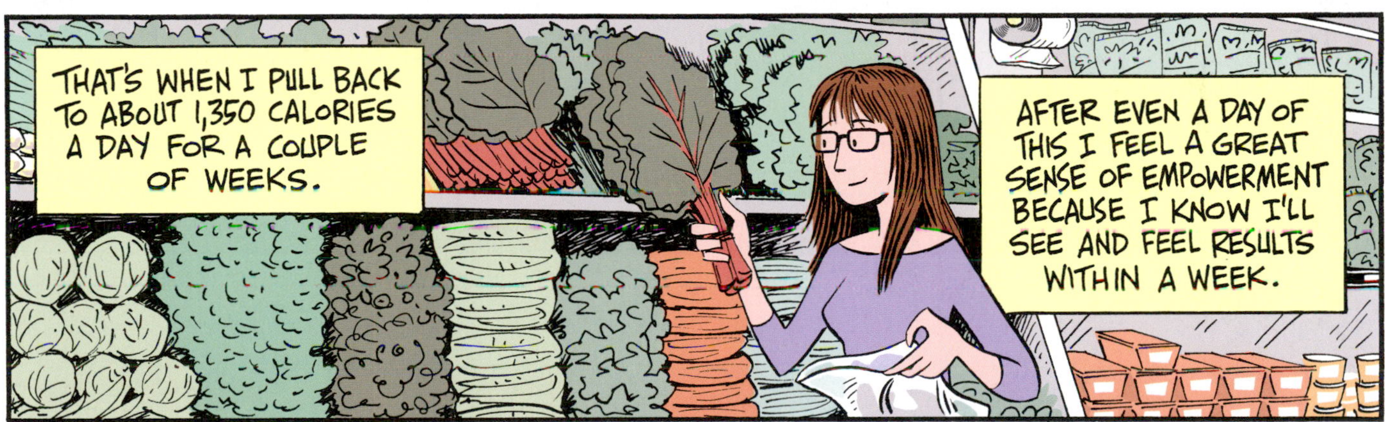

THAT'S WHEN I PULL BACK TO ABOUT 1,350 CALORIES A DAY FOR A COUPLE OF WEEKS.
AFTER EVEN A DAY OF THIS I FEEL A GREAT SENSE OF EMPOWERMENT BECAUSE I KNOW I'LL SEE AND FEEL RESULTS WITHIN A WEEK.

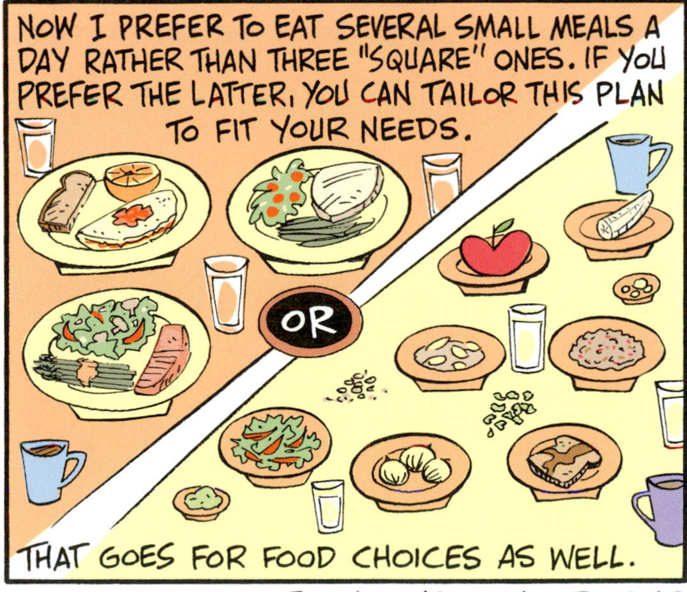

NOW I PREFER TO EAT SEVERAL SMALL MEALS A DAY RATHER THAN THREE "SQUARE" ONES. IF YOU PREFER THE LATTER, YOU CAN TAILOR THIS PLAN TO FIT YOUR NEEDS.
OR
THAT GOES FOR FOOD CHOICES AS WELL.

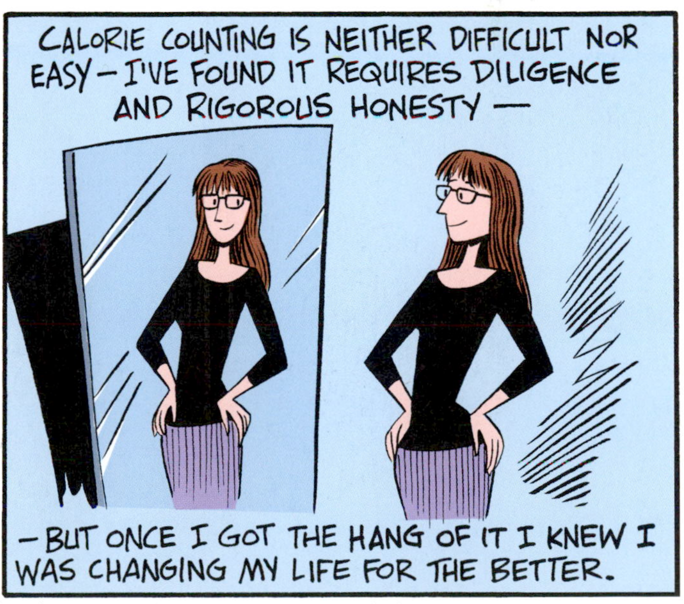

CALORIE COUNTING IS NEITHER DIFFICULT NOR EASY—I'VE FOUND IT REQUIRES DILIGENCE AND RIGOROUS HONESTY—
—BUT ONCE I GOT THE HANG OF IT I KNEW I WAS CHANGING MY LIFE FOR THE BETTER.

WHAT FOLLOWS IS MORE OR LESS HOW I DO IT, ONE DAY AT A TIME.

# A Day in the Diet

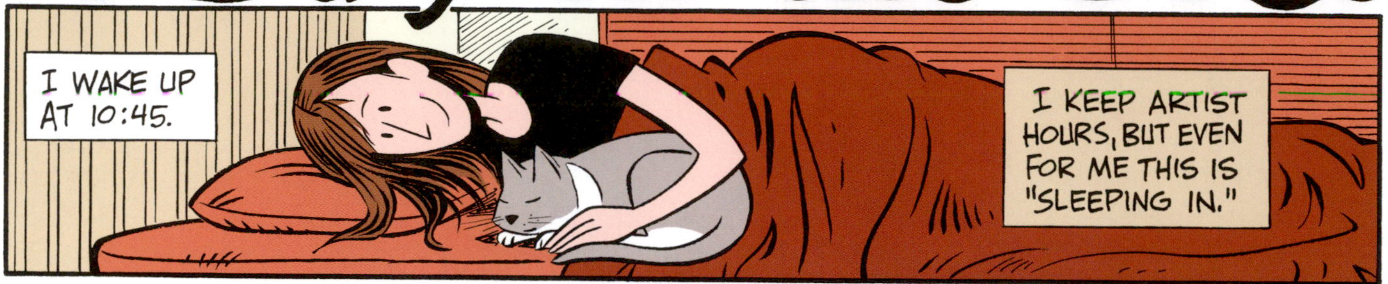

I WAKE UP AT 10:45.
I KEEP ARTIST HOURS, BUT EVEN FOR ME THIS IS "SLEEPING IN."


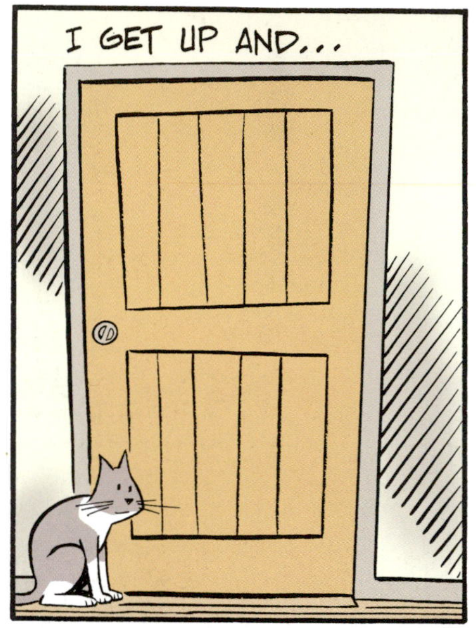

I GET UP AND...


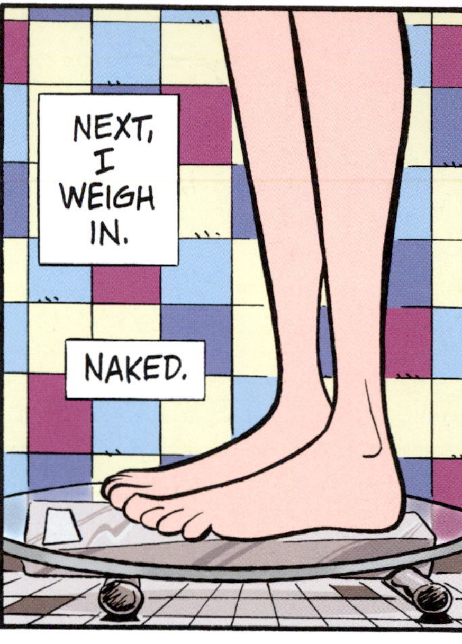

NEXT, I WEIGH IN.
NAKED.


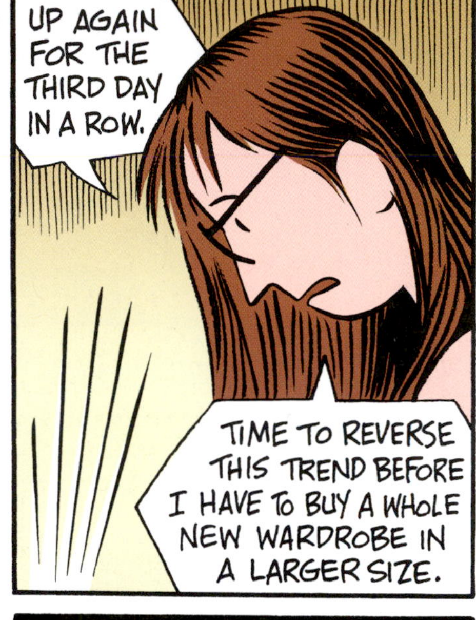

UP AGAIN FOR THE THIRD DAY IN A ROW.
TIME TO REVERSE THIS TREND BEFORE I HAVE TO BUY A WHOLE NEW WARDROBE IN A LARGER SIZE.


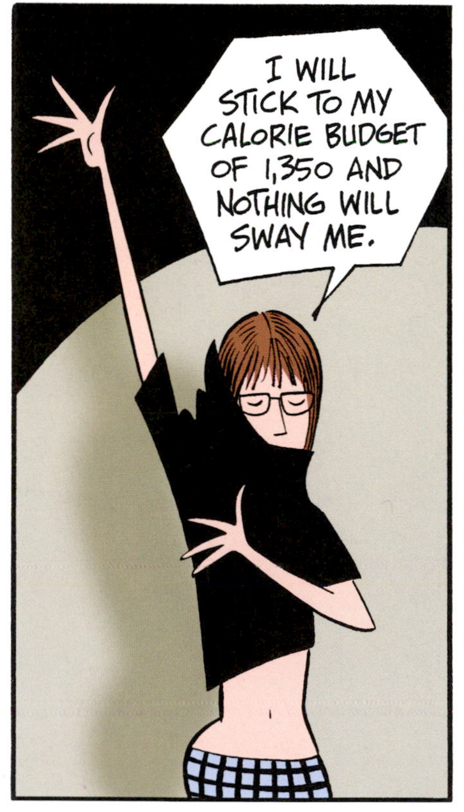

I WILL STICK TO MY CALORIE BUDGET OF 1,350 AND NOTHING WILL SWAY ME.


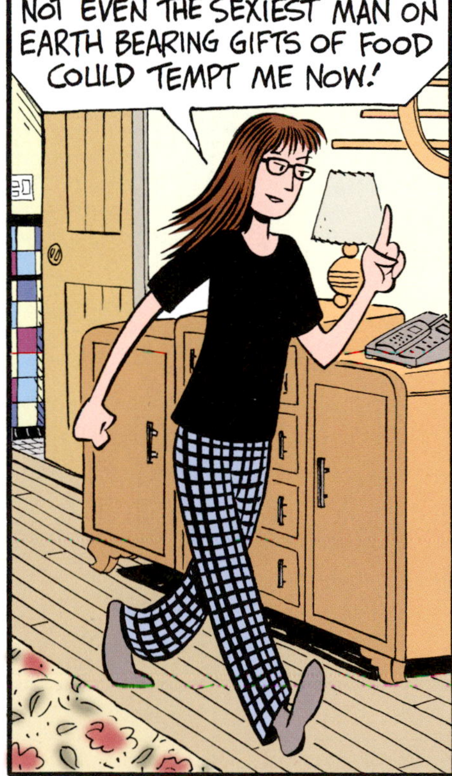

NOT EVEN THE SEXIEST MAN ON EARTH BEARING GIFTS OF FOOD COULD TEMPT ME NOW!


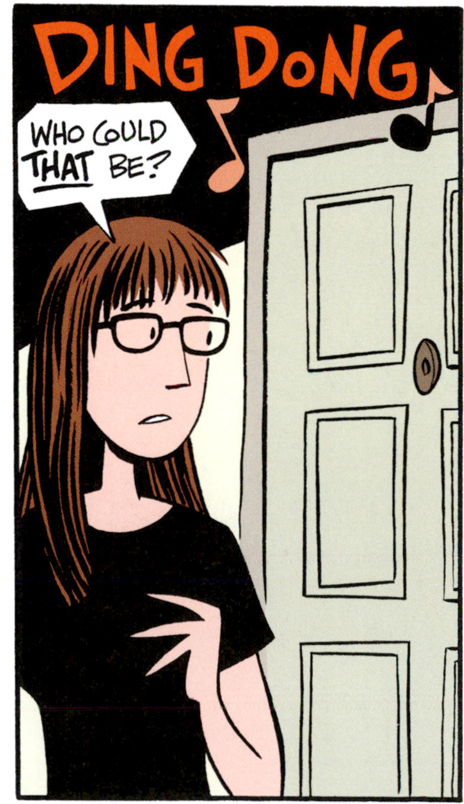

DING DONG
WHO COULD THAT BE?

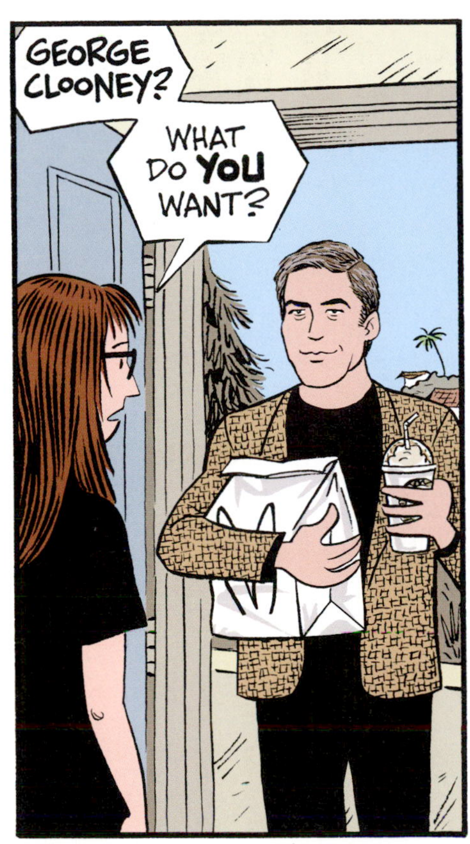
GEORGE CLOONEY?
WHAT DO YOU WANT?

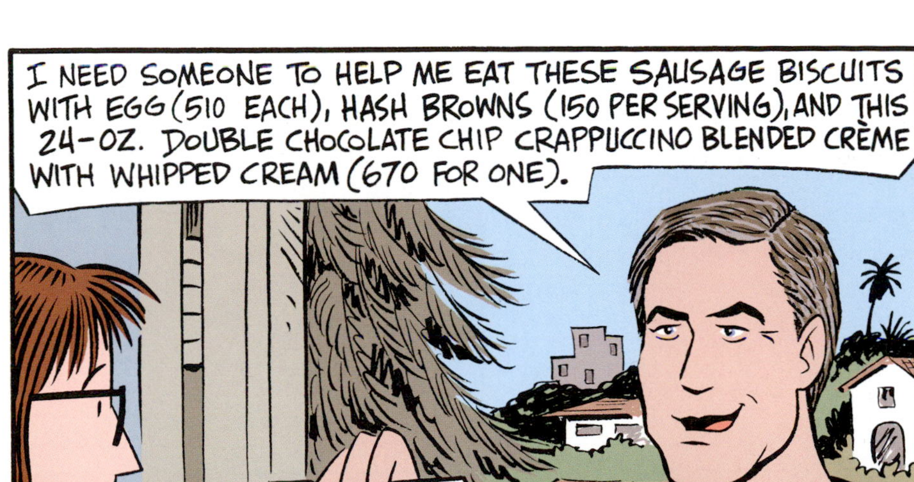
I NEED SOMEONE TO HELP ME EAT THESE SAUSAGE BISCUITS WITH EGG (510 EACH), HASH BROWNS (150 PER SERVING), AND THIS 24-OZ. DOUBLE CHOCOLATE CHIP CRAPPUCCINO BLENDED CRÈME WITH WHIPPED CREAM (670 FOR ONE).

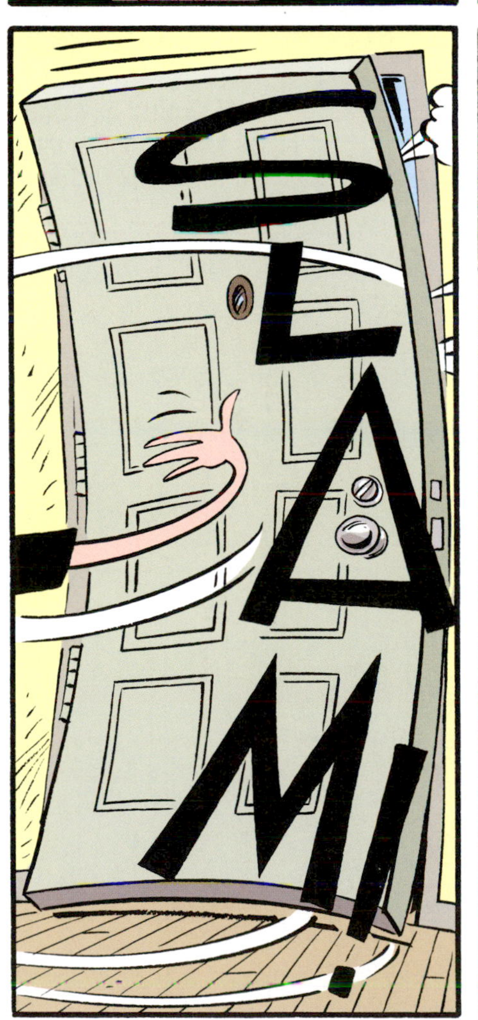
SLAM!

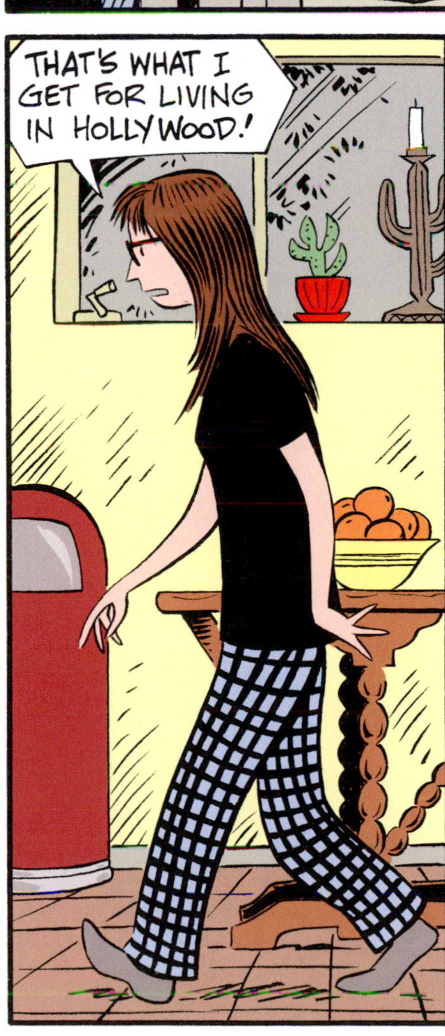
THAT'S WHAT I GET FOR LIVING IN HOLLYWOOD!

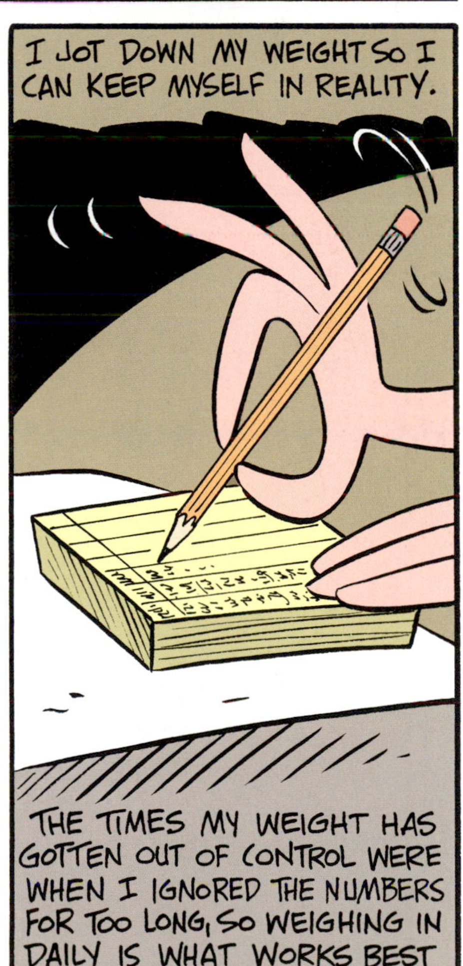
I JOT DOWN MY WEIGHT SO I CAN KEEP MYSELF IN REALITY.
THE TIMES MY WEIGHT HAS GOTTEN OUT OF CONTROL WERE WHEN I IGNORED THE NUMBERS FOR TOO LONG, SO WEIGHING IN DAILY IS WHAT WORKS BEST FOR ME.

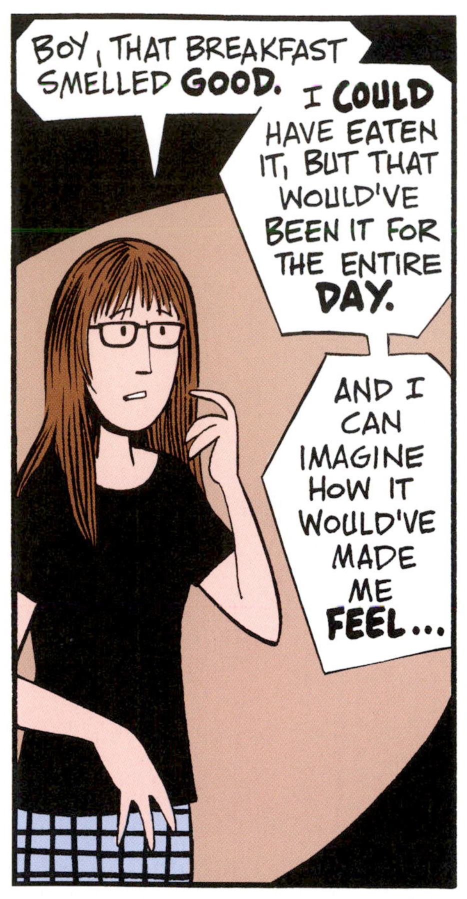
BOY, THAT BREAKFAST SMELLED GOOD.
I COULD HAVE EATEN IT, BUT THAT WOULD'VE BEEN IT FOR THE ENTIRE DAY.
AND I CAN IMAGINE HOW IT WOULD'VE MADE ME FEEL...
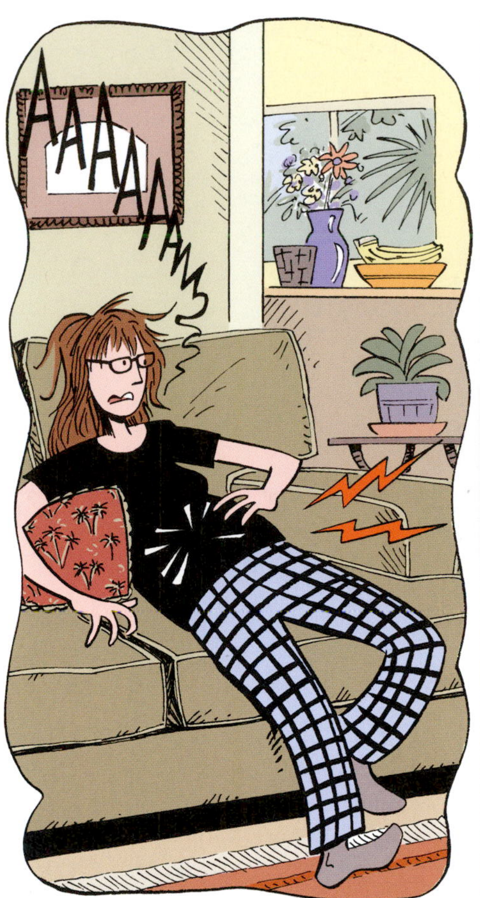
AAAAAAAWW
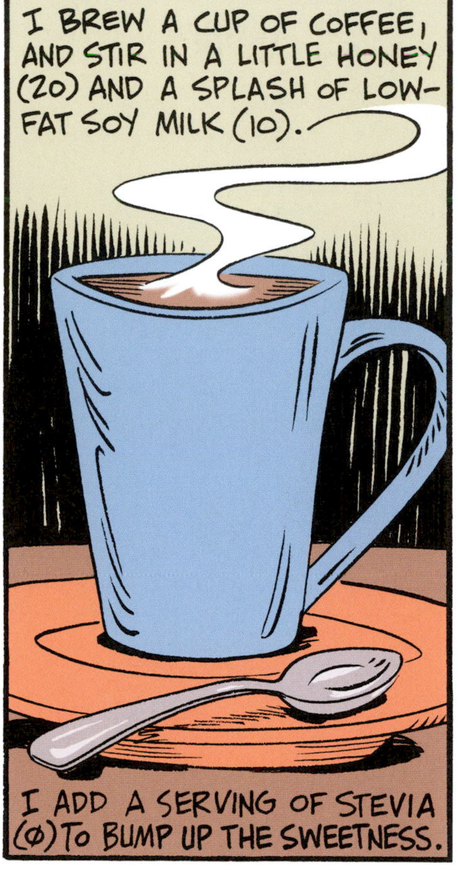
I BREW A CUP OF COFFEE, AND STIR IN A LITTLE HONEY (20) AND A SPLASH OF LOW-FAT SOY MILK (10).
I ADD A SERVING OF STEVIA (0) TO BUMP UP THE SWEETNESS.
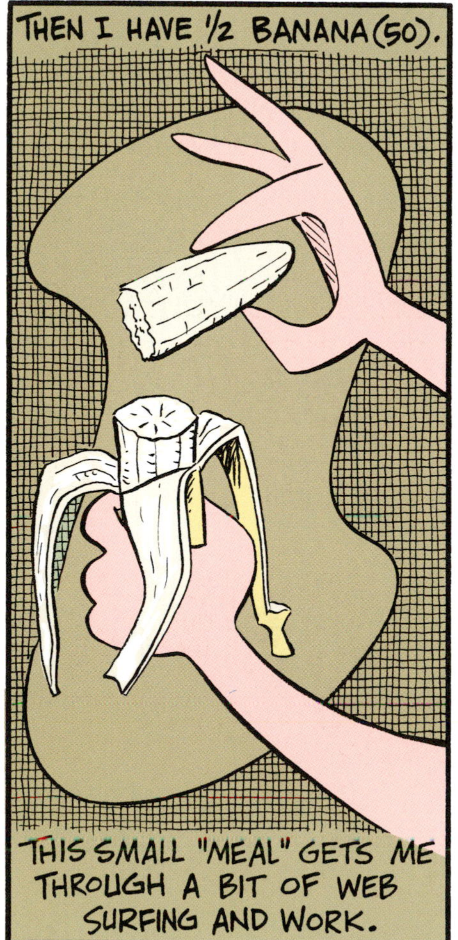
THEN I HAVE 1/2 BANANA (50).
THIS SMALL "MEAL" GETS ME THROUGH A BIT OF WEB SURFING AND WORK.
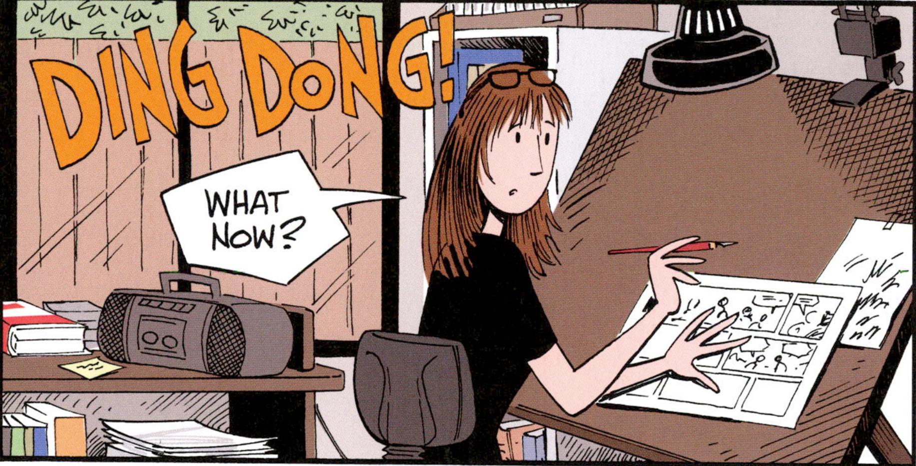
DING DONG!
WHAT NOW?
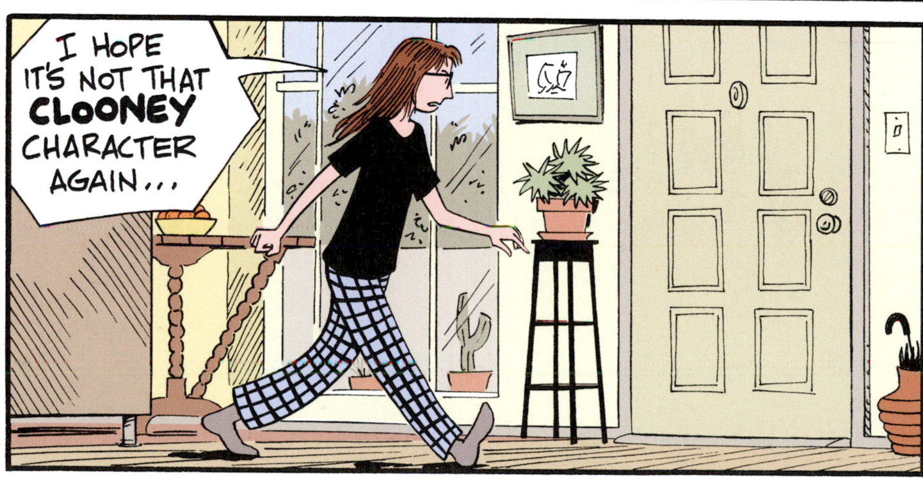
I HOPE IT'S NOT THAT CLONEY CHARACTER AGAIN...

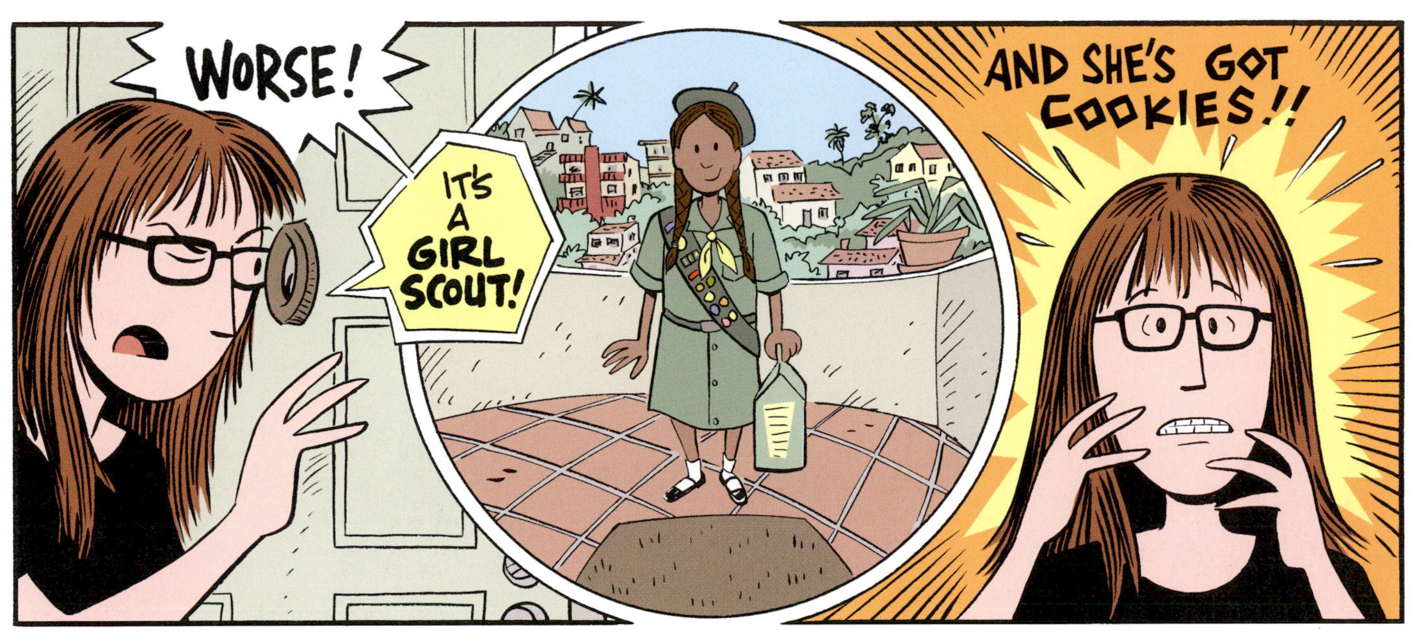
WORSE!
IT'S A GIRL SCOUT!
AND SHE'S GOT COOKIES!!
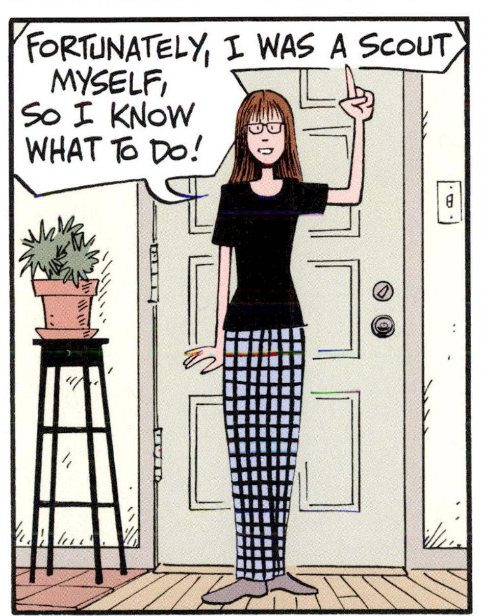
FORTUNATELY, I WAS A SCOUT MYSELF, SO I KNOW WHAT TO DO!
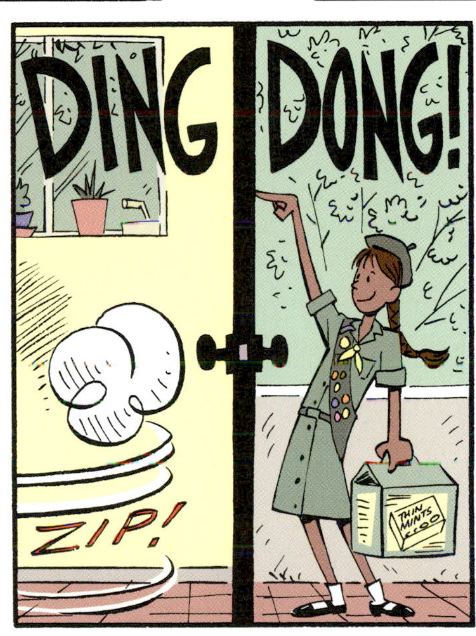
DING DONG!
ZIP!
THIN MINTS
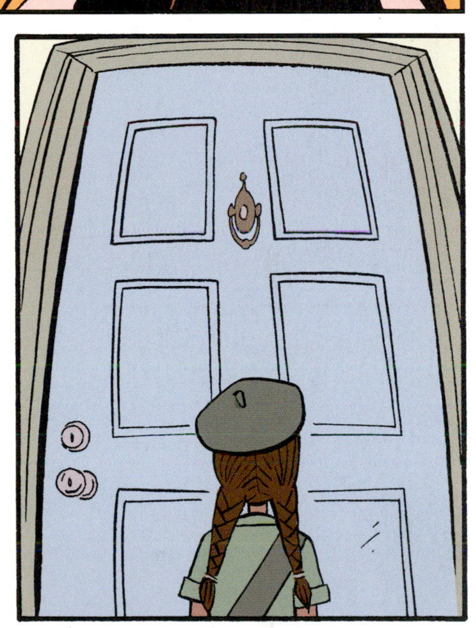
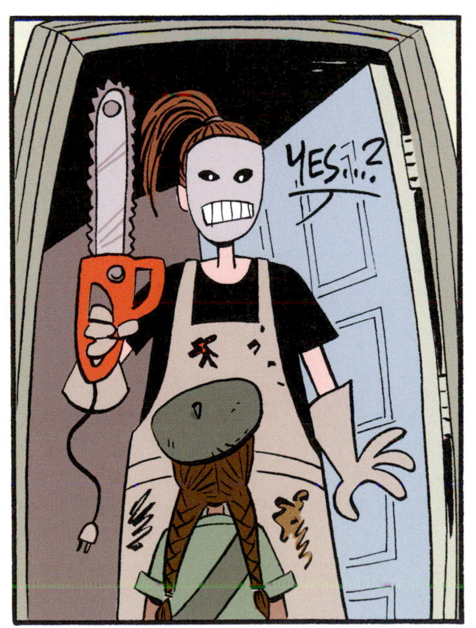
YES...?
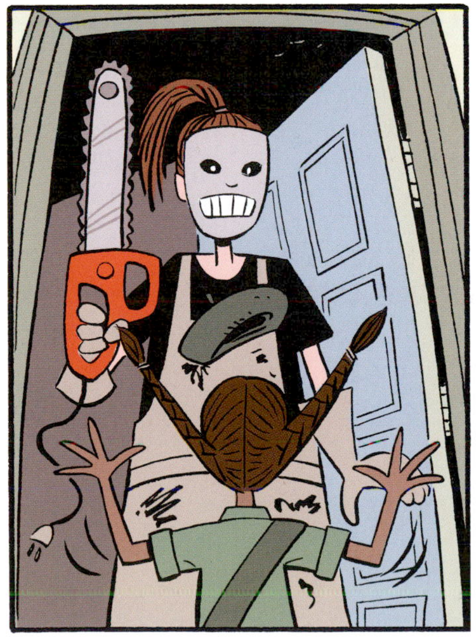
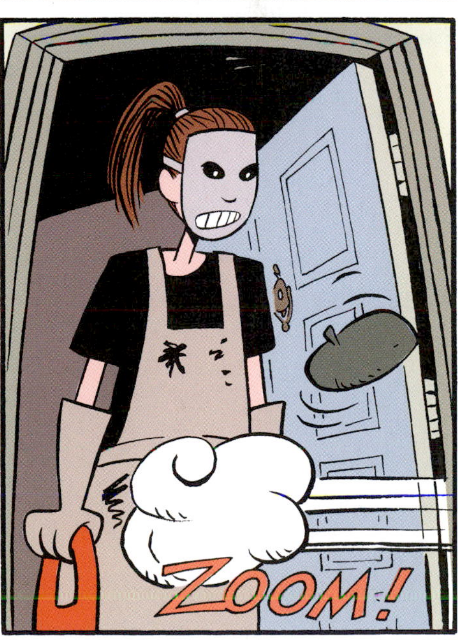
ZOOM!

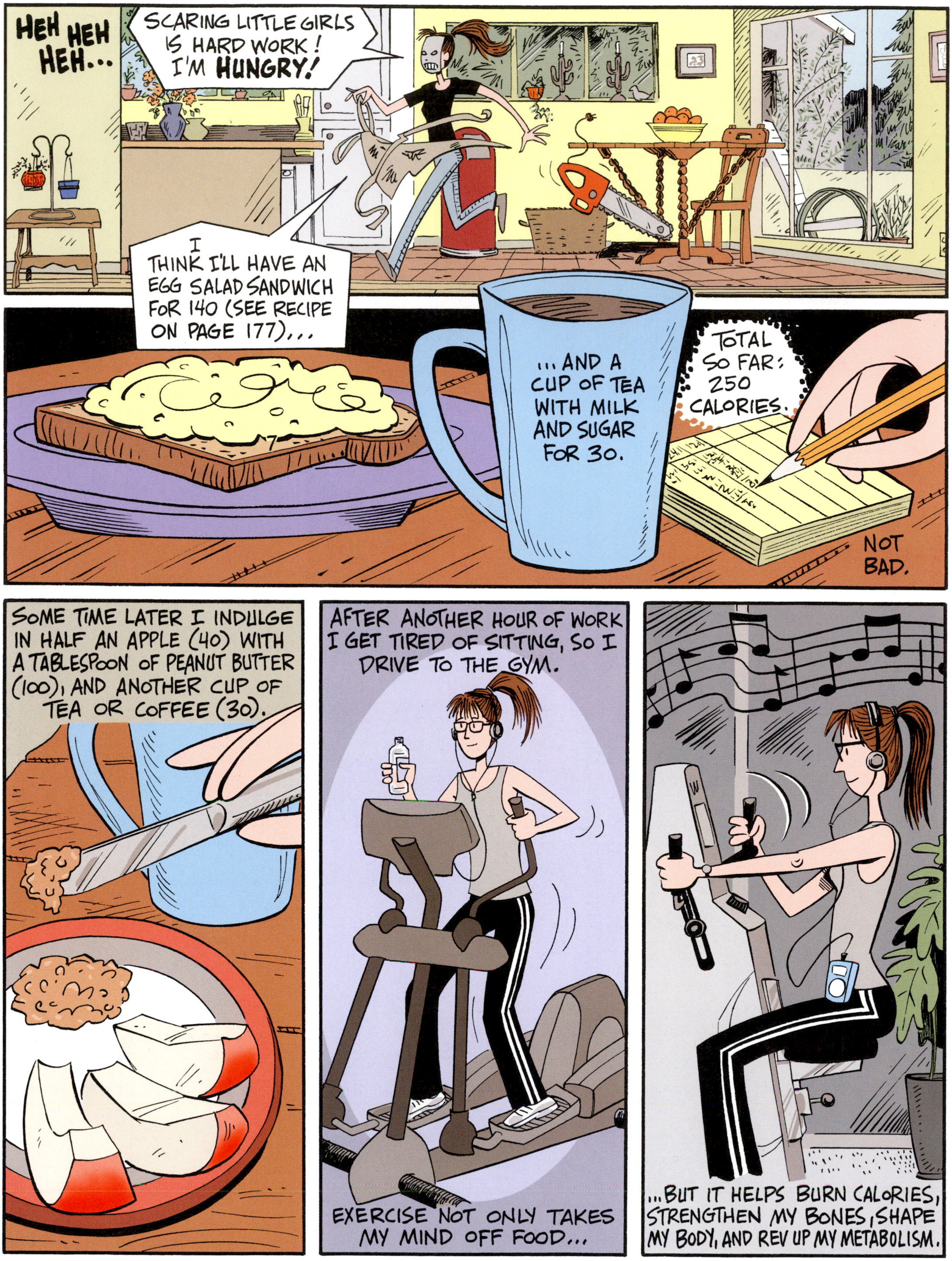

HEH HEH HEH...
SCARING LITTLE GIRLS IS HARD WORK! I'M **HUNGRY!**
I THINK I'LL HAVE AN EGG SALAD SANDWICH FOR 140 (SEE RECIPE ON PAGE 177)...
...AND A CUP OF TEA WITH MILK AND SUGAR FOR 30.
TOTAL SO FAR: 250 CALORIES.
NOT BAD.

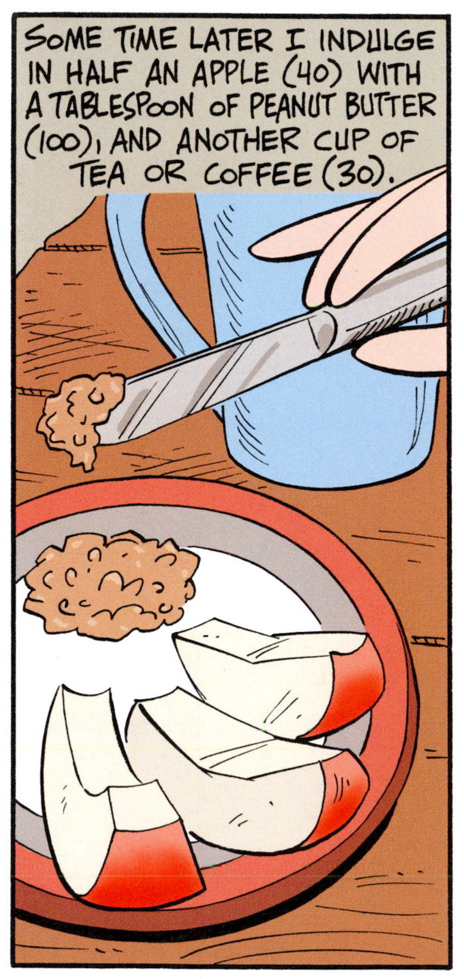


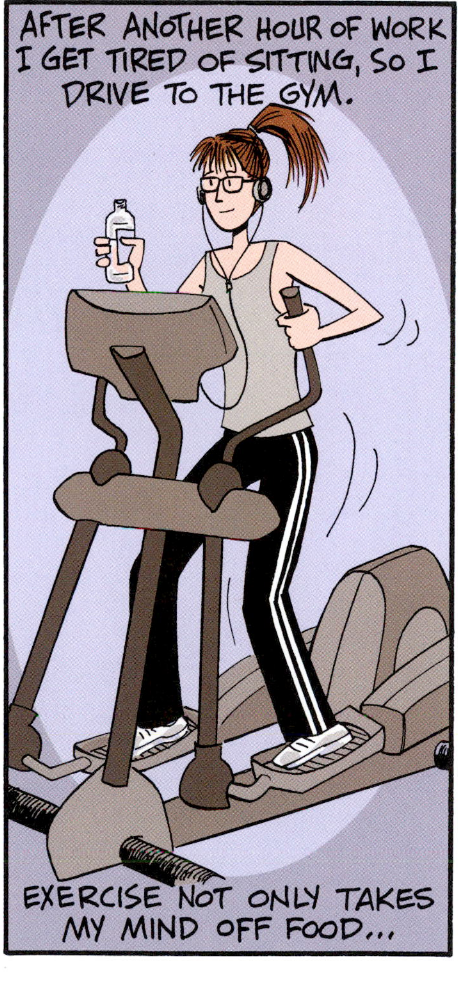
AFTER ANOTHER HOUR OF WORK I GET TIRED OF SITTING, SO I DRIVE TO THE GYM.
EXERCISE NOT ONLY TAKES MY MIND OFF FOOD...

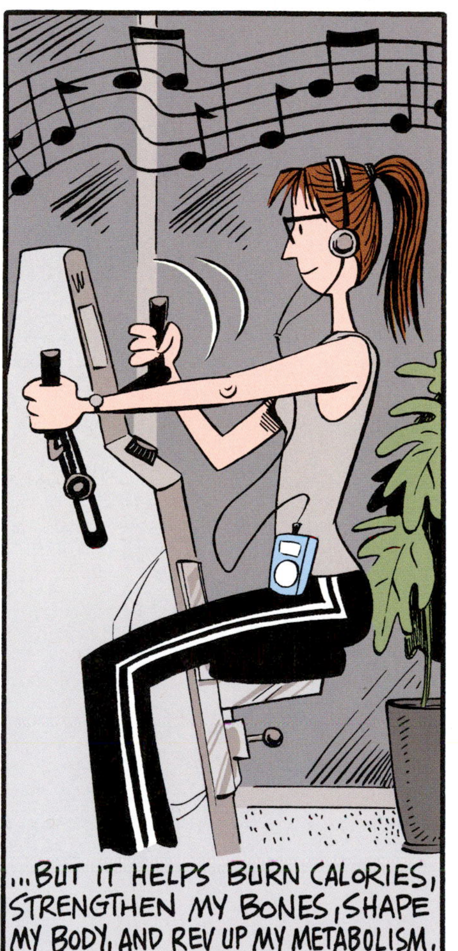
...BUT IT HELPS BURN CALORIES, STRENGTHEN MY BONES, SHAPE MY BODY, AND REV UP MY METABOLISM.

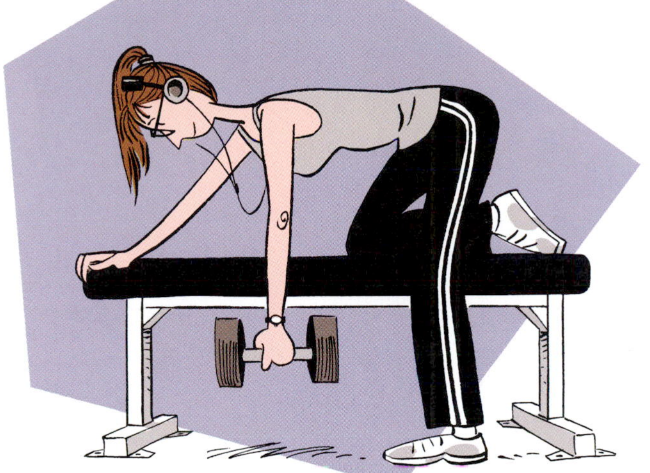
I TRY TO WORK OUT TWO OR THREE TIMES A WEEK, BUT WHEN THAT'S NOT POSSIBLE I MAKE SURE I WALK 20 MINUTES A DAY, AT THE VERY LEAST.

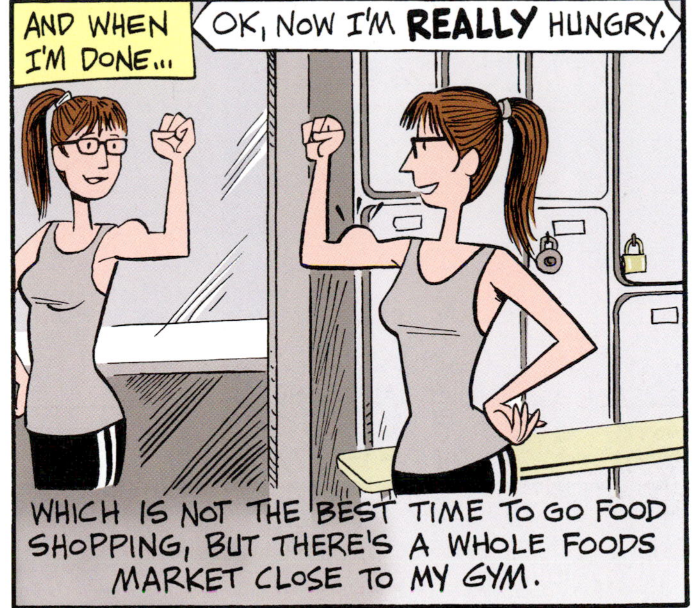
AND WHEN I'M DONE...
OK, NOW I'M **REALLY** HUNGRY.
WHICH IS NOT THE BEST TIME TO GO FOOD SHOPPING, BUT THERE'S A WHOLE FOODS MARKET CLOSE TO MY GYM.

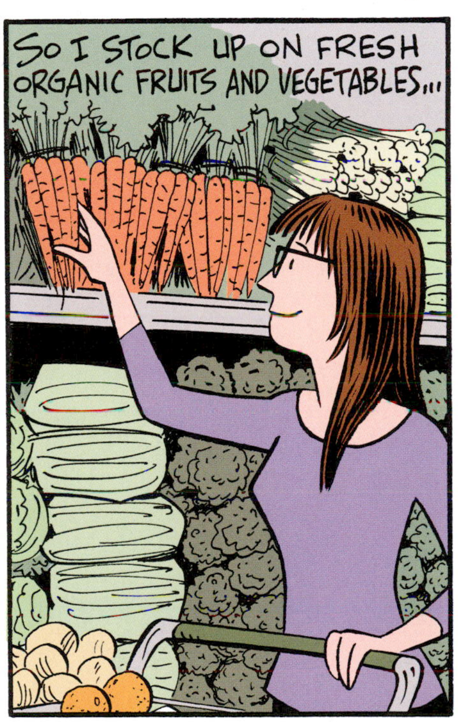
SO I STOCK UP ON FRESH ORGANIC FRUITS AND VEGETABLES...

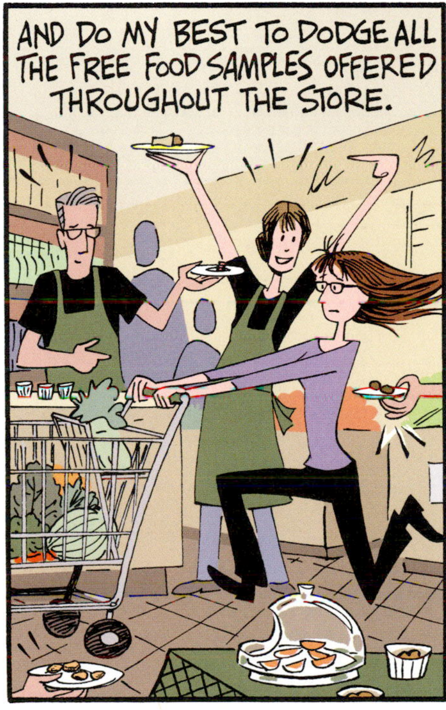
AND DO MY BEST TO DODGE ALL THE FREE FOOD SAMPLES OFFERED THROUGHOUT THE STORE.

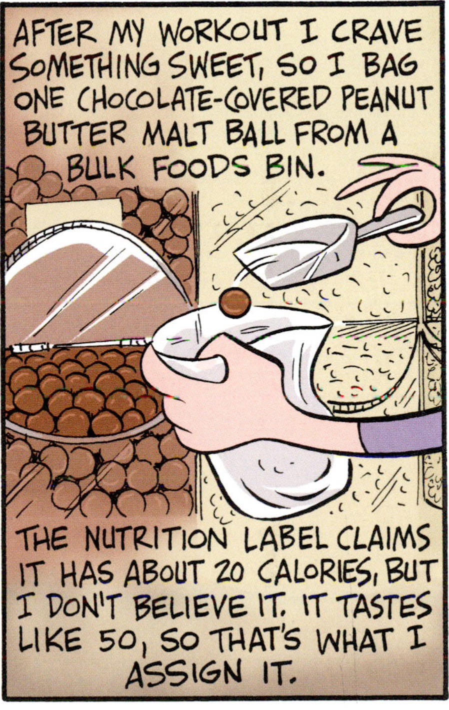
AFTER MY WORKOUT I CRAVE SOMETHING SWEET, SO I BAG ONE CHOCOLATE-COVERED PEANUT BUTTER MALT BALL FROM A BULK FOODS BIN.
THE NUTRITION LABEL CLAIMS IT HAS ABOUT 20 CALORIES, BUT I DON'T BELIEVE IT. IT TASTES LIKE 50, SO THAT'S WHAT I ASSIGN IT.

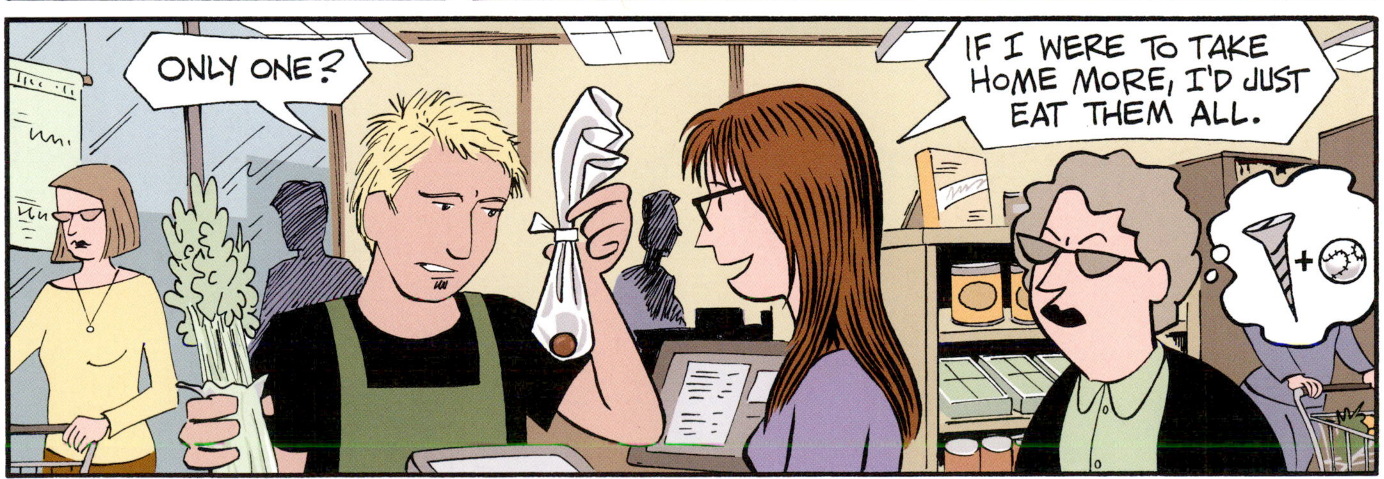
ONLY ONE?
IF I WERE TO TAKE HOME MORE, I'D JUST EAT THEM ALL.

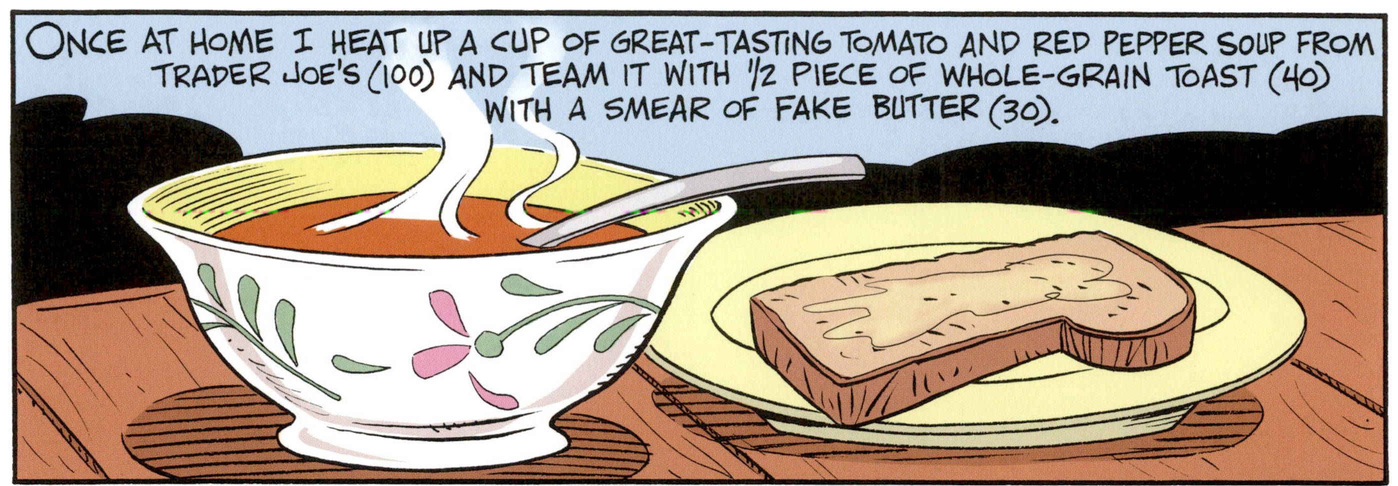
ONCE AT HOME I HEAT UP A CUP OF GREAT-TASTING TOMATO AND RED PEPPER SOUP FROM TRADER JOE'S (100) AND TEAM IT WITH 1/2 PIECE OF WHOLE-GRAIN TOAST (40) WITH A SMEAR OF FAKE BUTTER (30).

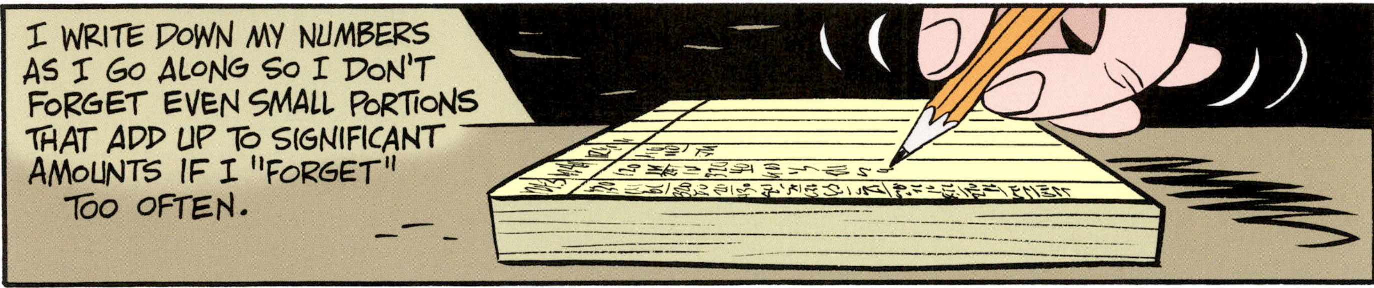
I WRITE DOWN MY NUMBERS AS I GO ALONG SO I DON'T FORGET EVEN SMALL PORTIONS THAT ADD UP TO SIGNIFICANT AMOUNTS IF I "FORGET" TOO OFTEN.

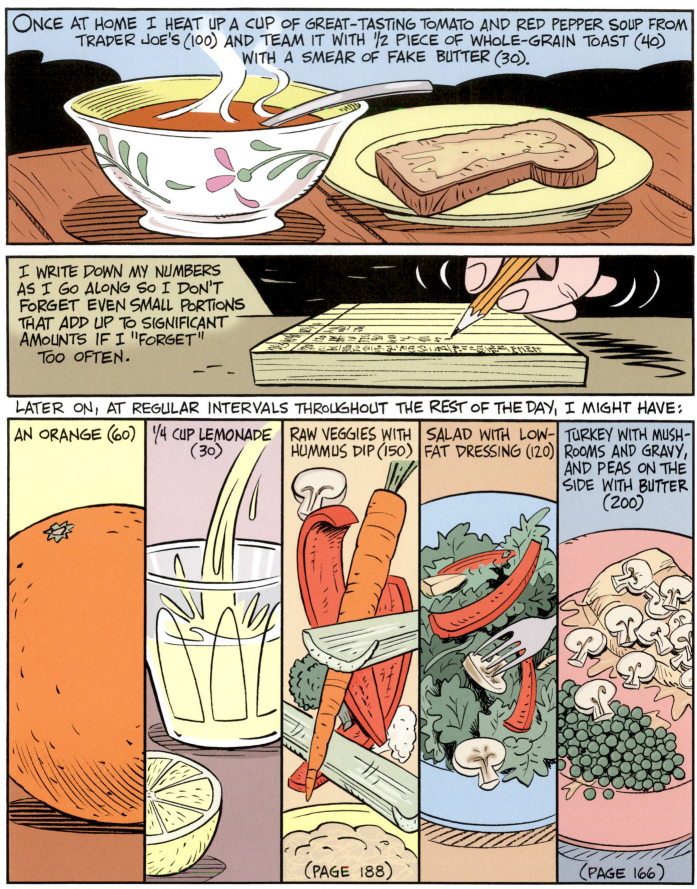

LATER ON, AT REGULAR INTERVALS THROUGHOUT THE REST OF THE DAY, I MIGHT HAVE:

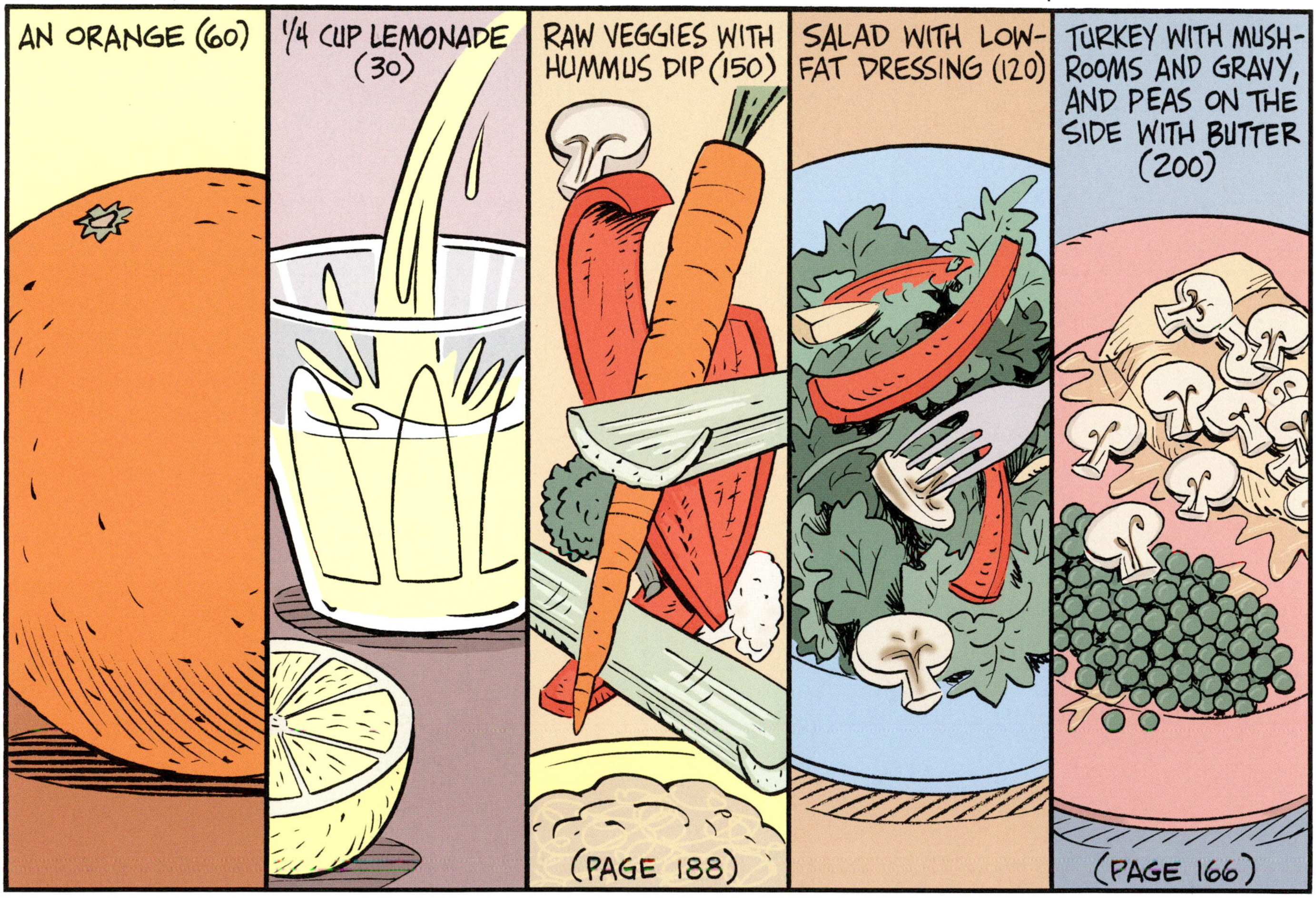

AN ORANGE (60)

1/4 CUP LEMONADE (30)

RAW VEGGIES WITH HUMMUS DIP (150)

(PAGE 188)

SALAD WITH LOW-FAT DRESSING (120)

TURKEY WITH MUSHROOMS AND GRAVY, AND PEAS ON THE SIDE WITH BUTTER (200)

(PAGE 166)

OR I MIGHT HAVE ANY OF A MYRIAD OF OTHER MEALS AND COMBINATIONS THAT ADD UP TO ROUGHLY THE SAME CALORIE AMOUNTS.

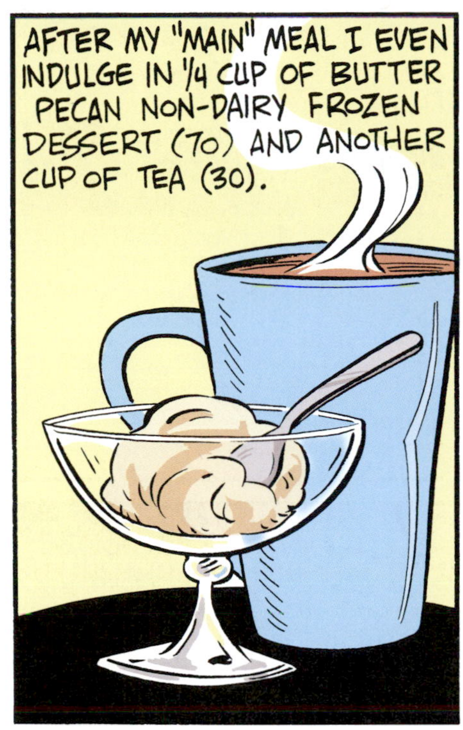
AFTER MY "MAIN" MEAL I EVEN INDULGE IN 1/4 CUP OF BUTTER PECAN NON-DAIRY FROZEN DESSERT (70) AND ANOTHER CUP OF TEA (30).

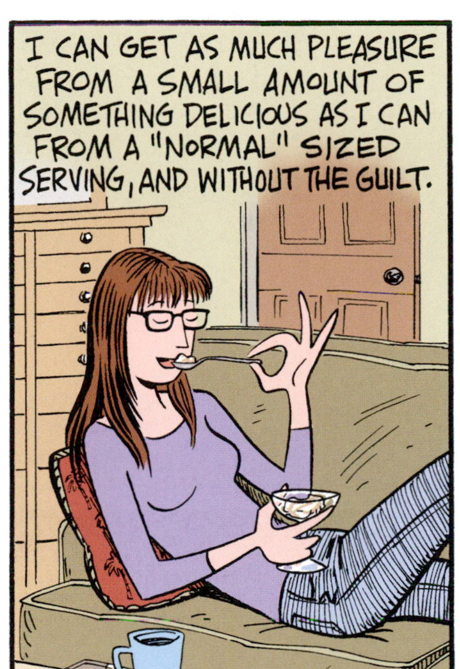
I CAN GET AS MUCH PLEASURE FROM A SMALL AMOUNT OF SOMETHING DELICIOUS AS I CAN FROM A "NORMAL" SIZED SERVING, AND WITHOUT THE GUILT.

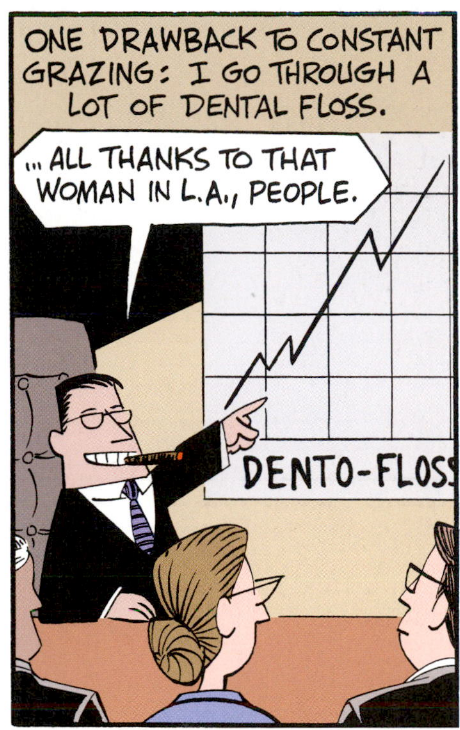
ONE DRAWBACK TO CONSTANT GRAZING: I GO THROUGH A LOT OF DENTAL FLOSS.
...ALL THANKS TO THAT WOMAN IN L.A., PEOPLE.
DENTO-FLOSS

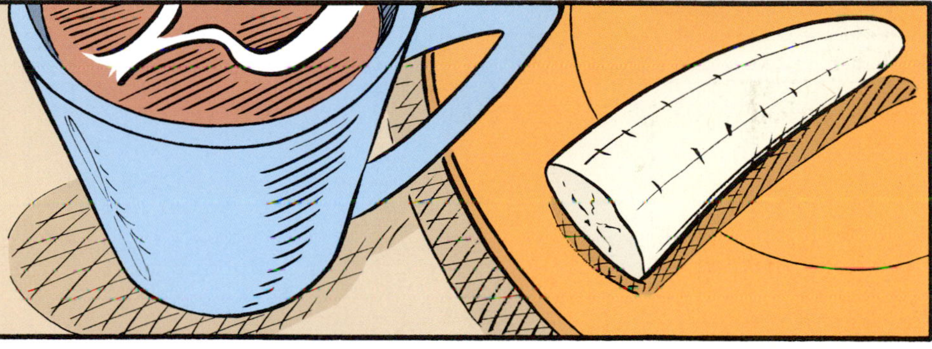
AROUND 1:00 AM (I GO TO SLEEP AROUND 2:00) I SNACK ON THE OTHER HALF OF THAT BANANA (50) AND ENJOY A LAST CUP OF HERBAL TEA (Ø).

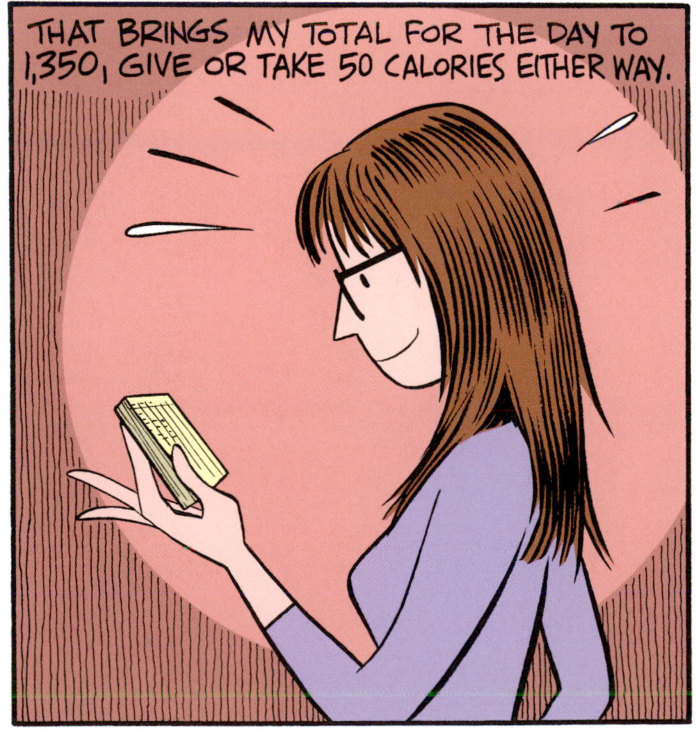
THAT BRINGS MY TOTAL FOR THE DAY TO 1,350, GIVE OR TAKE 50 CALORIES EITHER WAY.

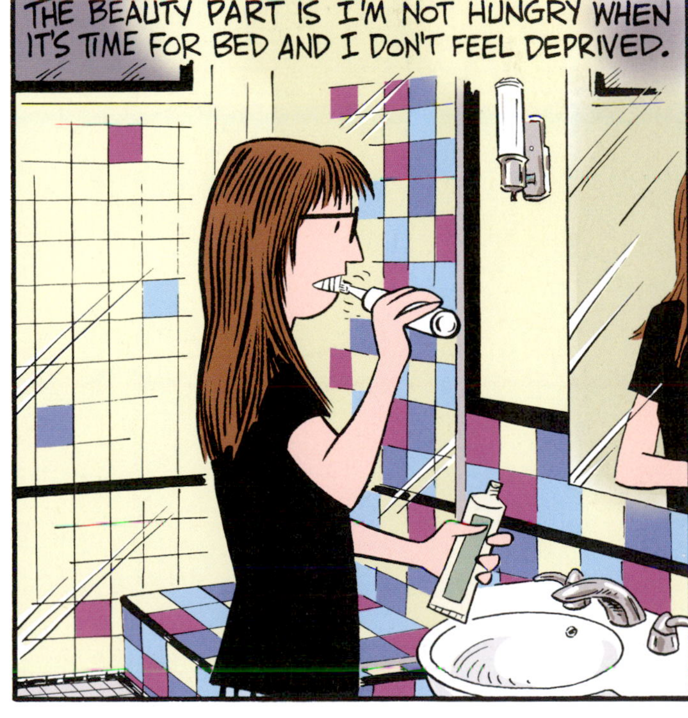
THE BEAUTY PART IS I'M NOT HUNGRY WHEN IT'S TIME FOR BED AND I DON'T FEEL DEPRIVED.

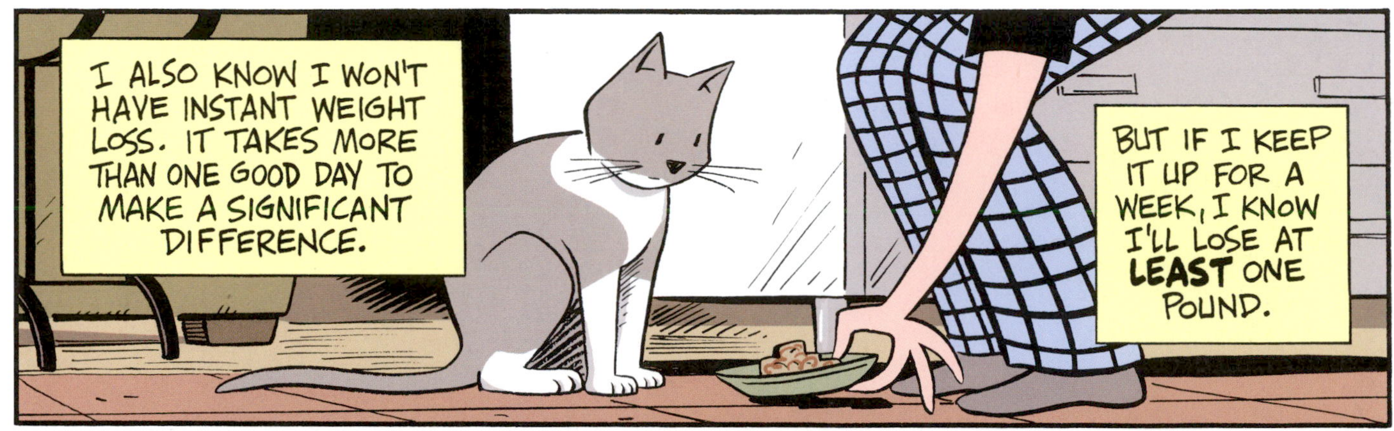
I ALSO KNOW I WON'T HAVE INSTANT WEIGHT LOSS. IT TAKES MORE THAN ONE GOOD DAY TO MAKE A SIGNIFICANT DIFFERENCE.
BUT IF I KEEP IT UP FOR A WEEK, I KNOW I'LL LOSE AT **LEAST** ONE POUND.

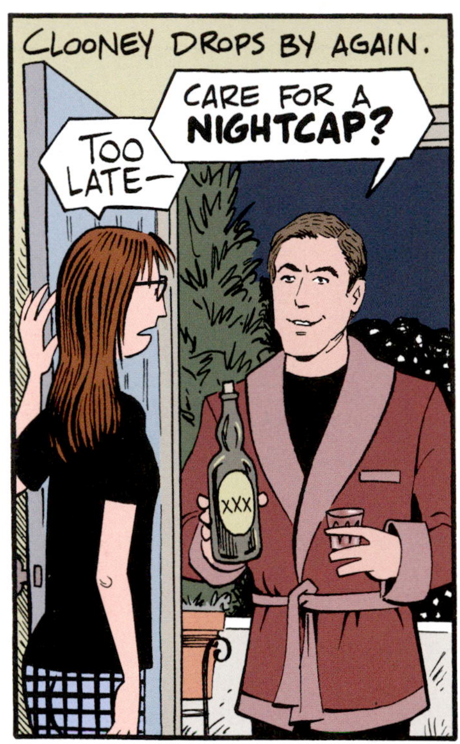
CLOONEY DROPS BY AGAIN.
CARE FOR A **NIGHTCAP?**
TOO LATE—
XXX

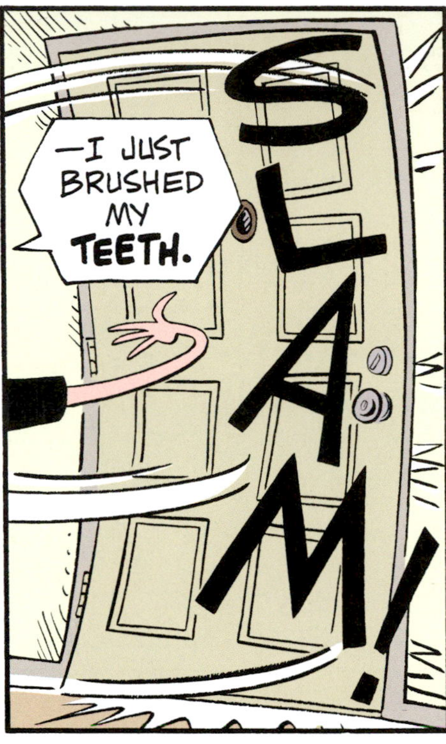
—I JUST BRUSHED MY **TEETH.**
SLAM!

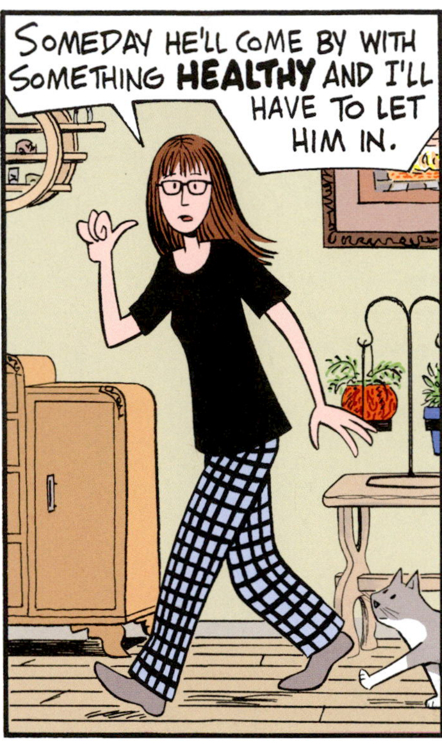
SOMEDAY HE'LL COME BY WITH SOMETHING **HEALTHY** AND I'LL HAVE TO LET HIM IN.

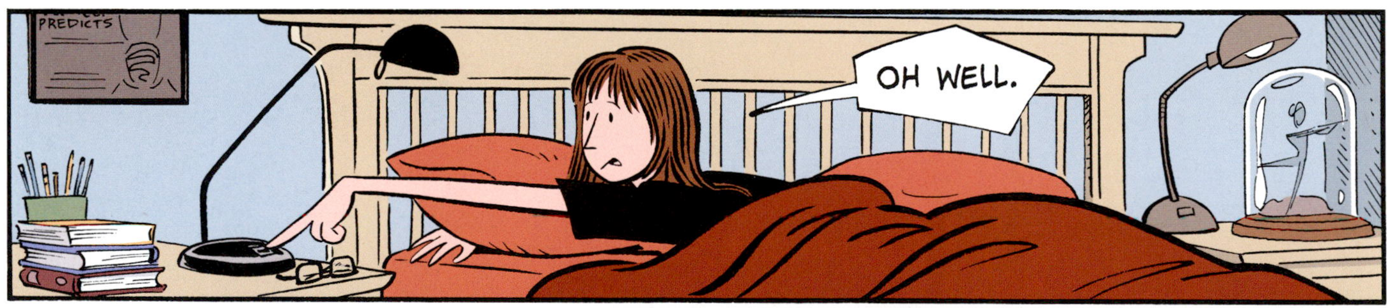
PREDICTS
OH WELL.

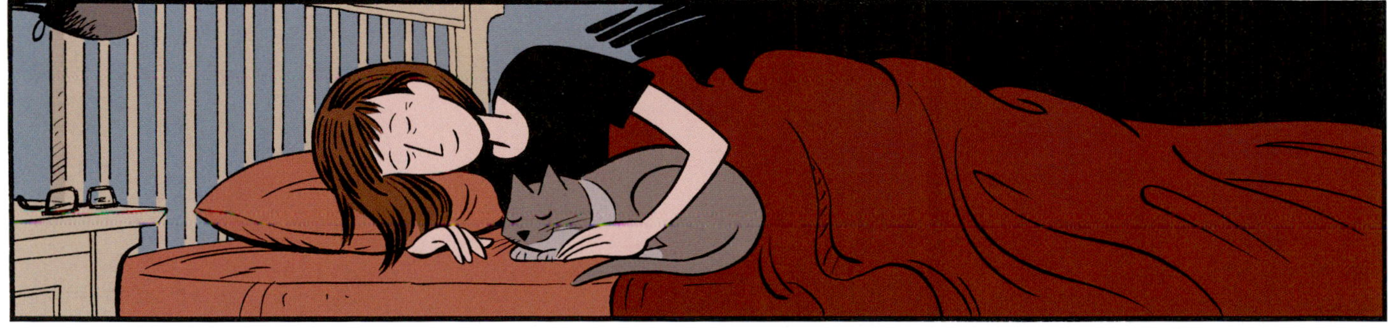

# THE NUMBERS GAME

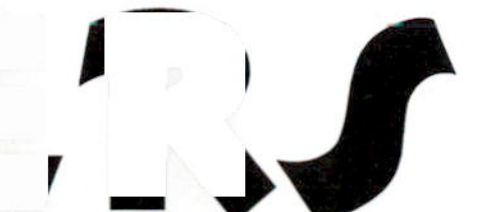

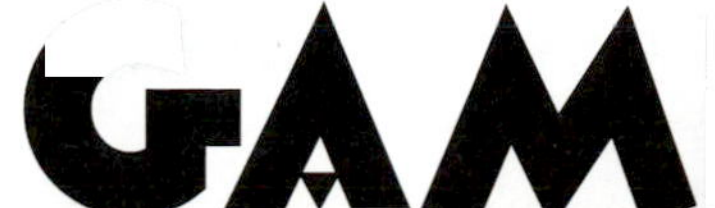

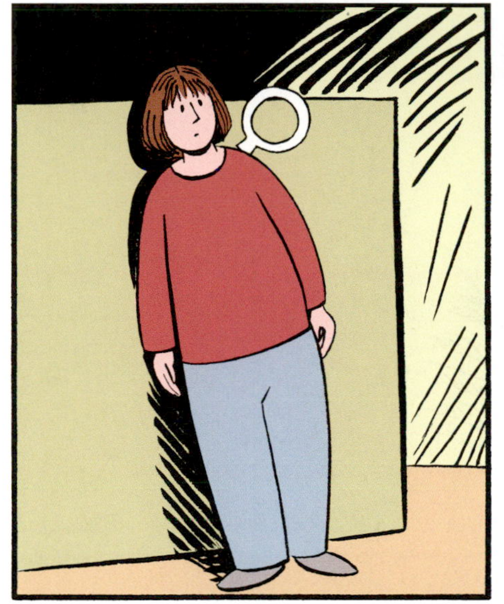

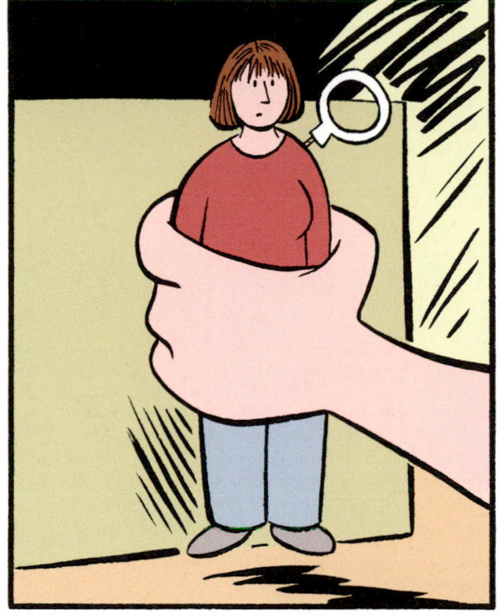

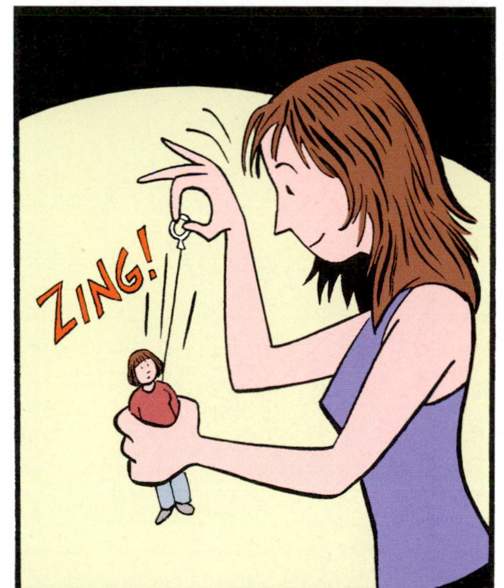
ZING!

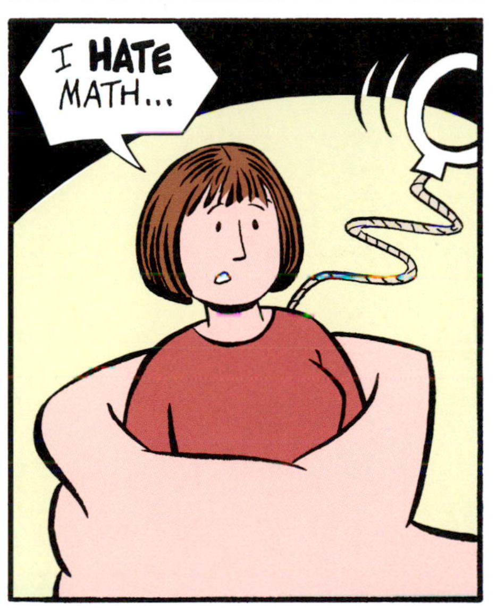
I **HATE** MATH...

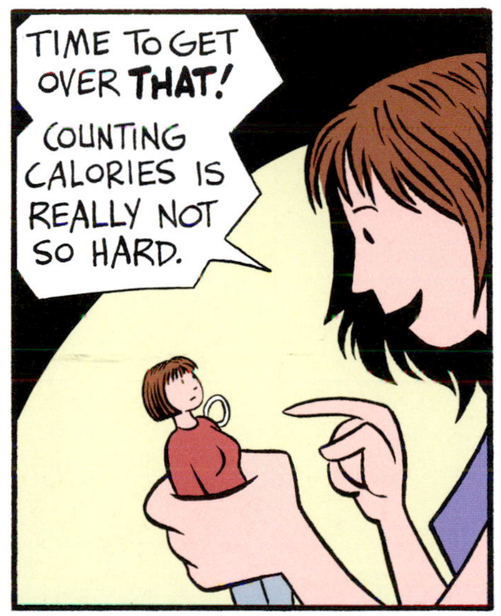
TIME TO GET OVER **THAT!**
COUNTING CALORIES IS REALLY NOT SO HARD.

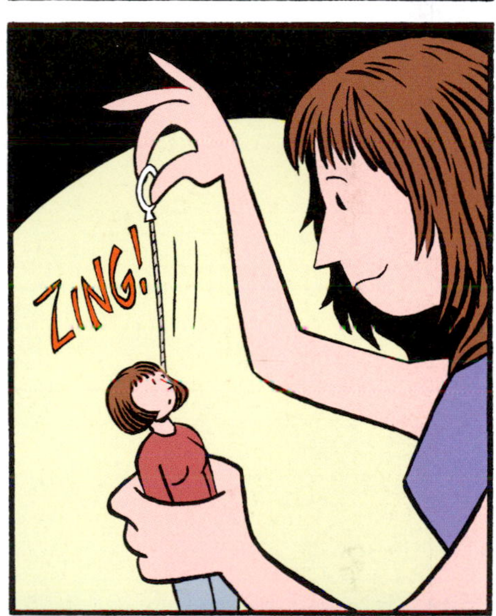
ZING!

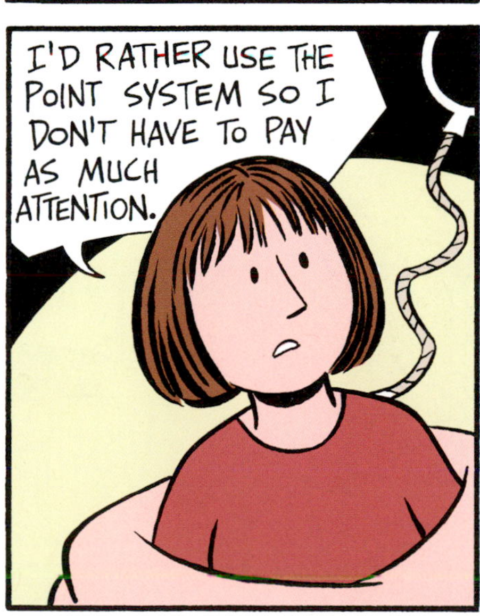
I'D RATHER USE THE POINT SYSTEM SO I DON'T HAVE TO PAY AS MUCH ATTENTION.

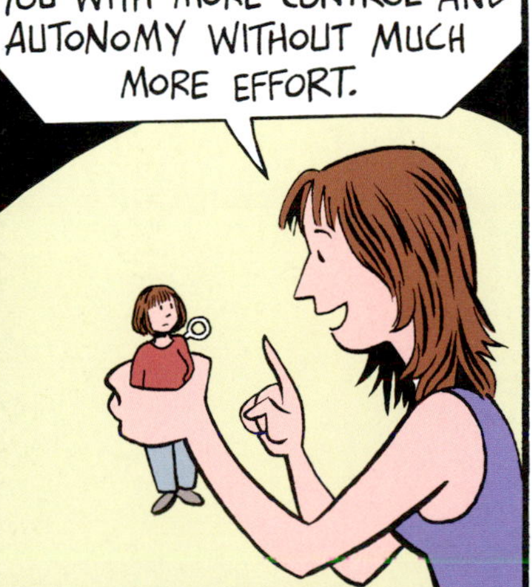
BUT THIS METHOD PROVIDES YOU WITH MORE CONTROL AND AUTONOMY WITHOUT MUCH MORE EFFORT.

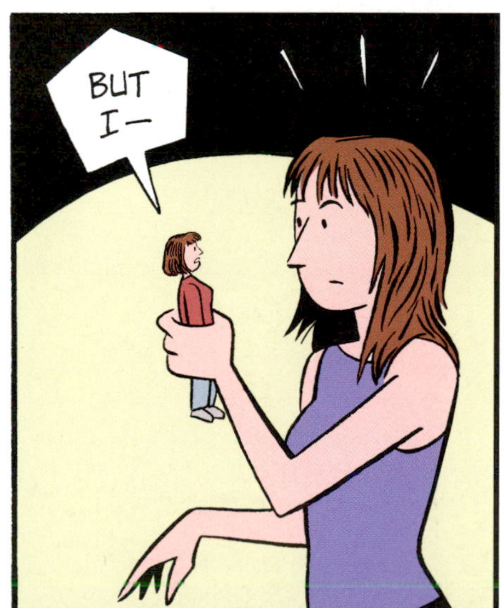
BUT I—

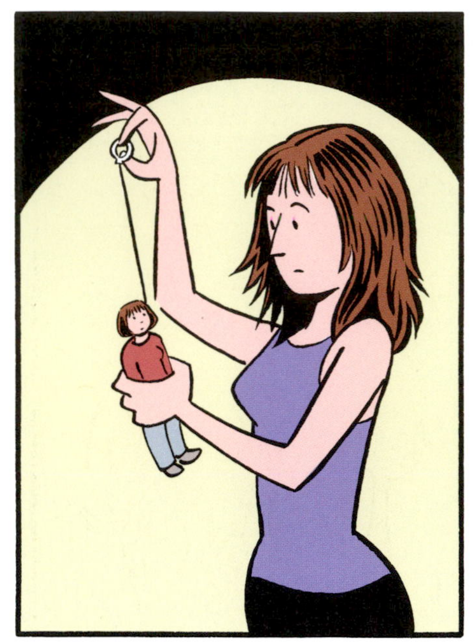

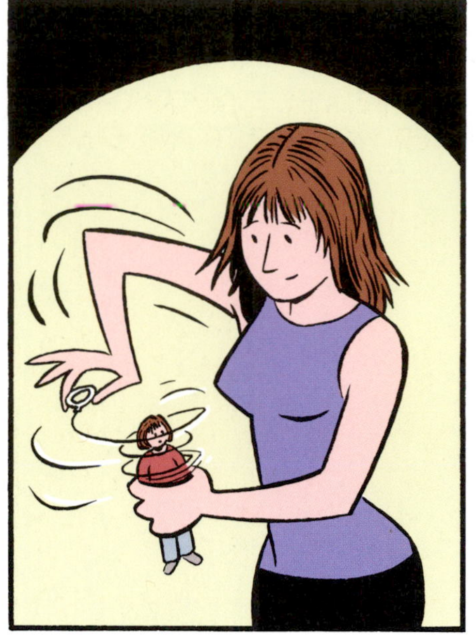

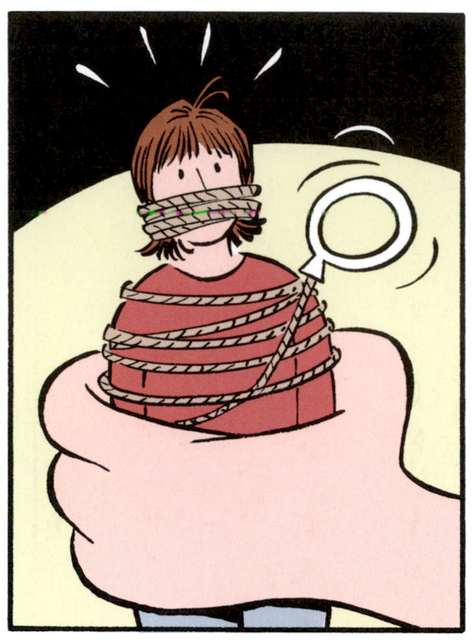

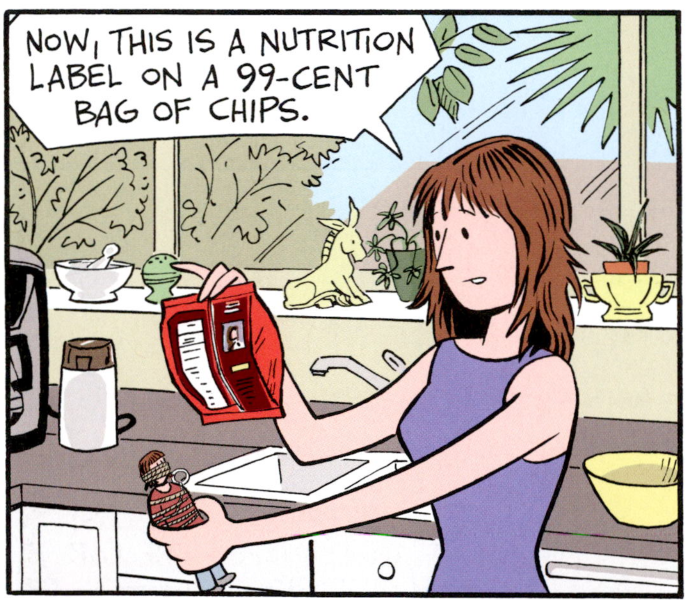

NOW, THIS IS A NUTRITION LABEL ON A 99-CENT BAG OF CHIPS.

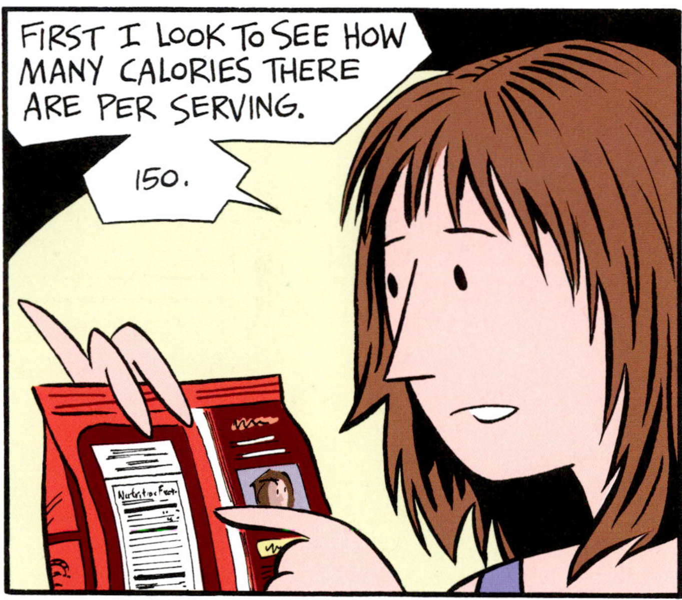

FIRST I LOOK TO SEE HOW MANY CALORIES THERE ARE PER SERVING.
150.

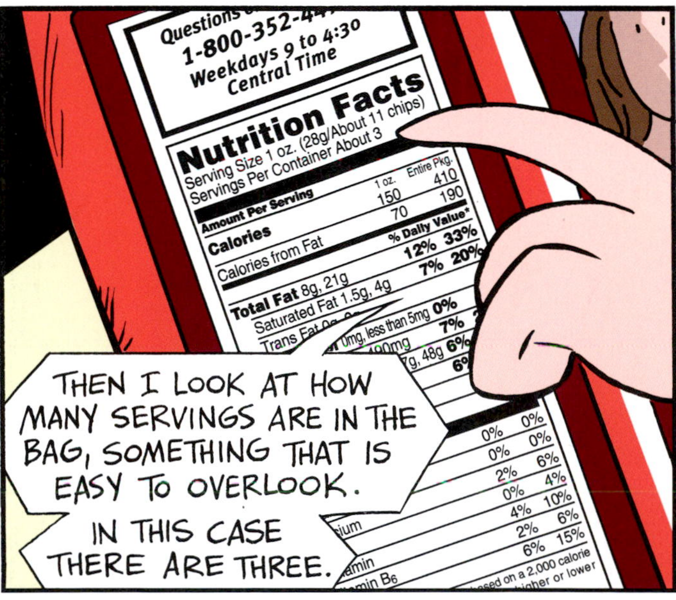

Weekdays 9 to 4:30
Central Time
Nutrition Facts
Serving Size 1 oz. (28g/About 11 chips)
Servings Per Container About 3
Amount Per Serving
Calories
Calories from Fat
Total Fat 8g, 21g
Saturated Fat 1.5g, 4g
THEN I LOOK AT HOW MANY SERVINGS ARE IN THE BAG, SOMETHING THAT IS EASY TO OVERLOOK.
IN THIS CASE THERE ARE THREE.

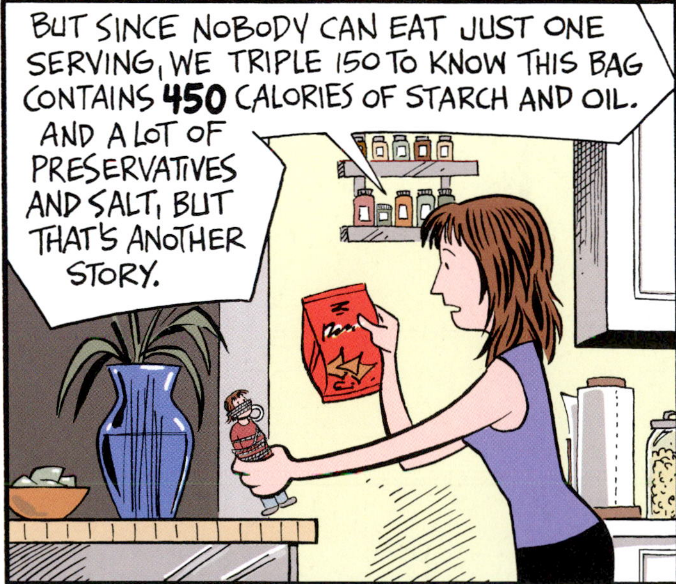

BUT SINCE NOBODY CAN EAT JUST ONE SERVING, WE TRIPLE 150 TO KNOW THIS BAG CONTAINS **450** CALORIES OF STARCH AND OIL.
AND A LOT OF PRESERVATIVES AND SALT, BUT THAT'S ANOTHER STORY.

BY THE WAY, A SIMPLE RULE FOR PROCESSED FOOD IS THIS: IF IT CONTAINS MORE THAN FIVE INGREDIENTS AND IF ANY OF THOSE ARE UNPRONOUNCEABLE, DON'T EAT IT.

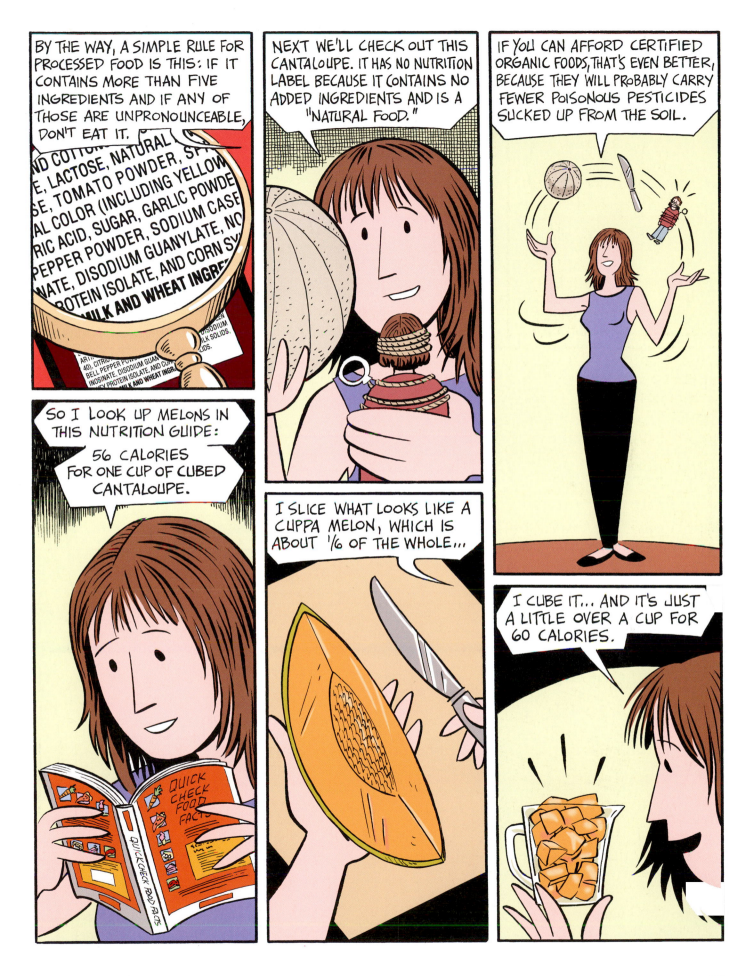

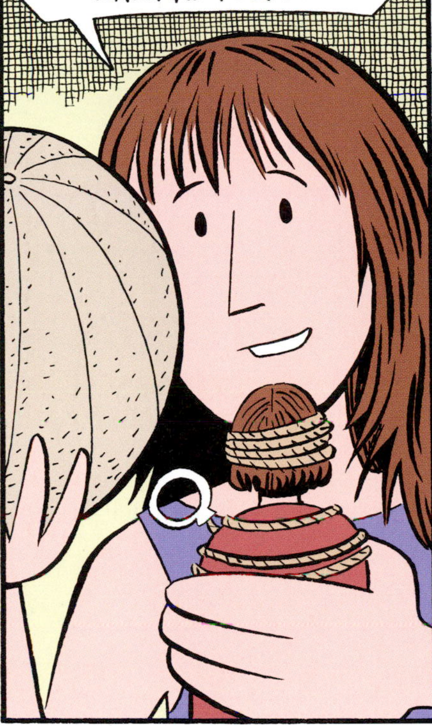
NEXT WE'LL CHECK OUT THIS CANTALOUPE. IT HAS NO NUTRITION LABEL BECAUSE IT CONTAINS NO ADDED INGREDIENTS AND IS A "NATURAL FOOD."

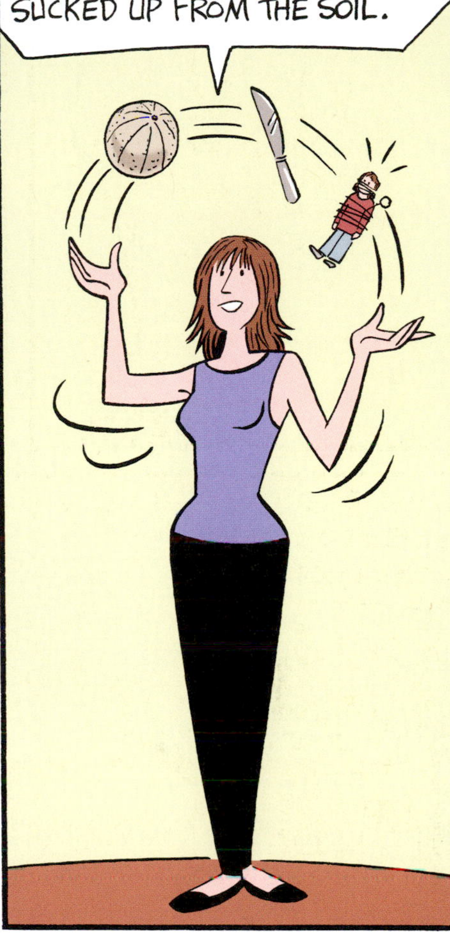
IF YOU CAN AFFORD CERTIFIED ORGANIC FOODS, THAT'S EVEN BETTER, BECAUSE THEY WILL PROBABLY CARRY FEWER POISONOUS PESTICIDES SUCKED UP FROM THE SOIL.

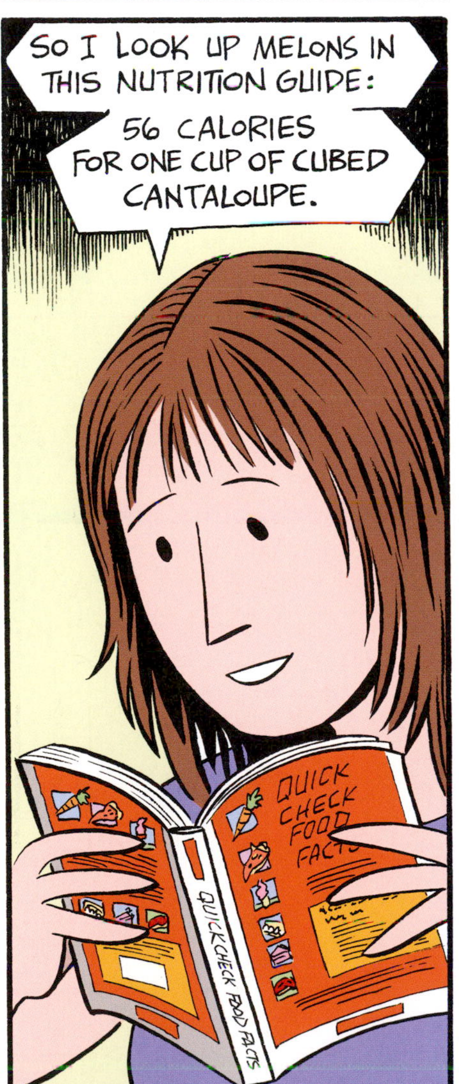
SO I LOOK UP MELONS IN THIS NUTRITION GUIDE:
56 CALORIES FOR ONE CUP OF CUBED CANTALOUPE.
QUICK CHECK FOOD FACTS
QUICKCHECK FOOD FACTS

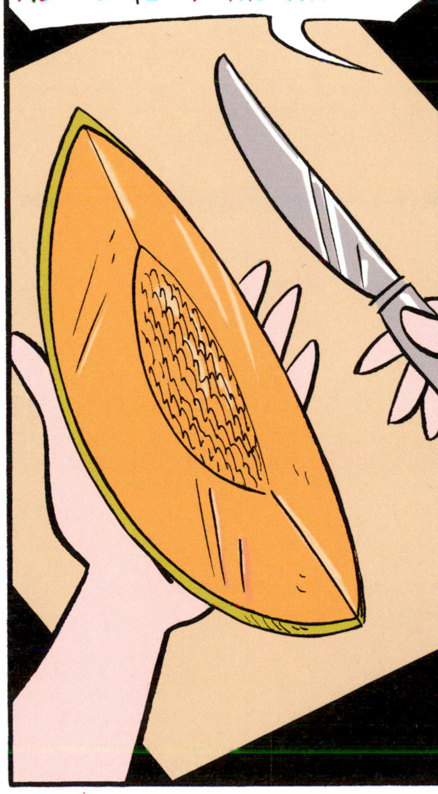
I SLICE WHAT LOOKS LIKE A CUPPA MELON, WHICH IS ABOUT 1/6 OF THE WHOLE...

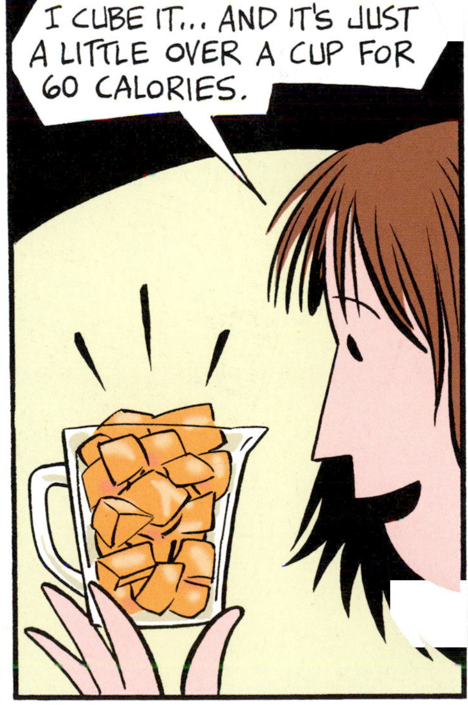
I CUBE IT... AND IT'S JUST A LITTLE OVER A CUP FOR 60 CALORIES.

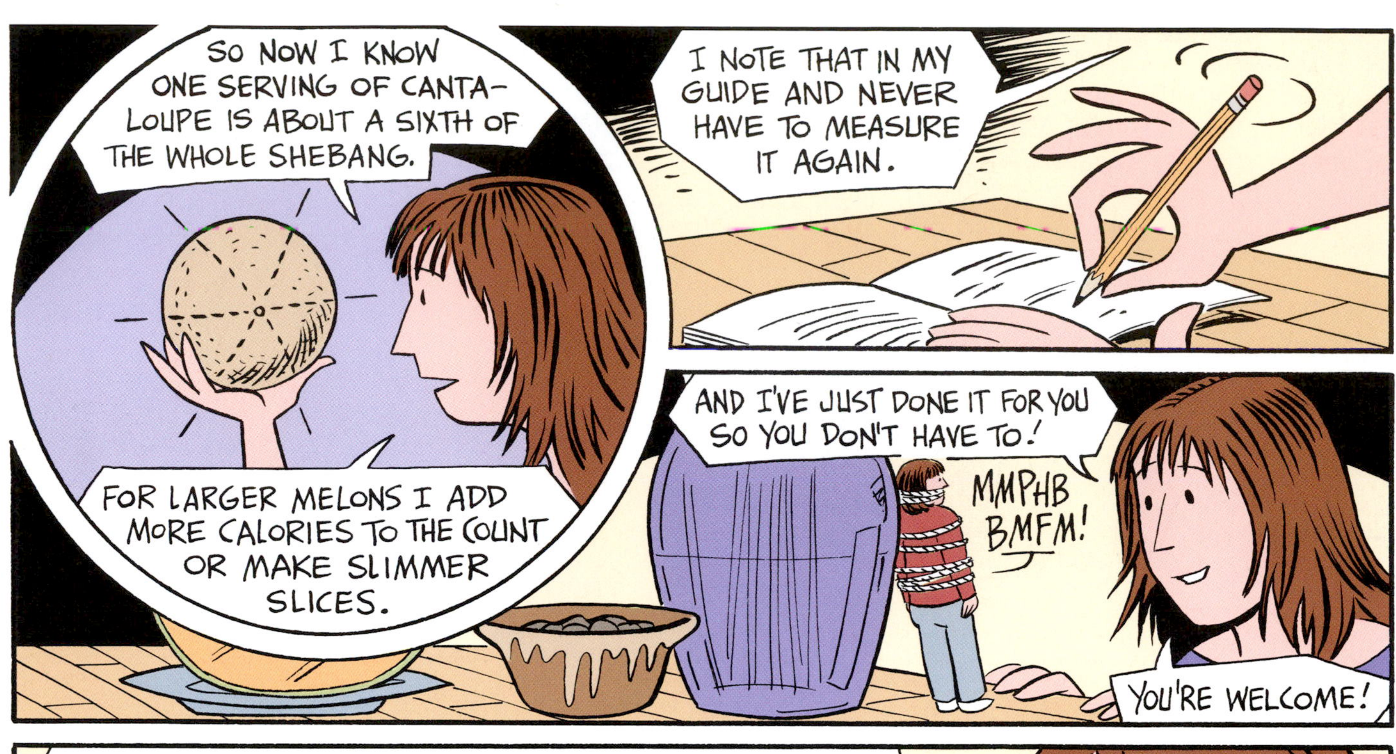
SO NOW I KNOW ONE SERVING OF CANTA-LOUPE IS ABOUT A SIXTH OF THE WHOLE SHEBANG.
FOR LARGER MELONS I ADD MORE CALORIES TO THE COUNT OR MAKE SLIMMER SLICES.
I NOTE THAT IN MY GUIDE AND NEVER HAVE TO MEASURE IT AGAIN.
AND I'VE JUST DONE IT FOR YOU SO YOU DON'T HAVE TO!
MMPHB BMFM!
YOU'RE WELCOME!

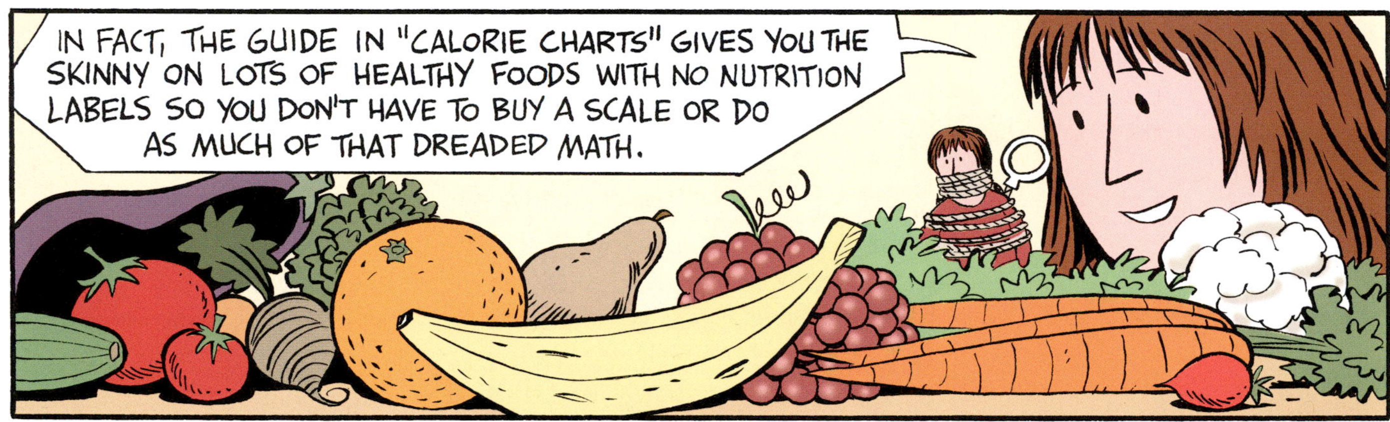
IN FACT, THE GUIDE IN "CALORIE CHARTS" GIVES YOU THE SKINNY ON LOTS OF HEALTHY FOODS WITH NO NUTRITION LABELS SO YOU DON'T HAVE TO BUY A SCALE OR DO AS MUCH OF THAT DREADED MATH.

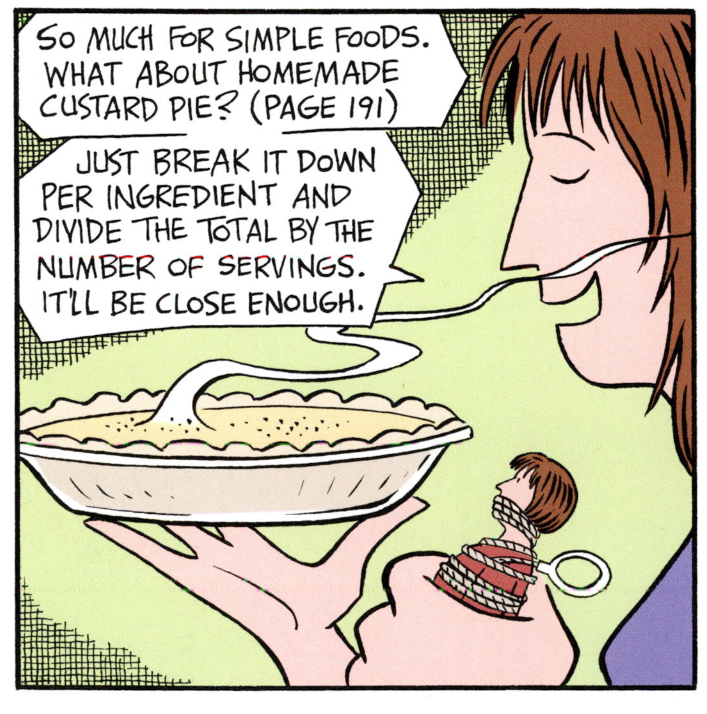
SO MUCH FOR SIMPLE FOODS. WHAT ABOUT HOMEMADE CUSTARD PIE? (PAGE 191)
JUST BREAK IT DOWN PER INGREDIENT AND DIVIDE THE TOTAL BY THE NUMBER OF SERVINGS. IT'LL BE CLOSE ENOUGH.

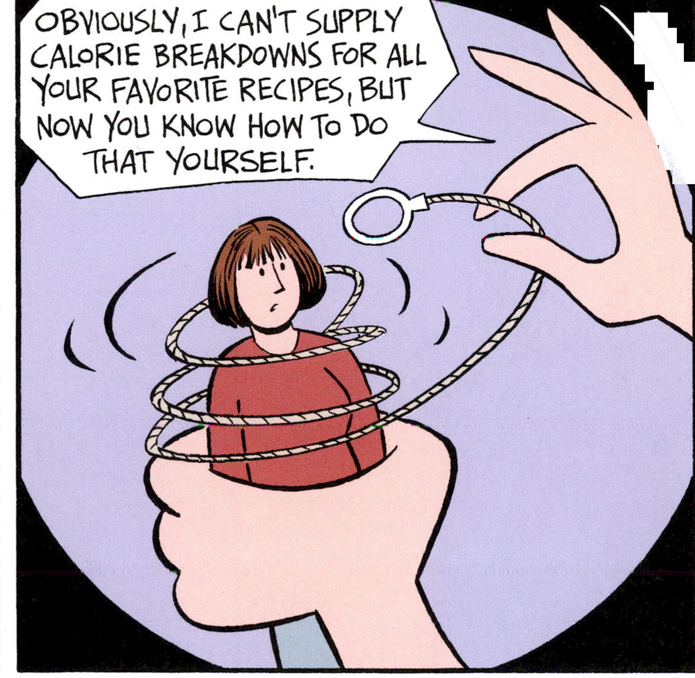
OBVIOUSLY, I CAN'T SUPPLY CALORIE BREAKDOWNS FOR ALL YOUR FAVORITE RECIPES, BUT NOW YOU KNOW HOW TO DO THAT YOURSELF.

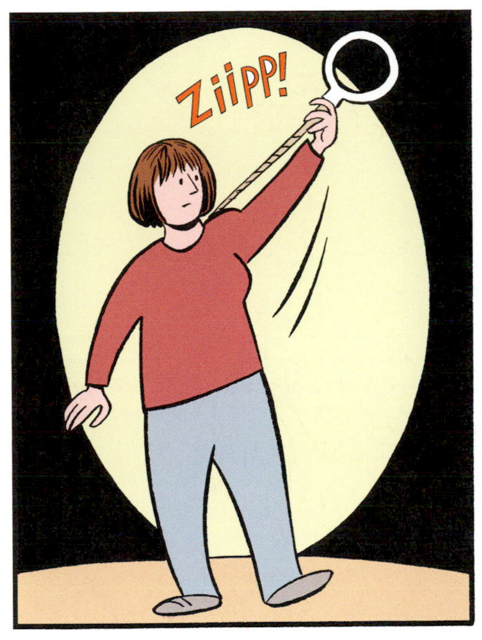
ZiiPP!

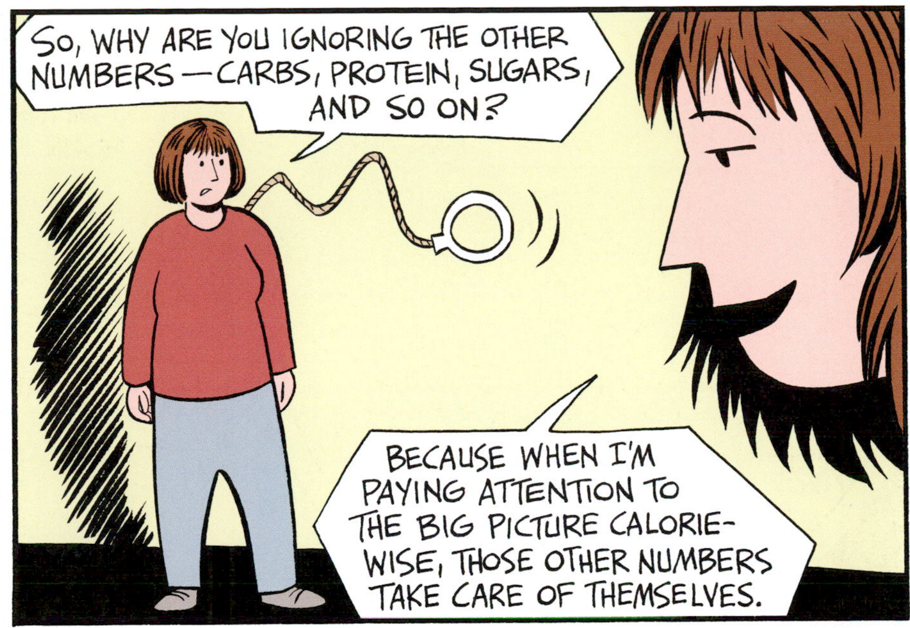
SO, WHY ARE YOU IGNORING THE OTHER NUMBERS — CARBS, PROTEIN, SUGARS, AND SO ON?
BECAUSE WHEN I'M PAYING ATTENTION TO THE BIG PICTURE CALORIE-WISE, THOSE OTHER NUMBERS TAKE CARE OF THEMSELVES.

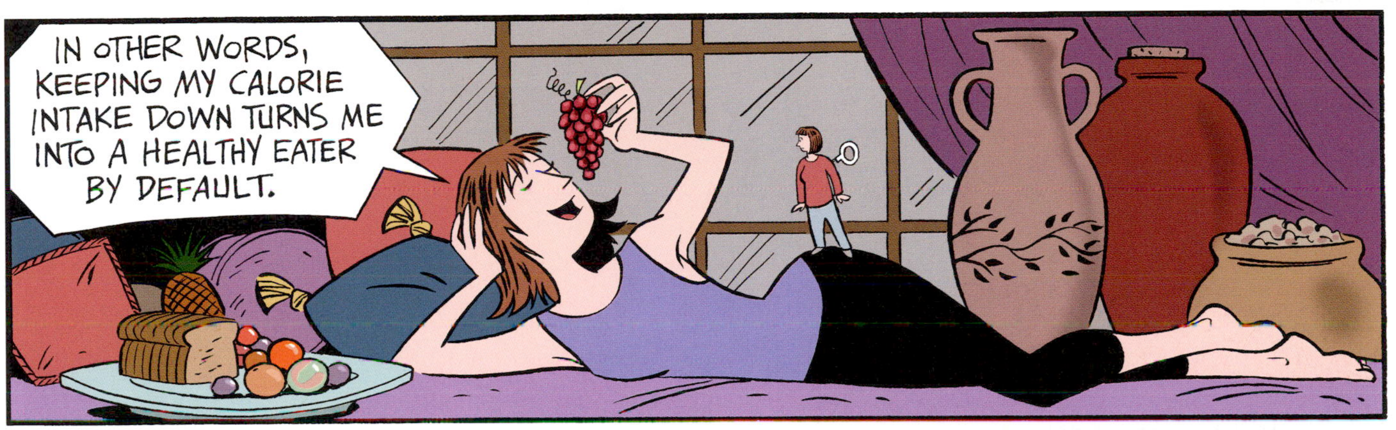
IN OTHER WORDS, KEEPING MY CALORIE INTAKE DOWN TURNS ME INTO A HEALTHY EATER BY DEFAULT.

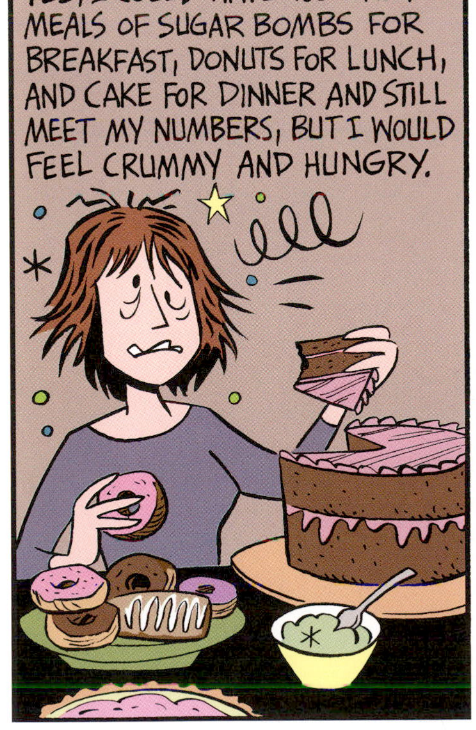
YES, I COULD HAVE 450-CALORIE MEALS OF SUGAR BOMBS FOR BREAKFAST, DONUTS FOR LUNCH, AND CAKE FOR DINNER AND STILL MEET MY NUMBERS, BUT I WOULD FEEL CRUMMY AND HUNGRY.

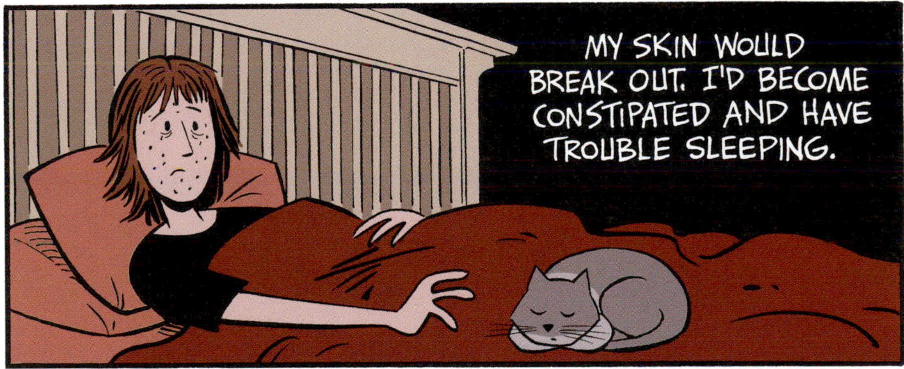
MY SKIN WOULD BREAK OUT. I'D BECOME CONSTIPATED AND HAVE TROUBLE SLEEPING.

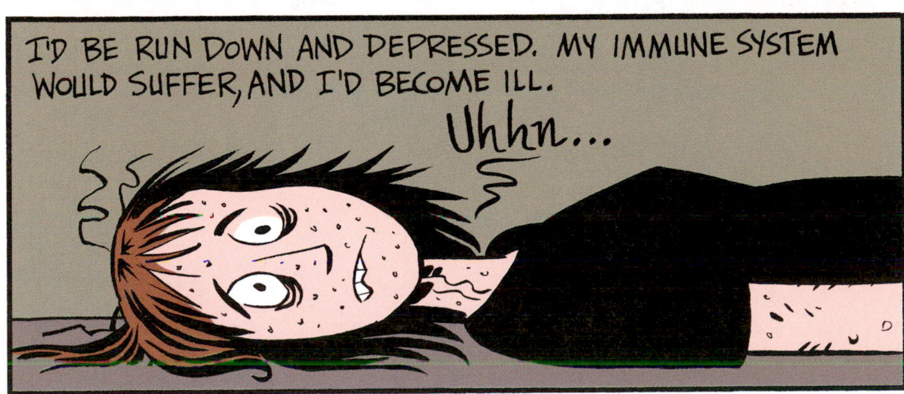
I'D BE RUN DOWN AND DEPRESSED. MY IMMUNE SYSTEM WOULD SUFFER, AND I'D BECOME ILL.
Uhhn...

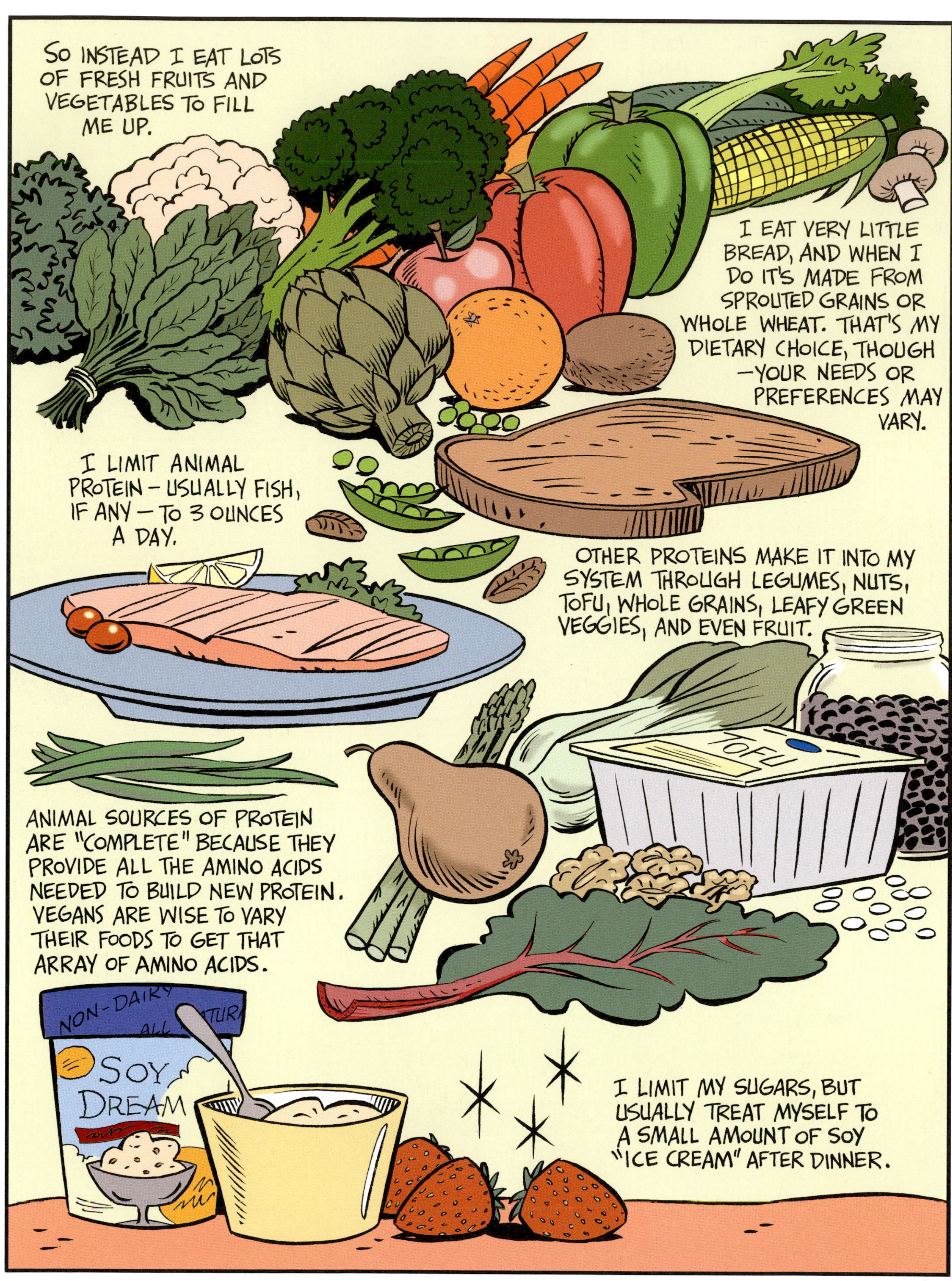
SO INSTEAD I EAT LOTS OF FRESH FRUITS AND VEGETABLES TO FILL ME UP.
I EAT VERY LITTLE BREAD, AND WHEN I DO IT'S MADE FROM SPROUTED GRAINS OR WHOLE WHEAT. THAT'S MY DIETARY CHOICE, THOUGH —YOUR NEEDS OR PREFERENCES MAY VARY.
I LIMIT ANIMAL PROTEIN — USUALLY FISH, IF ANY — TO 3 OUNCES A DAY.
OTHER PROTEINS MAKE IT INTO MY SYSTEM THROUGH LEGUMES, NUTS, TOFU, WHOLE GRAINS, LEAFY GREEN VEGGIES, AND EVEN FRUIT.
TOFU
ANIMAL SOURCES OF PROTEIN ARE "COMPLETE" BECAUSE THEY PROVIDE ALL THE AMINO ACIDS NEEDED TO BUILD NEW PROTEIN. VEGANS ARE WISE TO VARY THEIR FOODS TO GET THAT ARRAY OF AMINO ACIDS.
NON-DAIRY
SOY DREAM
I LIMIT MY SUGARS, BUT USUALLY TREAT MYSELF TO A SMALL AMOUNT OF SOY "ICE CREAM" AFTER DINNER.

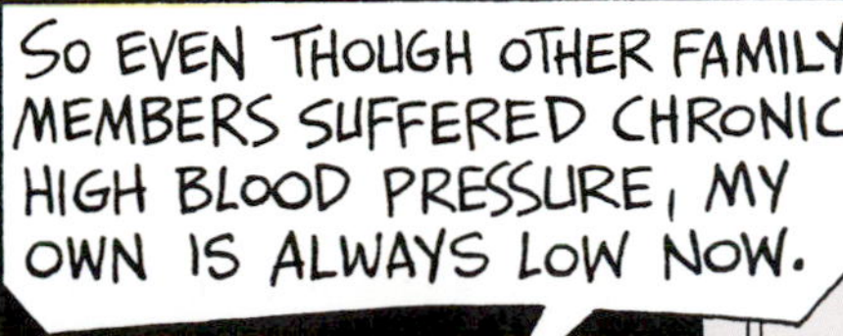
SO EVEN THOUGH OTHER FAMILY MEMBERS SUFFERED CHRONIC HIGH BLOOD PRESSURE, MY OWN IS ALWAYS LOW NOW.

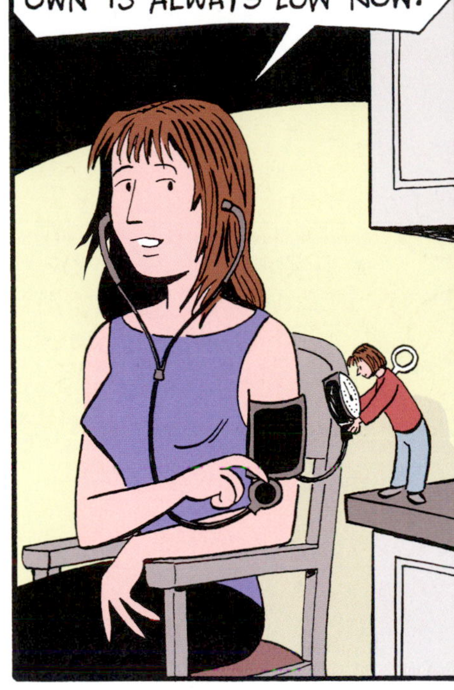

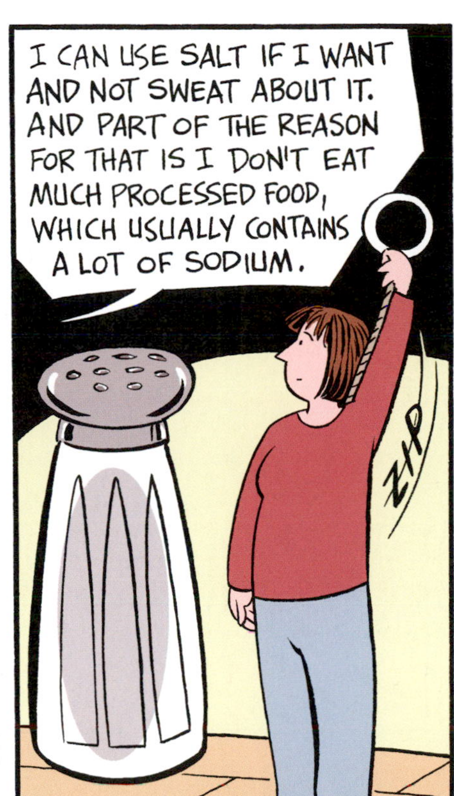
I CAN USE SALT IF I WANT AND NOT SWEAT ABOUT IT. AND PART OF THE REASON FOR THAT IS I DON'T EAT MUCH PROCESSED FOOD, WHICH USUALLY CONTAINS A LOT OF SODIUM.
ZIP

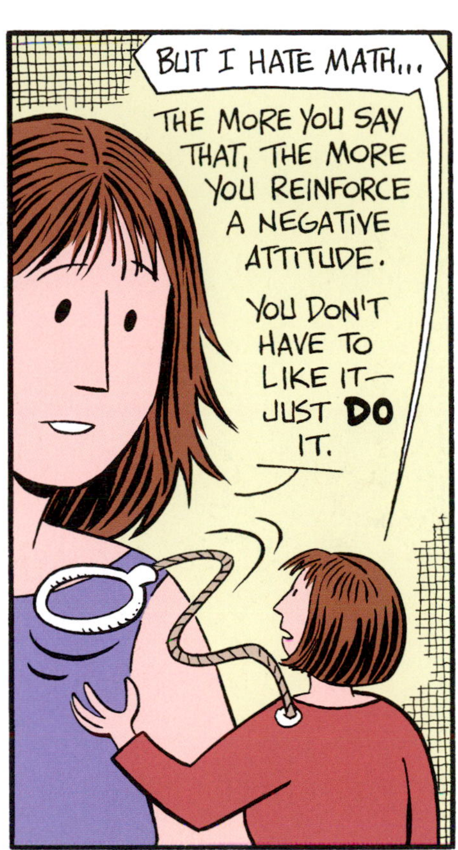
BUT I HATE MATH...
THE MORE YOU SAY THAT, THE MORE YOU REINFORCE A NEGATIVE ATTITUDE.
YOU DON'T HAVE TO LIKE IT— JUST **DO** IT.

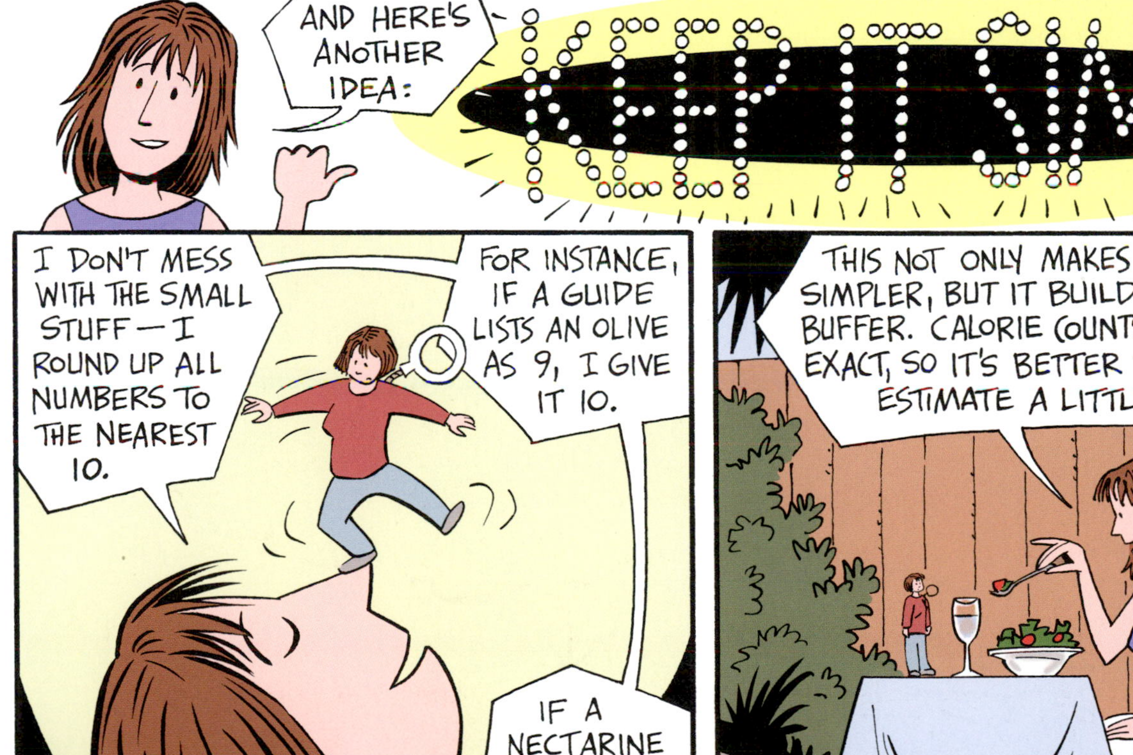
AND HERE'S ANOTHER IDEA:
KEEP IT SIMPLE
I DON'T MESS WITH THE SMALL STUFF — I ROUND UP ALL NUMBERS TO THE NEAREST 10.
FOR INSTANCE, IF A GUIDE LISTS AN OLIVE AS 9, I GIVE IT 10.
IF A NECTARINE IS 63, I GIVE IT 70.

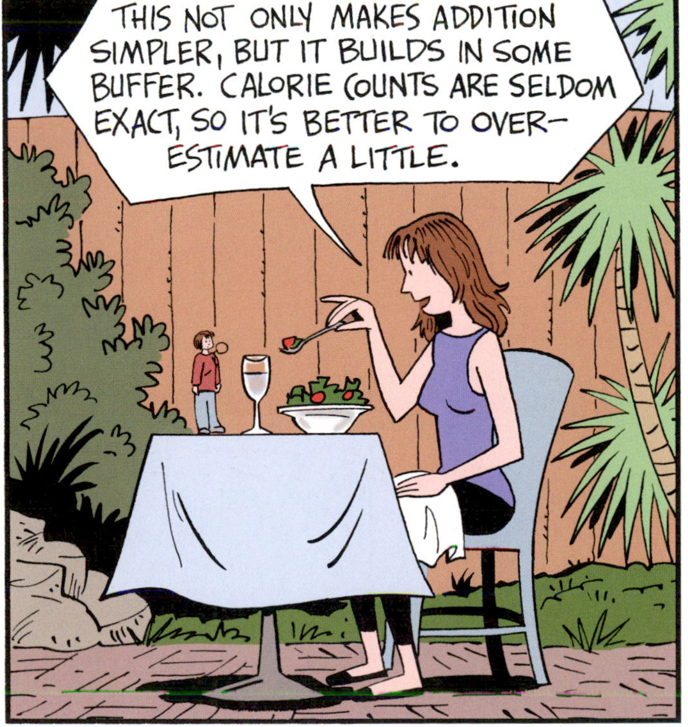
THIS NOT ONLY MAKES ADDITION SIMPLER, BUT IT BUILDS IN SOME BUFFER. CALORIE COUNTS ARE SELDOM EXACT, SO IT'S BETTER TO OVER-ESTIMATE A LITTLE.

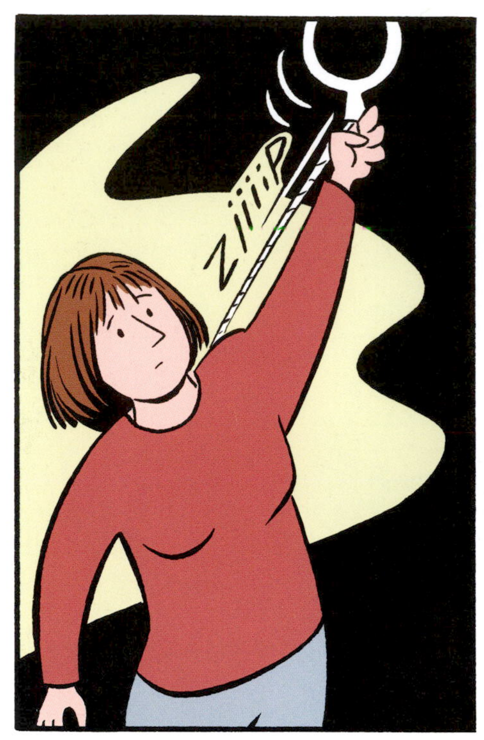
ZIIIIP

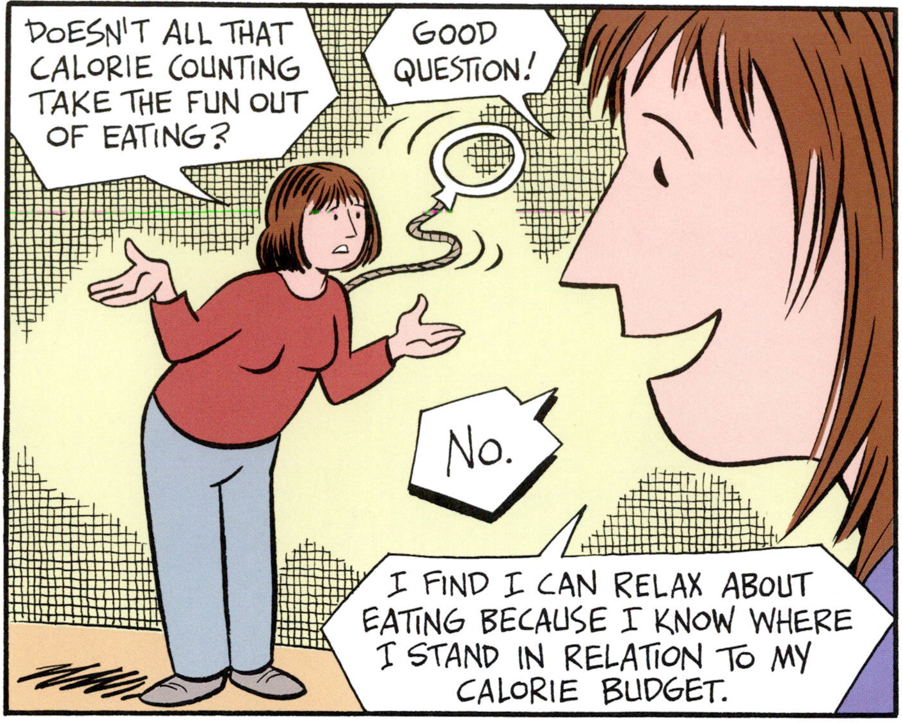
DOESN'T ALL THAT CALORIE COUNTING TAKE THE FUN OUT OF EATING?
GOOD QUESTION!
No.
I FIND I CAN RELAX ABOUT EATING BECAUSE I KNOW WHERE I STAND IN RELATION TO MY CALORIE BUDGET.

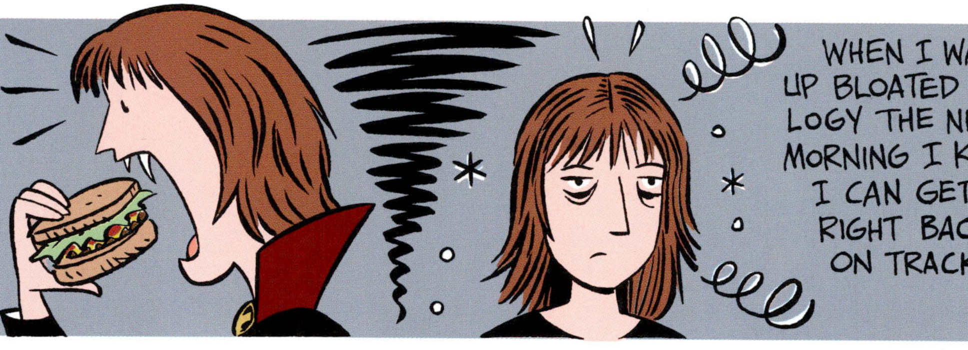
AND ONCE IN A WHILE, AFTER THE SUN GOES DOWN, I TURN INTO "HOGULA" AND GO NUTS WITH FOOD.
WHEN I WAKE UP BLOATED AND LOGY THE NEXT MORNING I KNOW I CAN GET RIGHT BACK ON TRACK.

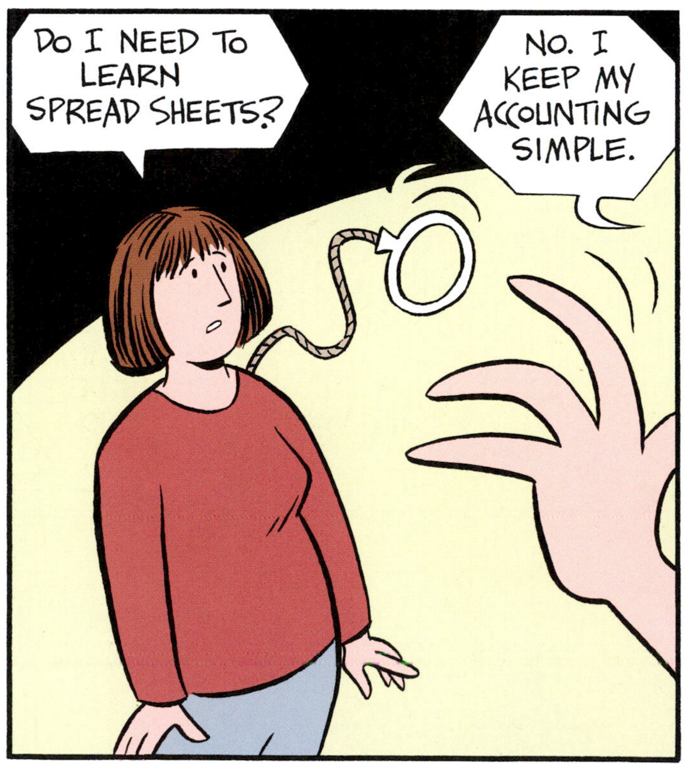
DO I NEED TO LEARN SPREAD SHEETS?
NO. I KEEP MY ACCOUNTING SIMPLE.

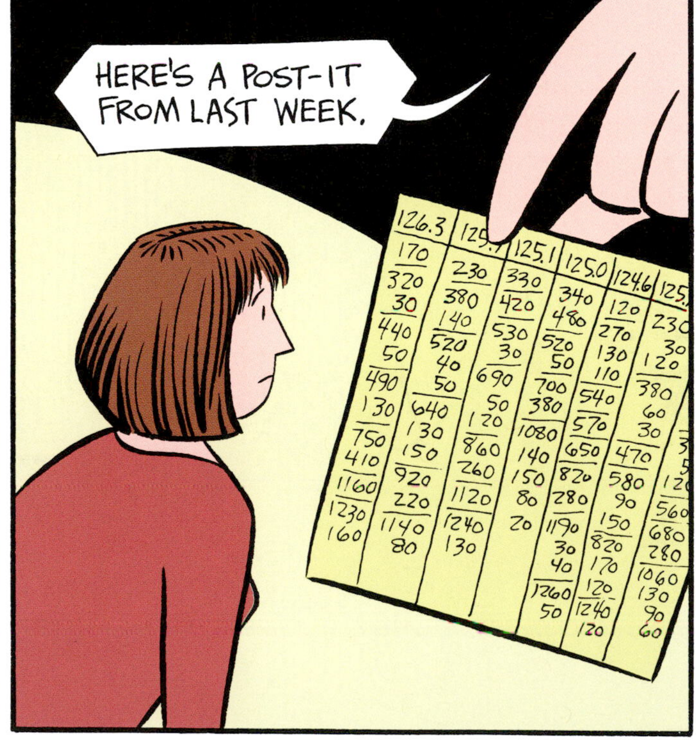
HERE'S A POST-IT FROM LAST WEEK.

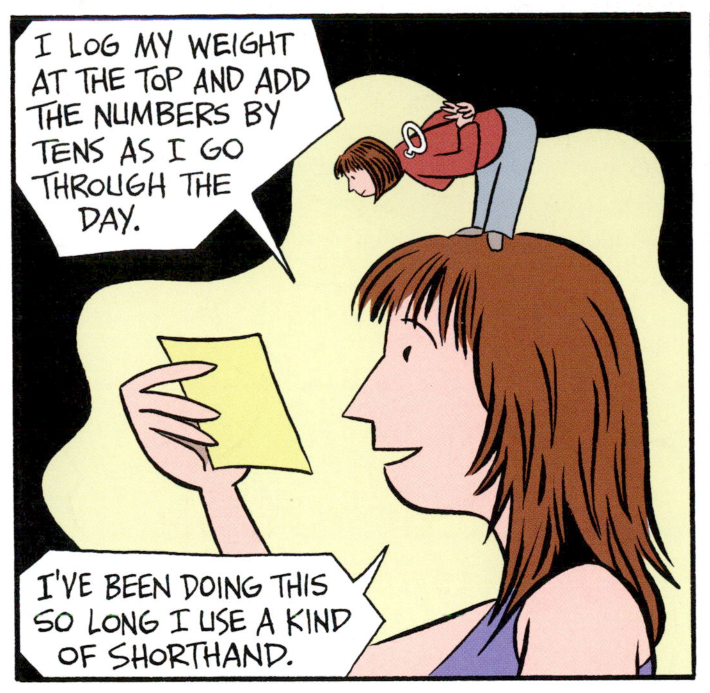
I LOG MY WEIGHT AT THE TOP AND ADD THE NUMBERS BY TENS AS I GO THROUGH THE DAY.
I'VE BEEN DOING THIS SO LONG I USE A KIND OF SHORTHAND.

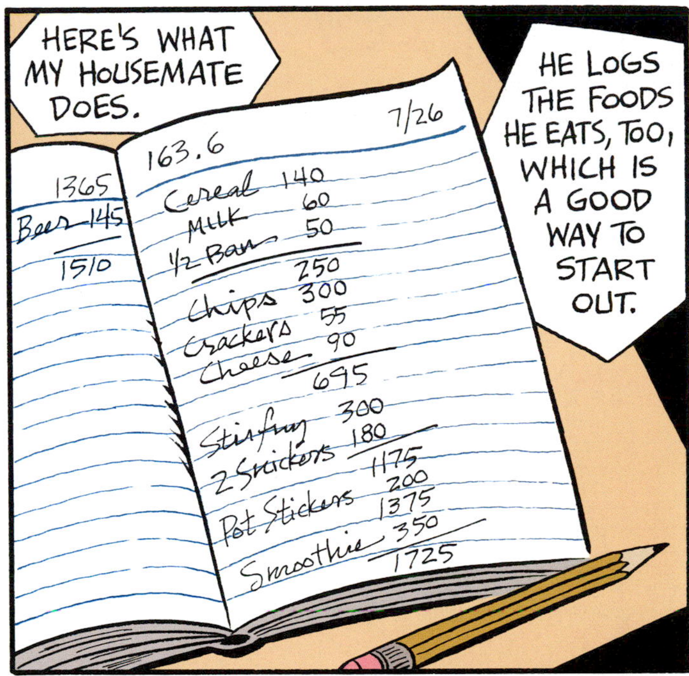
HERE'S WHAT MY HOUSEMATE DOES.
HE LOGS THE FOODS HE EATS, TOO, WHICH IS A GOOD WAY TO START OUT.
1365
Beer 145
1510
163.6
7/26
Cereal 140
Milk 60
1/2 Bar 50
250
Chips 300
Crackers 55
Cheese 90
695
Stirfry 300
2 Snickers 180
1175
Pot Stickers 200
1375
Smoothie 350
1725

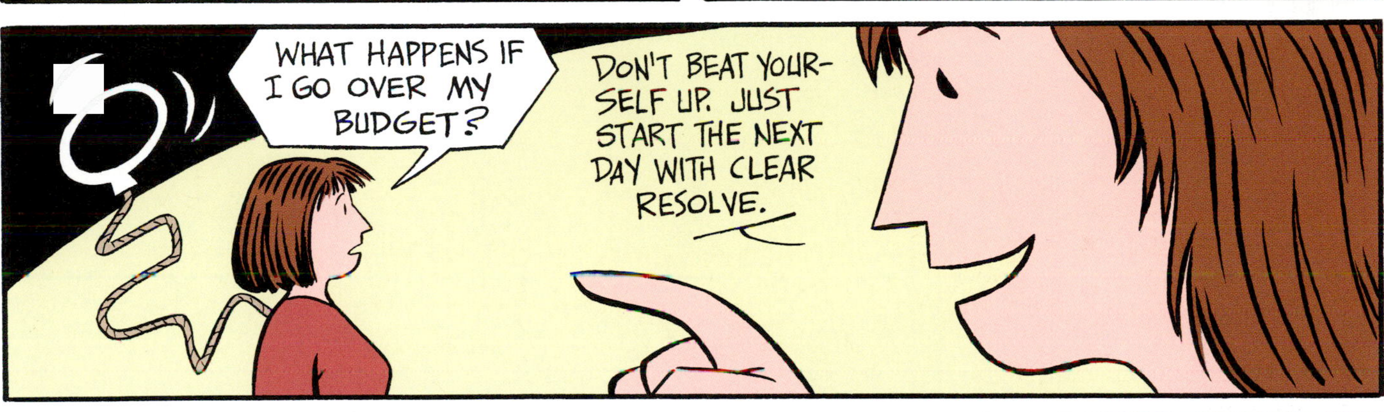
WHAT HAPPENS IF I GO OVER MY BUDGET?
DON'T BEAT YOURSELF UP. JUST START THE NEXT DAY WITH CLEAR RESOLVE.

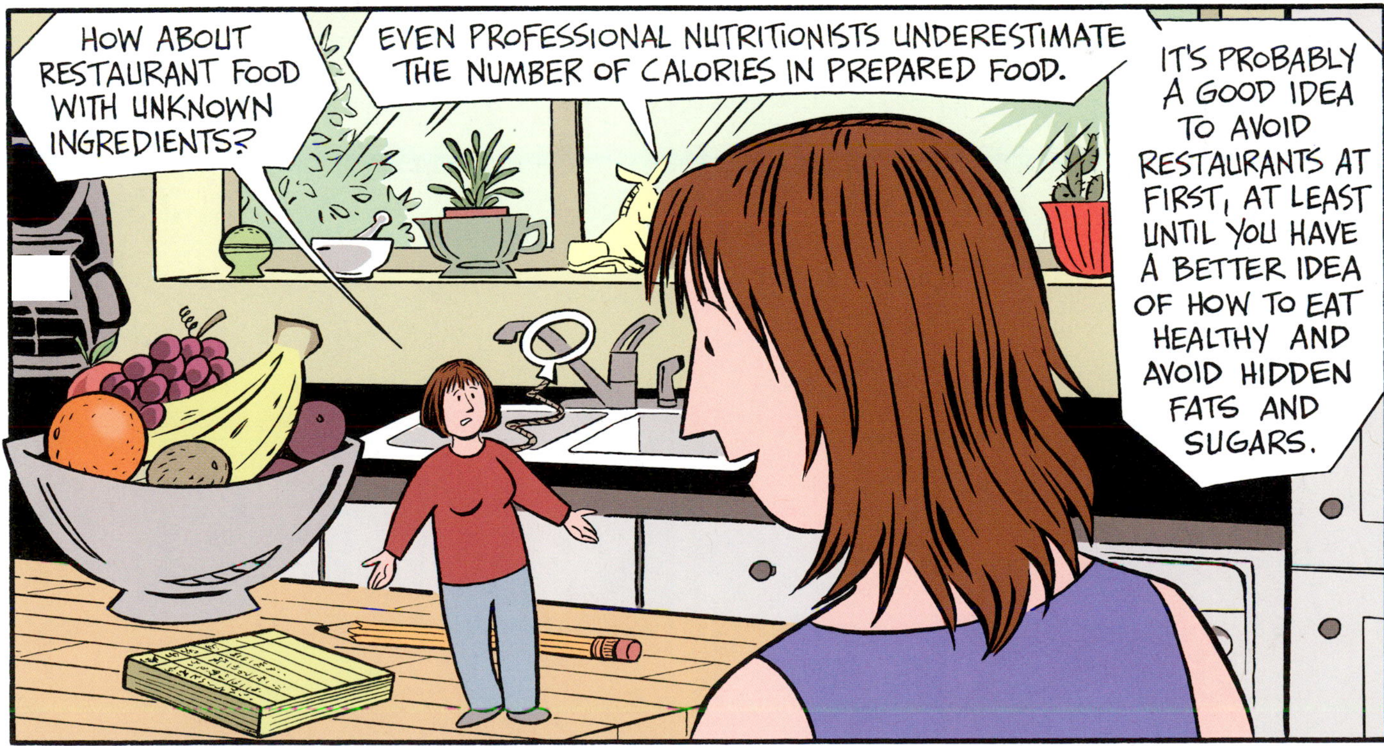
HOW ABOUT RESTAURANT FOOD WITH UNKNOWN INGREDIENTS?
EVEN PROFESSIONAL NUTRITIONISTS UNDERESTIMATE THE NUMBER OF CALORIES IN PREPARED FOOD.
IT'S PROBABLY A GOOD IDEA TO AVOID RESTAURANTS AT FIRST, AT LEAST UNTIL YOU HAVE A BETTER IDEA OF HOW TO EAT HEALTHY AND AVOID HIDDEN FATS AND SUGARS.

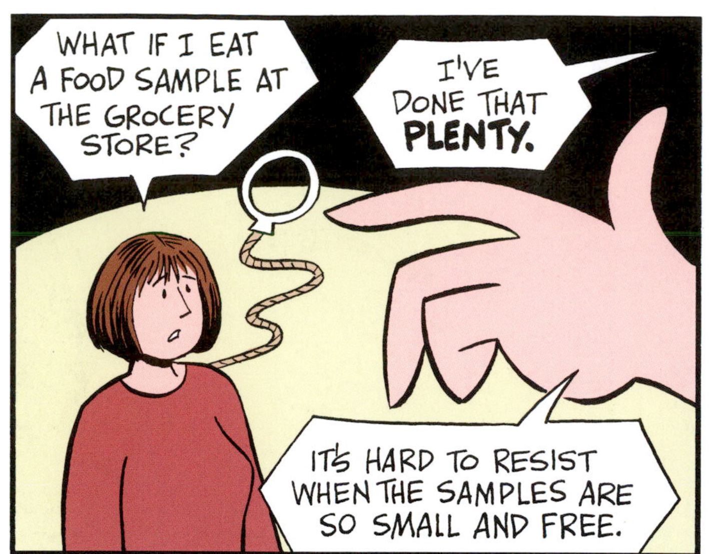
WHAT IF I EAT A FOOD SAMPLE AT THE GROCERY STORE?
I'VE DONE THAT **PLENTY.**
IT'S HARD TO RESIST WHEN THE SAMPLES ARE SO SMALL AND FREE.

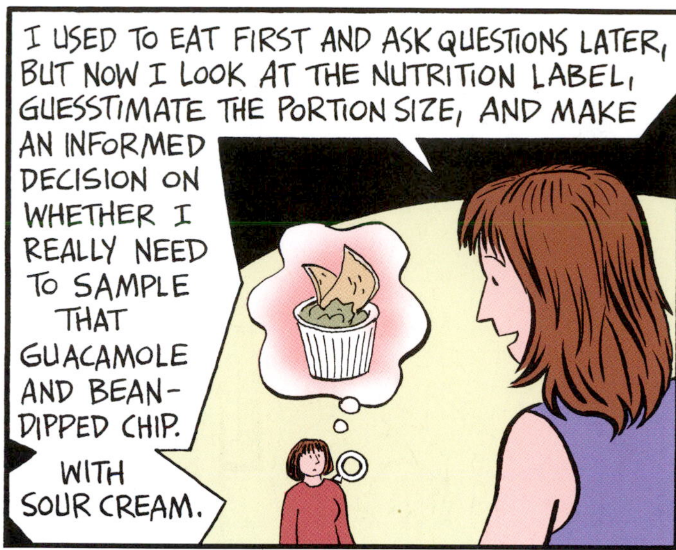
I USED TO EAT FIRST AND ASK QUESTIONS LATER, BUT NOW I LOOK AT THE NUTRITION LABEL, GUESSTIMATE THE PORTION SIZE, AND MAKE AN INFORMED DECISION ON WHETHER I REALLY NEED TO SAMPLE THAT GUACAMOLE AND BEAN-DIPPED CHIP.
WITH SOUR CREAM.

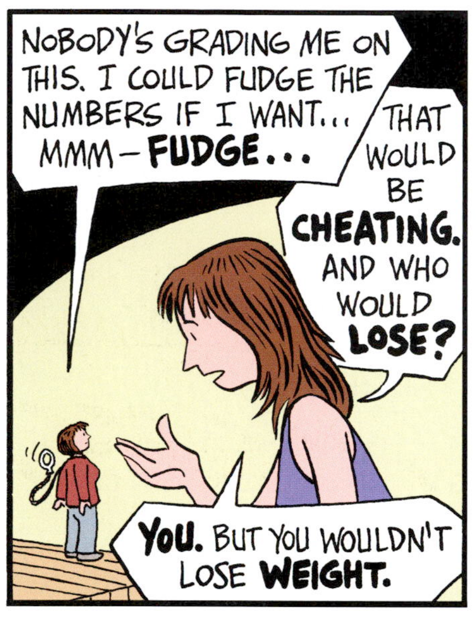
NOBODY'S GRADING ME ON THIS. I COULD FUDGE THE NUMBERS IF I WANT... MMM—**FUDGE...**
THAT WOULD BE **CHEATING.** AND WHO WOULD **LOSE?**
**YOU.** BUT YOU WOULDN'T LOSE **WEIGHT.**

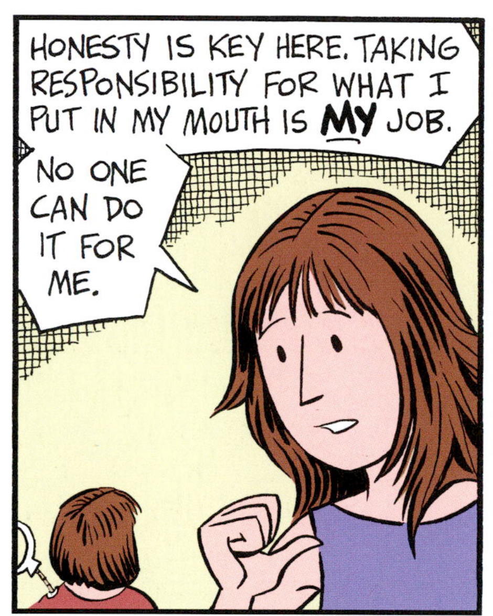
HONESTY IS KEY HERE. TAKING RESPONSIBILITY FOR WHAT I PUT IN MY MOUTH IS **MY** JOB.
NO ONE CAN DO IT FOR ME.

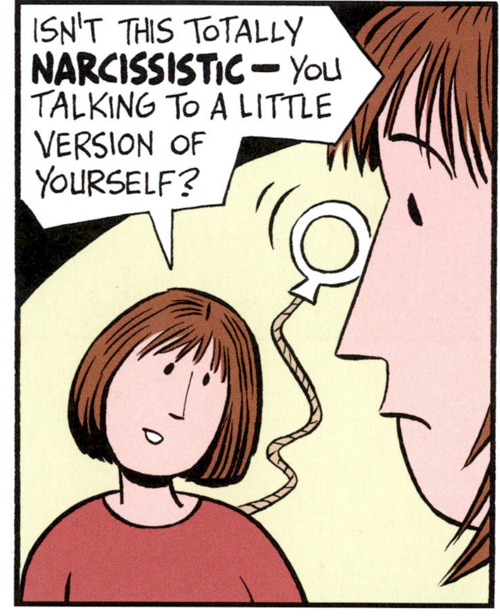
ISN'T THIS TOTALLY **NARCISSISTIC**—YOU TALKING TO A LITTLE VERSION OF YOURSELF?

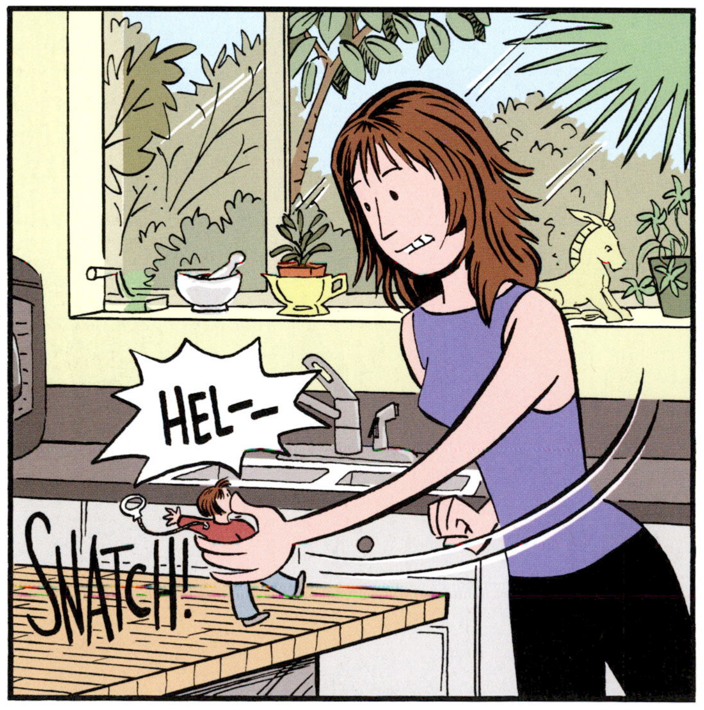
HEL-–
SNATCH!

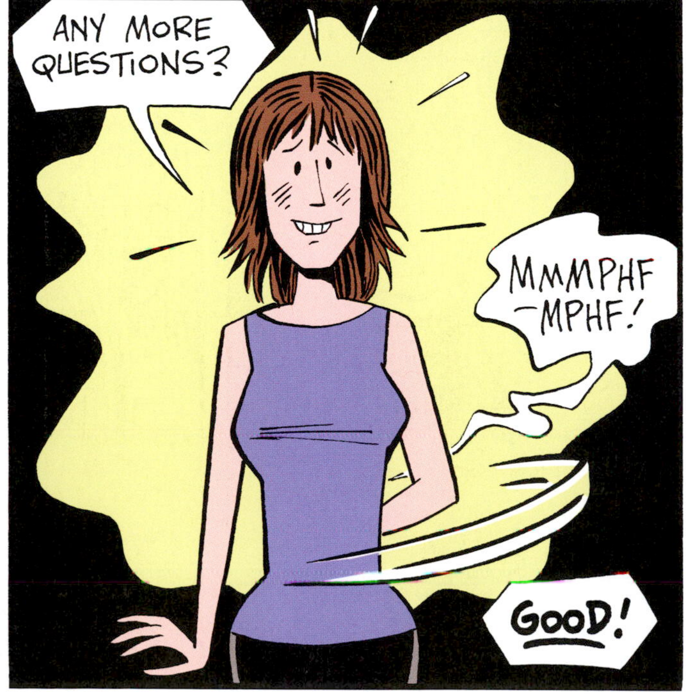
ANY MORE QUESTIONS?
MMMPHF —MPHF!
GOOD!

# Spray Oil Exposé!

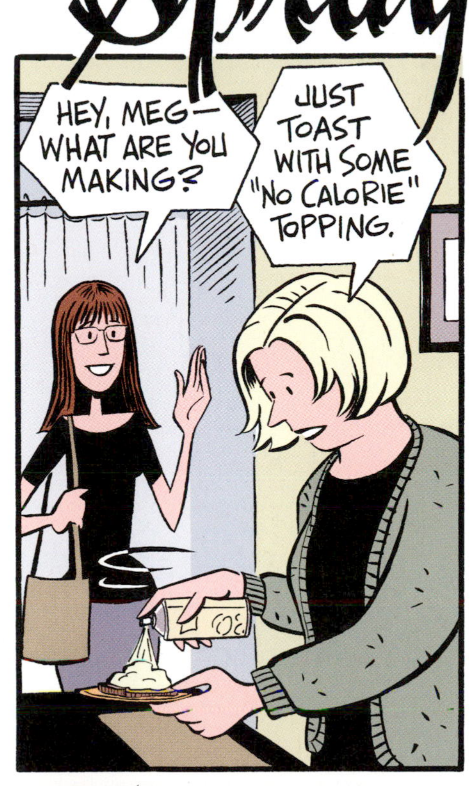
HEY, MEG— WHAT ARE YOU MAKING?
JUST TOAST WITH SOME "NO CALORIE" TOPPING.

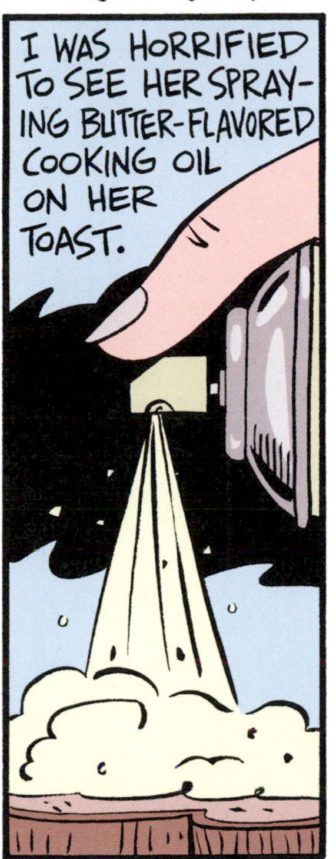
I WAS HORRIFIED TO SEE HER SPRAYING BUTTER-FLAVORED COOKING OIL ON HER TOAST.

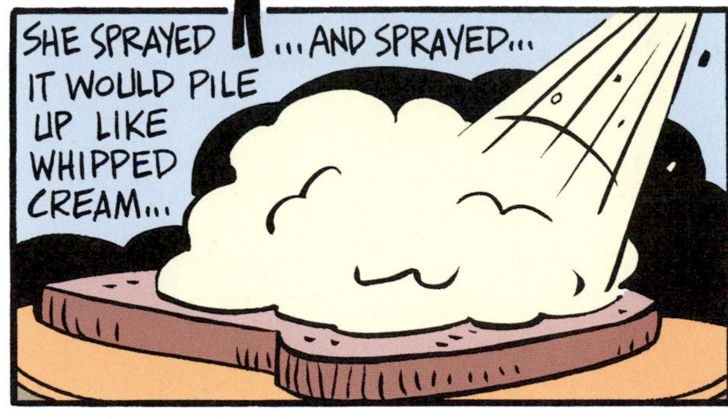
SHE SPRAYED
...AND SPRAYED...
IT WOULD PILE UP LIKE WHIPPED CREAM...

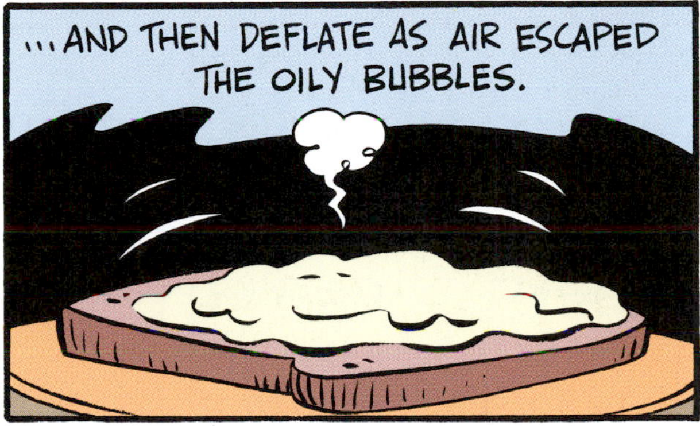
...AND THEN DEFLATE AS AIR ESCAPED THE OILY BUBBLES.

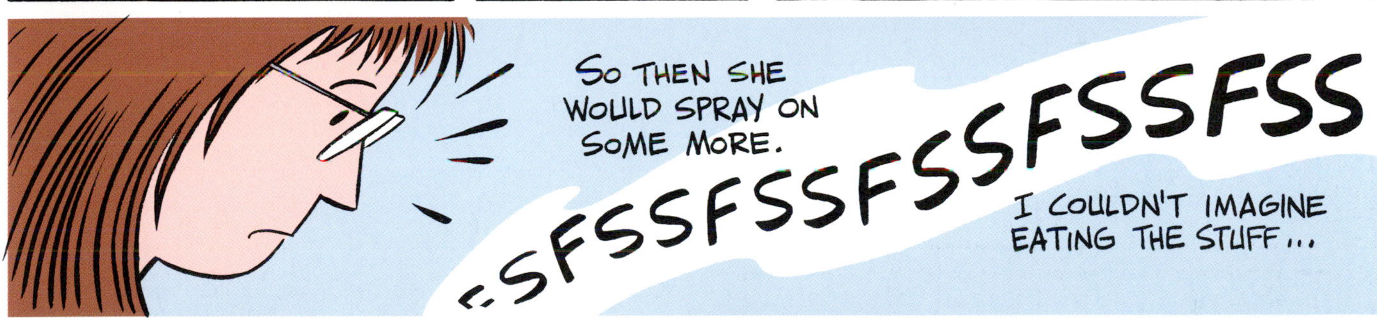
SO THEN SHE WOULD SPRAY ON SOME MORE.
FSSFSSFSSFSSFSSFSS
I COULDN'T IMAGINE EATING THE STUFF...

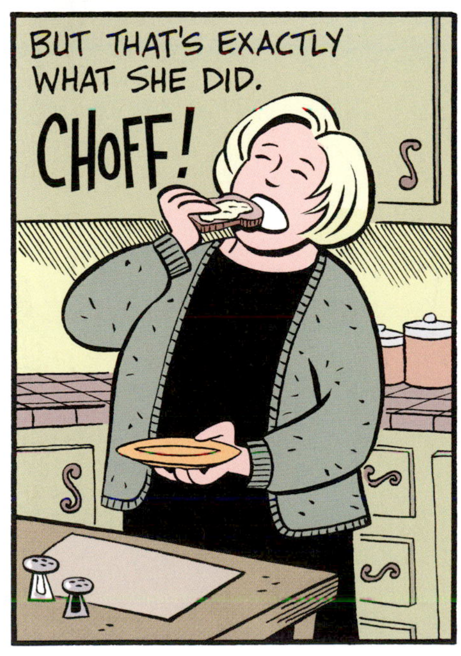
BUT THAT'S EXACTLY WHAT SHE DID.
CHOFF!

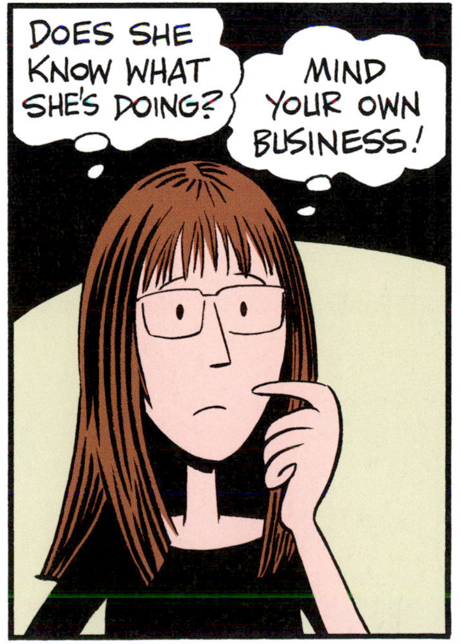
DOES SHE KNOW WHAT SHE'S DOING?
MIND YOUR OWN BUSINESS!

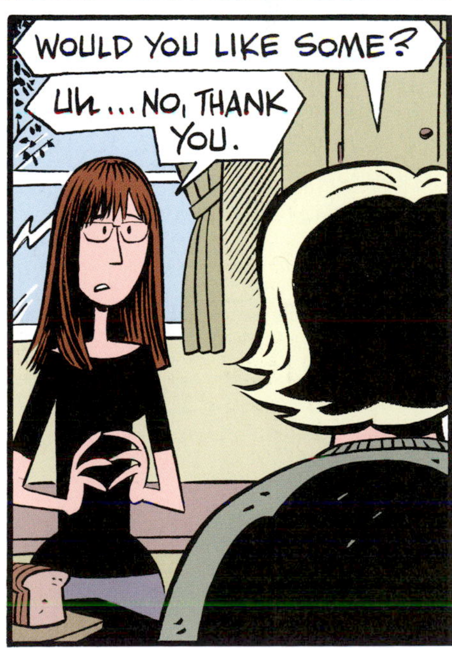
WOULD YOU LIKE SOME?
UH... NO, THANK YOU.

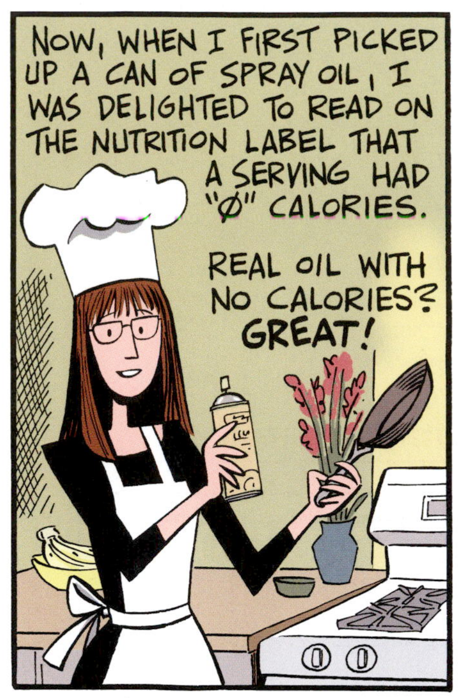
NOW, WHEN I FIRST PICKED UP A CAN OF SPRAY OIL, I WAS DELIGHTED TO READ ON THE NUTRITION LABEL THAT A SERVING HAD "Ø" CALORIES.
REAL OIL WITH NO CALORIES? GREAT!

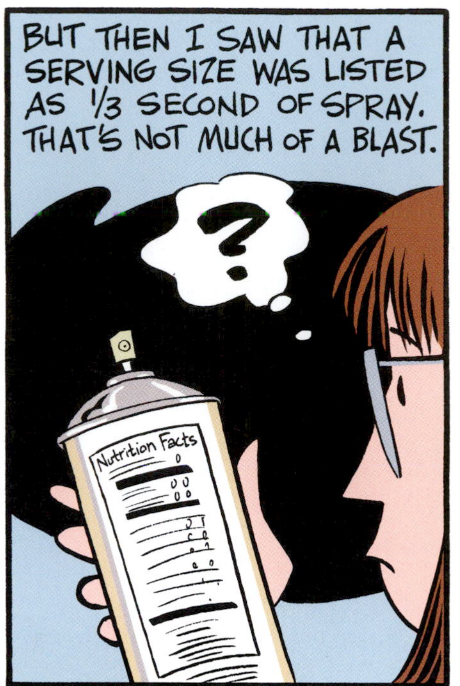
BUT THEN I SAW THAT A SERVING SIZE WAS LISTED AS 1/3 SECOND OF SPRAY. THAT'S NOT MUCH OF A BLAST.
?
Nutrition Facts

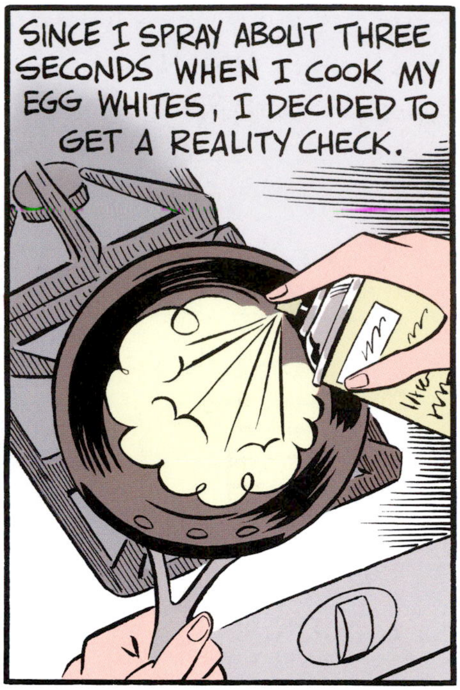
SINCE I SPRAY ABOUT THREE SECONDS WHEN I COOK MY EGG WHITES, I DECIDED TO GET A REALITY CHECK.

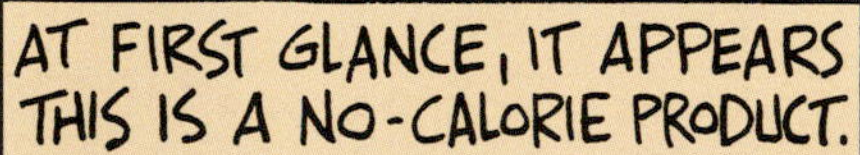


**Nutrition Facts**

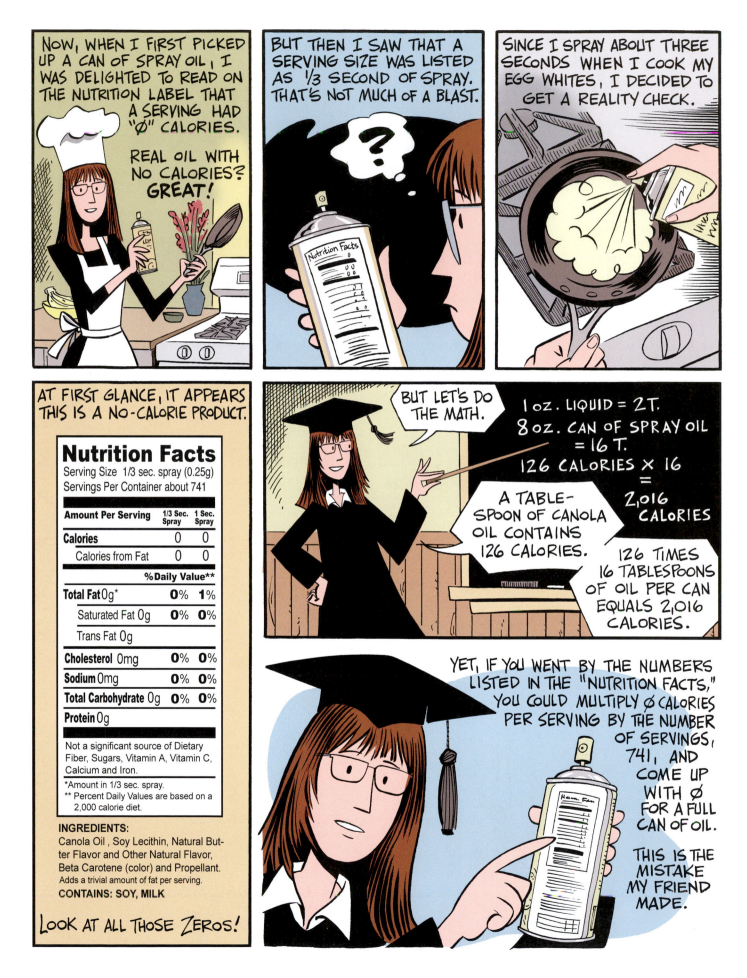

Serving Size 1/3 sec. spray (0.25g)
Servings Per Container about 741

| Amount Per Serving | 1/3 Sec. Spray | 1 Sec. Spray |
|---|---|---|
| **Calories** | 0 | 0 |
| Calories from Fat | 0 | 0 |
| | **%Daily Value**** | |
| **Total Fat** 0g* | **0**% | **1**% |
| Saturated Fat 0g | **0**% | **0**% |
| Trans Fat 0g | | |
| **Cholesterol** 0mg | **0**% | **0**% |
| **Sodium** 0mg | **0**% | **0**% |
| **Total Carbohydrate** 0g | **0**% | **0**% |
| **Protein** 0g | | |

Not a significant source of Dietary Fiber, Sugars, Vitamin A, Vitamin C, Calcium and Iron.

*Amount in 1/3 sec. spray.
** Percent Daily Values are based on a 2,000 calorie diet.

**INGREDIENTS:**
Canola Oil , Soy Lecithin, Natural Butter Flavor and Other Natural Flavor, Beta Carotene (color) and Propellant.
Adds a trivial amount of fat per serving.
**CONTAINS: SOY, MILK**

LOOK AT ALL THOSE ZEROS!

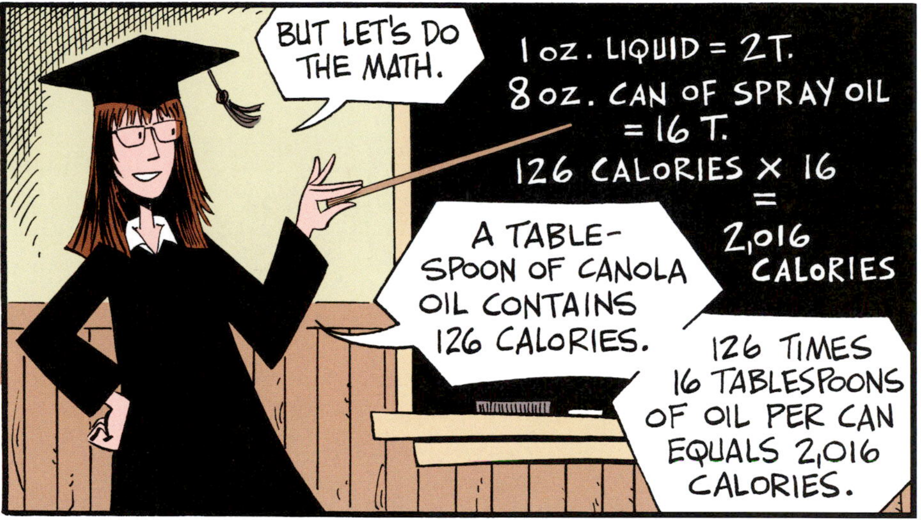
BUT LET'S DO THE MATH.
1 oz. LIQUID = 2T.
8 oz. CAN OF SPRAY OIL = 16 T.
126 CALORIES × 16 = 2,016 CALORIES
A TABLESPOON OF CANOLA OIL CONTAINS 126 CALORIES.
126 TIMES 16 TABLESPOONS OF OIL PER CAN EQUALS 2,016 CALORIES.

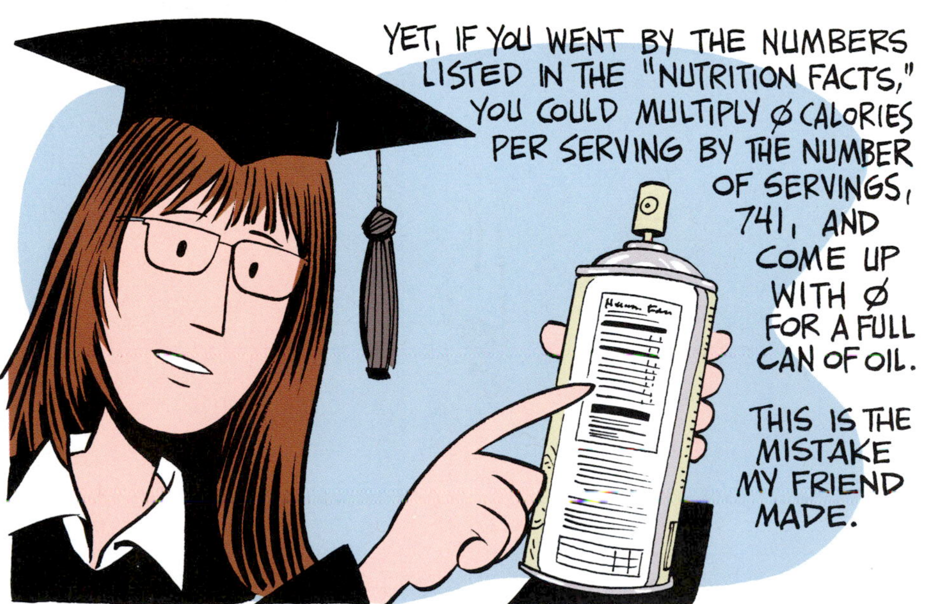
YET, IF YOU WENT BY THE NUMBERS LISTED IN THE "NUTRITION FACTS," YOU COULD MULTIPLY Ø CALORIES PER SERVING BY THE NUMBER OF SERVINGS, 741, AND COME UP WITH Ø FOR A FULL CAN OF OIL.
THIS IS THE MISTAKE MY FRIEND MADE.

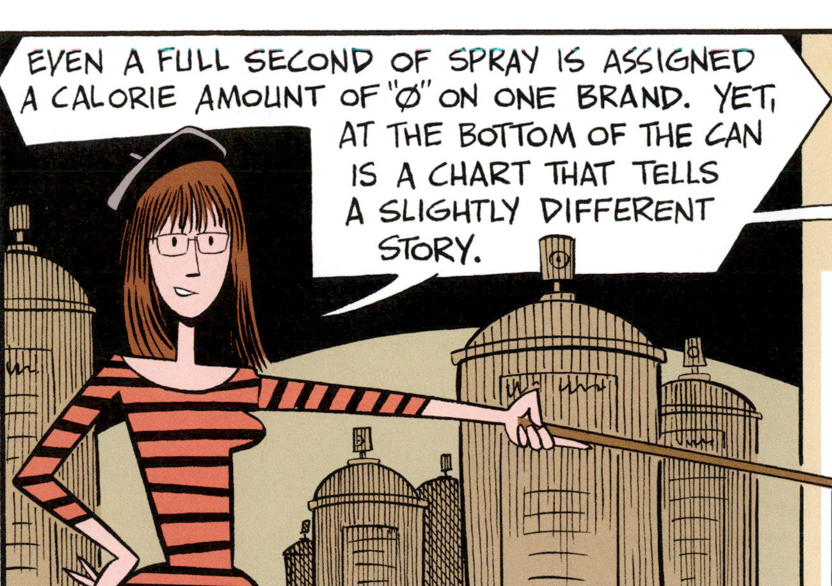


EVEN A FULL SECOND OF SPRAY IS ASSIGNED A CALORIE AMOUNT OF "Ø" ON ONE BRAND. YET, AT THE BOTTOM OF THE CAN IS A CHART THAT TELLS A SLIGHTLY DIFFERENT STORY.
NOTICE HOW THE AMOUNTS COMPARE: WHOLE TABLESPOONS OF BUTTER OR OIL VERSUS A TINY AMOUNT OF SPRAY OIL.

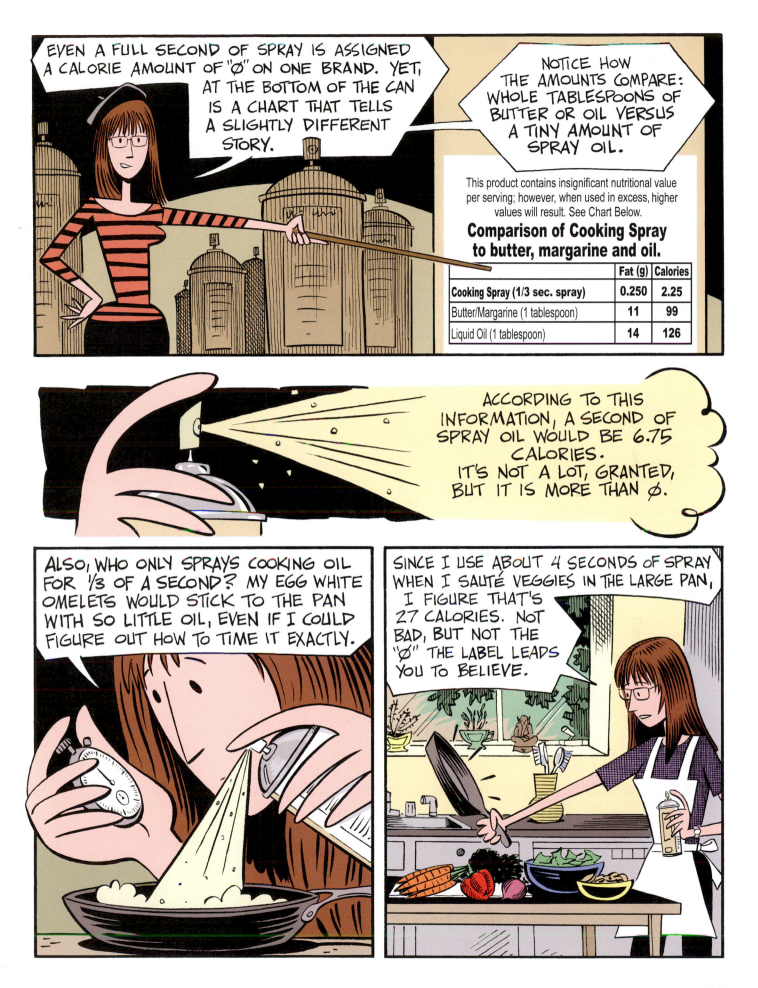

This product contains insignificant nutritional value per serving; however, when used in excess, higher values will result. See Chart Below.

**Comparison of Cooking Spray to butter, margarine and oil.**

| | Fat (g) | Calories |
|---|---|---|
| **Cooking Spray (1/3 sec. spray)** | **0.250** | **2.25** |
| Butter/Margarine (1 tablespoon) | **11** | **99** |
| Liquid Oil (1 tablespoon) | **14** | **126** |

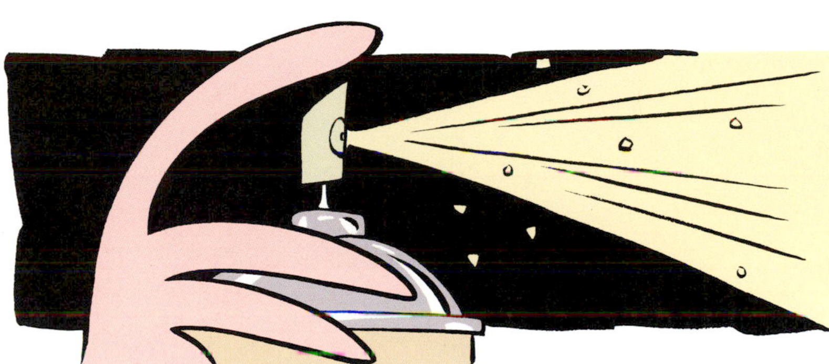

ACCORDING TO THIS INFORMATION, A SECOND OF SPRAY OIL WOULD BE 6.75 CALORIES. IT'S NOT A LOT, GRANTED, BUT IT IS MORE THAN Ø.

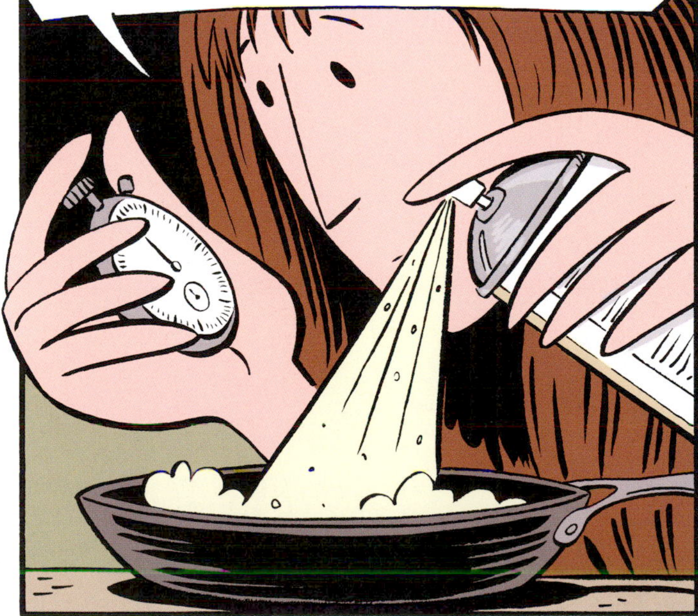

ALSO, WHO ONLY SPRAYS COOKING OIL FOR 1/3 OF A SECOND? MY EGG WHITE OMELETS WOULD STICK TO THE PAN WITH SO LITTLE OIL, EVEN IF I COULD FIGURE OUT HOW TO TIME IT EXACTLY.

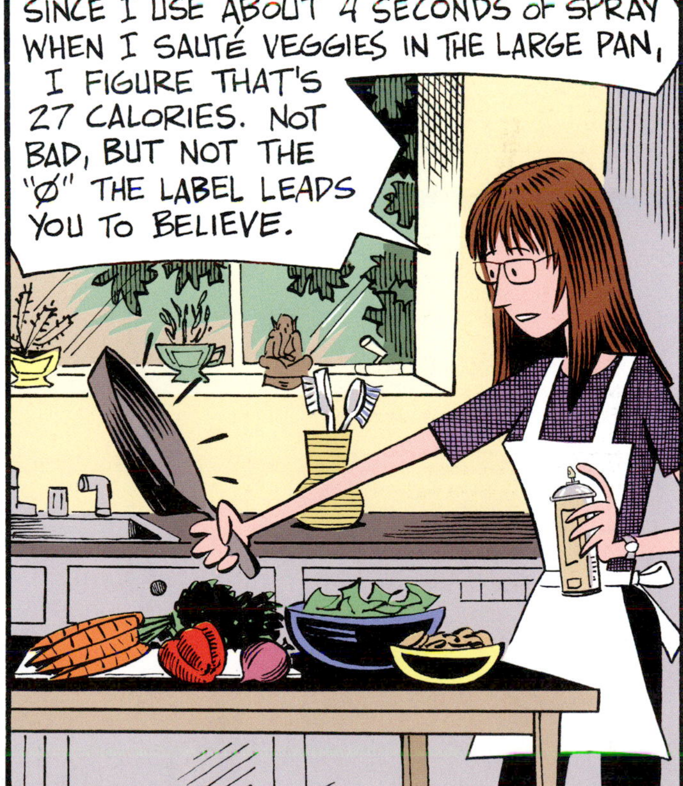

SINCE I USE ABOUT 4 SECONDS OF SPRAY WHEN I SAUTÉ VEGGIES IN THE LARGE PAN, I FIGURE THAT'S 27 CALORIES. NOT BAD, BUT NOT THE "Ø" THE LABEL LEADS YOU TO BELIEVE.

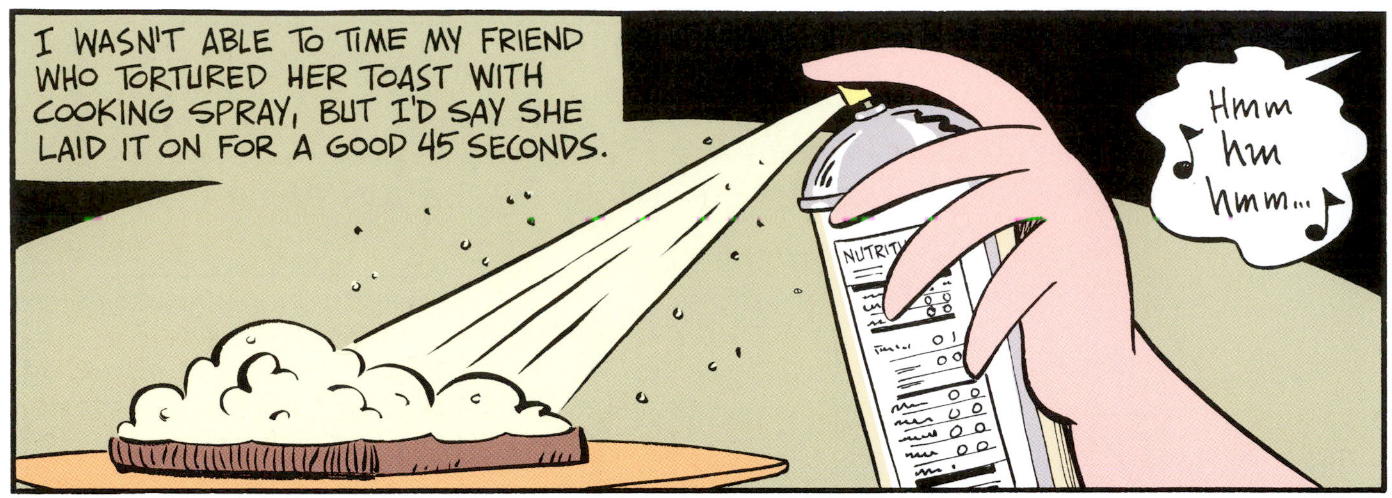
I WASN'T ABLE TO TIME MY FRIEND WHO TORTURED HER TOAST WITH COOKING SPRAY, BUT I'D SAY SHE LAID IT ON FOR A GOOD 45 SECONDS.
Hmm hm hmm...
NUTRITI

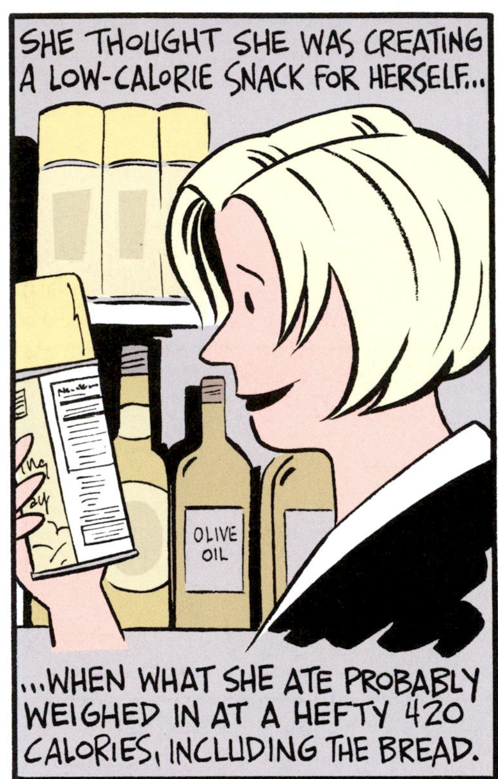
SHE THOUGHT SHE WAS CREATING A LOW-CALORIE SNACK FOR HERSELF...
OLIVE OIL
...WHEN WHAT SHE ATE PROBABLY WEIGHED IN AT A HEFTY 420 CALORIES, INCLUDING THE BREAD.

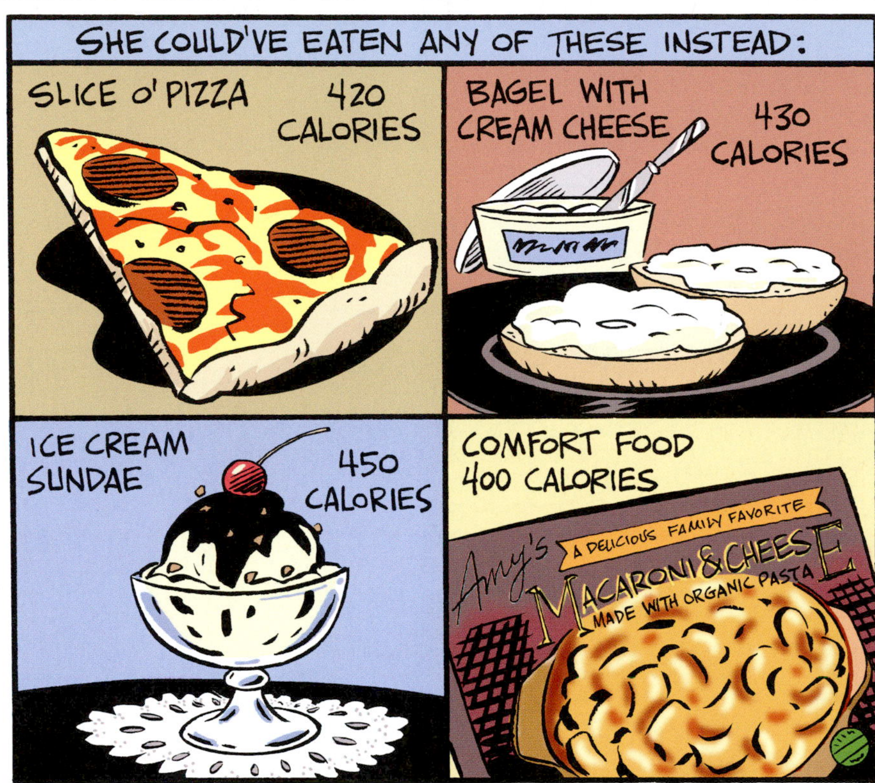
SHE COULD'VE EATEN ANY OF THESE INSTEAD:
SLICE O' PIZZA 420 CALORIES
BAGEL WITH CREAM CHEESE 430 CALORIES
ICE CREAM SUNDAE 450 CALORIES
COMFORT FOOD 400 CALORIES
A DELICIOUS FAMILY FAVORITE
Amy's
MACARONI & CHEESE
MADE WITH ORGANIC PASTA

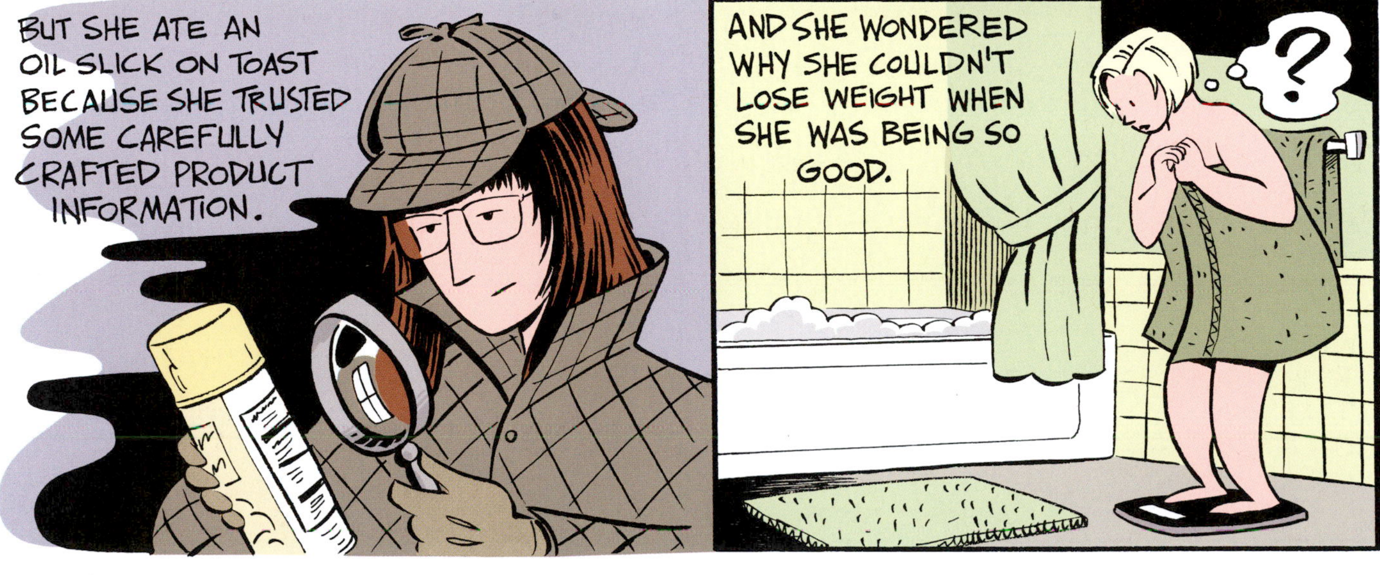
BUT SHE ATE AN OIL SLICK ON TOAST BECAUSE SHE TRUSTED SOME CAREFULLY CRAFTED PRODUCT INFORMATION.
AND SHE WONDERED WHY SHE COULDN'T LOSE WEIGHT WHEN SHE WAS BEING SO GOOD.
?

# MISSION: IMPROBABLE

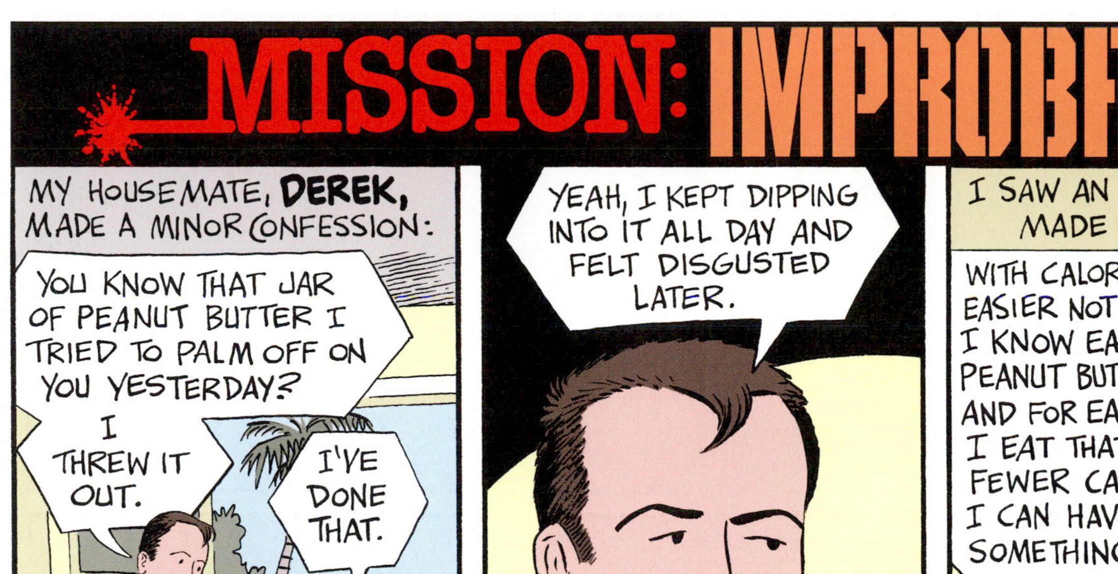

MY HOUSEMATE, **DEREK,** MADE A MINOR CONFESSION:
YOU KNOW THAT JAR OF PEANUT BUTTER I TRIED TO PALM OFF ON YOU YESTERDAY?
I THREW IT OUT.
I'VE DONE THAT.
YEAH, I KEPT DIPPING INTO IT ALL DAY AND FELT DISGUSTED LATER.


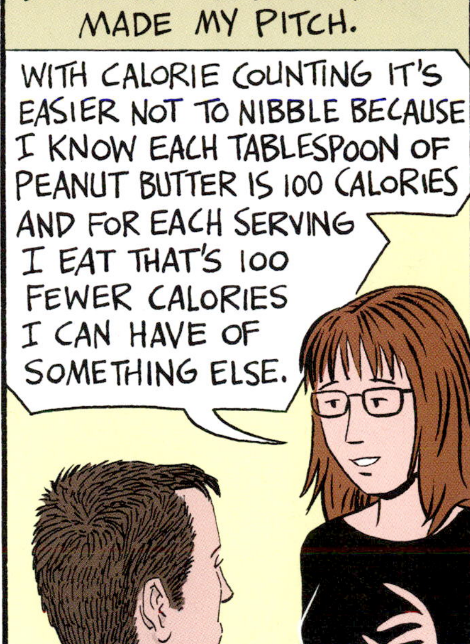

I SAW AN OPENING AND MADE MY PITCH.
WITH CALORIE COUNTING IT'S EASIER NOT TO NIBBLE BECAUSE I KNOW EACH TABLESPOON OF PEANUT BUTTER IS 100 CALORIES AND FOR EACH SERVING I EAT THAT'S 100 FEWER CALORIES I CAN HAVE OF SOMETHING ELSE.


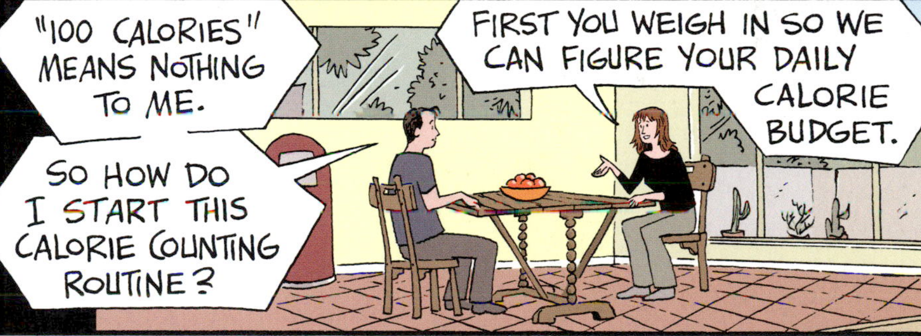

HE'D BEEN OBSERVING MY METHOD FOR A COUPLE OF YEARS BY THEN AND DIDN'T WANT TO GET INTO IT HIMSELF, BUT A HARD SLOG OF FILM EDITING HAD PUDGED HIM OUT.
"100 CALORIES" MEANS NOTHING TO ME.
SO HOW DO I START THIS CALORIE COUNTING ROUTINE?
FIRST YOU WEIGH IN SO WE CAN FIGURE YOUR DAILY CALORIE BUDGET.


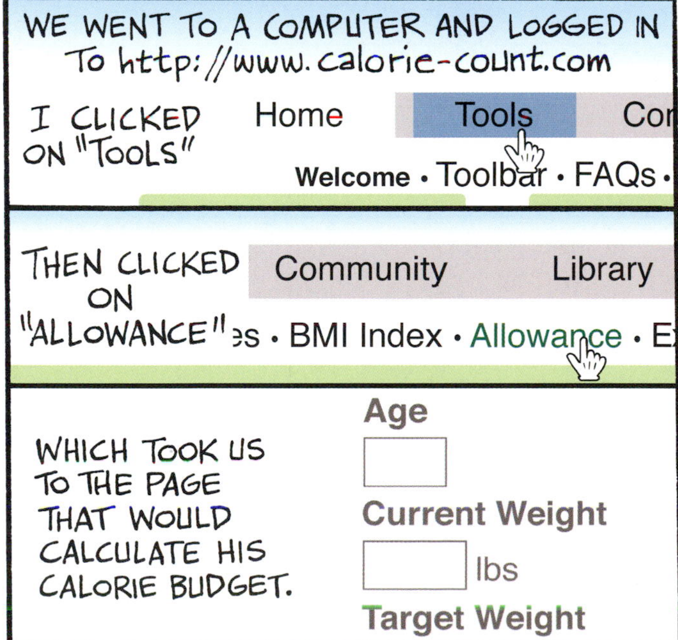

WE WENT TO A COMPUTER AND LOGGED IN TO http://www.calorie-count.com
I CLICKED ON "TOOLS"
Home
Tools
Co
Welcome • Toolbar • FAQs •
THEN CLICKED ON "ALLOWANCE"
Community
Library
es • BMI Index • Allowance • E
WHICH TOOK US TO THE PAGE THAT WOULD CALCULATE HIS CALORIE BUDGET.
Age
Current Weight
lbs
Target Weight


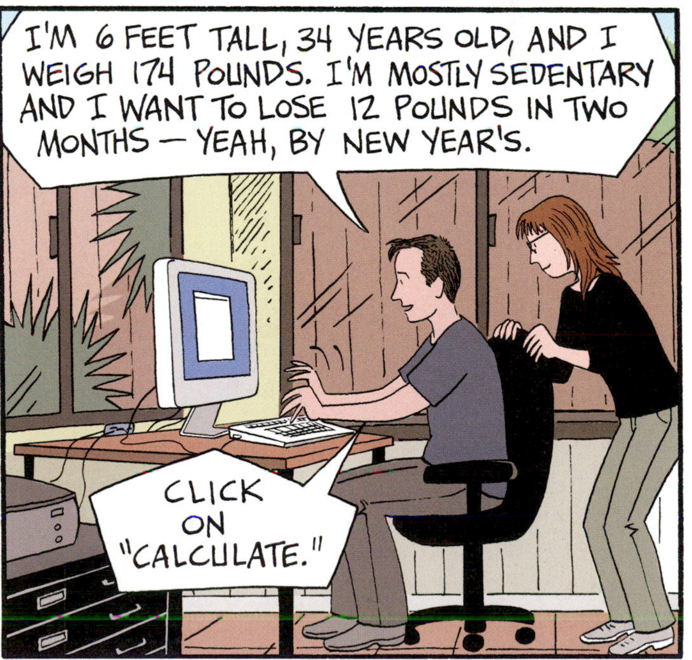

I'M 6 FEET TALL, 34 YEARS OLD, AND I WEIGH 174 POUNDS. I'M MOSTLY SEDENTARY AND I WANT TO LOSE 12 POUNDS IN TWO MONTHS — YEAH, BY NEW YEAR'S.
CLICK ON "CALCULATE."

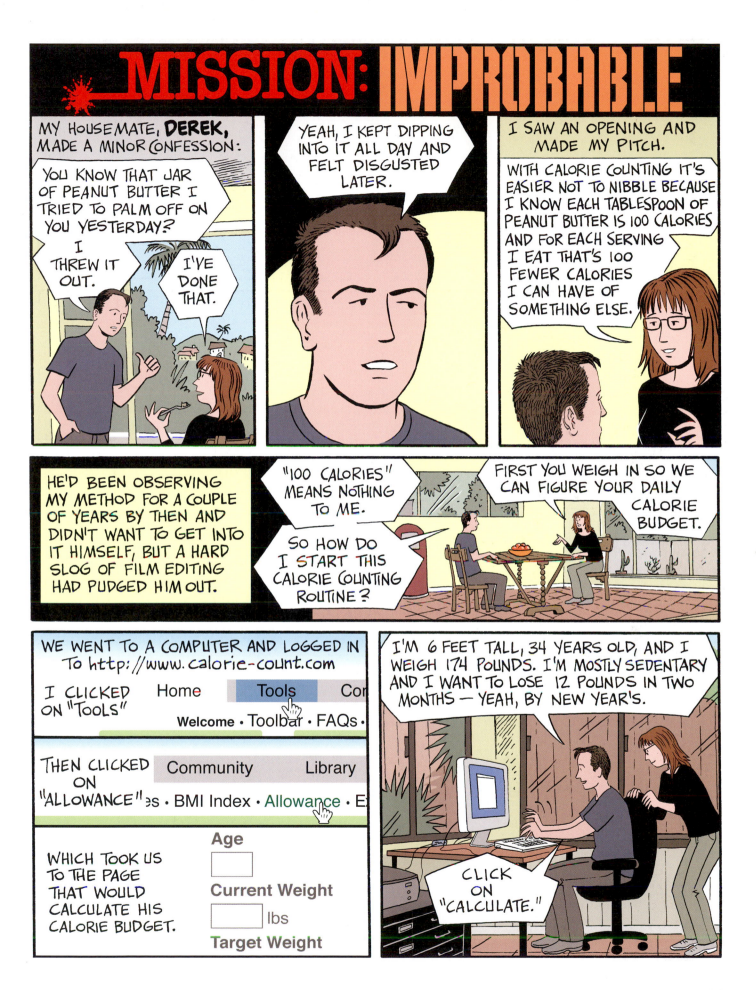

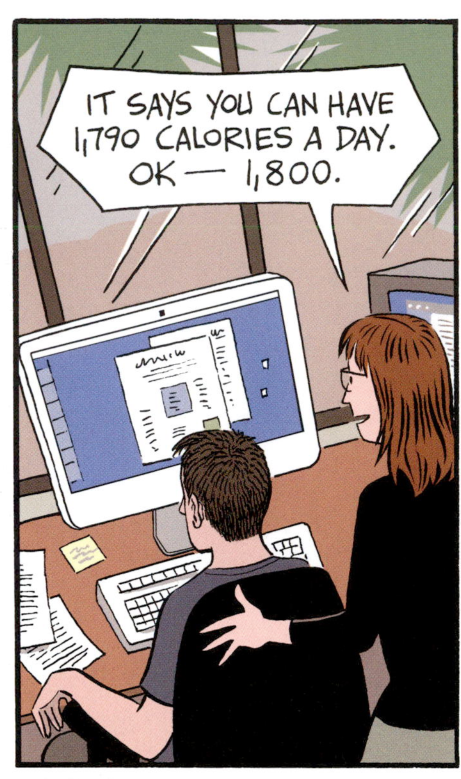
IT SAYS YOU CAN HAVE 1,790 CALORIES A DAY. OK — 1,800.

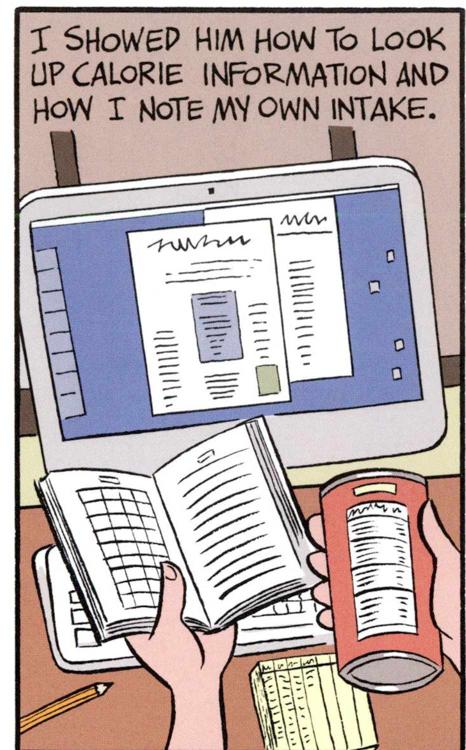
I SHOWED HIM HOW TO LOOK UP CALORIE INFORMATION AND HOW I NOTE MY OWN INTAKE.

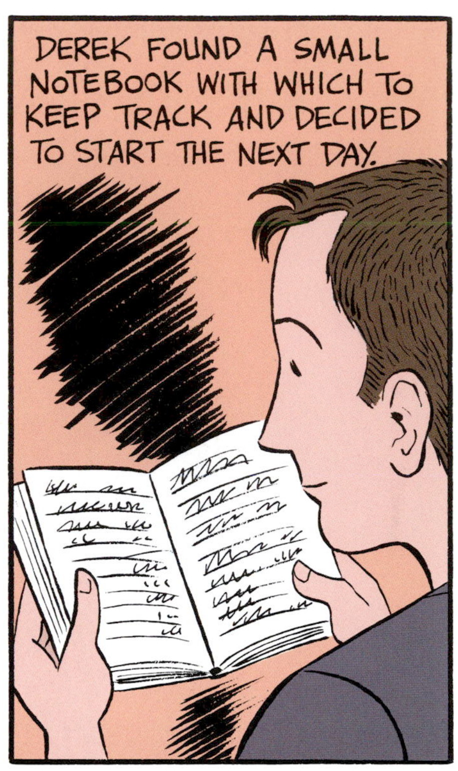
DEREK FOUND A SMALL NOTEBOOK WITH WHICH TO KEEP TRACK AND DECIDED TO START THE NEXT DAY.

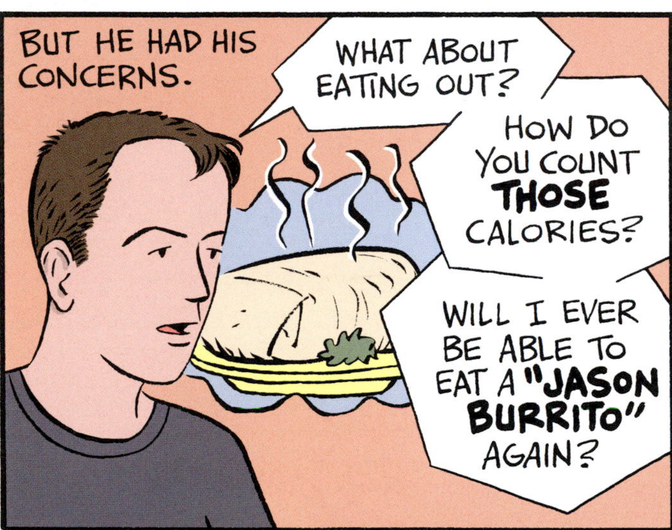
BUT HE HAD HIS CONCERNS.
WHAT ABOUT EATING OUT?
HOW DO YOU COUNT **THOSE** CALORIES?
WILL I EVER BE ABLE TO EAT A **"JASON BURRITO"** AGAIN?

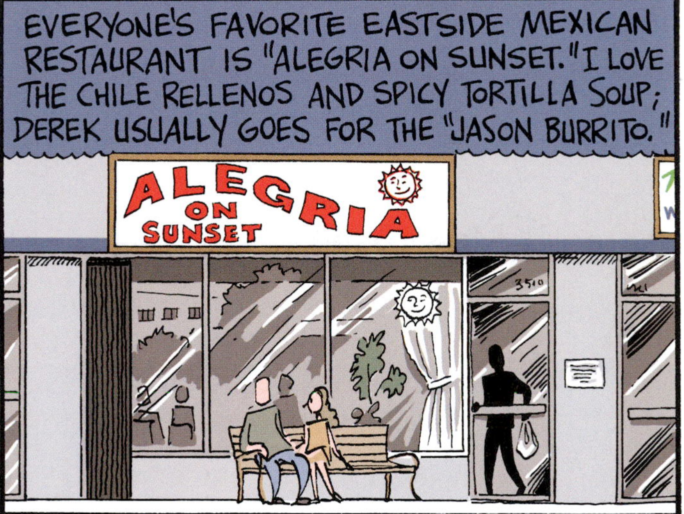
EVERYONE'S FAVORITE EASTSIDE MEXICAN RESTAURANT IS "ALEGRIA ON SUNSET." I LOVE THE CHILE RELLENOS AND SPICY TORTILLA SOUP; DEREK USUALLY GOES FOR THE "JASON BURRITO."
ALEGRIA ON SUNSET
3510

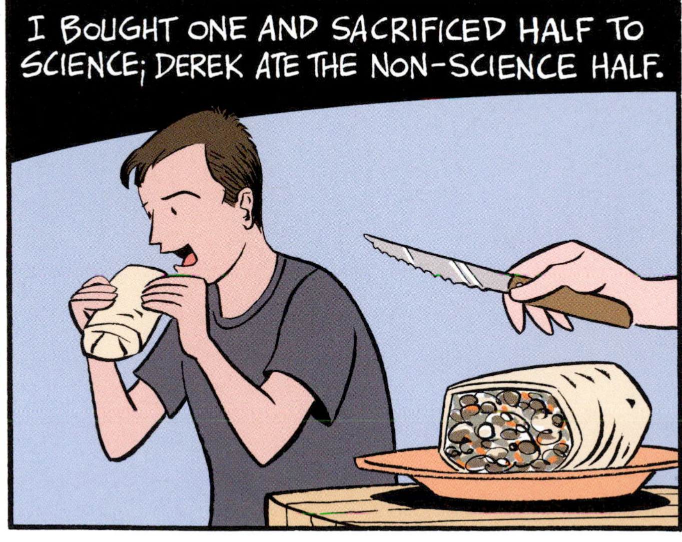
I BOUGHT ONE AND SACRIFICED HALF TO SCIENCE; DEREK ATE THE NON-SCIENCE HALF.

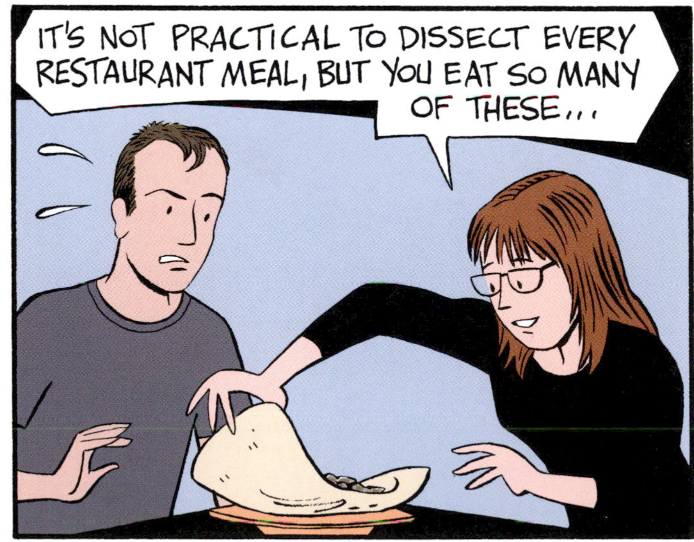
IT'S NOT PRACTICAL TO DISSECT EVERY RESTAURANT MEAL, BUT YOU EAT SO MANY OF THESE...

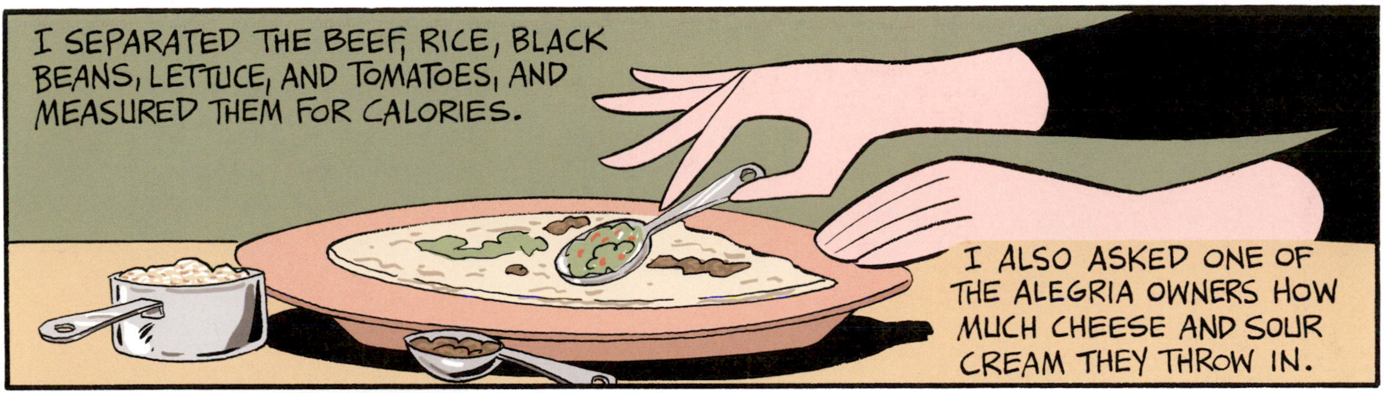
I SEPARATED THE BEEF, RICE, BLACK BEANS, LETTUCE, AND TOMATOES, AND MEASURED THEM FOR CALORIES.
I ALSO ASKED ONE OF THE ALEGRIA OWNERS HOW MUCH CHEESE AND SOUR CREAM THEY THROW IN.

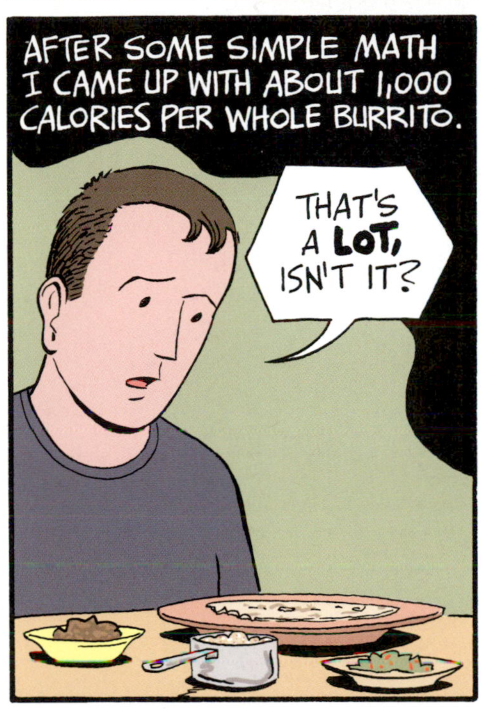
AFTER SOME SIMPLE MATH I CAME UP WITH ABOUT 1,000 CALORIES PER WHOLE BURRITO.
THAT'S A **LOT,** ISN'T IT?

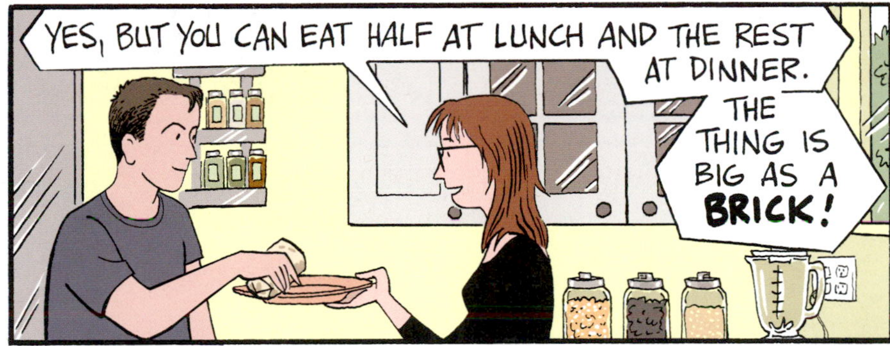
YES, BUT YOU CAN EAT HALF AT LUNCH AND THE REST AT DINNER.
THE THING IS BIG AS A **BRICK!**

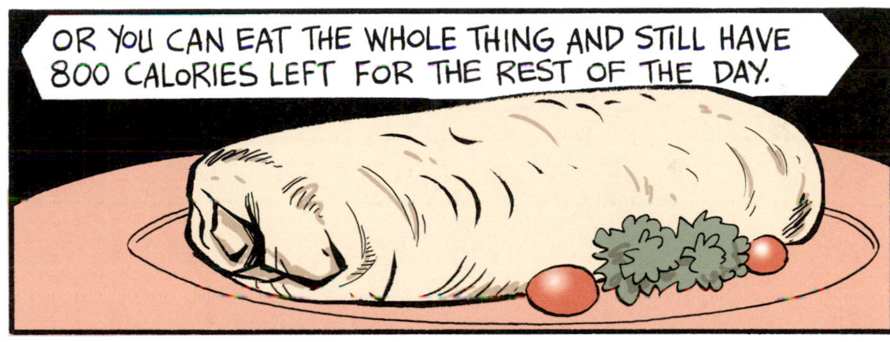
OR YOU CAN EAT THE WHOLE THING AND STILL HAVE 800 CALORIES LEFT FOR THE REST OF THE DAY.

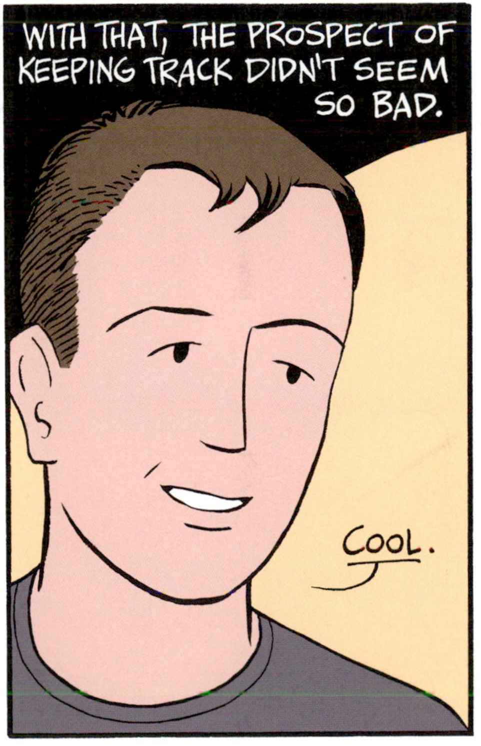
WITH THAT, THE PROSPECT OF KEEPING TRACK DIDN'T SEEM SO BAD.
COOL.

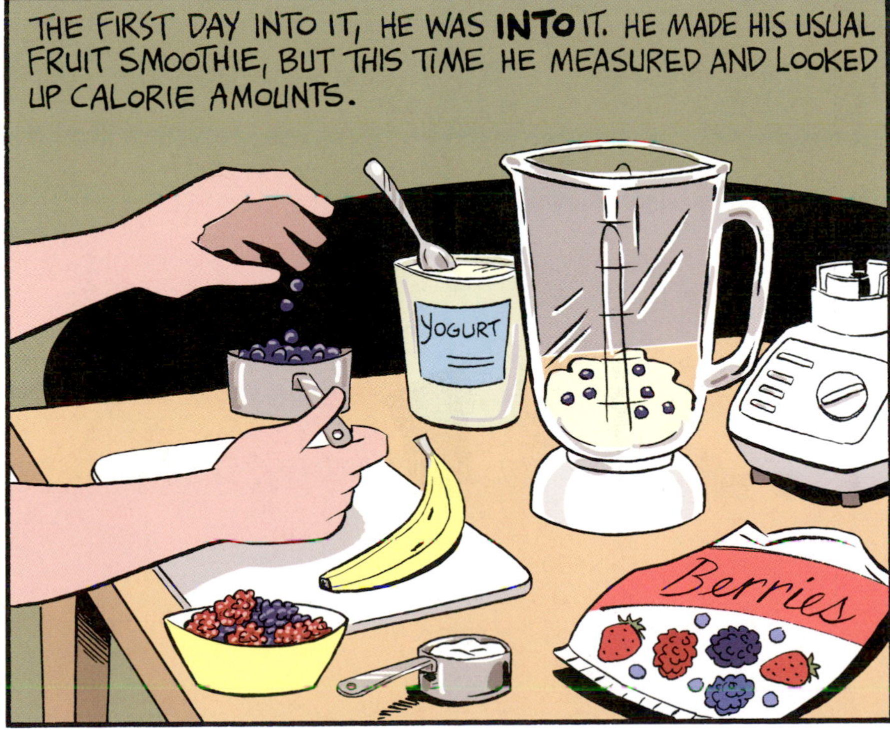
THE FIRST DAY INTO IT, HE WAS **INTO** IT. HE MADE HIS USUAL FRUIT SMOOTHIE, BUT THIS TIME HE MEASURED AND LOOKED UP CALORIE AMOUNTS.
YOGURT
Berries

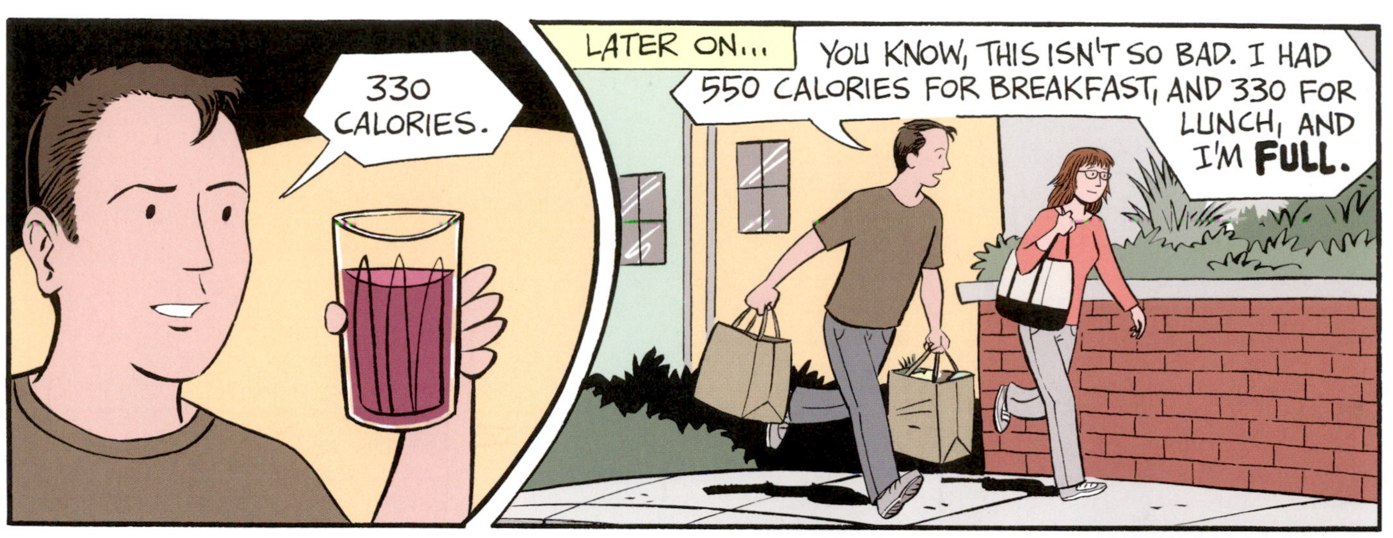
330 CALORIES.
LATER ON...
YOU KNOW, THIS ISN'T SO BAD. I HAD 550 CALORIES FOR BREAKFAST, AND 330 FOR LUNCH, AND I'M **FULL**.

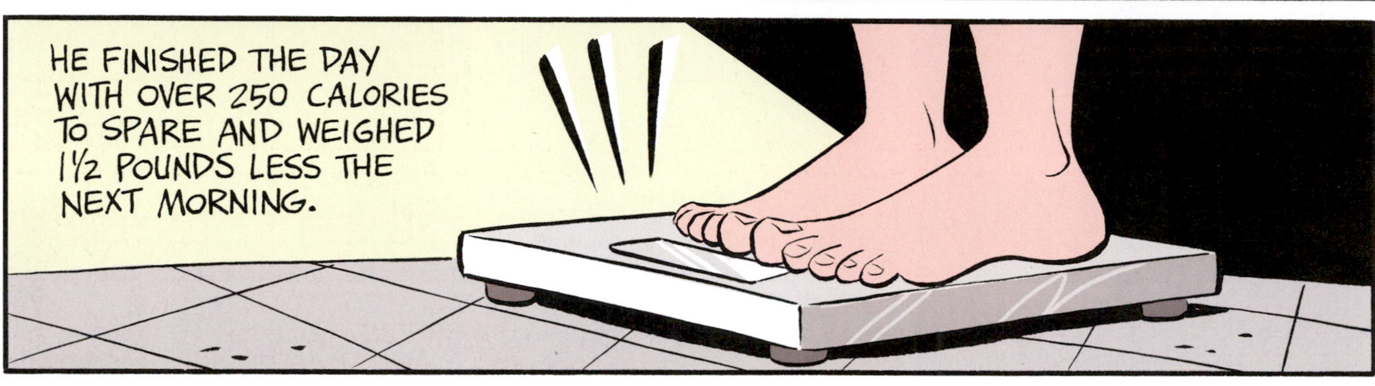
HE FINISHED THE DAY WITH OVER 250 CALORIES TO SPARE AND WEIGHED 1½ POUNDS LESS THE NEXT MORNING.

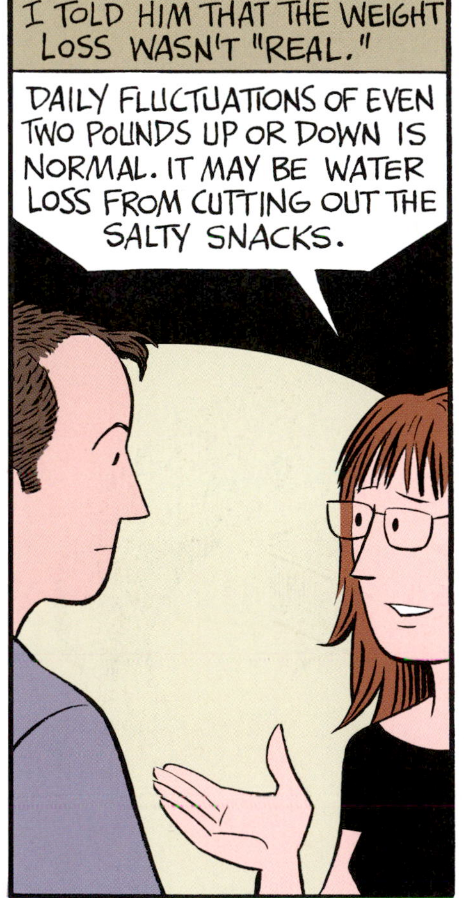
I TOLD HIM THAT THE WEIGHT LOSS WASN'T "REAL."
DAILY FLUCTUATIONS OF EVEN TWO POUNDS UP OR DOWN IS NORMAL. IT MAY BE WATER LOSS FROM CUTTING OUT THE SALTY SNACKS.

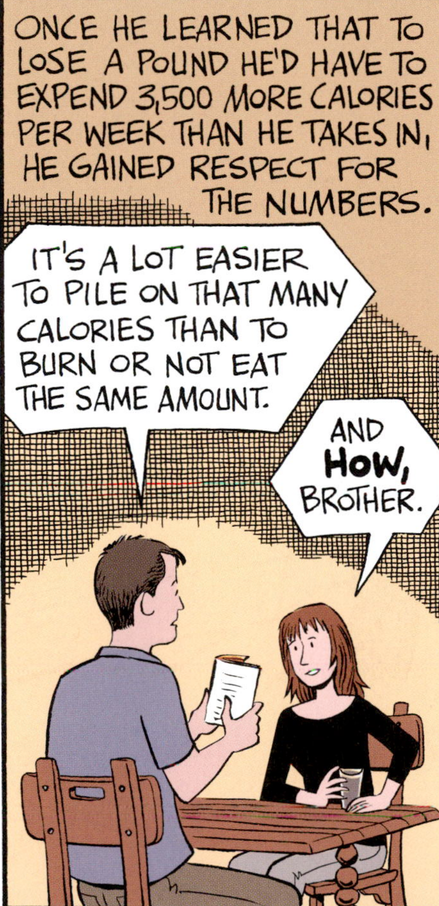
ONCE HE LEARNED THAT TO LOSE A POUND HE'D HAVE TO EXPEND 3,500 MORE CALORIES PER WEEK THAN HE TAKES IN, HE GAINED RESPECT FOR THE NUMBERS.
IT'S A LOT EASIER TO PILE ON THAT MANY CALORIES THAN TO BURN OR NOT EAT THE SAME AMOUNT.
AND **HOW**, BROTHER.

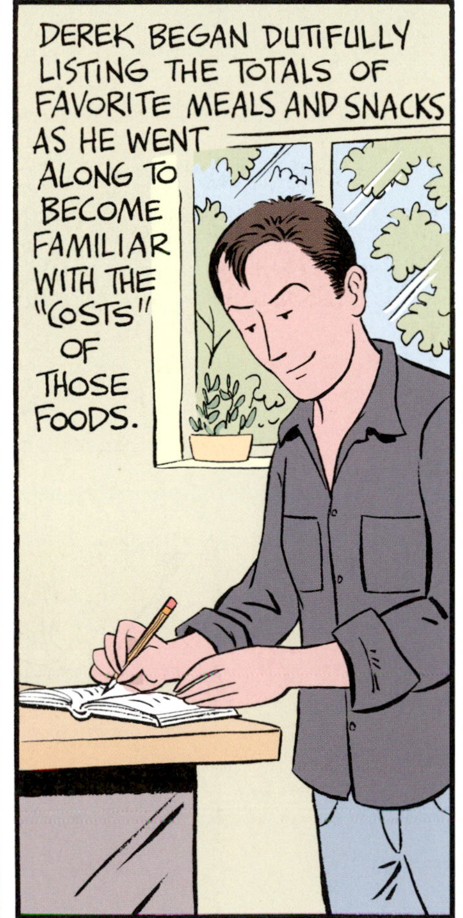
DEREK BEGAN DUTIFULLY LISTING THE TOTALS OF FAVORITE MEALS AND SNACKS AS HE WENT ALONG TO BECOME FAMILIAR WITH THE "COSTS" OF THOSE FOODS.

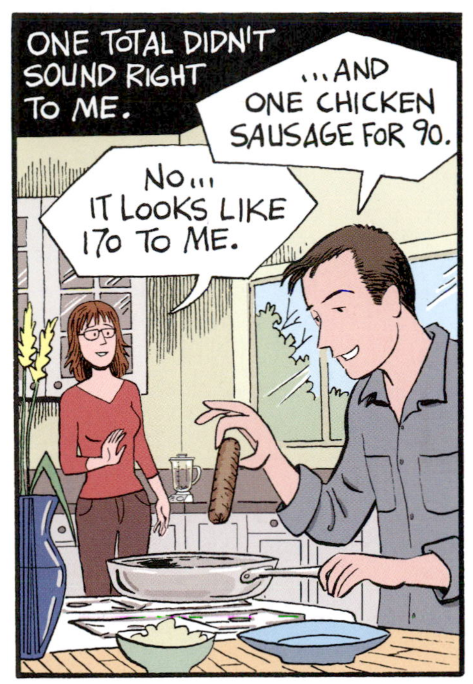
ONE TOTAL DIDN'T SOUND RIGHT TO ME.
...AND ONE CHICKEN SAUSAGE FOR 90.
NO... IT LOOKS LIKE 170 TO ME.

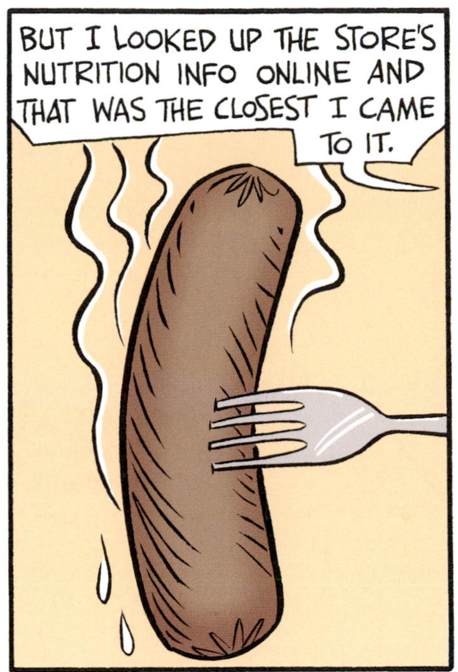
BUT I LOOKED UP THE STORE'S NUTRITION INFO ONLINE AND THAT WAS THE CLOSEST I CAME TO IT.

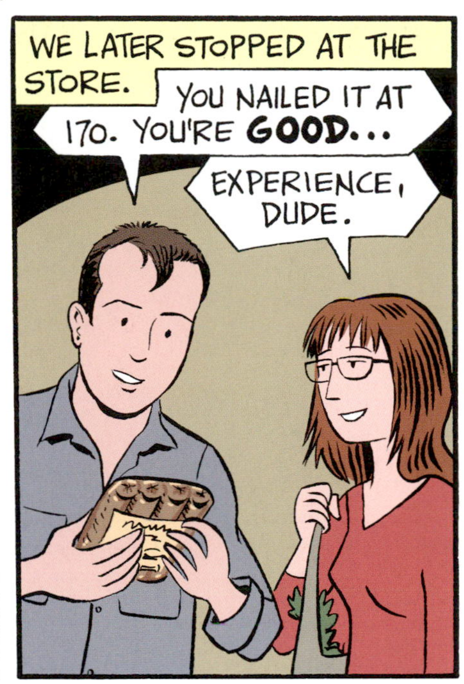
WE LATER STOPPED AT THE STORE.
YOU NAILED IT AT 170. YOU'RE **GOOD...**
EXPERIENCE, DUDE.

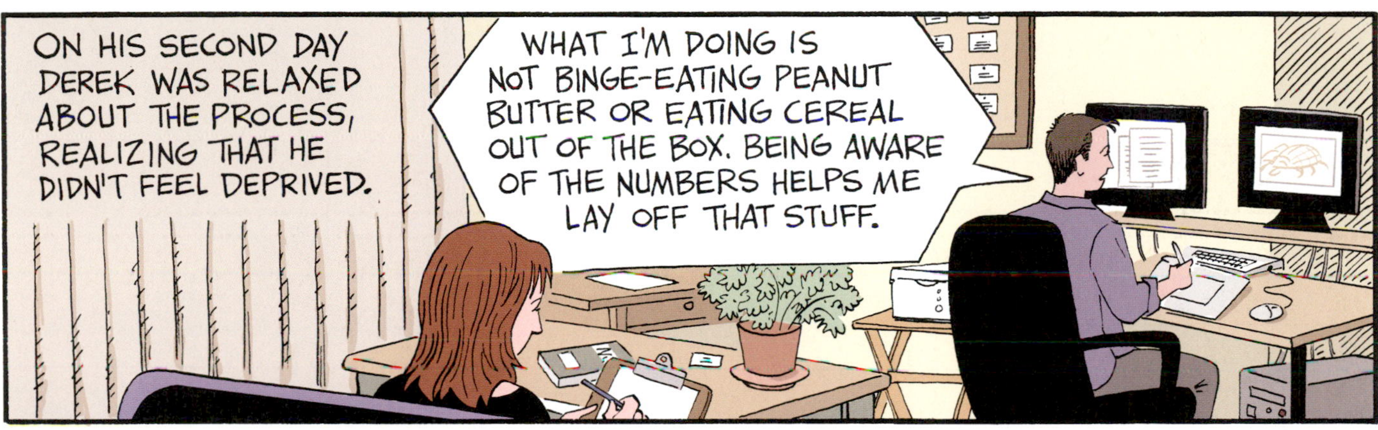
ON HIS SECOND DAY DEREK WAS RELAXED ABOUT THE PROCESS, REALIZING THAT HE DIDN'T FEEL DEPRIVED.
WHAT I'M DOING IS NOT BINGE-EATING PEANUT BUTTER OR EATING CEREAL OUT OF THE BOX. BEING AWARE OF THE NUMBERS HELPS ME LAY OFF THAT STUFF.

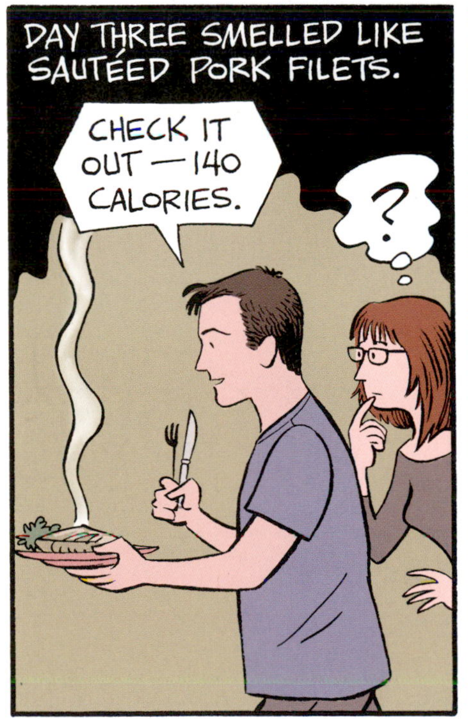
DAY THREE SMELLED LIKE SAUTÉED PORK FILETS.
CHECK IT OUT — 140 CALORIES.
?

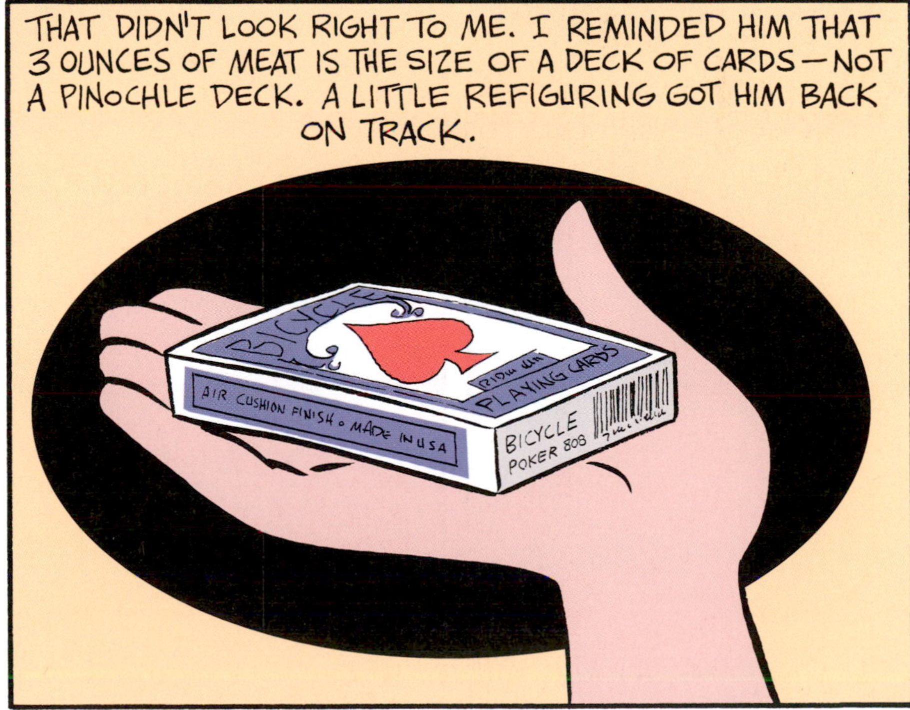
THAT DIDN'T LOOK RIGHT TO ME. I REMINDED HIM THAT 3 OUNCES OF MEAT IS THE SIZE OF A DECK OF CARDS — NOT A PINOCHLE DECK. A LITTLE REFIGURING GOT HIM BACK ON TRACK.
BICYCLE
PLAYING CARDS
AIR CUSHION FINISH • MADE IN USA
BICYCLE
POKER 808

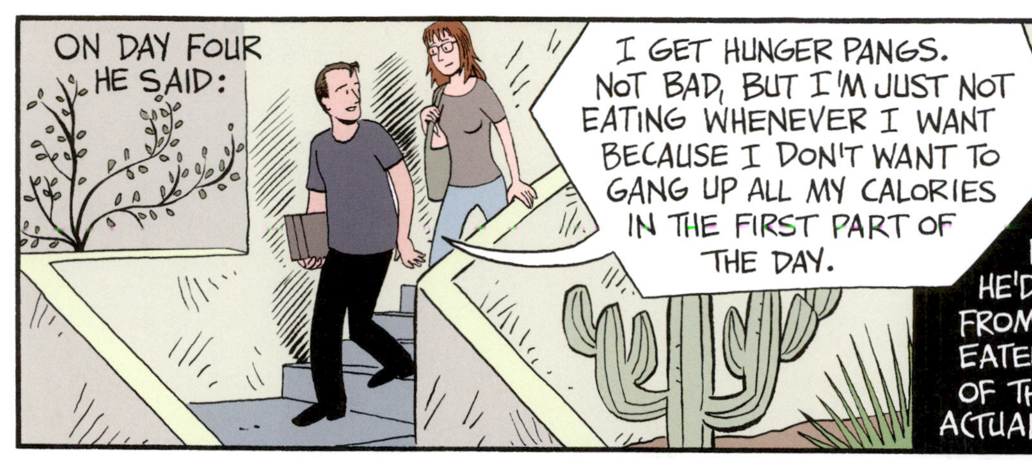
ON DAY FOUR HE SAID:
I GET HUNGER PANGS. NOT BAD, BUT I'M JUST NOT EATING WHENEVER I WANT BECAUSE I DON'T WANT TO GANG UP ALL MY CALORIES IN THE FIRST PART OF THE DAY.

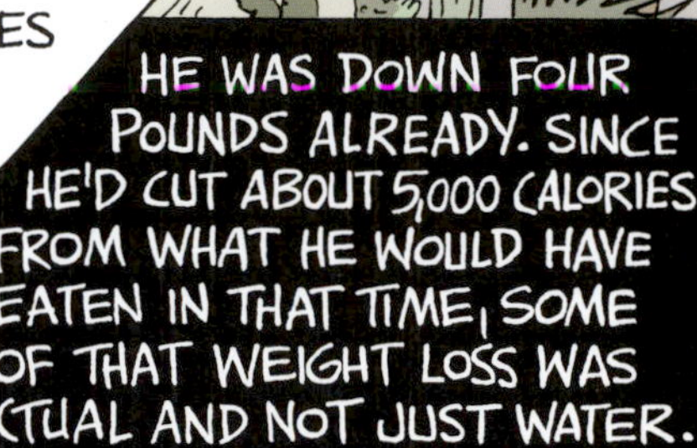
HE WAS DOWN FOUR POUNDS ALREADY. SINCE HE'D CUT ABOUT 5,000 CALORIES FROM WHAT HE WOULD HAVE EATEN IN THAT TIME, SOME OF THAT WEIGHT LOSS WAS ACTUAL AND NOT JUST WATER.

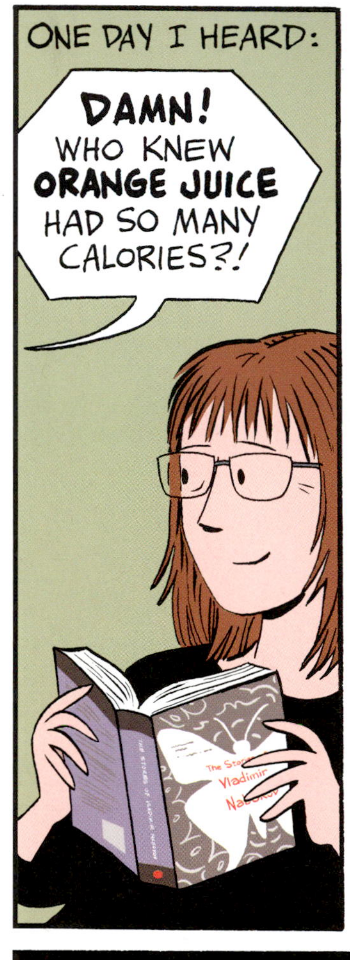
ONE DAY I HEARD:
DAMN! WHO KNEW ORANGE JUICE HAD SO MANY CALORIES?!

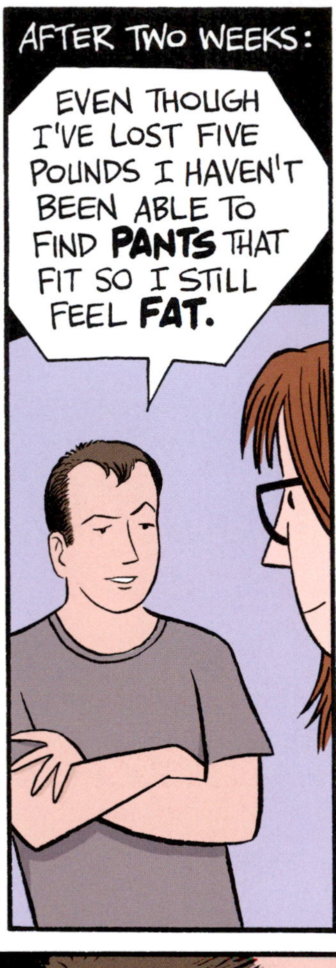
AFTER TWO WEEKS:
EVEN THOUGH I'VE LOST FIVE POUNDS I HAVEN'T BEEN ABLE TO FIND PANTS THAT FIT SO I STILL FEEL FAT.

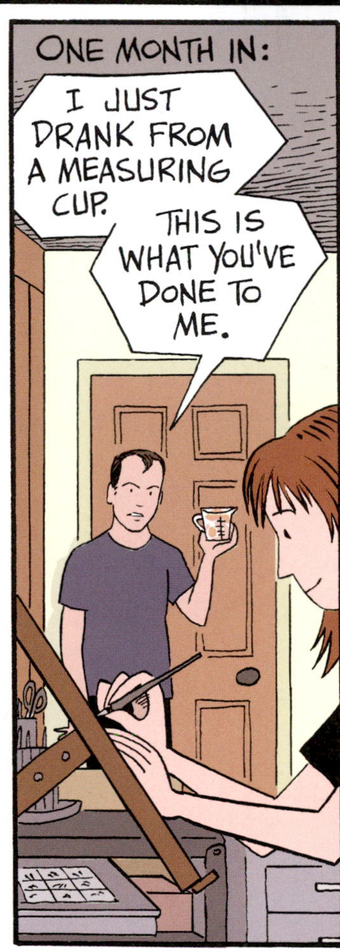
ONE MONTH IN:
I JUST DRANK FROM A MEASURING CUP.
THIS IS WHAT YOU'VE DONE TO ME.

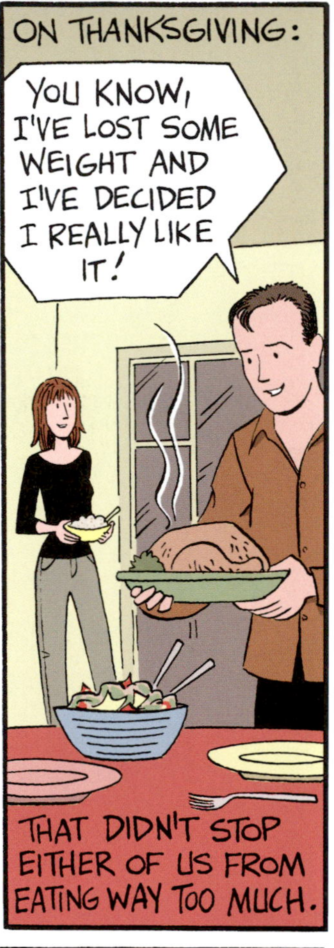
ON THANKSGIVING:
YOU KNOW, I'VE LOST SOME WEIGHT AND I'VE DECIDED I REALLY LIKE IT!
THAT DIDN'T STOP EITHER OF US FROM EATING WAY TOO MUCH.

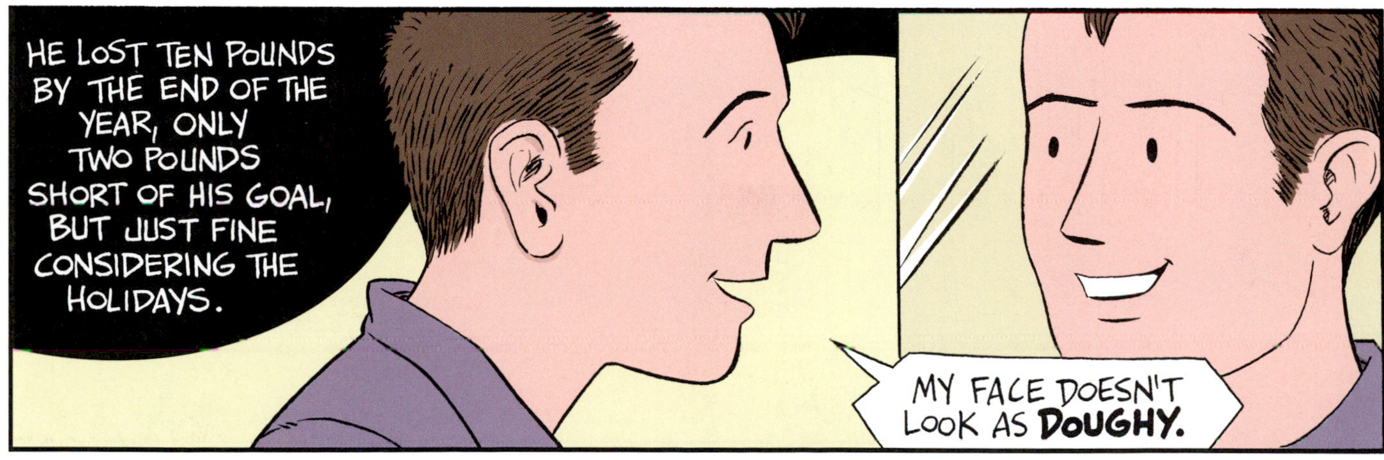
HE LOST TEN POUNDS BY THE END OF THE YEAR, ONLY TWO POUNDS SHORT OF HIS GOAL, BUT JUST FINE CONSIDERING THE HOLIDAYS.
MY FACE DOESN'T LOOK AS DOUGHY.

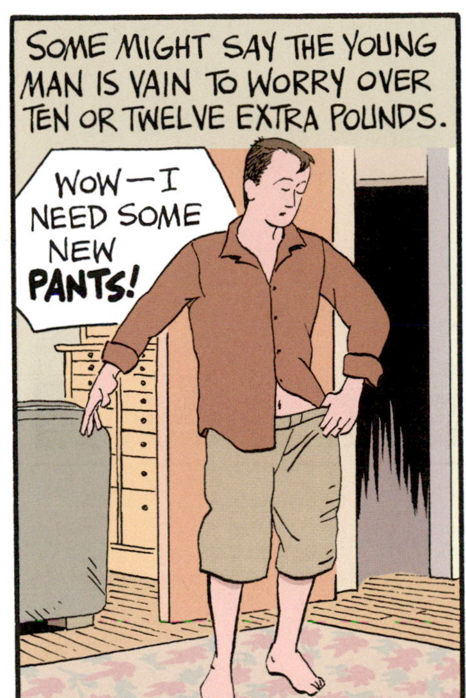
SOME MIGHT SAY THE YOUNG MAN IS VAIN TO WORRY OVER TEN OR TWELVE EXTRA POUNDS.
WOW—I NEED SOME NEW **PANTS!**

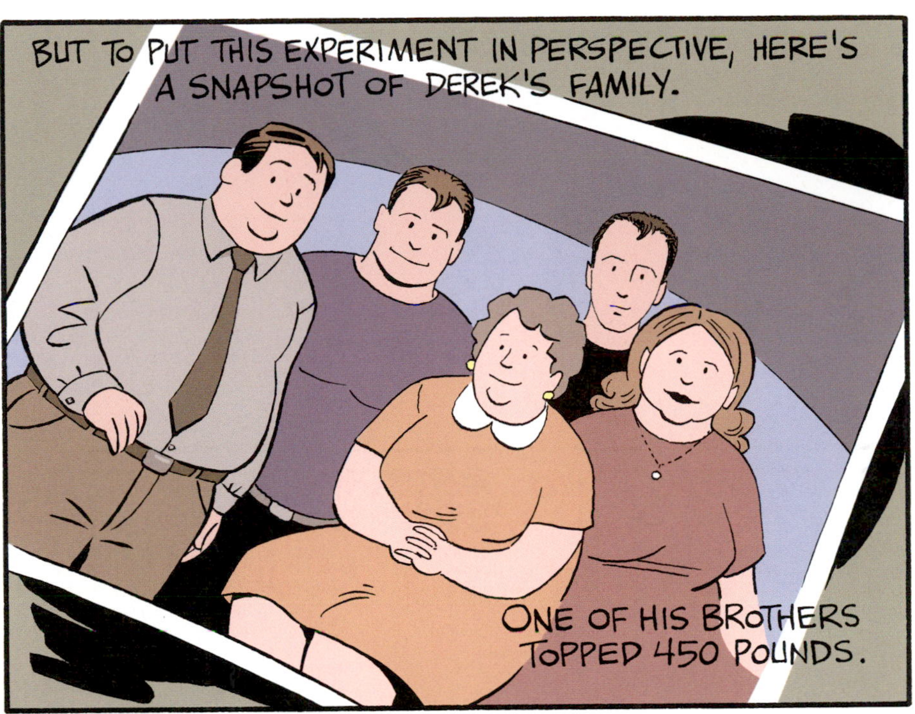
BUT TO PUT THIS EXPERIMENT IN PERSPECTIVE, HERE'S A SNAPSHOT OF DEREK'S FAMILY.
ONE OF HIS BROTHERS TOPPED 450 POUNDS.

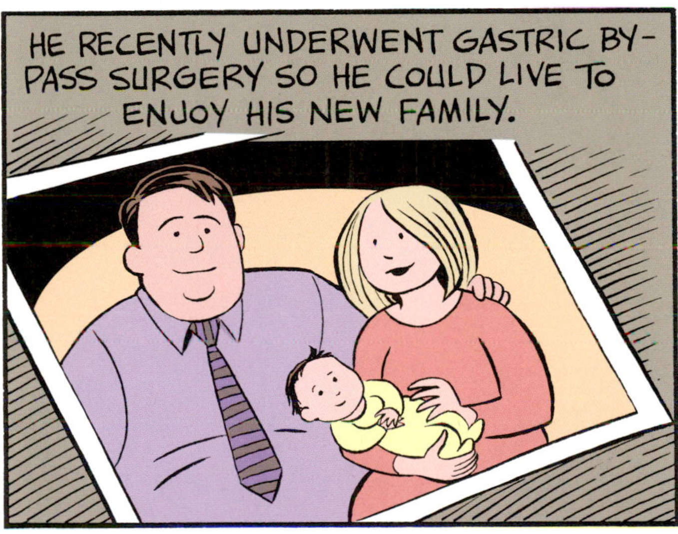
HE RECENTLY UNDERWENT GASTRIC BY-PASS SURGERY SO HE COULD LIVE TO ENJOY HIS NEW FAMILY.

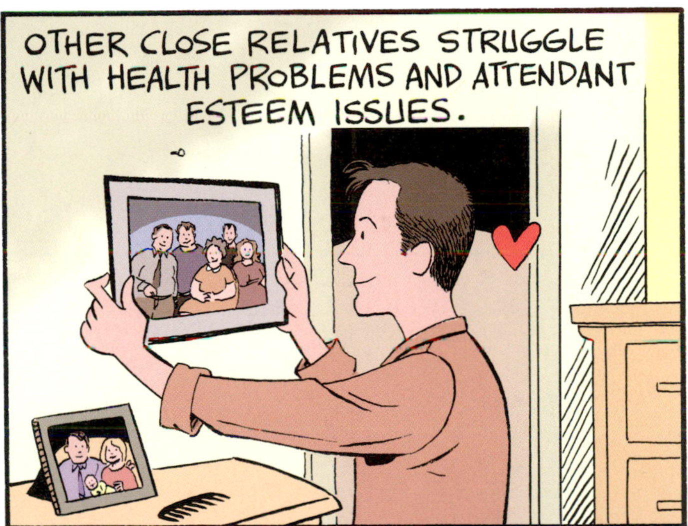
OTHER CLOSE RELATIVES STRUGGLE WITH HEALTH PROBLEMS AND ATTENDANT ESTEEM ISSUES.

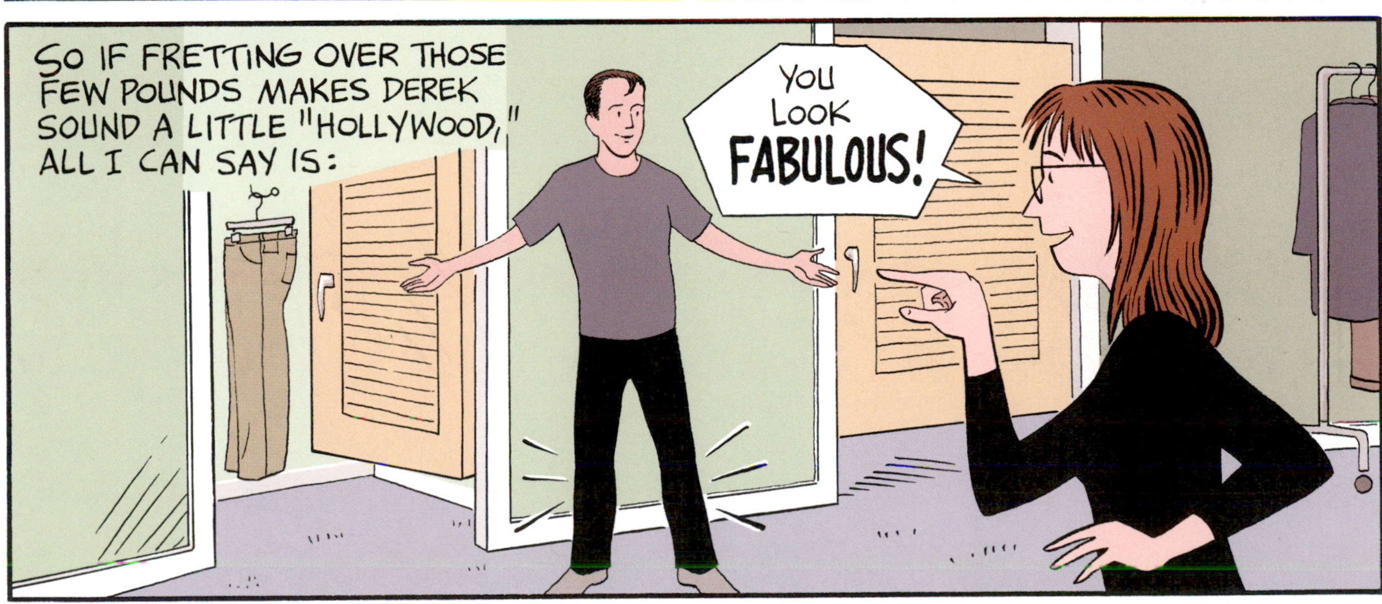
SO IF FRETTING OVER THOSE FEW POUNDS MAKES DEREK SOUND A LITTLE "HOLLYWOOD," ALL I CAN SAY IS:
YOU LOOK **FABULOUS!**

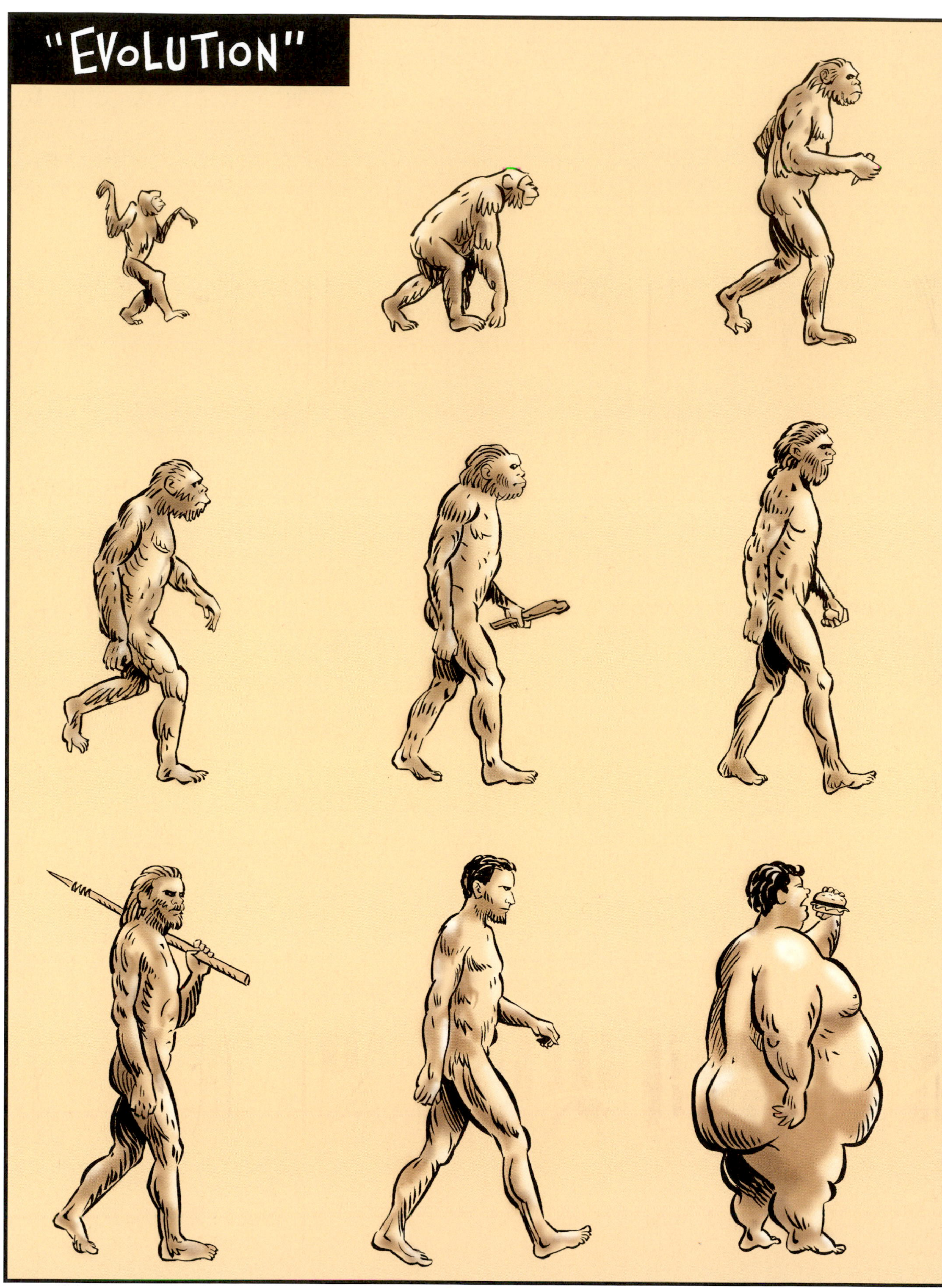
"EVOLUTION"

# Jane's Addiction

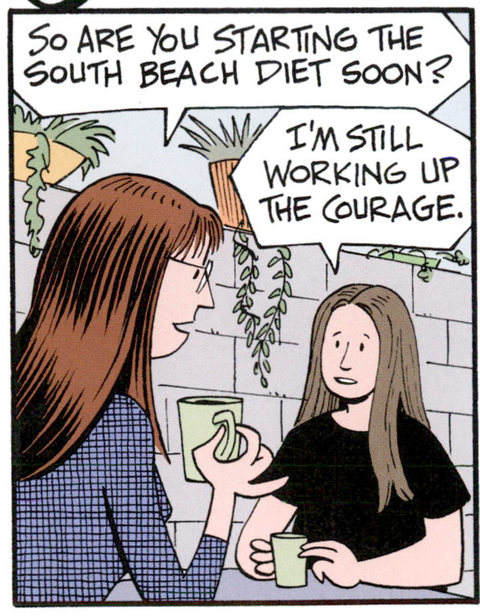
So are you starting the South Beach diet soon?
I'm still working up the courage.

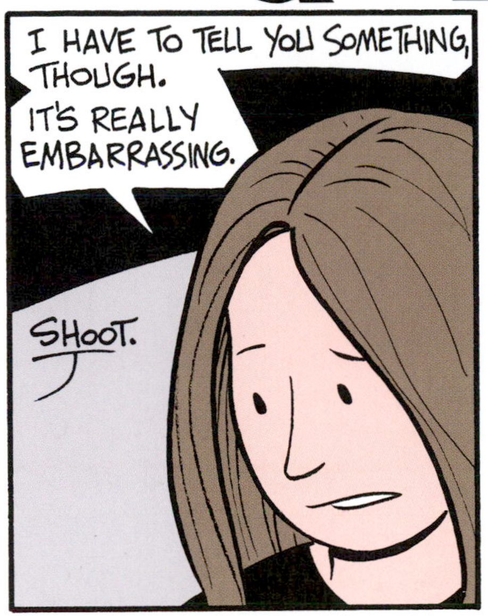
I have to tell you something, though.
It's really embarrassing.
Shoot.

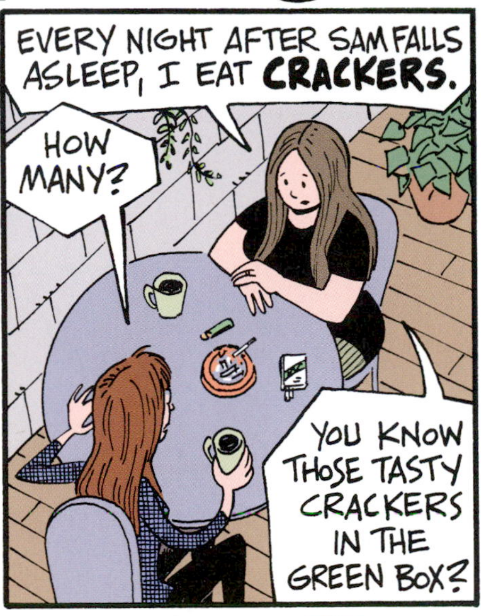
Every night after Sam falls asleep, I eat **crackers.**
How many?
You know those tasty crackers in the green box?

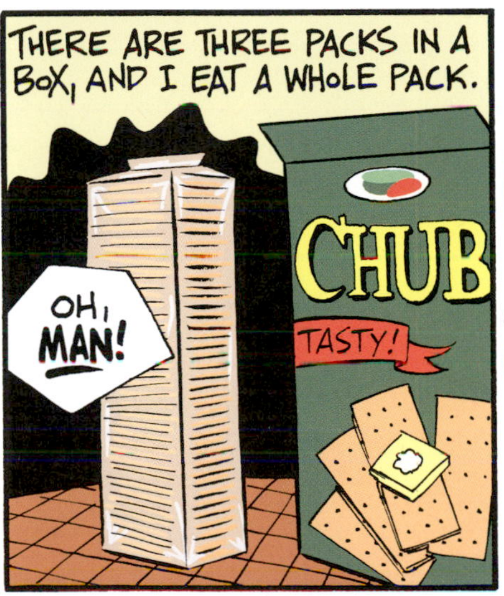
There are three packs in a box, and I eat a whole pack.
Oh, man!
CHUB
TASTY!

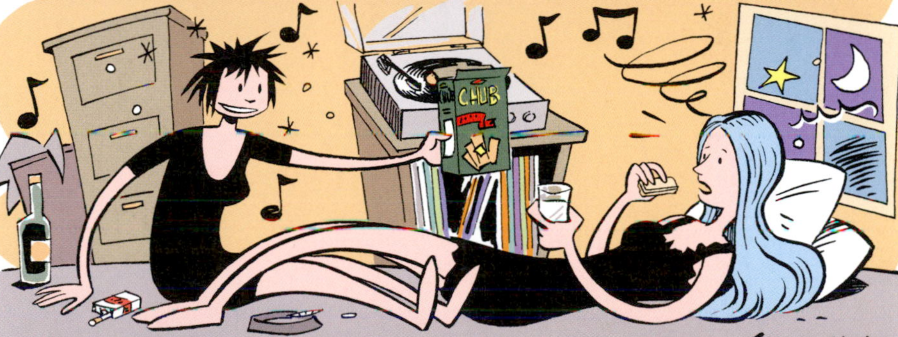
It all started when a friend of mine reminded me how we used crackers and milk as comfort foods back when we were in the punk scene and addicted to drugs.
CHUB
A few months ago, when I was going through something stressful, that information popped back into my head — crackers and milk would calm me down.

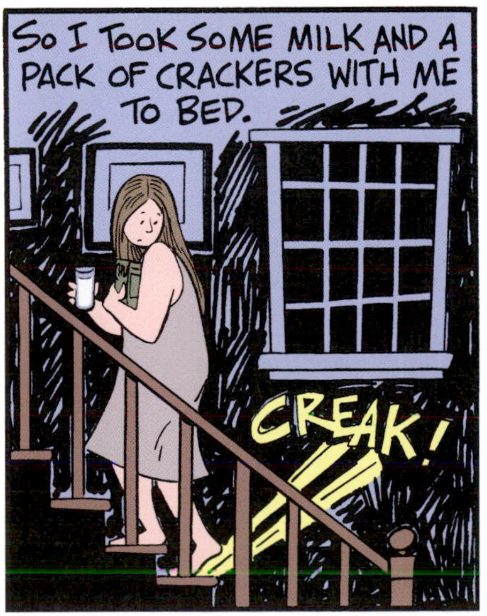
So I took some milk and a pack of crackers with me to bed.
CREAK!

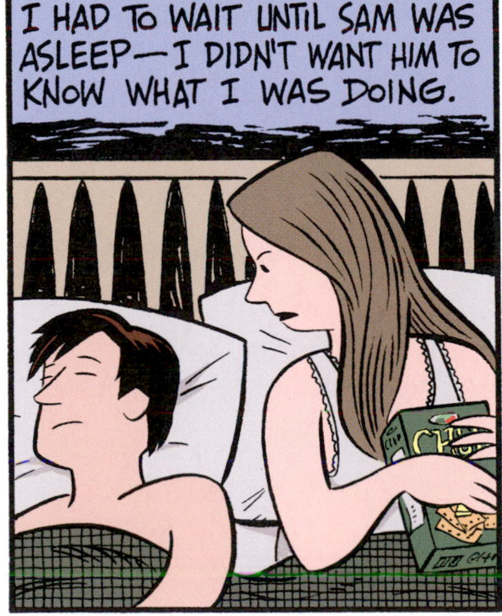
I had to wait until Sam was asleep—I didn't want him to know what I was doing.

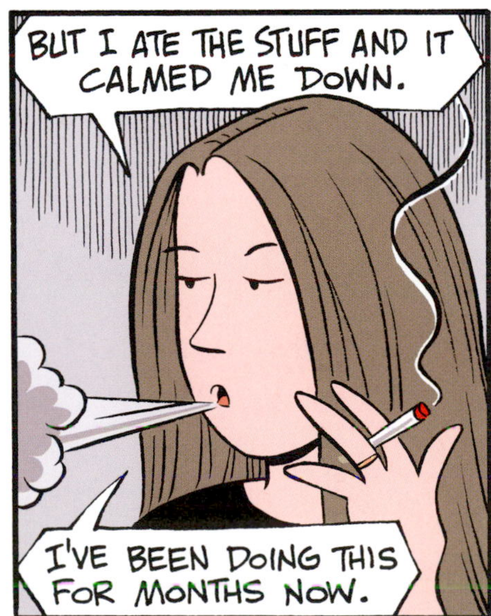
But I ate the stuff and it calmed me down.
I've been doing this for months now.

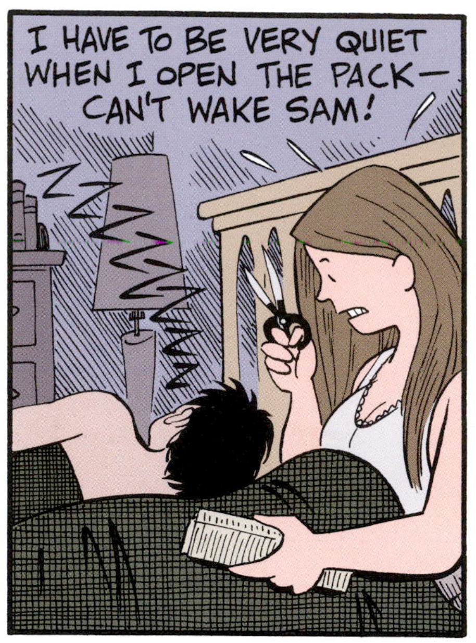
I HAVE TO BE VERY QUIET WHEN I OPEN THE PACK—CAN'T WAKE SAM!

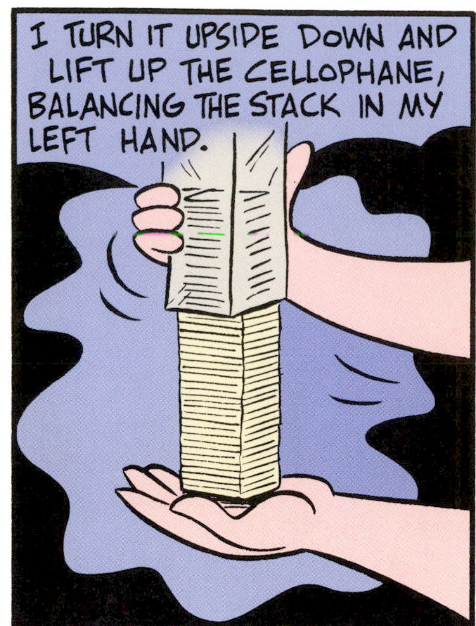
I TURN IT UPSIDE DOWN AND LIFT UP THE CELLOPHANE, BALANCING THE STACK IN MY LEFT HAND.

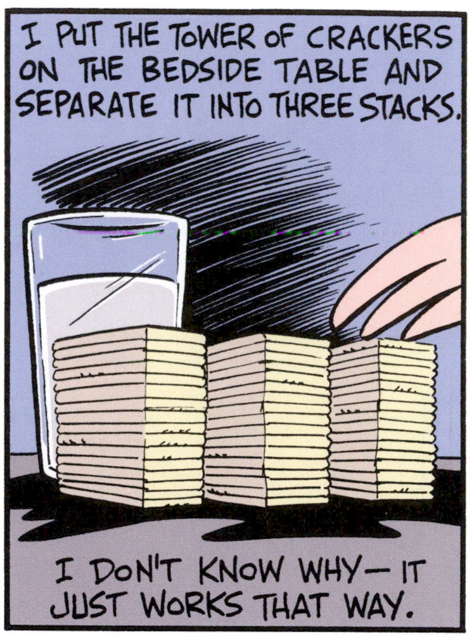
I PUT THE TOWER OF CRACKERS ON THE BEDSIDE TABLE AND SEPARATE IT INTO THREE STACKS.
I DON'T KNOW WHY—IT JUST WORKS THAT WAY.

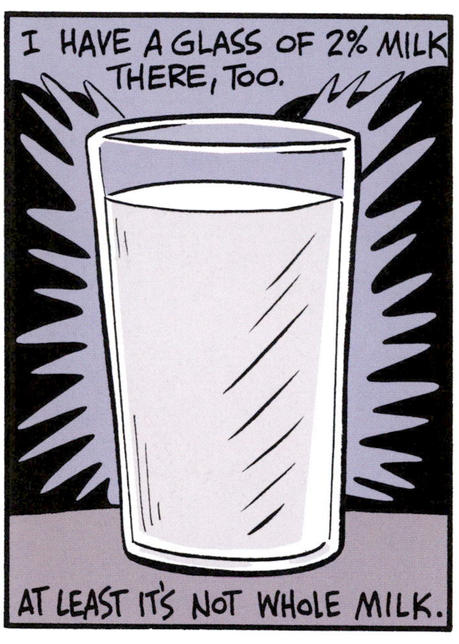
I HAVE A GLASS OF 2% MILK THERE, TOO.
AT LEAST IT'S NOT WHOLE MILK.

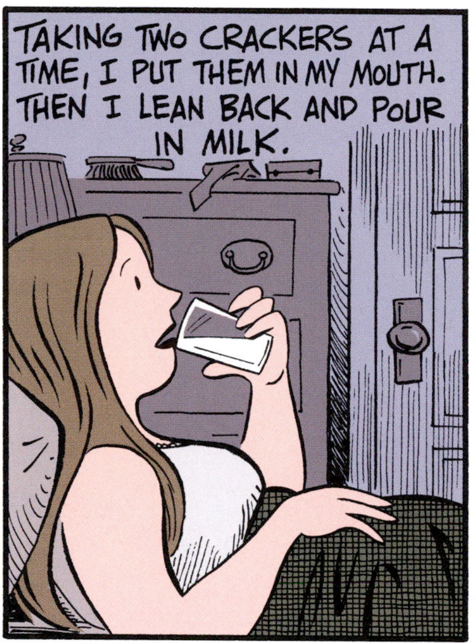
TAKING TWO CRACKERS AT A TIME, I PUT THEM IN MY MOUTH. THEN I LEAN BACK AND POUR IN MILK.

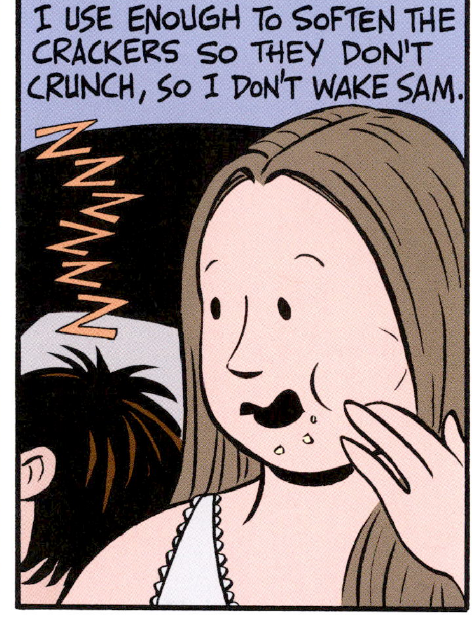
I USE ENOUGH TO SOFTEN THE CRACKERS SO THEY DON'T CRUNCH, SO I DON'T WAKE SAM.

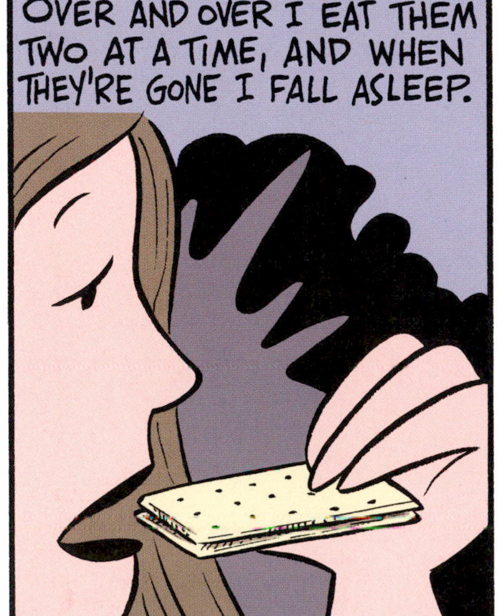
OVER AND OVER I EAT THEM TWO AT A TIME, AND WHEN THEY'RE GONE I FALL ASLEEP.

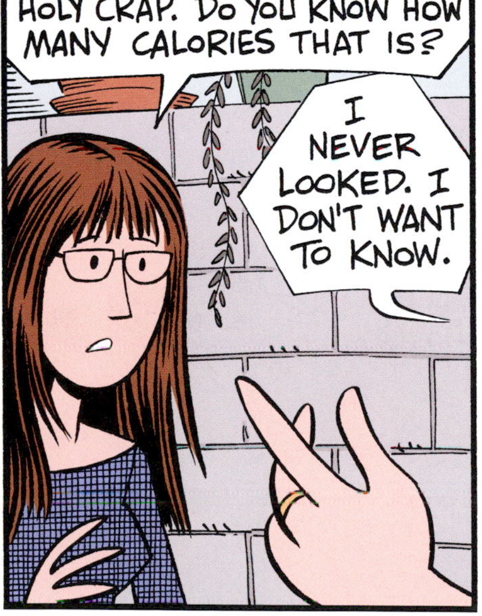
HOLY CRAP. DO YOU KNOW HOW MANY CALORIES THAT IS?
I NEVER LOOKED. I DON'T WANT TO KNOW.

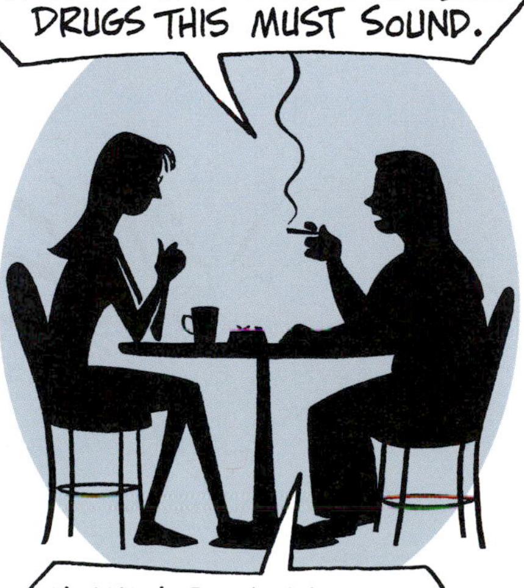
JUST TELLING YOU THIS, I REALIZE HOW MUCH LIKE USING DRUGS THIS MUST SOUND.
HIGHLY RITUALIZED.

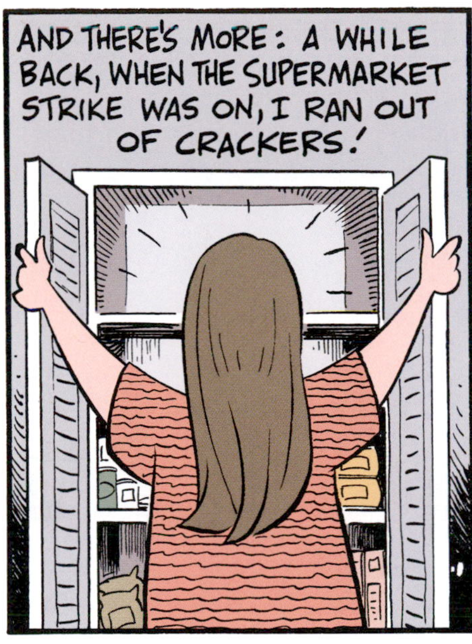
AND THERE'S MORE: A WHILE BACK, WHEN THE SUPERMARKET STRIKE WAS ON, I RAN OUT OF CRACKERS!

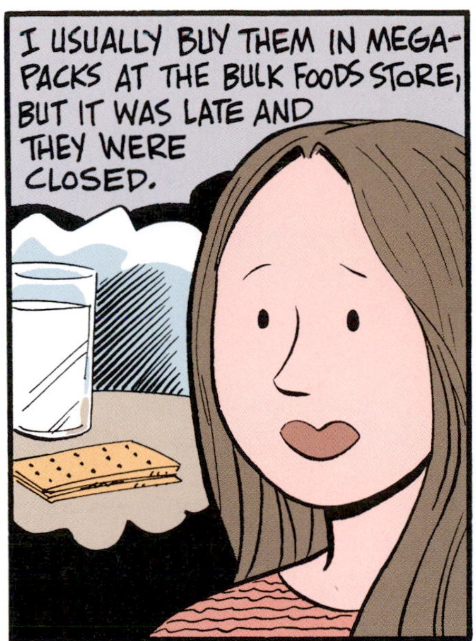
I USUALLY BUY THEM IN MEGA-PACKS AT THE BULK FOODS STORE, BUT IT WAS LATE AND THEY WERE CLOSED.

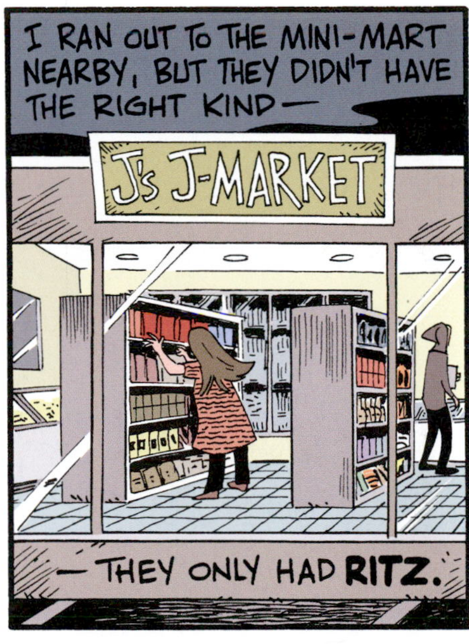
I RAN OUT TO THE MINI-MART NEARBY, BUT THEY DIDN'T HAVE THE RIGHT KIND—
J's J-MARKET
—THEY ONLY HAD **RITZ.**

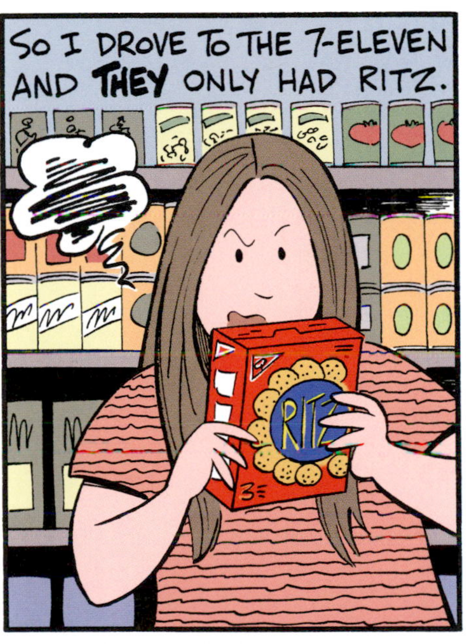
SO I DROVE TO THE 7-ELEVEN AND **THEY** ONLY HAD RITZ.
RITZ

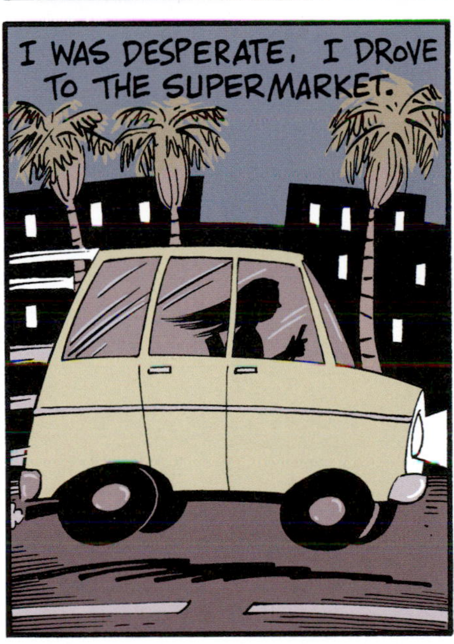
I WAS DESPERATE. I DROVE TO THE SUPERMARKET.

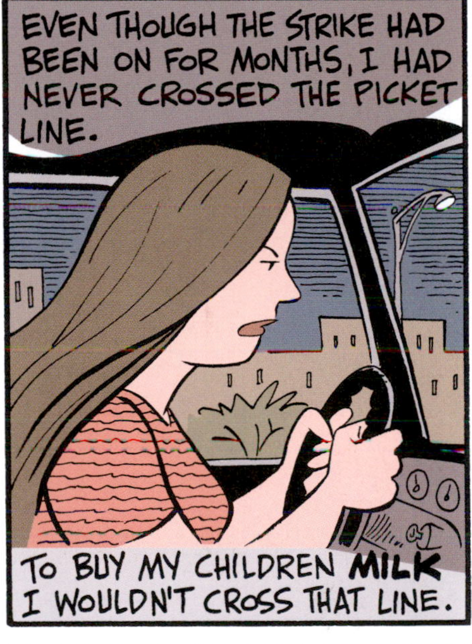
EVEN THOUGH THE STRIKE HAD BEEN ON FOR MONTHS, I HAD NEVER CROSSED THE PICKET LINE.
TO BUY MY CHILDREN **MILK** I WOULDN'T CROSS THAT LINE.

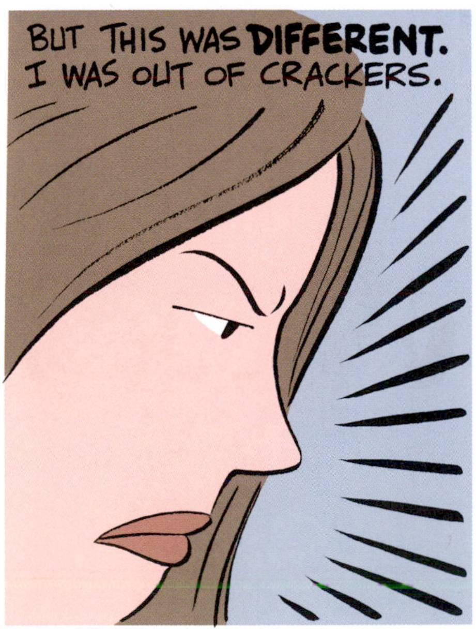
BUT THIS WAS **DIFFERENT.** I WAS OUT OF CRACKERS.

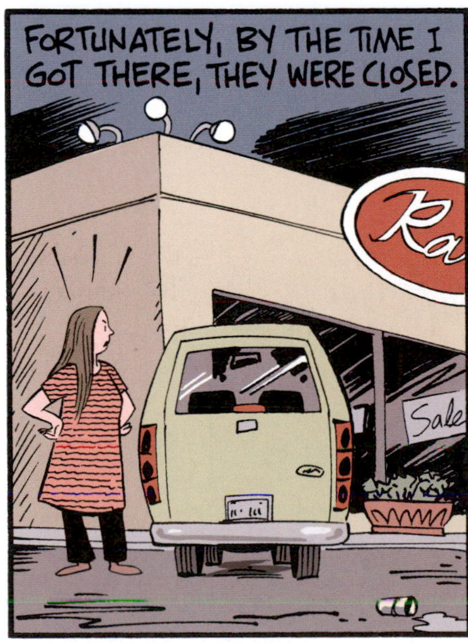
FORTUNATELY, BY THE TIME I GOT THERE, THEY WERE CLOSED.
Sale

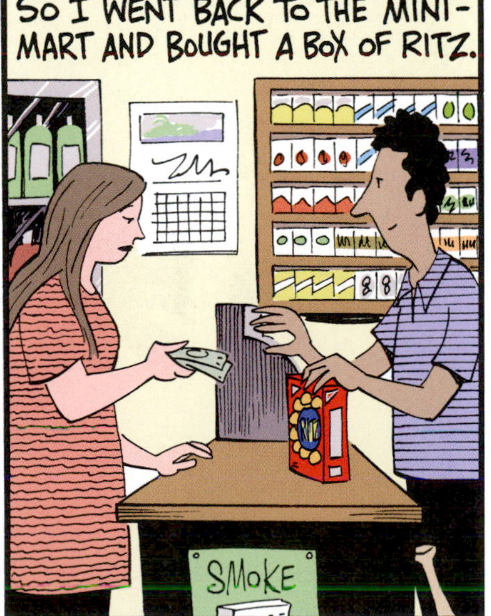
SO I WENT BACK TO THE MINI-MART AND BOUGHT A BOX OF RITZ.
SMOKE

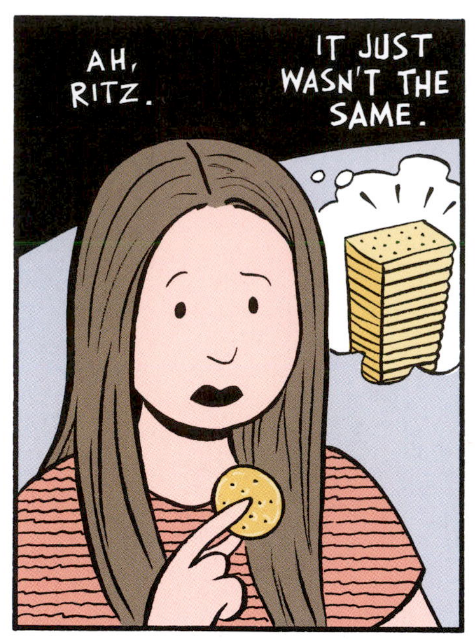
AH, RITZ.
IT JUST WASN'T THE SAME.

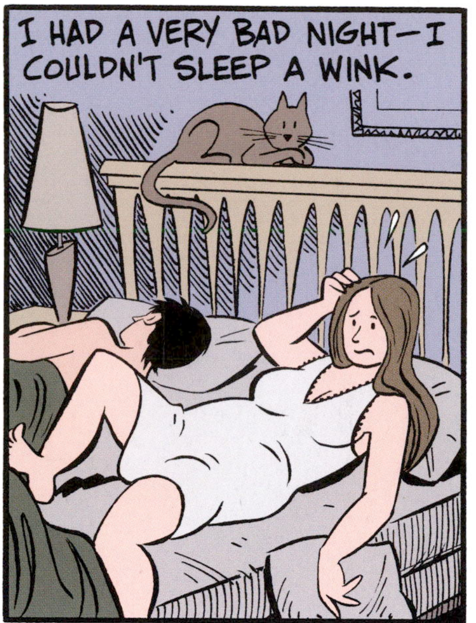
I HAD A VERY BAD NIGHT—I COULDN'T SLEEP A WINK.

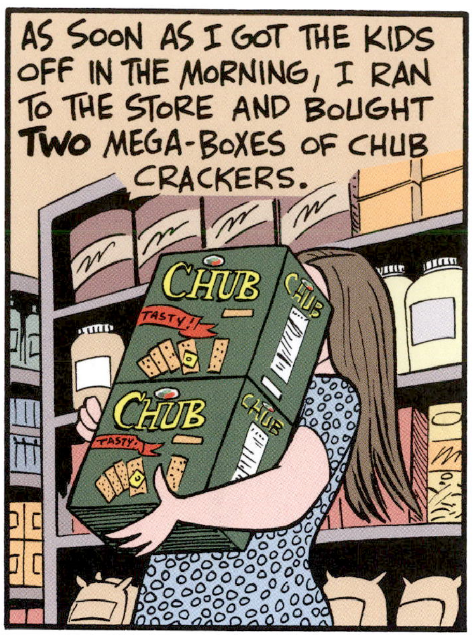
AS SOON AS I GOT THE KIDS OFF IN THE MORNING, I RAN TO THE STORE AND BOUGHT TWO MEGA-BOXES OF CHUB CRACKERS.
CHUB
TASTY!
CHUB
TASTY!

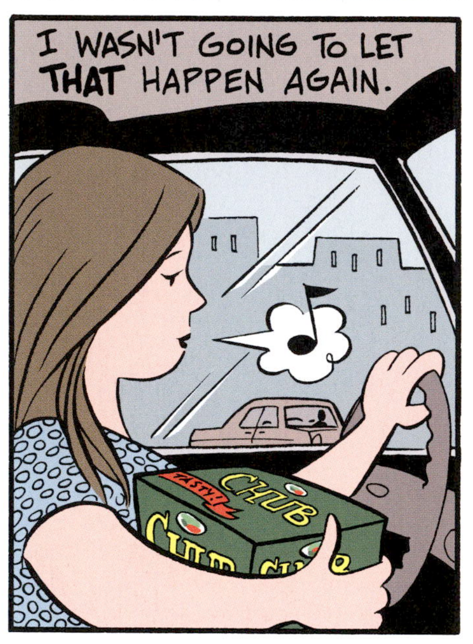
I WASN'T GOING TO LET THAT HAPPEN AGAIN.
TASTY!
CHUB

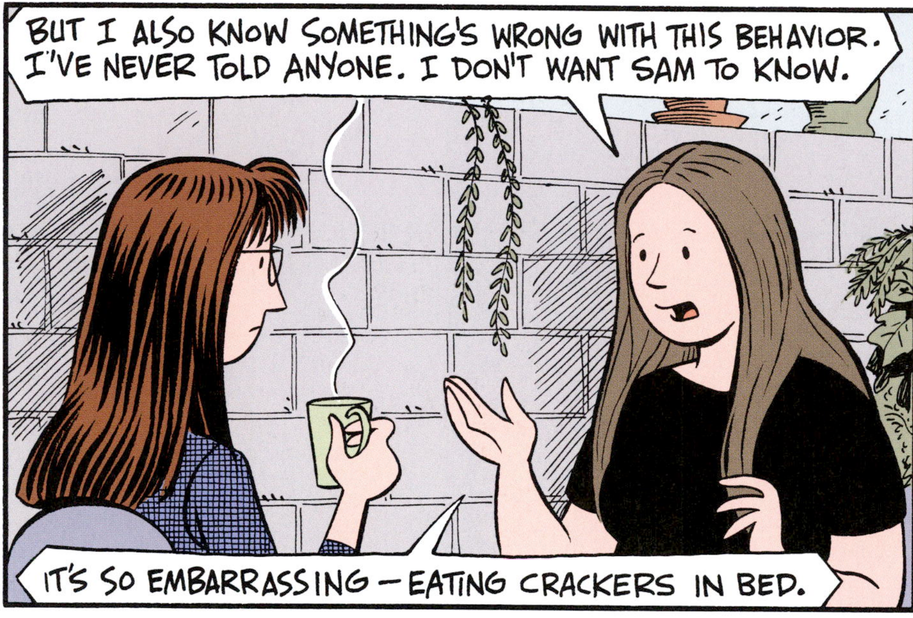
BUT I ALSO KNOW SOMETHING'S WRONG WITH THIS BEHAVIOR. I'VE NEVER TOLD ANYONE. I DON'T WANT SAM TO KNOW.
IT'S SO EMBARRASSING—EATING CRACKERS IN BED.

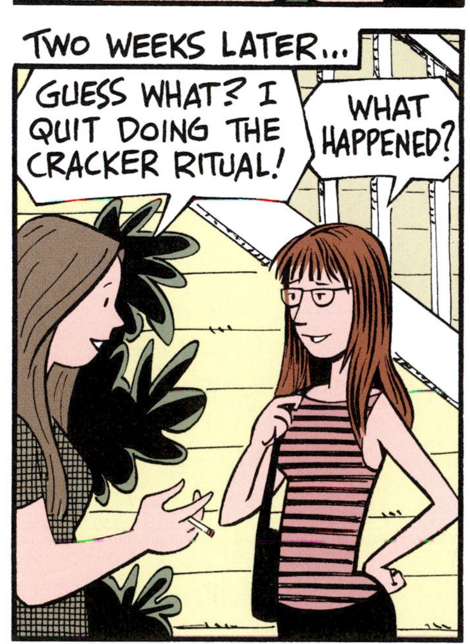
TWO WEEKS LATER...
GUESS WHAT? I QUIT DOING THE CRACKER RITUAL!
WHAT HAPPENED?

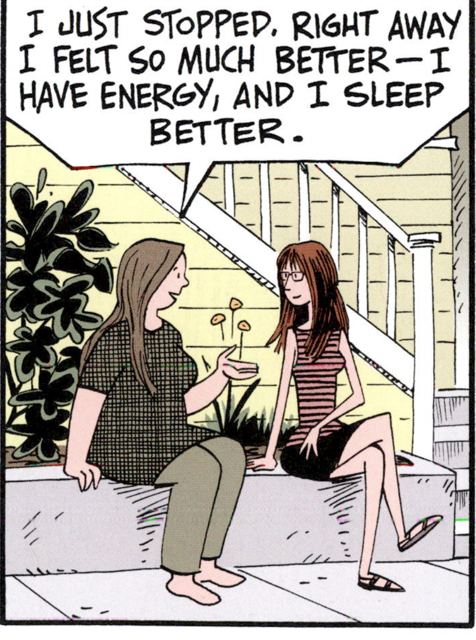
I JUST STOPPED. RIGHT AWAY I FELT SO MUCH BETTER—I HAVE ENERGY, AND I SLEEP BETTER.

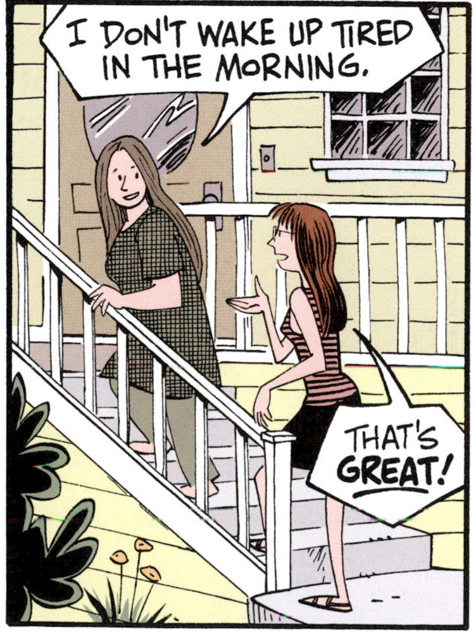
I DON'T WAKE UP TIRED IN THE MORNING.
THAT'S GREAT!

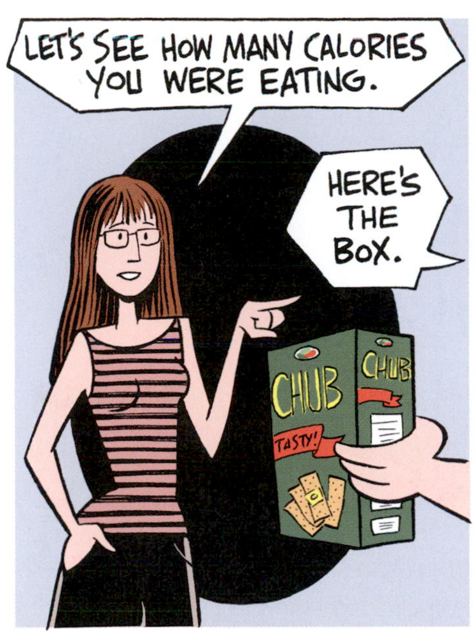
LET'S SEE HOW MANY CALORIES YOU WERE EATING.
HERE'S THE BOX.
CHUB
CHUB
TASTY!

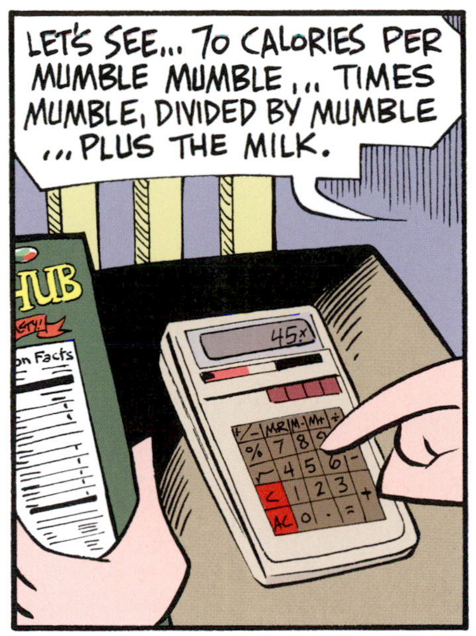
LET'S SEE... 70 CALORIES PER MUMBLE MUMBLE... TIMES MUMBLE, DIVIDED BY MUMBLE ...PLUS THE MILK.

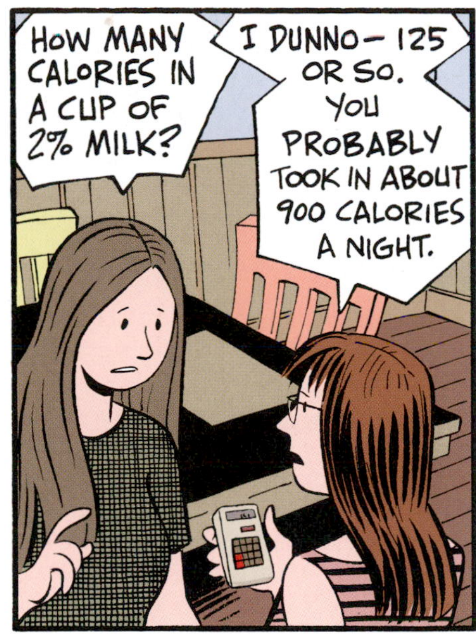
HOW MANY CALORIES IN A CUP OF 2% MILK?
I DUNNO– 125 OR SO.
YOU PROBABLY TOOK IN ABOUT 900 CALORIES A NIGHT.

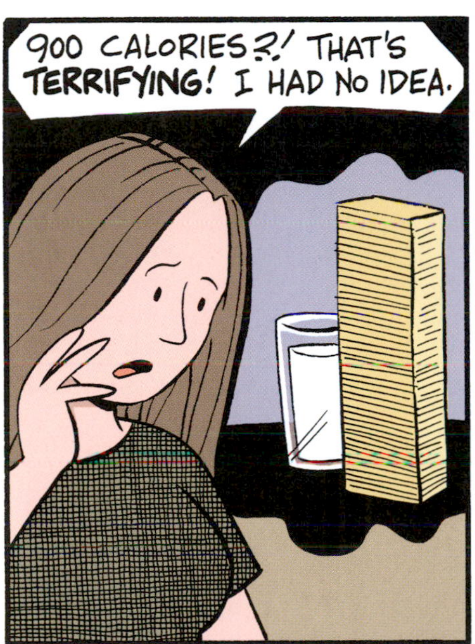
900 CALORIES?! THAT'S **TERRIFYING**! I HAD NO IDEA.

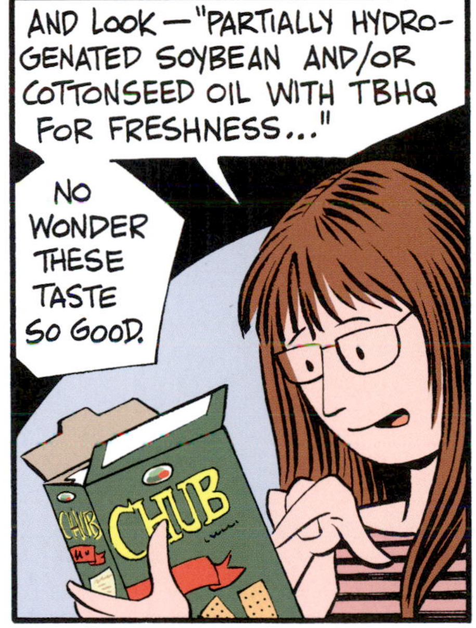
AND LOOK—"PARTIALLY HYDROGENATED SOYBEAN AND/OR COTTONSEED OIL WITH TBHQ FOR FRESHNESS..."
NO WONDER THESE TASTE SO GOOD.
CHUB

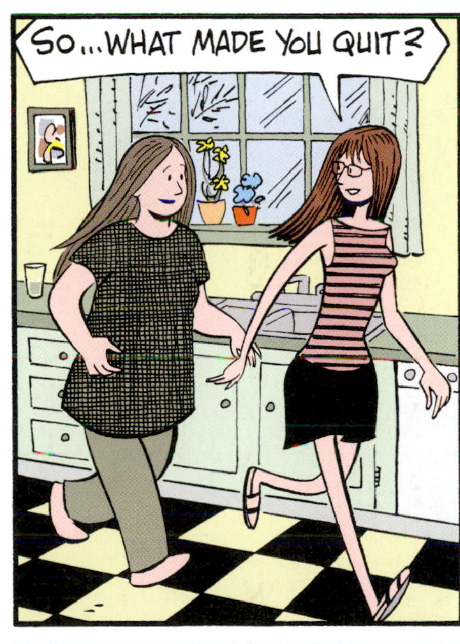
SO...WHAT MADE YOU QUIT?

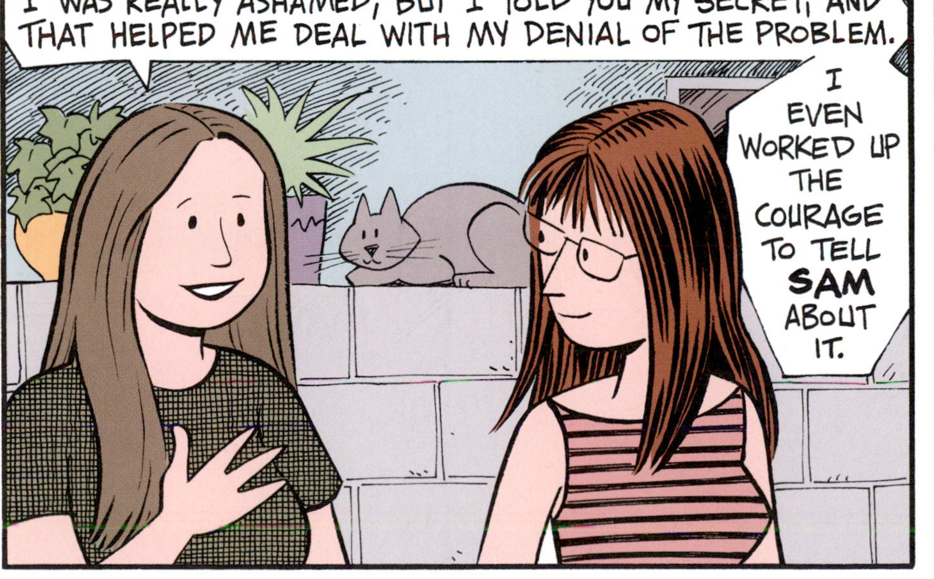
I WAS REALLY ASHAMED, BUT I TOLD YOU MY SECRET, AND THAT HELPED ME DEAL WITH MY DENIAL OF THE PROBLEM.
I EVEN WORKED UP THE COURAGE TO TELL **SAM** ABOUT IT.

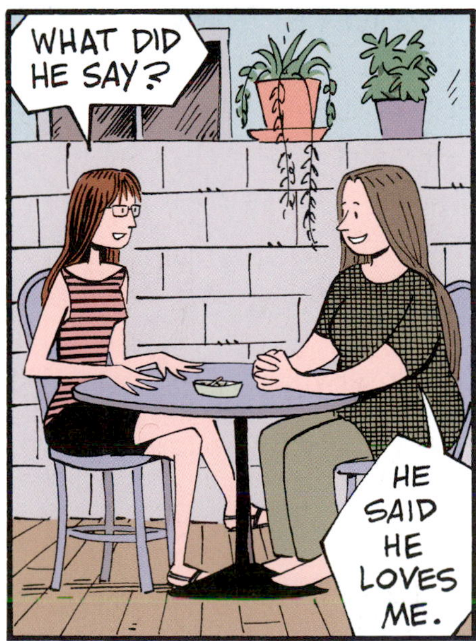
WHAT DID HE SAY?
HE SAID HE LOVES ME.

# ¡MUSICA!

A RECENT NEWS ARTICLE FOCUSED ON **MUSIC** AND HOW STUDIES SHOW THAT PEOPLE WHO LISTEN TO MUSIC WHILE THEY EXERCISE WORK HARDER AND LONGER THAN THOSE WHO DON'T.

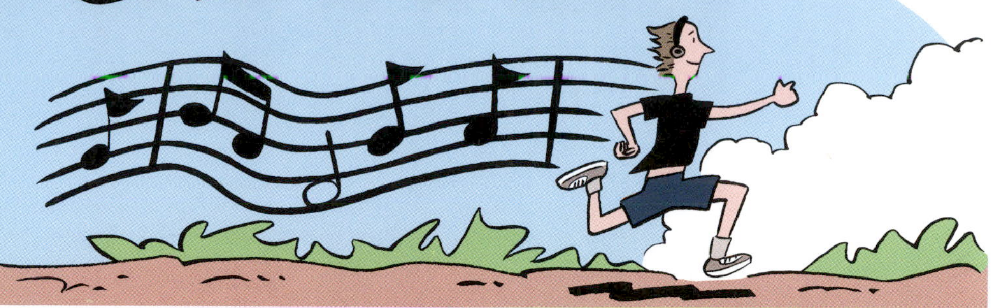

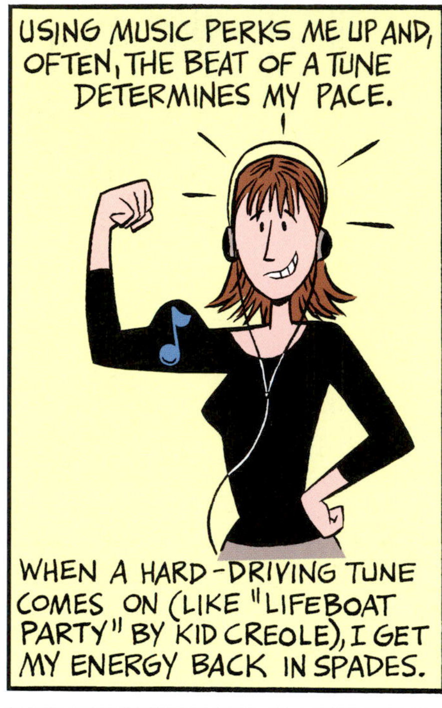

USING MUSIC PERKS ME UP AND, OFTEN, THE BEAT OF A TUNE DETERMINES MY PACE.
WHEN A HARD-DRIVING TUNE COMES ON (LIKE "LIFEBOAT PARTY" BY KID CREOLE), I GET MY ENERGY BACK IN SPADES.

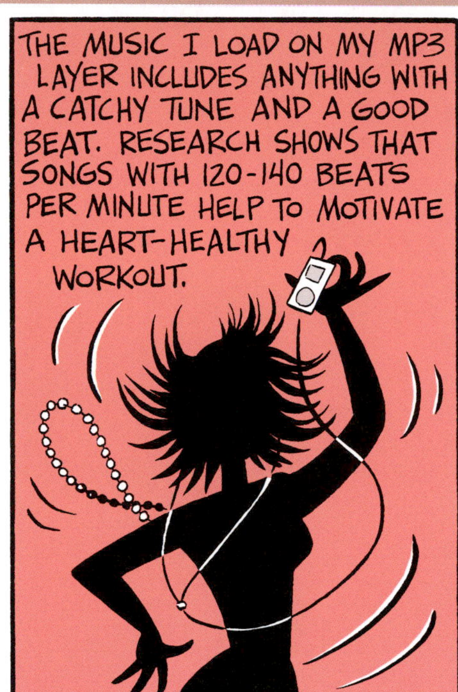

THE MUSIC I LOAD ON MY MP3 LAYER INCLUDES ANYTHING WITH A CATCHY TUNE AND A GOOD BEAT. RESEARCH SHOWS THAT SONGS WITH 120-140 BEATS PER MINUTE HELP TO MOTIVATE A HEART-HEALTHY WORKOUT.

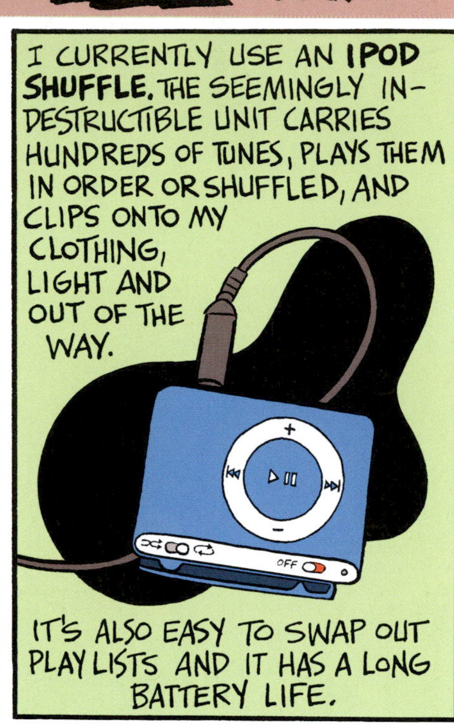

I CURRENTLY USE AN **IPOD SHUFFLE.** THE SEEMINGLY INDESTRUCTIBLE UNIT CARRIES HUNDREDS OF TUNES, PLAYS THEM IN ORDER OR SHUFFLED, AND CLIPS ONTO MY CLOTHING, LIGHT AND OUT OF THE WAY.
OFF
IT'S ALSO EASY TO SWAP OUT PLAYLISTS AND IT HAS A LONG BATTERY LIFE.

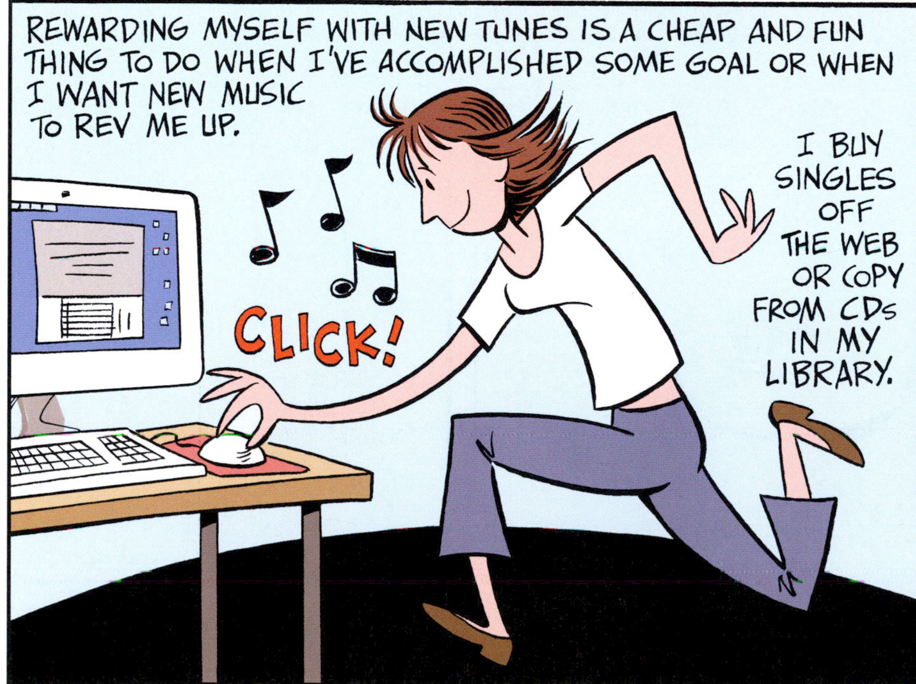

REWARDING MYSELF WITH NEW TUNES IS A CHEAP AND FUN THING TO DO WHEN I'VE ACCOMPLISHED SOME GOAL OR WHEN I WANT NEW MUSIC TO REV ME UP.
CLICK!
I BUY SINGLES OFF THE WEB OR COPY FROM CDs IN MY LIBRARY.

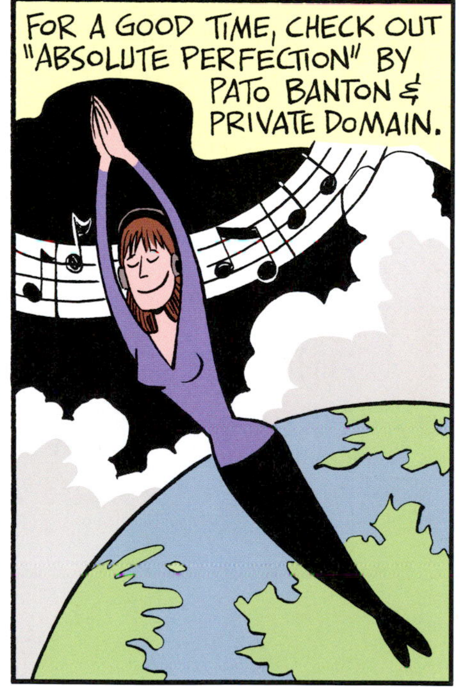

FOR A GOOD TIME, CHECK OUT "ABSOLUTE PERFECTION" BY PATO BANTON & PRIVATE DOMAIN.

# Emotional Triggers

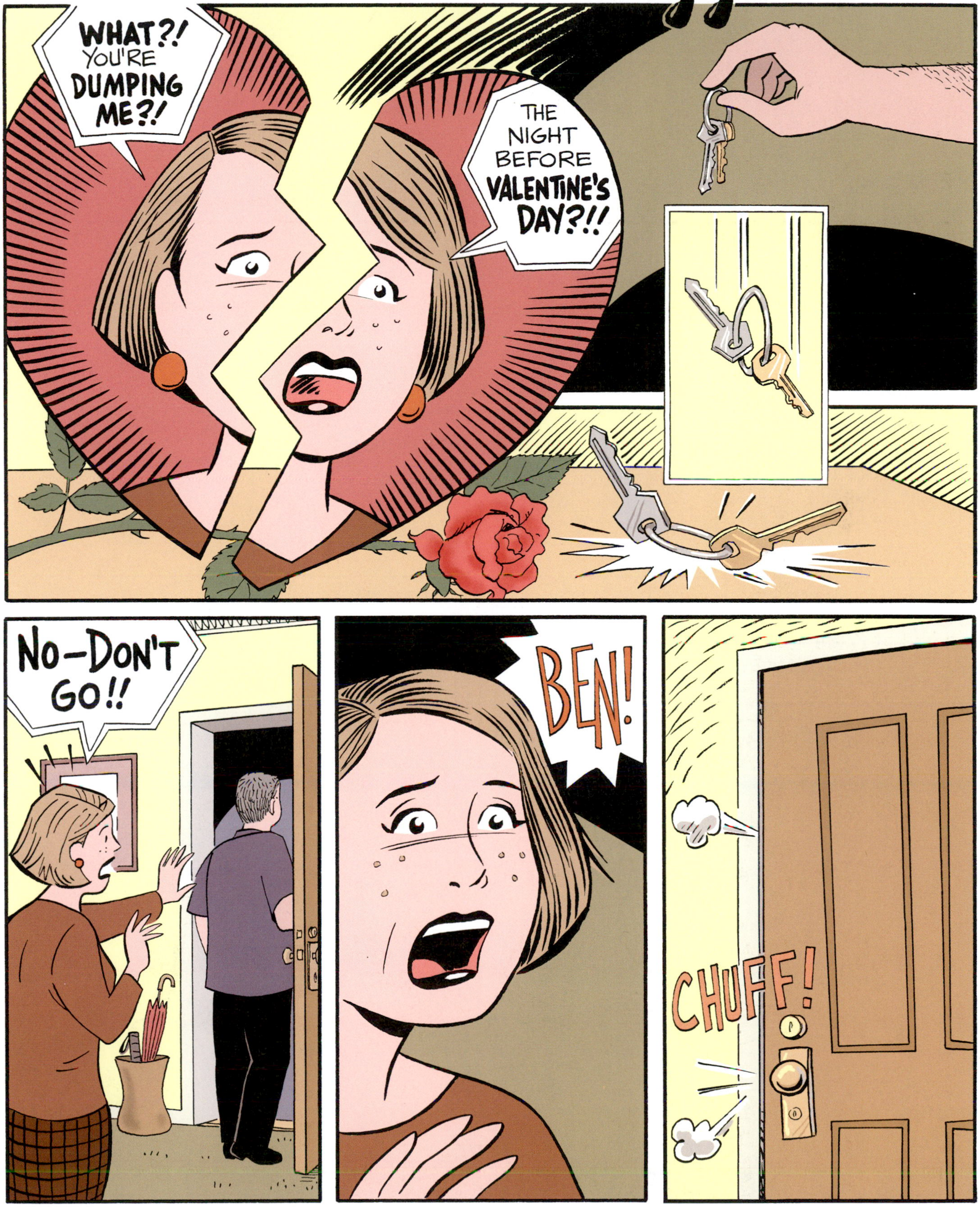

WHAT?! YOU'RE DUMPING ME?!

THE NIGHT BEFORE VALENTINE'S DAY?!!

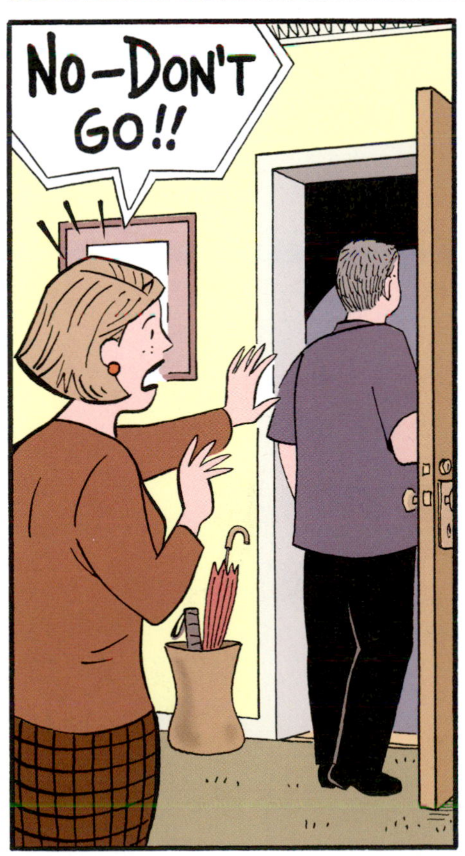


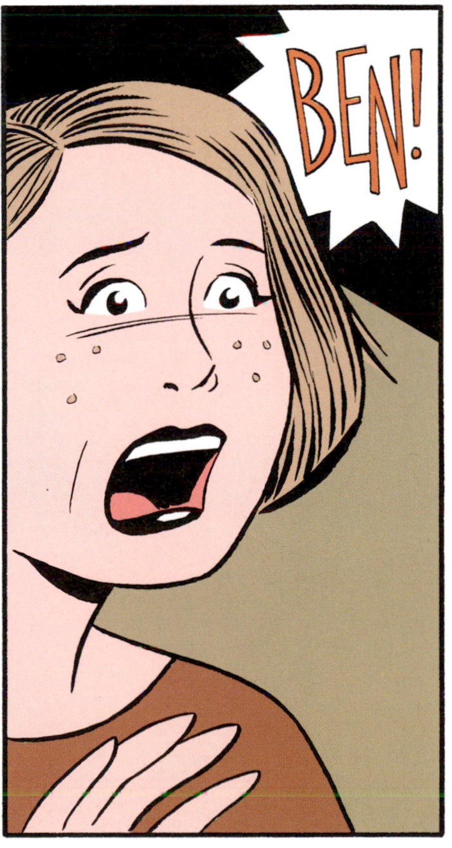


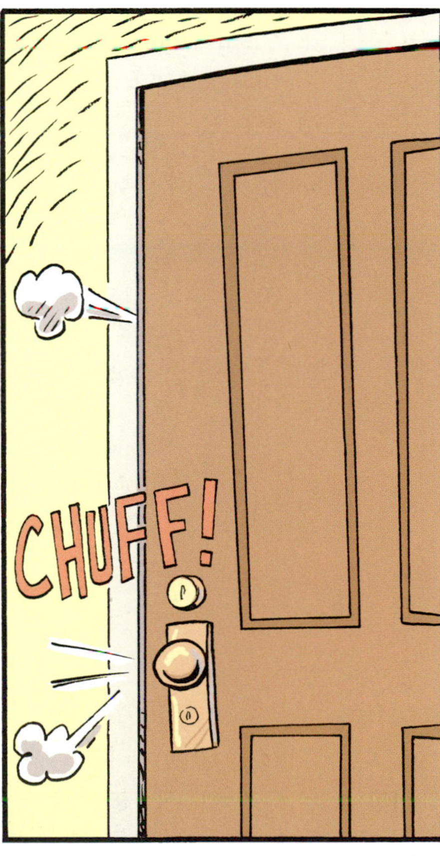

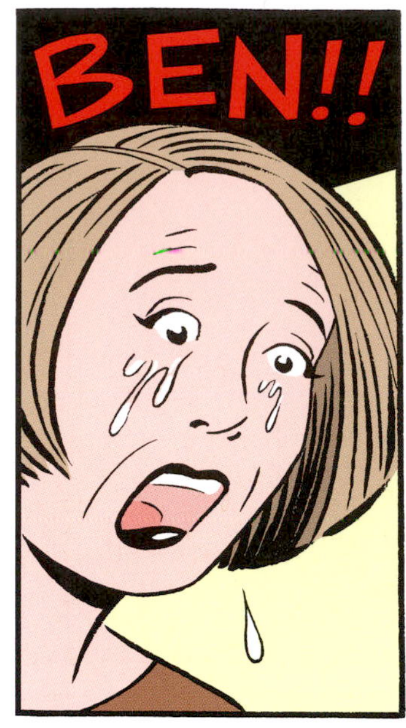
BEN!!
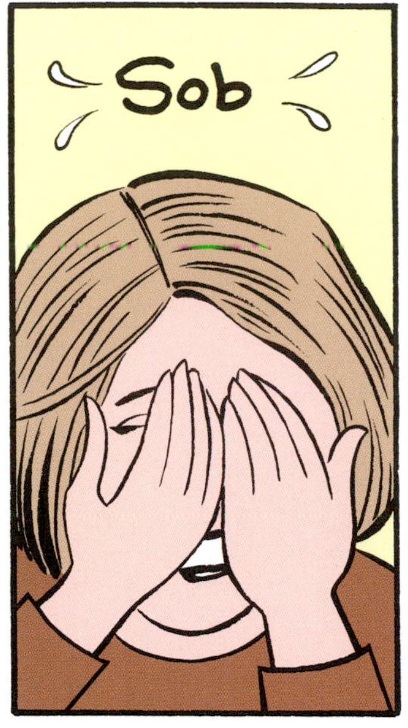
Sob
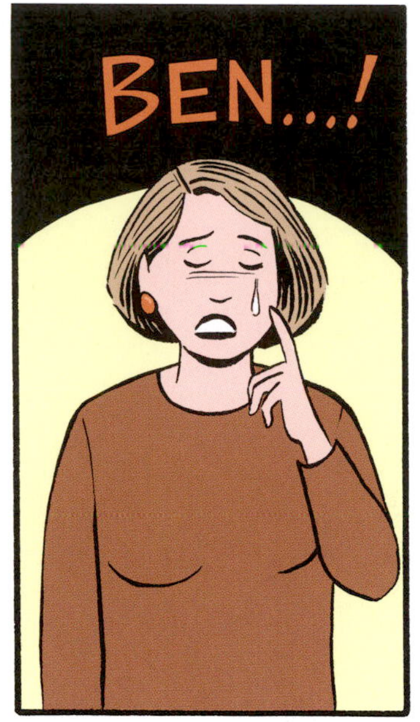
BEN...!
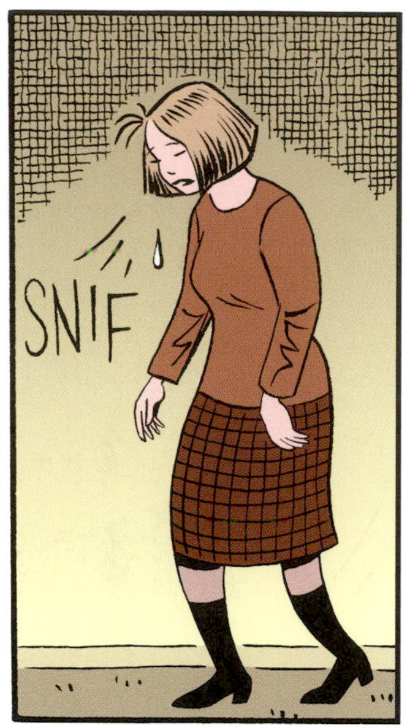
SNIF
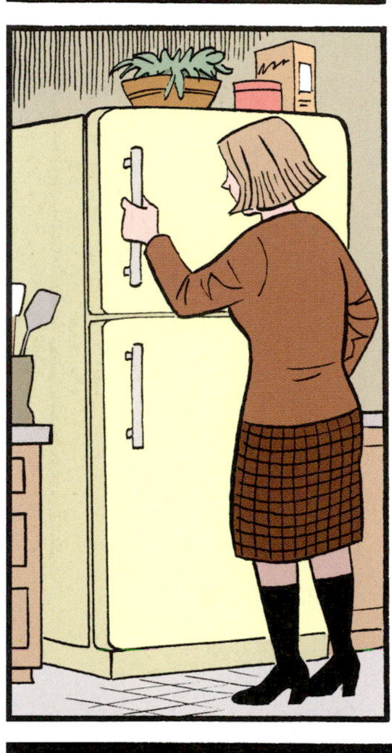
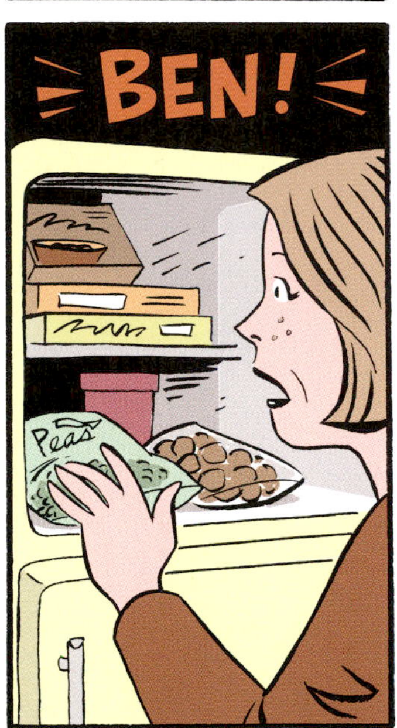
BEN!
Peas
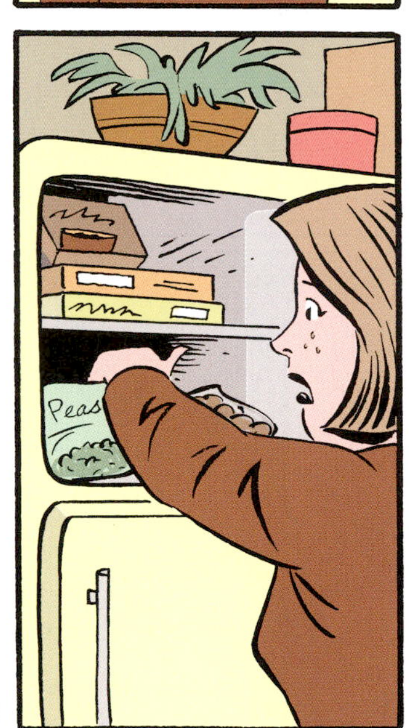
Peas
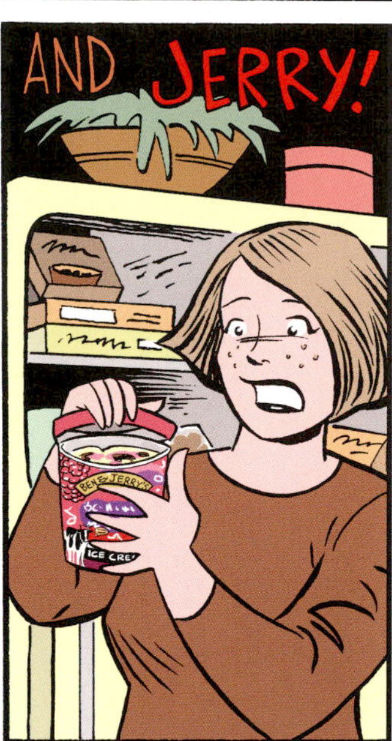
AND JERRY!
ICE CREAM
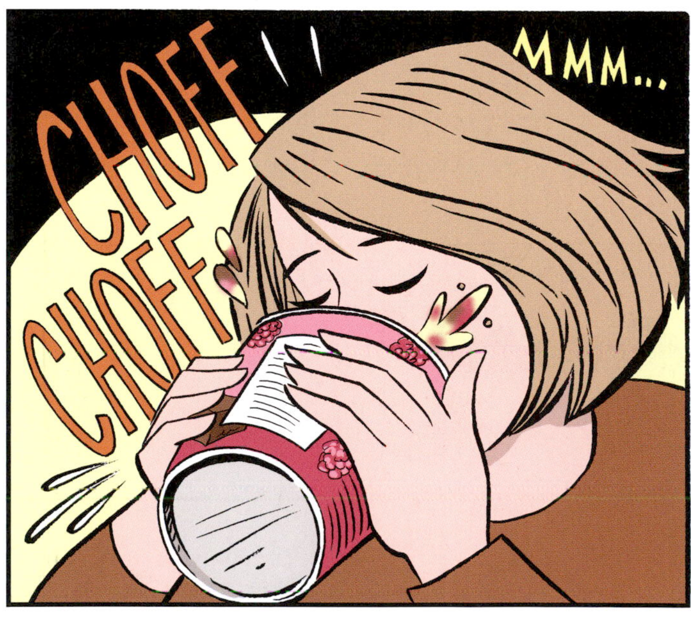
CHOFF
CHOFF
MMM...
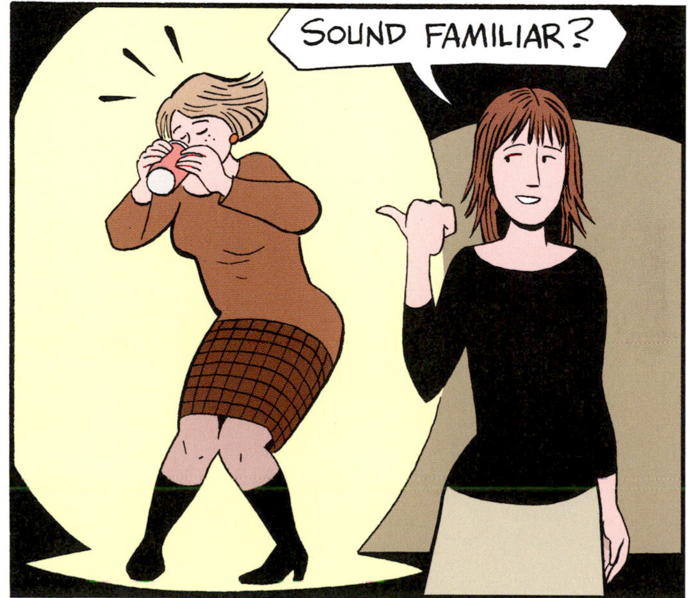
SOUND FAMILIAR?

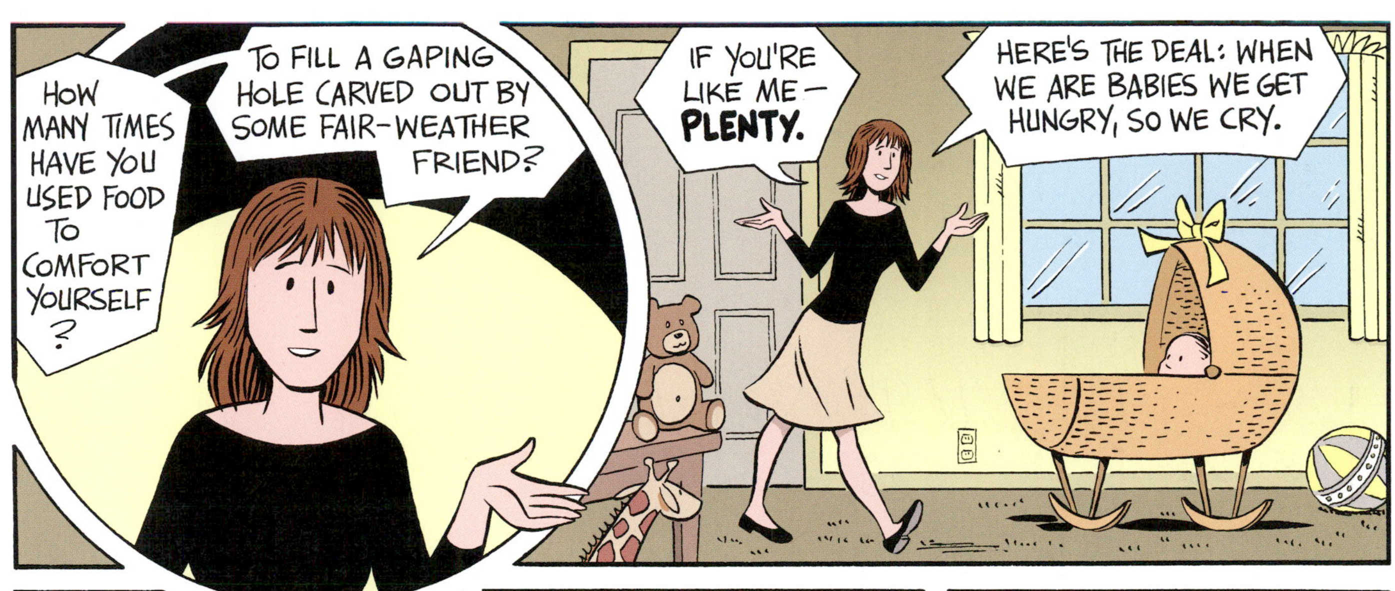
HOW MANY TIMES HAVE YOU USED FOOD TO COMFORT YOURSELF?
TO FILL A GAPING HOLE CARVED OUT BY SOME FAIR-WEATHER FRIEND?
IF YOU'RE LIKE ME— **PLENTY.**
HERE'S THE DEAL: WHEN WE ARE BABIES WE GET HUNGRY, SO WE CRY.

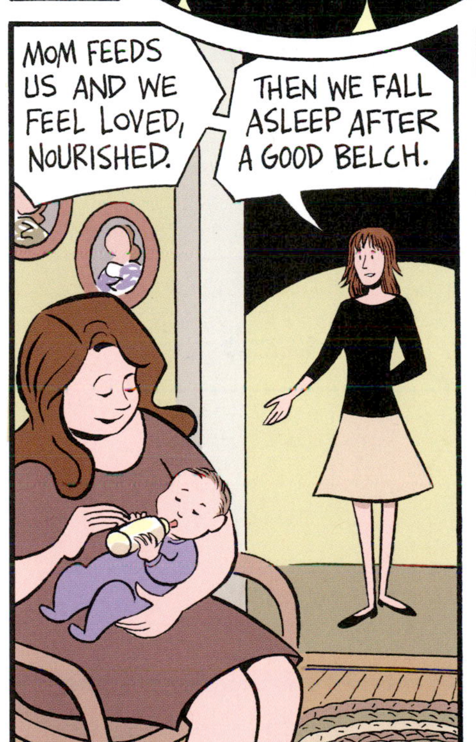
MOM FEEDS US AND WE FEEL LOVED, NOURISHED.
THEN WE FALL ASLEEP AFTER A GOOD BELCH.

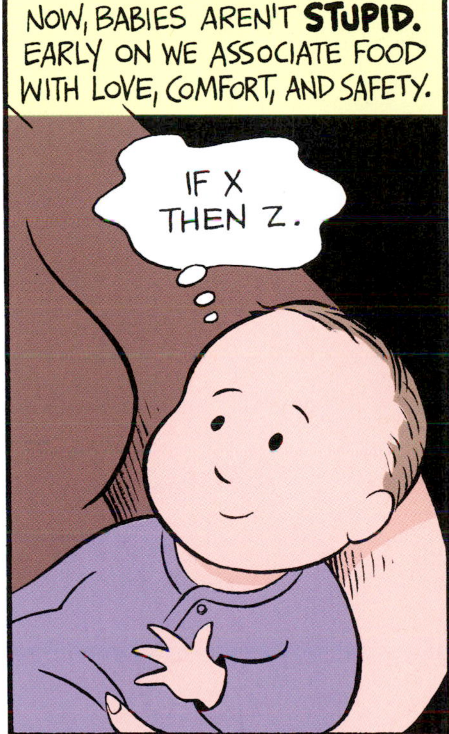
NOW, BABIES AREN'T **STUPID.** EARLY ON WE ASSOCIATE FOOD WITH LOVE, COMFORT, AND SAFETY.
IF X THEN Z.

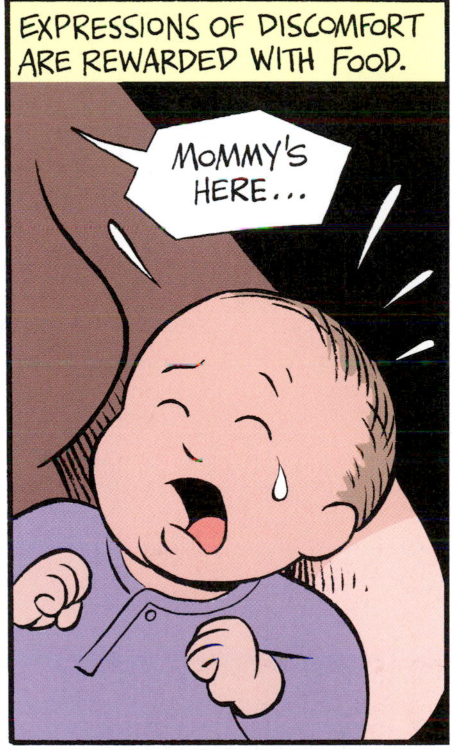
EXPRESSIONS OF DISCOMFORT ARE REWARDED WITH FOOD.
MOMMY'S HERE...

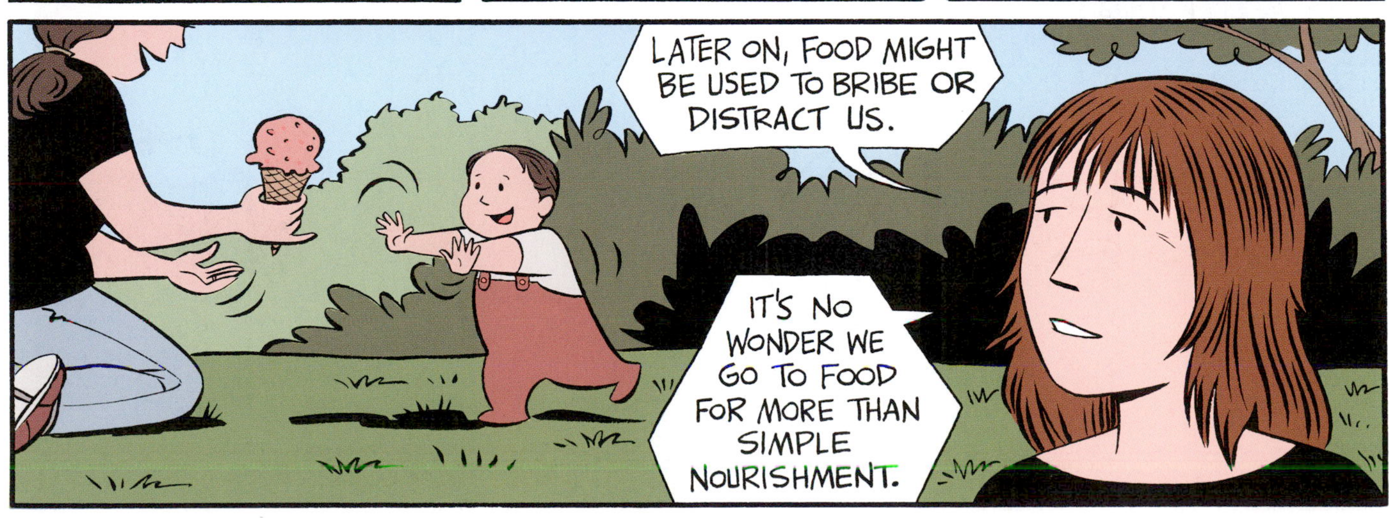
LATER ON, FOOD MIGHT BE USED TO BRIBE OR DISTRACT US.
IT'S NO WONDER WE GO TO FOOD FOR MORE THAN SIMPLE NOURISHMENT.

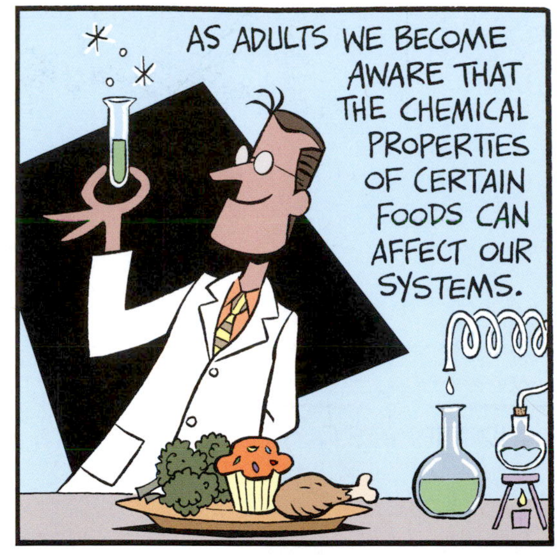
AS ADULTS WE BECOME AWARE THAT THE CHEMICAL PROPERTIES OF CERTAIN FOODS CAN AFFECT OUR SYSTEMS.

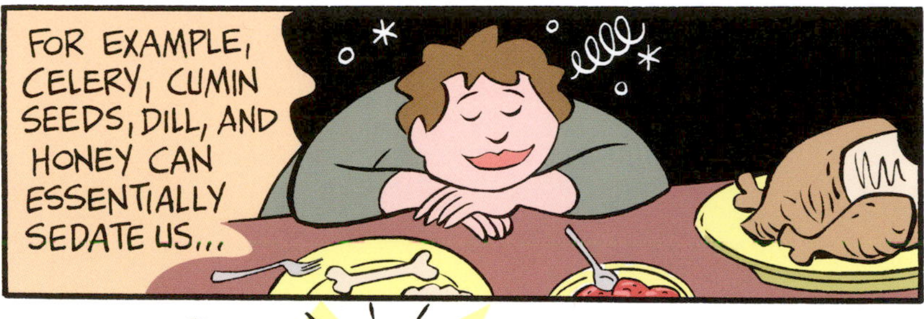
FOR EXAMPLE, CELERY, CUMIN SEEDS, DILL, AND HONEY CAN ESSENTIALLY SEDATE US...

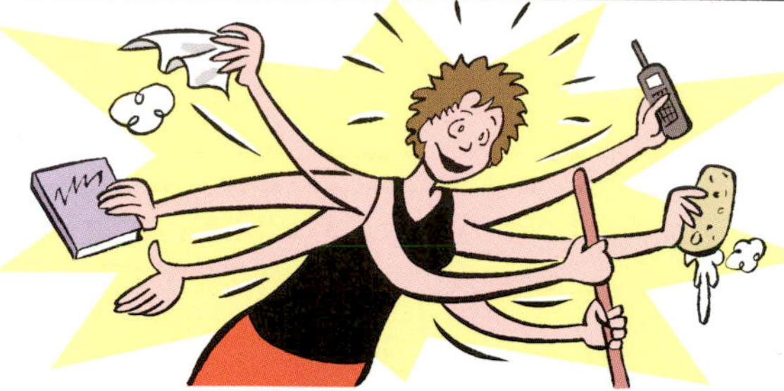
...AND SUGARY FOODS CAN REV US UP, WHICH FEELS GOOD WHILE IT LASTS.

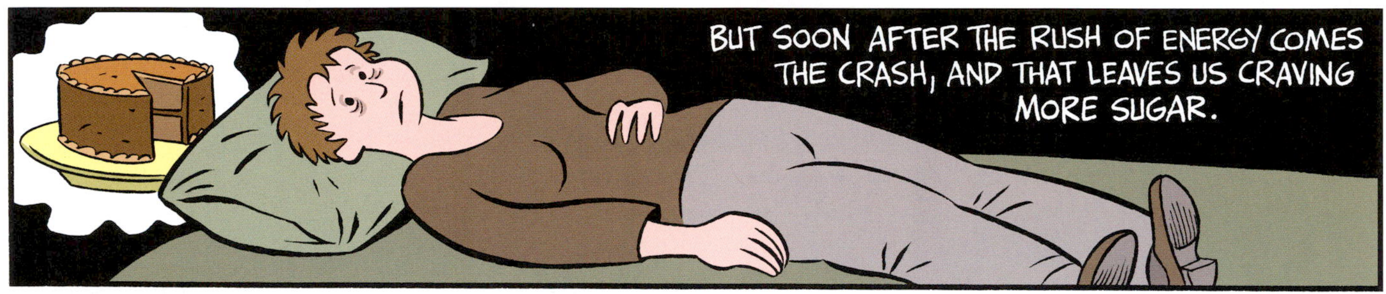
BUT SOON AFTER THE RUSH OF ENERGY COMES THE CRASH, AND THAT LEAVES US CRAVING MORE SUGAR.

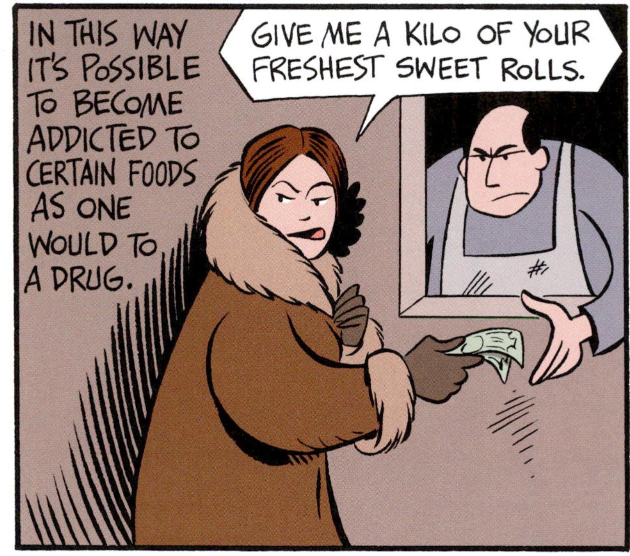
IN THIS WAY IT'S POSSIBLE TO BECOME ADDICTED TO CERTAIN FOODS AS ONE WOULD TO A DRUG.
GIVE ME A KILO OF YOUR FRESHEST SWEET ROLLS.

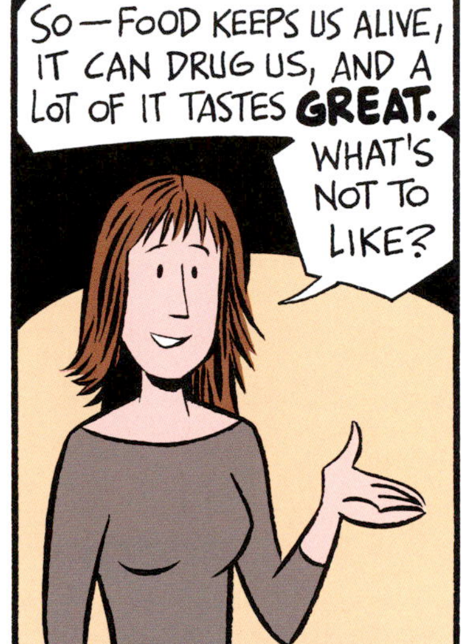
SO—FOOD KEEPS US ALIVE, IT CAN DRUG US, AND A LOT OF IT TASTES **GREAT.**
WHAT'S NOT TO LIKE?

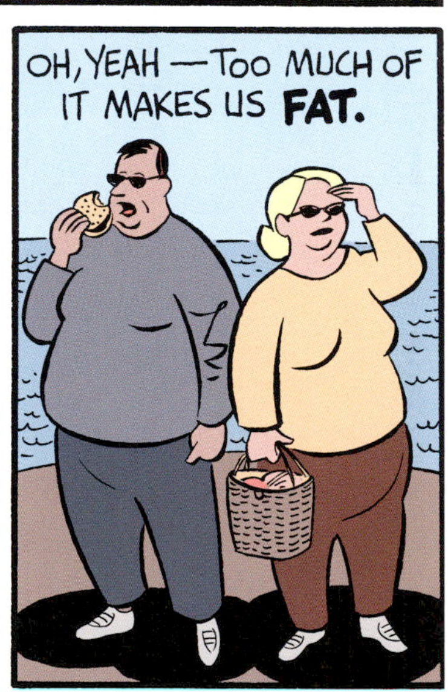
OH, YEAH—TOO MUCH OF IT MAKES US **FAT.**

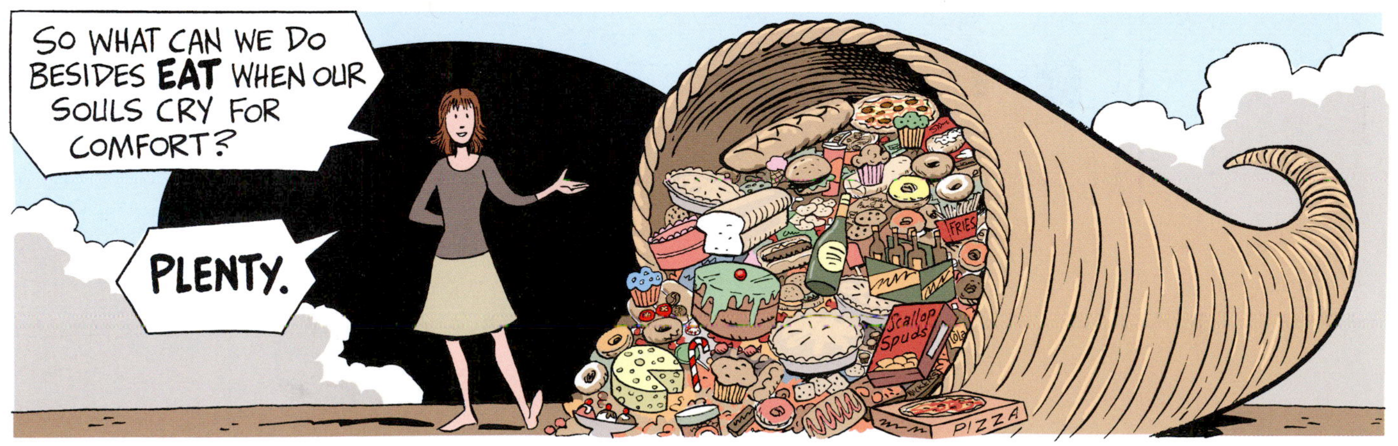
SO WHAT CAN WE DO BESIDES **EAT** WHEN OUR SOULS CRY FOR COMFORT?
PLENTY.
FRIES
Scallop Spuds
PIZZA

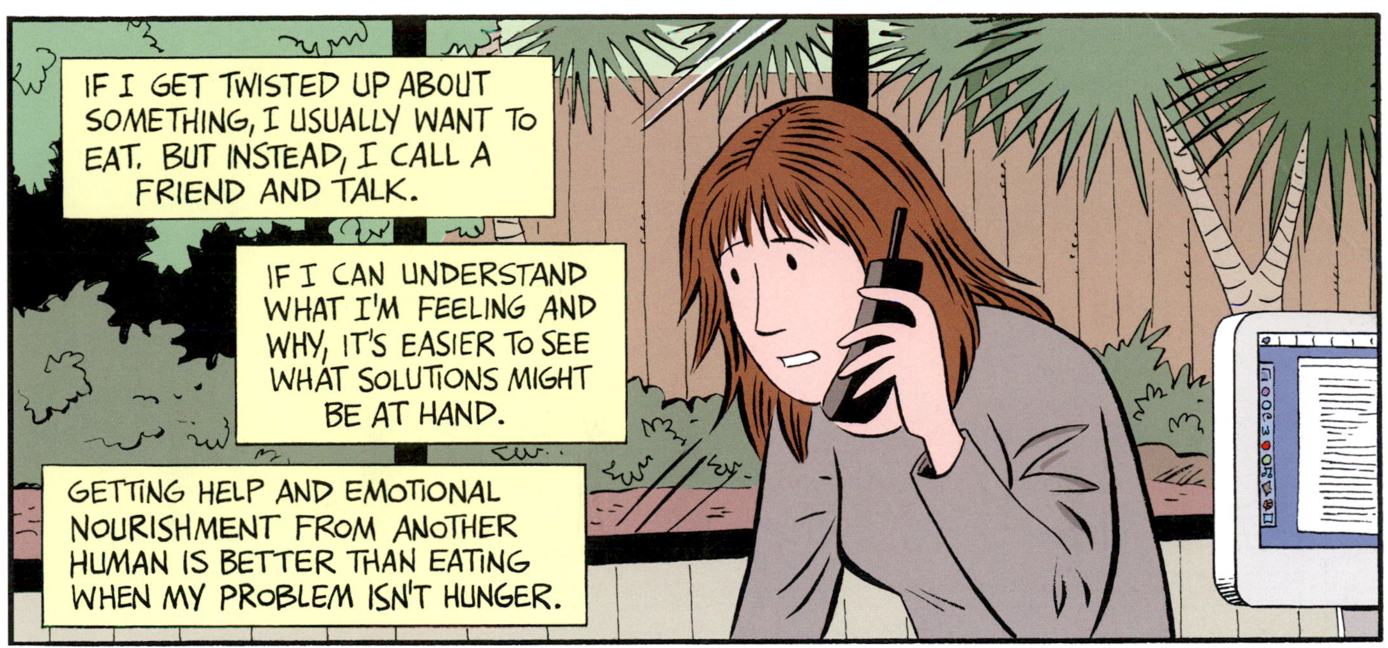
IF I GET TWISTED UP ABOUT SOMETHING, I USUALLY WANT TO EAT. BUT INSTEAD, I CALL A FRIEND AND TALK.
IF I CAN UNDERSTAND WHAT I'M FEELING AND WHY, IT'S EASIER TO SEE WHAT SOLUTIONS MIGHT BE AT HAND.
GETTING HELP AND EMOTIONAL NOURISHMENT FROM ANOTHER HUMAN IS BETTER THAN EATING WHEN MY PROBLEM ISN'T HUNGER.

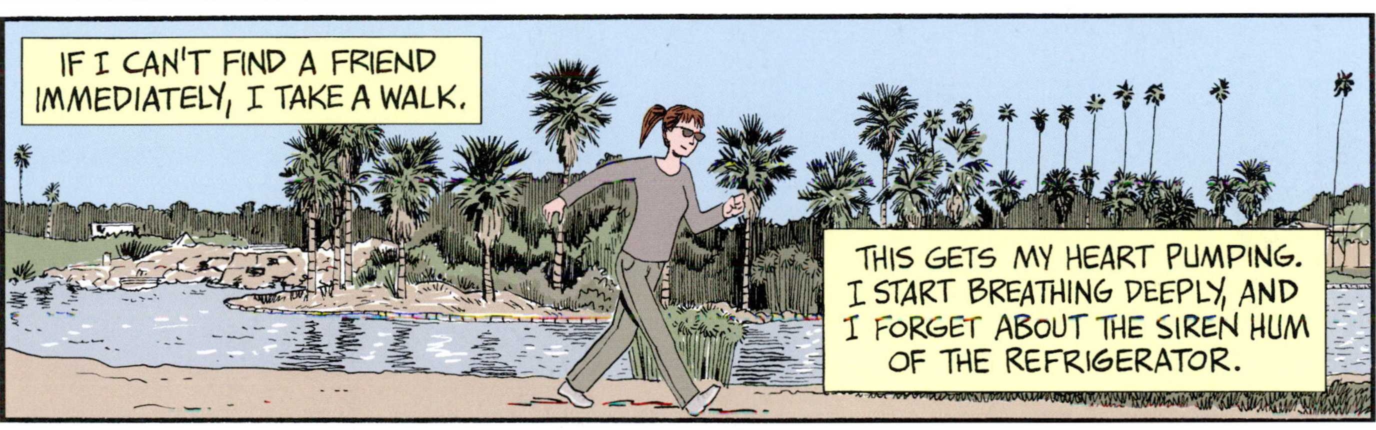
IF I CAN'T FIND A FRIEND IMMEDIATELY, I TAKE A WALK.
THIS GETS MY HEART PUMPING. I START BREATHING DEEPLY, AND I FORGET ABOUT THE SIREN HUM OF THE REFRIGERATOR.

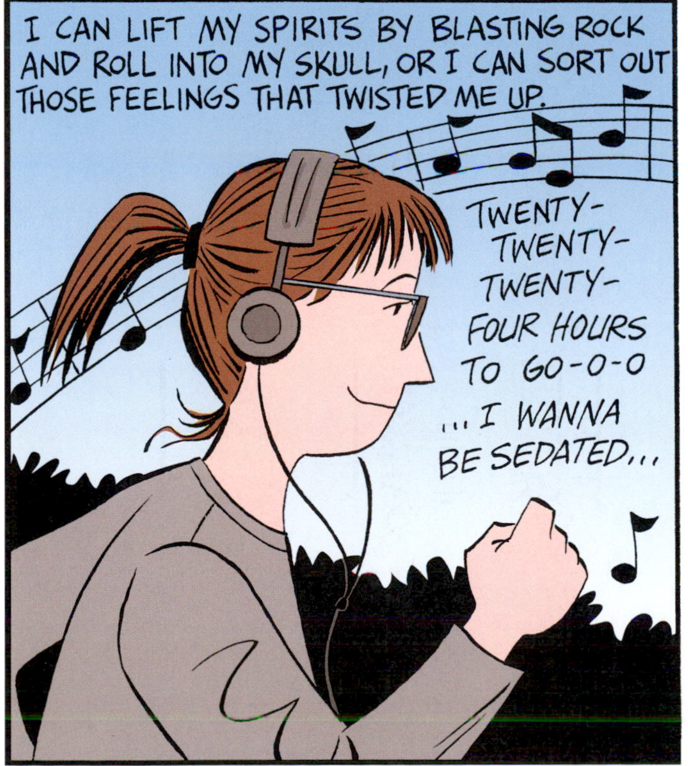
I CAN LIFT MY SPIRITS BY BLASTING ROCK AND ROLL INTO MY SKULL, OR I CAN SORT OUT THOSE FEELINGS THAT TWISTED ME UP.
TWENTY-TWENTY-TWENTY-FOUR HOURS TO GO-O-O ...I WANNA BE SEDATED...

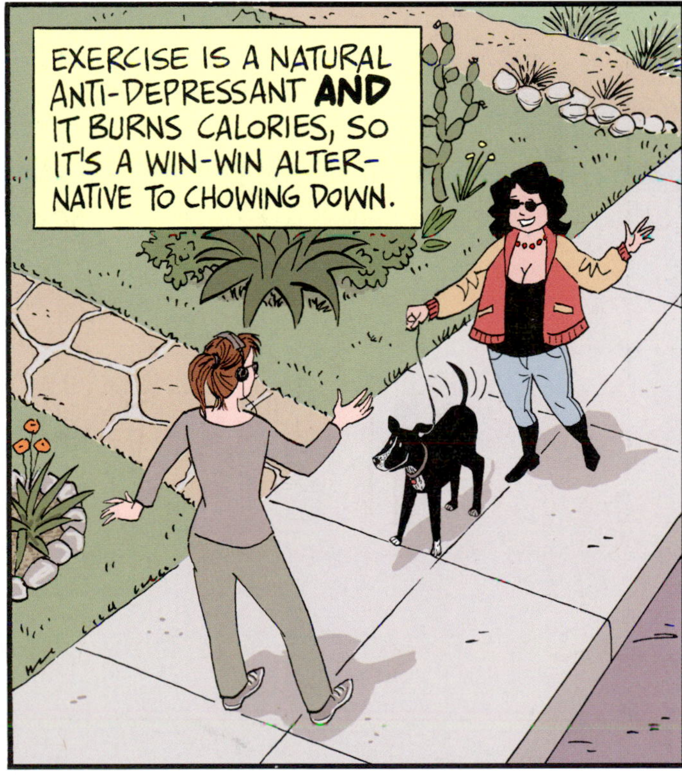
EXERCISE IS A NATURAL ANTI-DEPRESSANT **AND** IT BURNS CALORIES, SO IT'S A WIN-WIN ALTERNATIVE TO CHOWING DOWN.

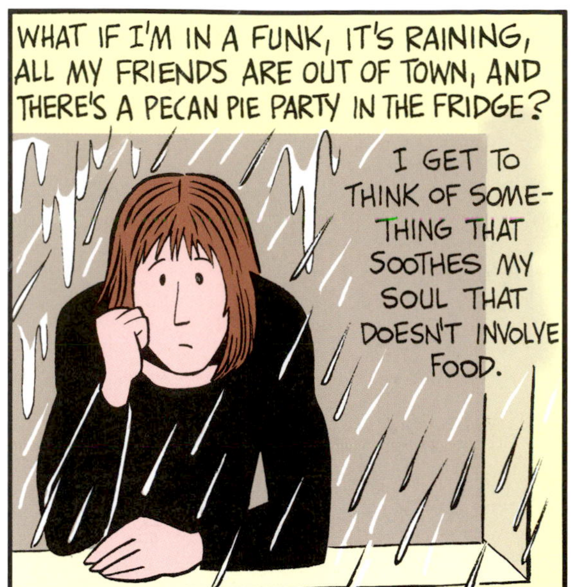
WHAT IF I'M IN A FUNK, IT'S RAINING, ALL MY FRIENDS ARE OUT OF TOWN, AND THERE'S A PECAN PIE PARTY IN THE FRIDGE?
I GET TO THINK OF SOME-THING THAT SOOTHES MY SOUL THAT DOESN'T INVOLVE FOOD.

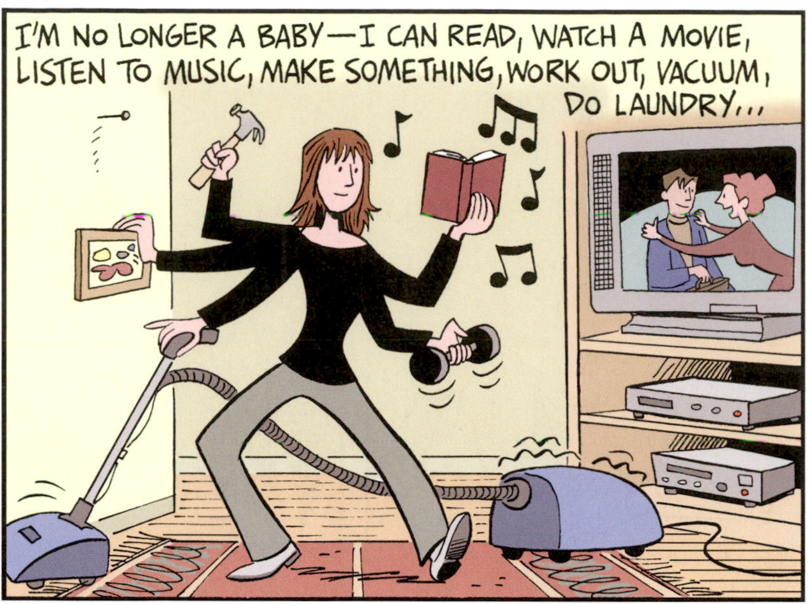
I'M NO LONGER A BABY—I CAN READ, WATCH A MOVIE, LISTEN TO MUSIC, MAKE SOMETHING, WORK OUT, VACUUM, DO LAUNDRY...

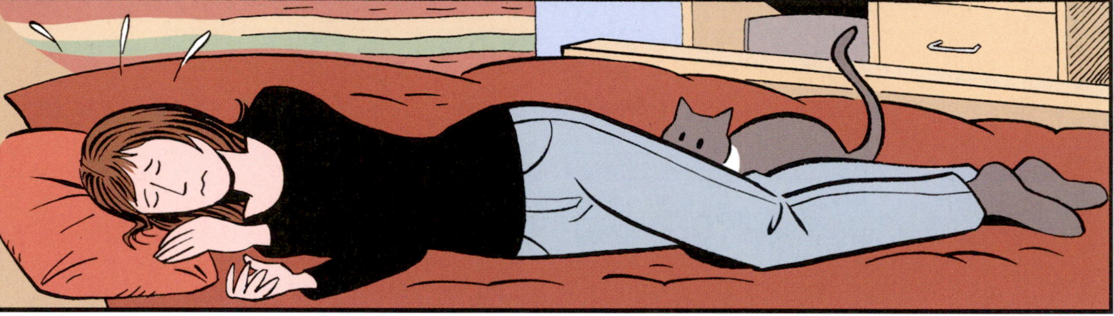
IF I'M **REALLY** STRESSED OUT I CAN HAVE A GOOD CRY. BUT NO WALLOWING! —FIVE OR TEN MINUTES TOPS.

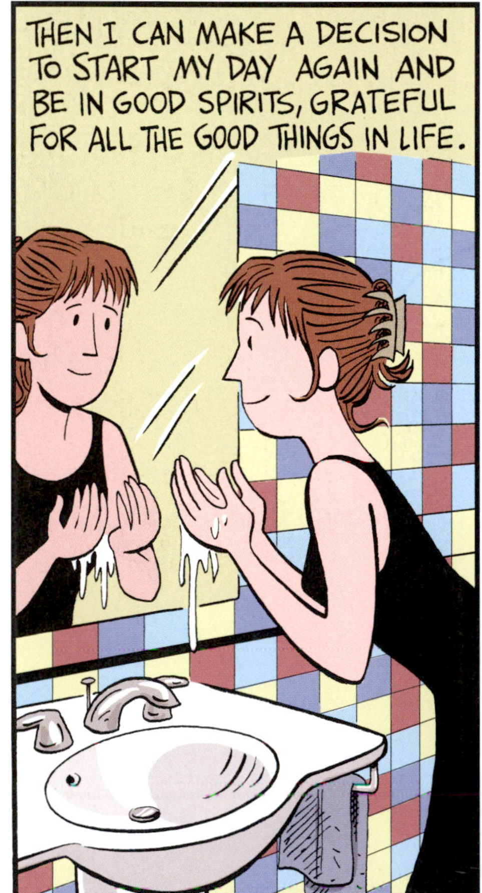
THEN I CAN MAKE A DECISION TO START MY DAY AGAIN AND BE IN GOOD SPIRITS, GRATEFUL FOR ALL THE GOOD THINGS IN LIFE.

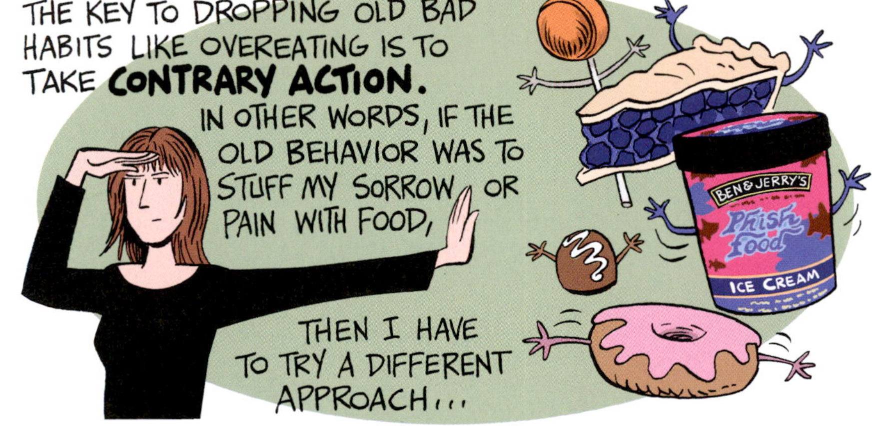
THE KEY TO DROPPING OLD BAD HABITS LIKE OVEREATING IS TO TAKE **CONTRARY ACTION.**
IN OTHER WORDS, IF THE OLD BEHAVIOR WAS TO STUFF MY SORROW OR PAIN WITH FOOD,
THEN I HAVE TO TRY A DIFFERENT APPROACH...
BEN & JERRY'S
Phish Food
ICE CREAM

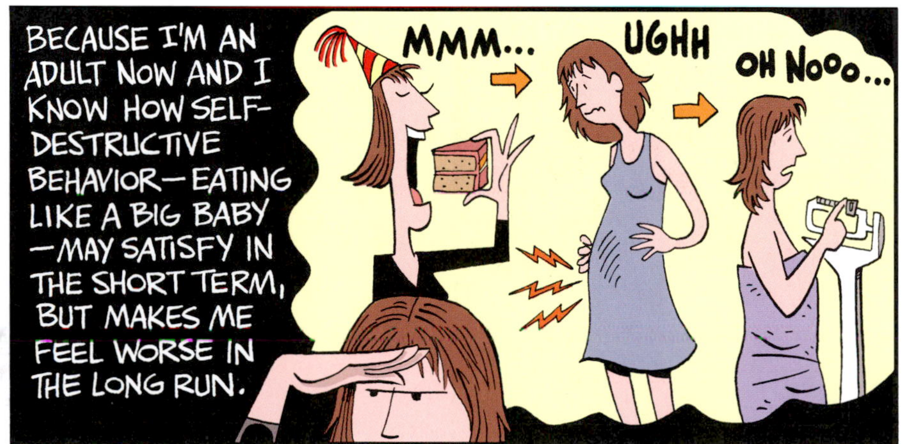
BECAUSE I'M AN ADULT NOW AND I KNOW HOW SELF-DESTRUCTIVE BEHAVIOR—EATING LIKE A BIG BABY—MAY SATISFY IN THE SHORT TERM, BUT MAKES ME FEEL WORSE IN THE LONG RUN.
MMM...
UGHH
OH NOoo...

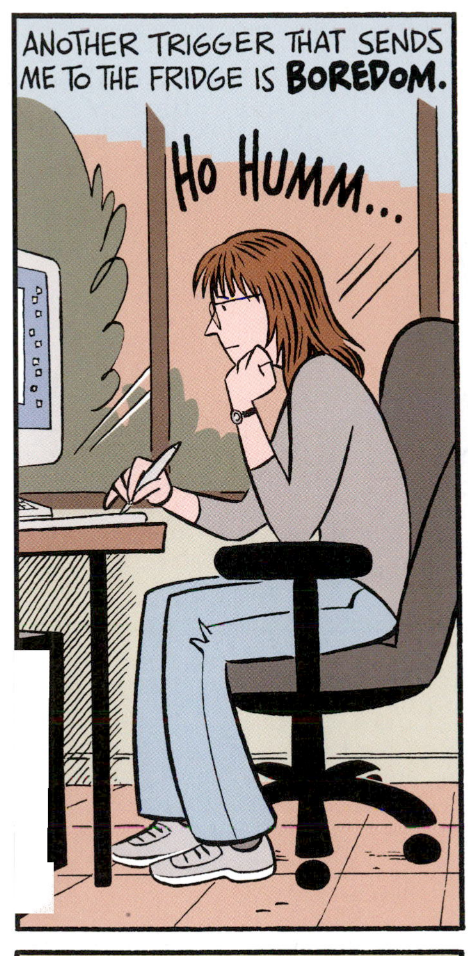
ANOTHER TRIGGER THAT SENDS ME TO THE FRIDGE IS **BOREDOM.**
HO HUMM...

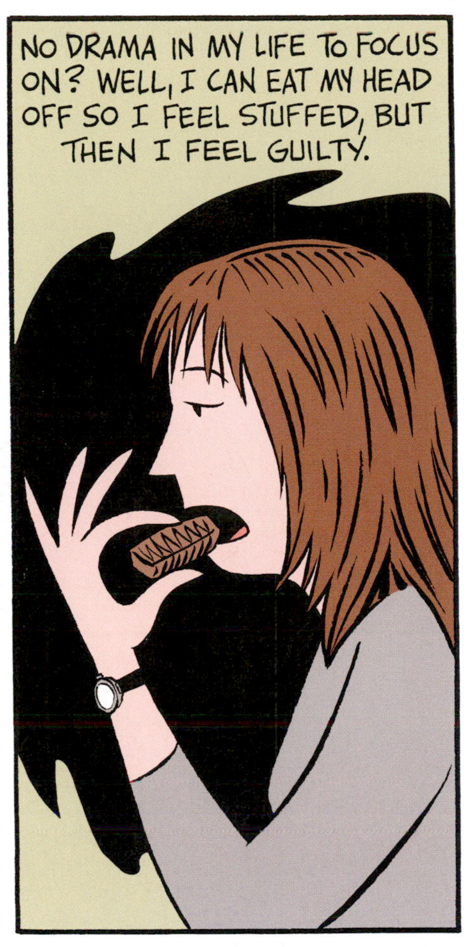
NO DRAMA IN MY LIFE TO FOCUS ON? WELL, I CAN EAT MY HEAD OFF SO I FEEL STUFFED, BUT THEN I FEEL GUILTY.

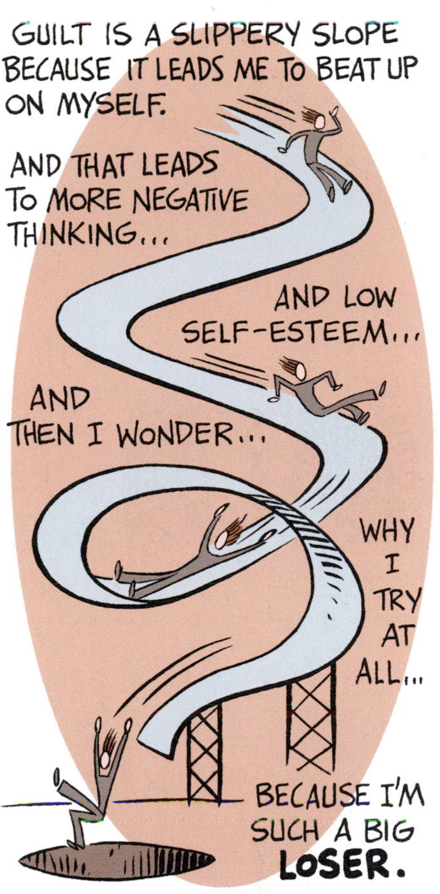
GUILT IS A SLIPPERY SLOPE BECAUSE IT LEADS ME TO BEAT UP ON MYSELF.
AND THAT LEADS TO MORE NEGATIVE THINKING...
AND LOW SELF-ESTEEM...
AND THEN I WONDER...
WHY I TRY AT ALL...
BECAUSE I'M SUCH A BIG **LOSER.**

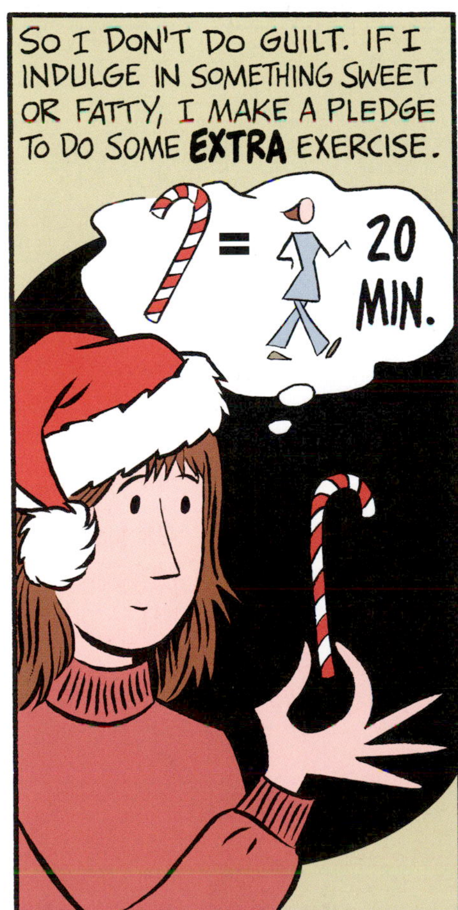
SO I DON'T DO GUILT. IF I INDULGE IN SOMETHING SWEET OR FATTY, I MAKE A PLEDGE TO DO SOME **EXTRA** EXERCISE.
= 20 MIN.

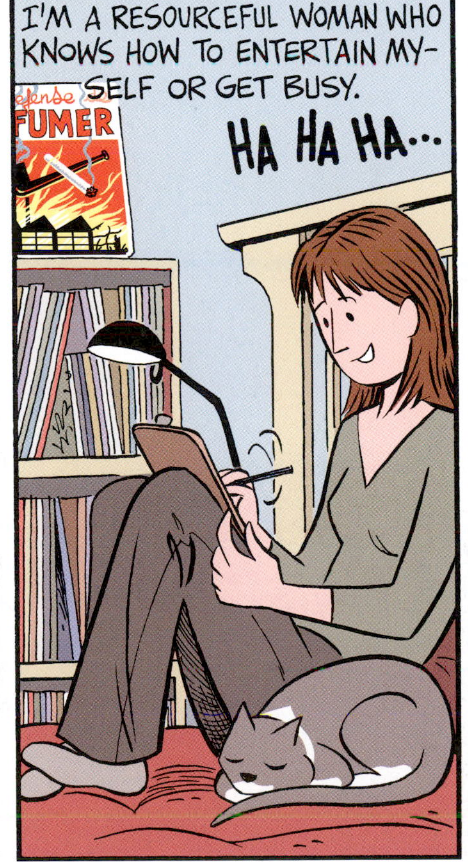
AND I STAY OUT OF BOREDOM. I'M A RESOURCEFUL WOMAN WHO KNOWS HOW TO ENTERTAIN MYSELF OR GET BUSY.
FUMER
HA HA HA...

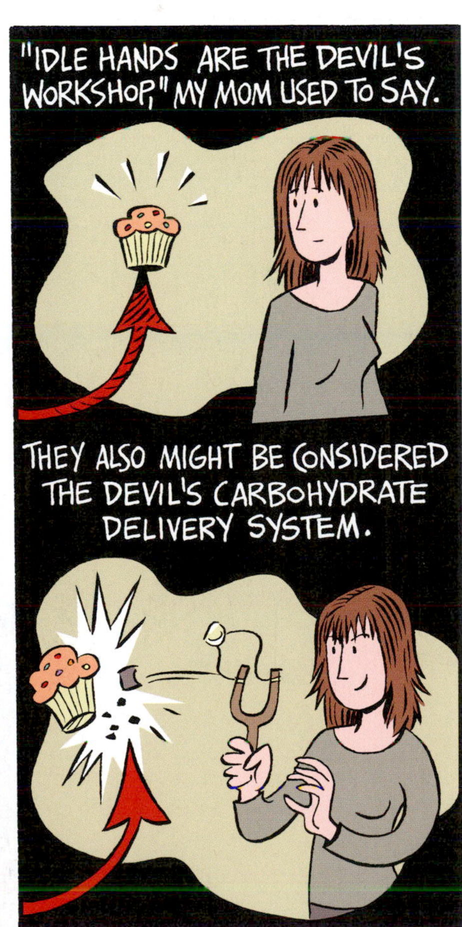
"IDLE HANDS ARE THE DEVIL'S WORKSHOP," MY MOM USED TO SAY.
THEY ALSO MIGHT BE CONSIDERED THE DEVIL'S CARBOHYDRATE DELIVERY SYSTEM.

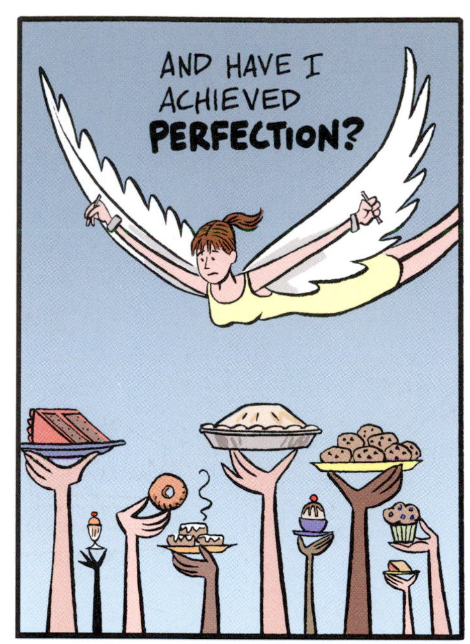
AND HAVE I ACHIEVED **PERFECTION?**

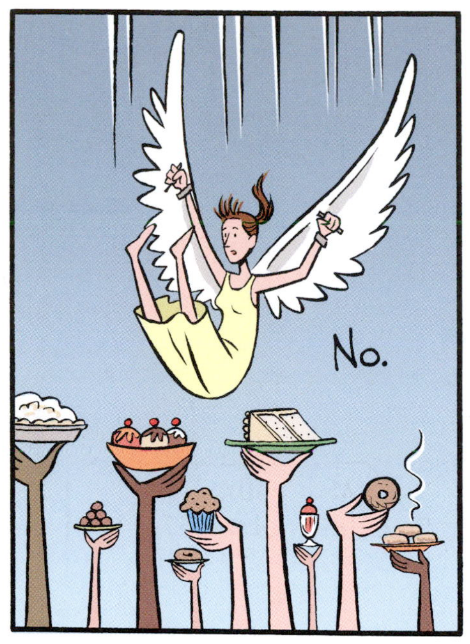
No.

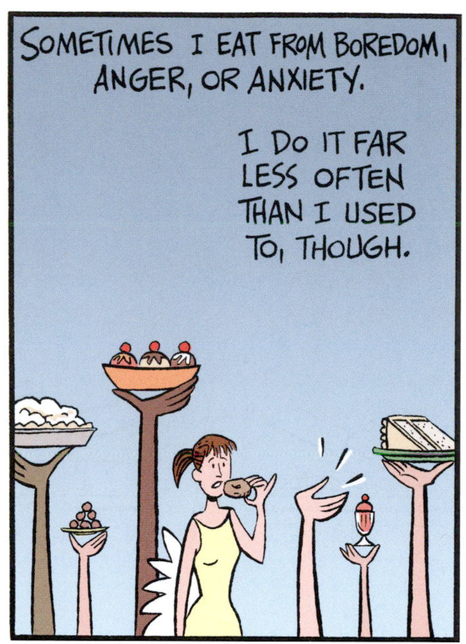
SOMETIMES I EAT FROM BOREDOM, ANGER, OR ANXIETY.
I DO IT FAR LESS OFTEN THAN I USED TO, THOUGH.

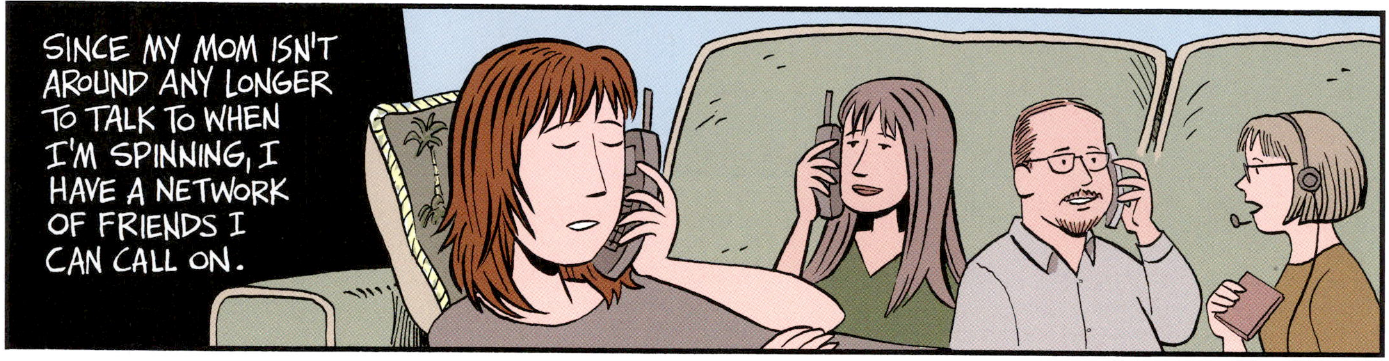
SINCE MY MOM ISN'T AROUND ANY LONGER TO TALK TO WHEN I'M SPINNING, I HAVE A NETWORK OF FRIENDS I CAN CALL ON.

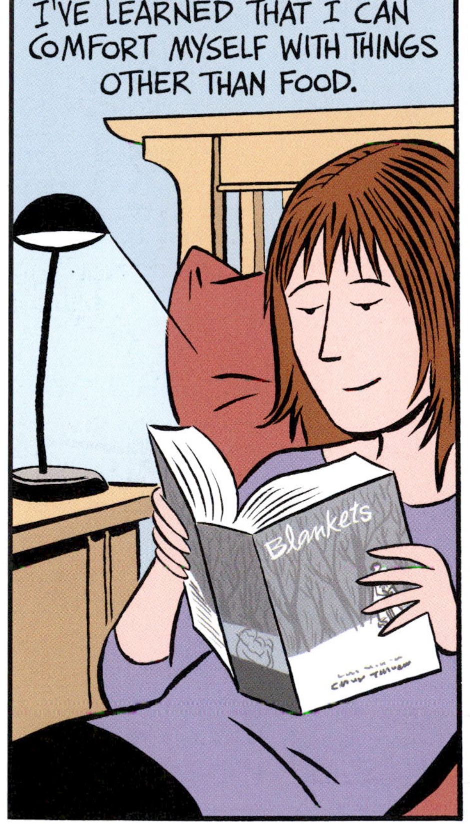
I'VE LEARNED THAT I CAN COMFORT MYSELF WITH THINGS OTHER THAN FOOD.
Blankets

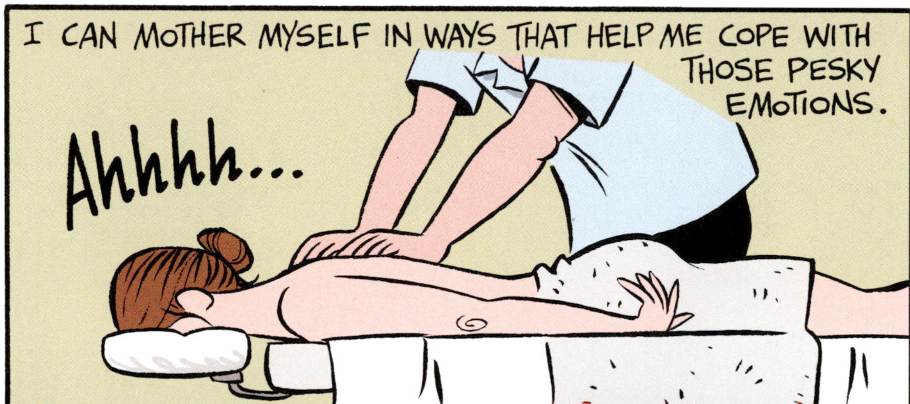
I CAN MOTHER MYSELF IN WAYS THAT HELP ME COPE WITH THOSE PESKY EMOTIONS.
Ahhhh...

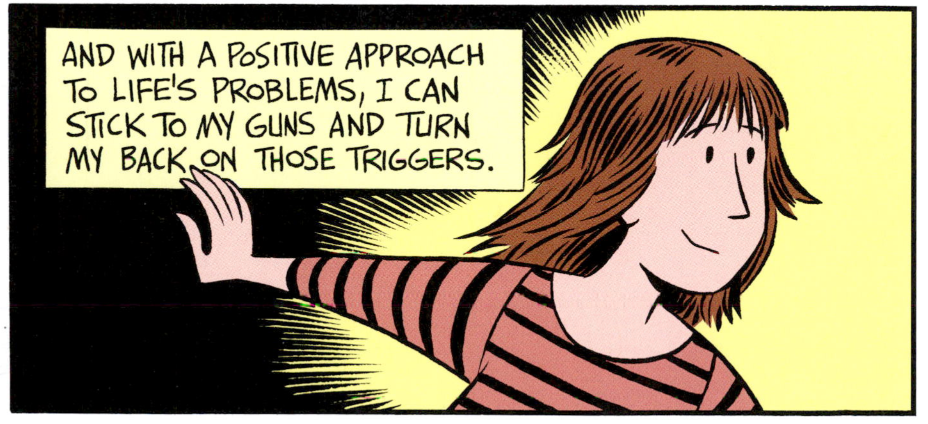
AND WITH A POSITIVE APPROACH TO LIFE'S PROBLEMS, I CAN STICK TO MY GUNS AND TURN MY BACK ON THOSE TRIGGERS.

# the ANTHROPOLOGIZER

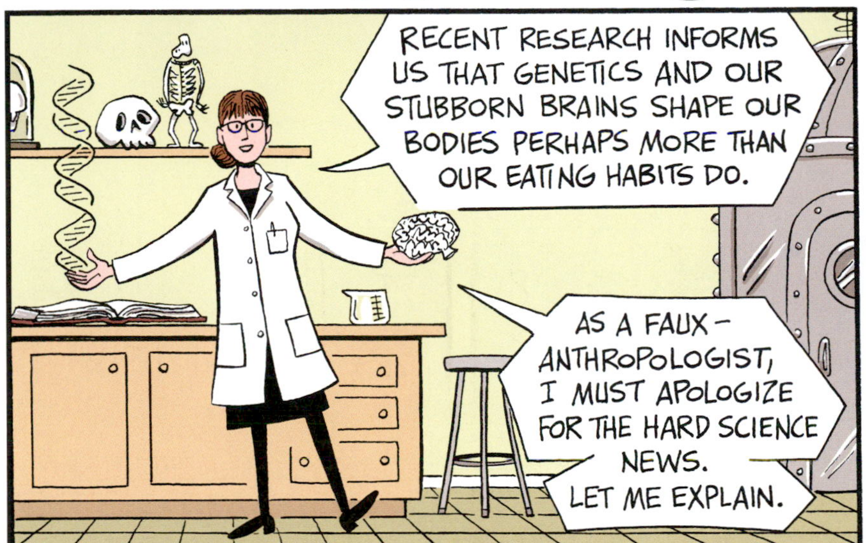

RECENT RESEARCH INFORMS US THAT GENETICS AND OUR STUBBORN BRAINS SHAPE OUR BODIES PERHAPS MORE THAN OUR EATING HABITS DO.
AS A FAUX-ANTHROPOLOGIST, I MUST APOLOGIZE FOR THE HARD SCIENCE NEWS. LET ME EXPLAIN.


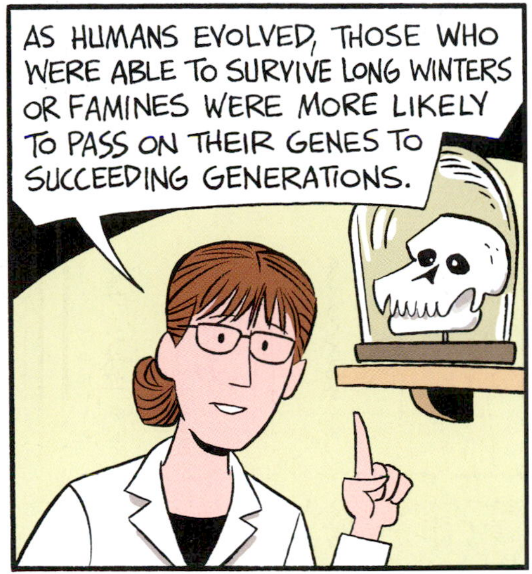

AS HUMANS EVOLVED, THOSE WHO WERE ABLE TO SURVIVE LONG WINTERS OR FAMINES WERE MORE LIKELY TO PASS ON THEIR GENES TO SUCCEEDING GENERATIONS.


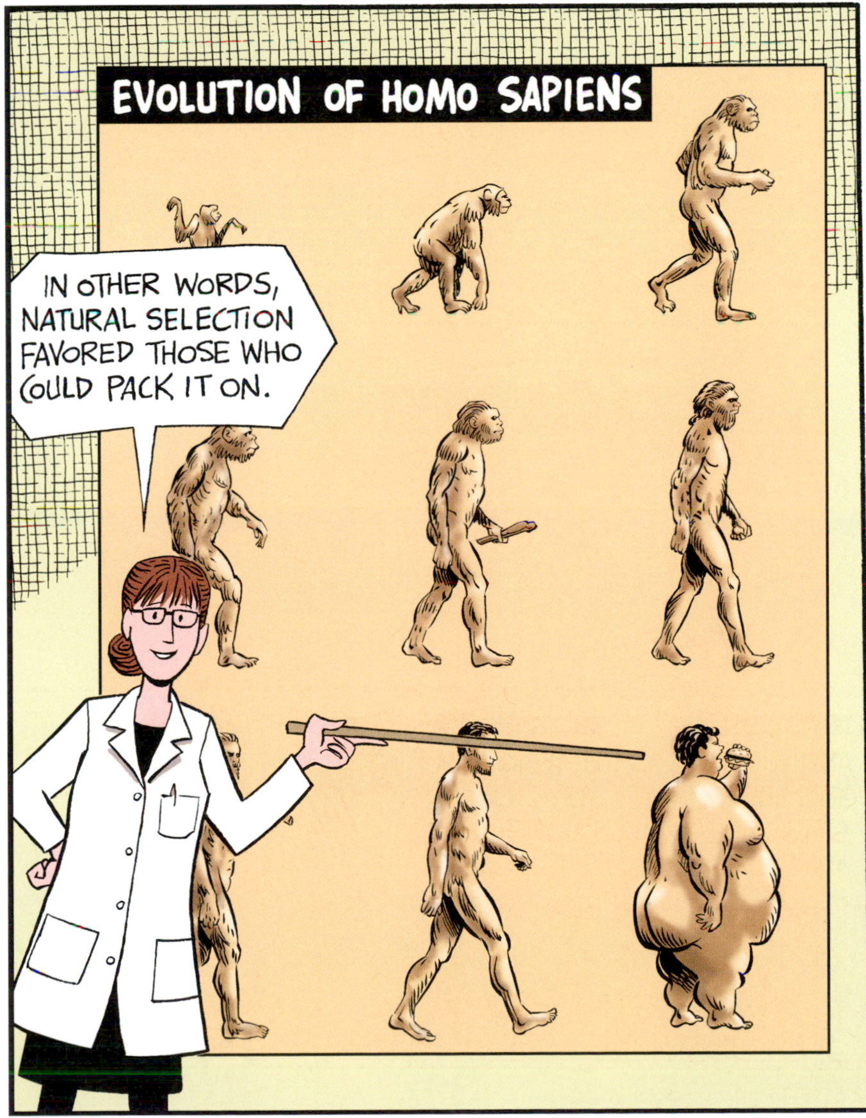

EVOLUTION OF HOMO SAPIENS
IN OTHER WORDS, NATURAL SELECTION FAVORED THOSE WHO COULD PACK IT ON.


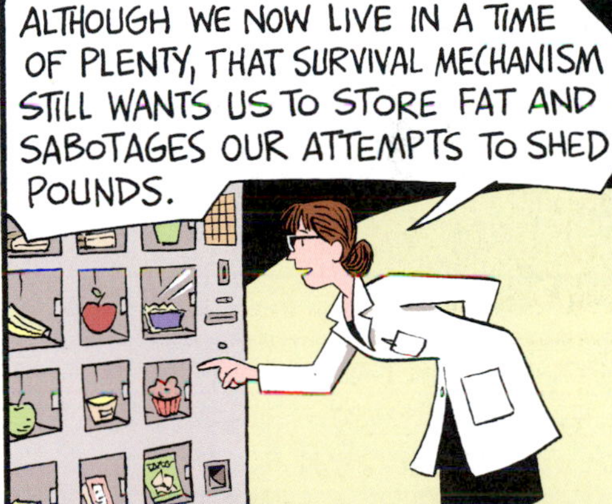

ALTHOUGH WE NOW LIVE IN A TIME OF PLENTY, THAT SURVIVAL MECHANISM STILL WANTS US TO STORE FAT AND SABOTAGES OUR ATTEMPTS TO SHED POUNDS.


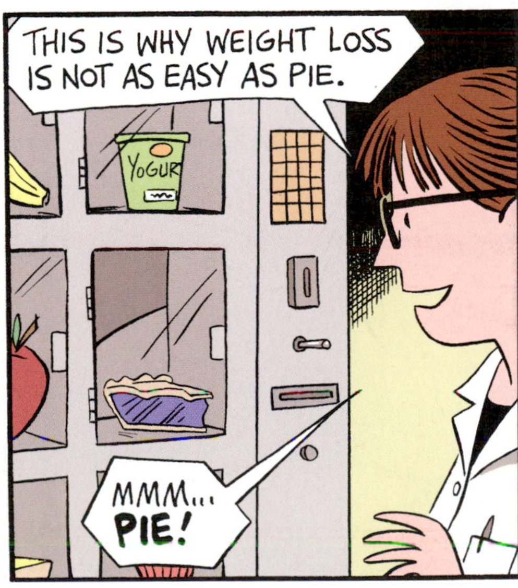

THIS IS WHY WEIGHT LOSS IS NOT AS EASY AS PIE.
YOGUR
MMM... PIE!

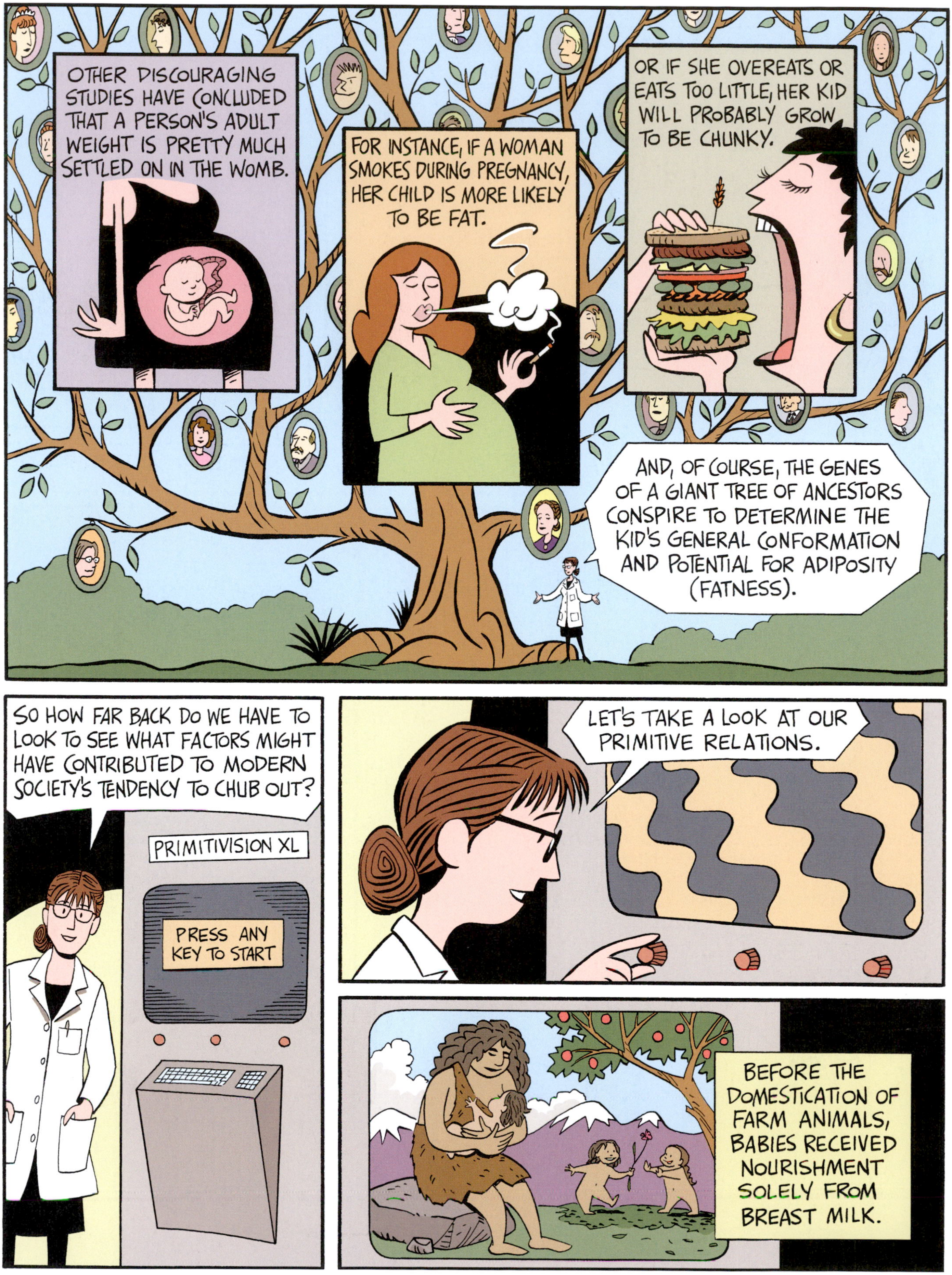

OTHER DISCOURAGING STUDIES HAVE CONCLUDED THAT A PERSON'S ADULT WEIGHT IS PRETTY MUCH SETTLED ON IN THE WOMB.

FOR INSTANCE, IF A WOMAN SMOKES DURING PREGNANCY, HER CHILD IS MORE LIKELY TO BE FAT.

OR IF SHE OVEREATS OR EATS TOO LITTLE, HER KID WILL PROBABLY GROW TO BE CHUNKY.

AND, OF COURSE, THE GENES OF A GIANT TREE OF ANCESTORS CONSPIRE TO DETERMINE THE KID'S GENERAL CONFORMATION AND POTENTIAL FOR ADIPOSITY (FATNESS).

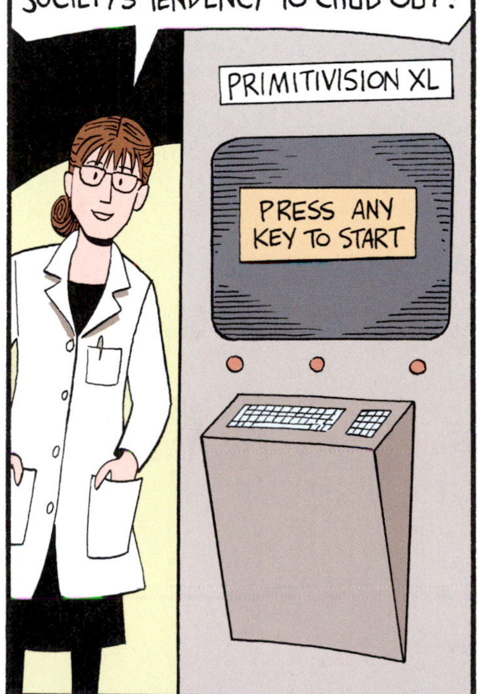

SO HOW FAR BACK DO WE HAVE TO LOOK TO SEE WHAT FACTORS MIGHT HAVE CONTRIBUTED TO MODERN SOCIETY'S TENDENCY TO CHUB OUT?
PRIMITIVISION XL
PRESS ANY KEY TO START

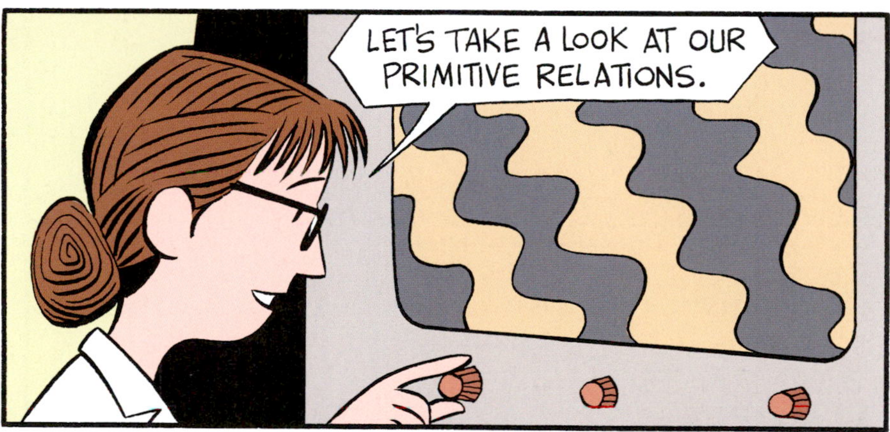

LET'S TAKE A LOOK AT OUR PRIMITIVE RELATIONS.

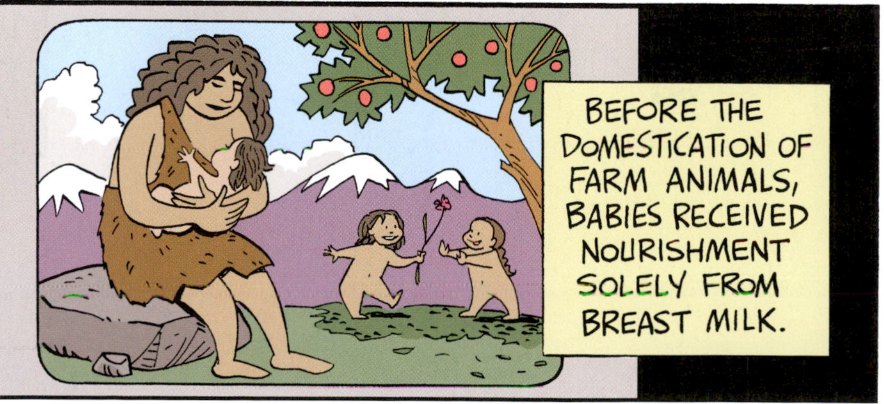

BEFORE THE DOMESTICATION OF FARM ANIMALS, BABIES RECEIVED NOURISHMENT SOLELY FROM BREAST MILK.

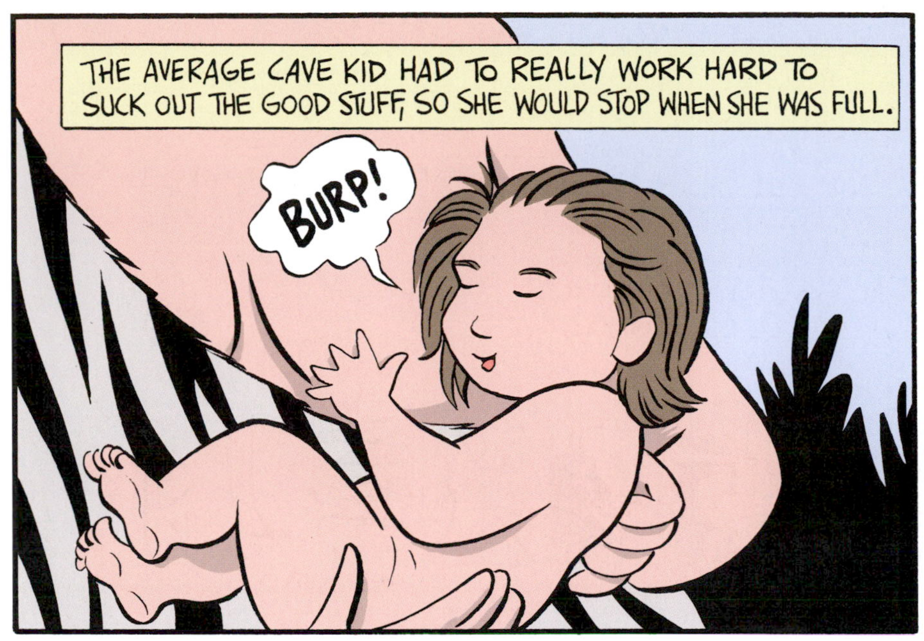
THE AVERAGE CAVE KID HAD TO REALLY WORK HARD TO SUCK OUT THE GOOD STUFF, SO SHE WOULD STOP WHEN SHE WAS FULL.
BURP!

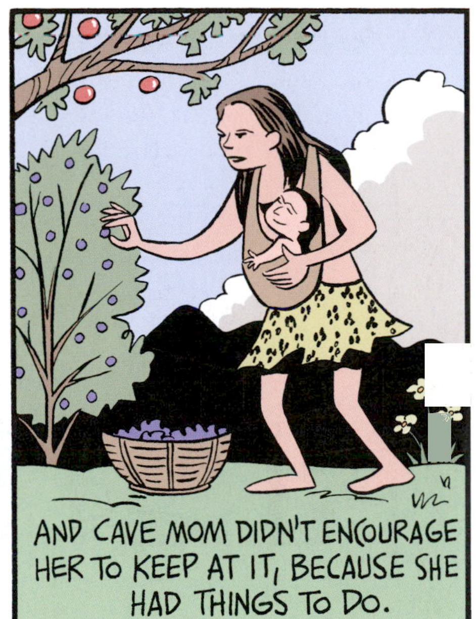
AND CAVE MOM DIDN'T ENCOURAGE HER TO KEEP AT IT, BECAUSE SHE HAD THINGS TO DO.

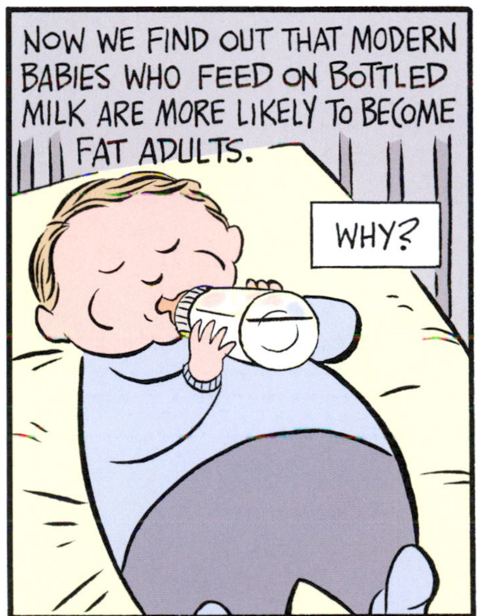
NOW WE FIND OUT THAT MODERN BABIES WHO FEED ON BOTTLED MILK ARE MORE LIKELY TO BECOME FAT ADULTS.
WHY?

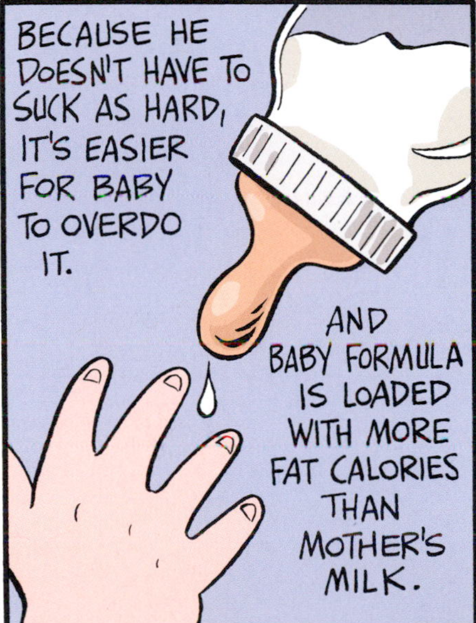
BECAUSE HE DOESN'T HAVE TO SUCK AS HARD, IT'S EASIER FOR BABY TO OVERDO IT.
AND BABY FORMULA IS LOADED WITH MORE FAT CALORIES THAN MOTHER'S MILK.

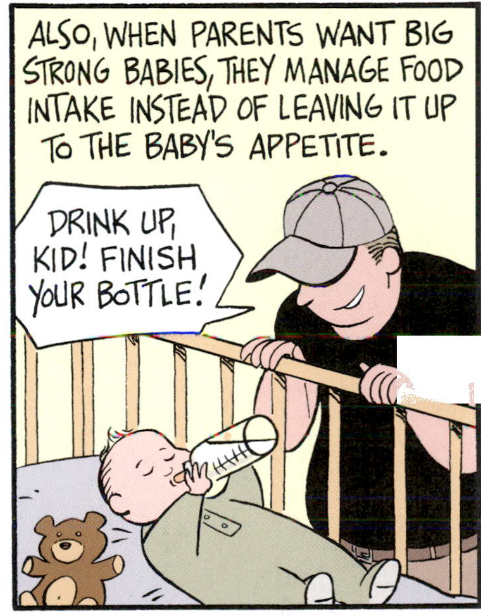
ALSO, WHEN PARENTS WANT BIG STRONG BABIES, THEY MANAGE FOOD INTAKE INSTEAD OF LEAVING IT UP TO THE BABY'S APPETITE.
DRINK UP, KID! FINISH YOUR BOTTLE!

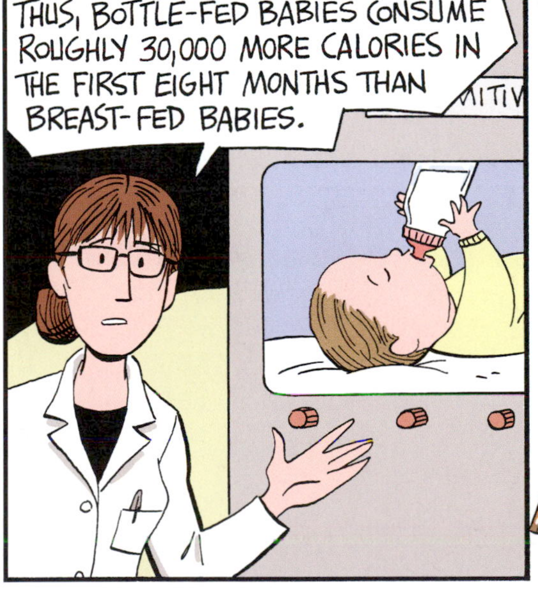
THUS, BOTTLE-FED BABIES CONSUME ROUGHLY 30,000 MORE CALORIES IN THE FIRST EIGHT MONTHS THAN BREAST-FED BABIES.

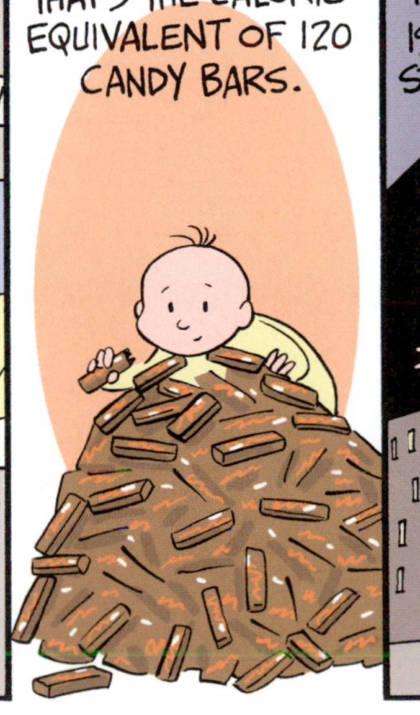
THAT'S THE CALORIC EQUIVALENT OF 120 CANDY BARS.

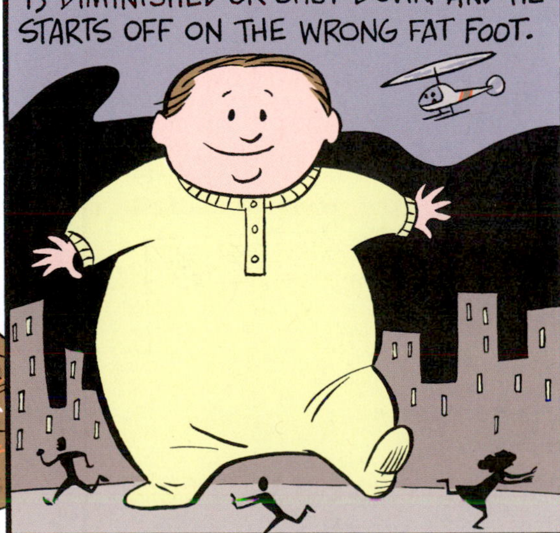
THE KID'S NATURAL APPETITE CONTROL IS DIMINISHED OR SHUT DOWN AND HE STARTS OFF ON THE WRONG FAT FOOT.

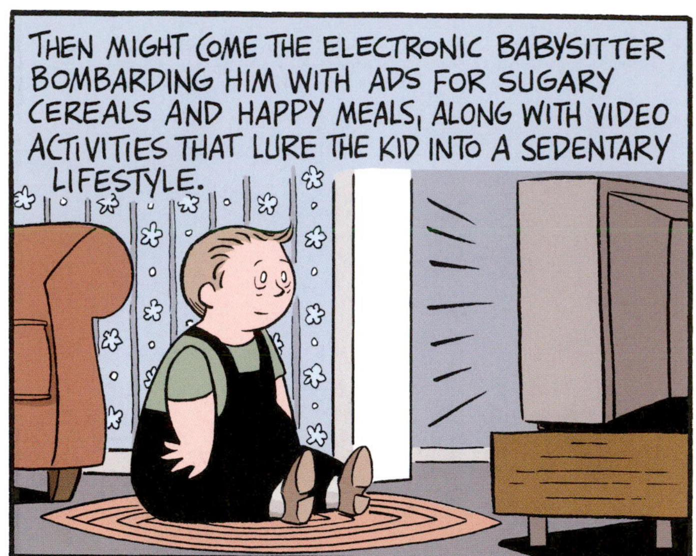
THEN MIGHT COME THE ELECTRONIC BABYSITTER BOMBARDING HIM WITH ADS FOR SUGARY CEREALS AND HAPPY MEALS, ALONG WITH VIDEO ACTIVITIES THAT LURE THE KID INTO A SEDENTARY LIFESTYLE.

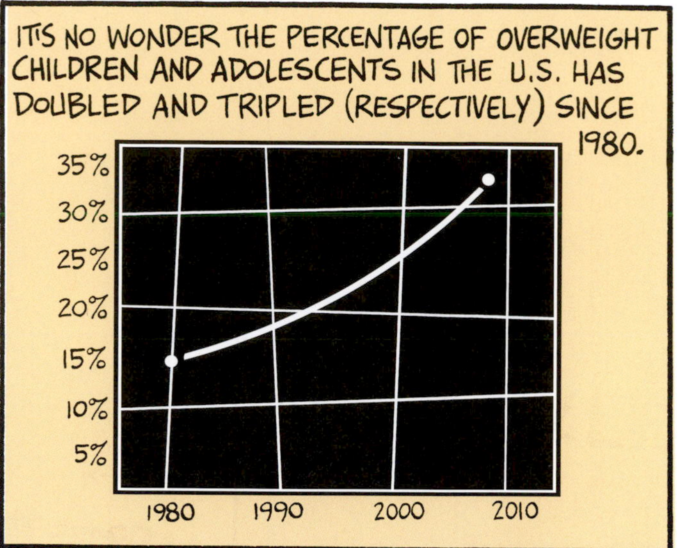
IT'S NO WONDER THE PERCENTAGE OF OVERWEIGHT CHILDREN AND ADOLESCENTS IN THE U.S. HAS DOUBLED AND TRIPLED (RESPECTIVELY) SINCE 1980.
35%
30%
25%
20%
15%
10%
5%
1980
1990
2000
2010

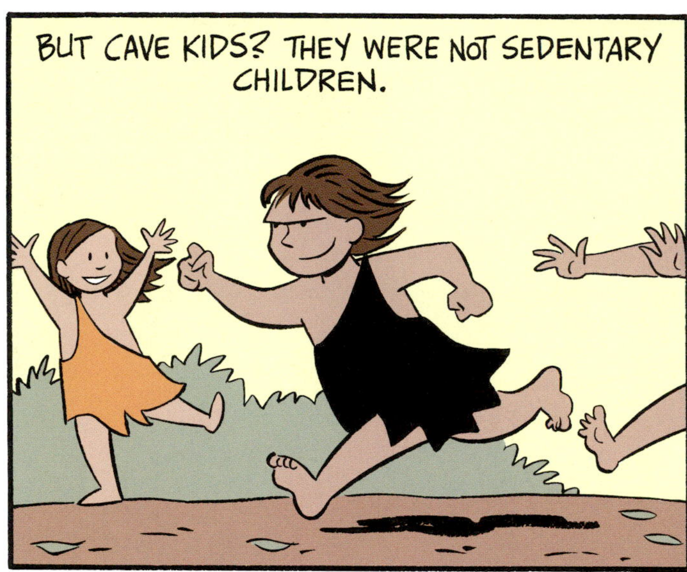
BUT CAVE KIDS? THEY WERE NOT SEDENTARY CHILDREN.

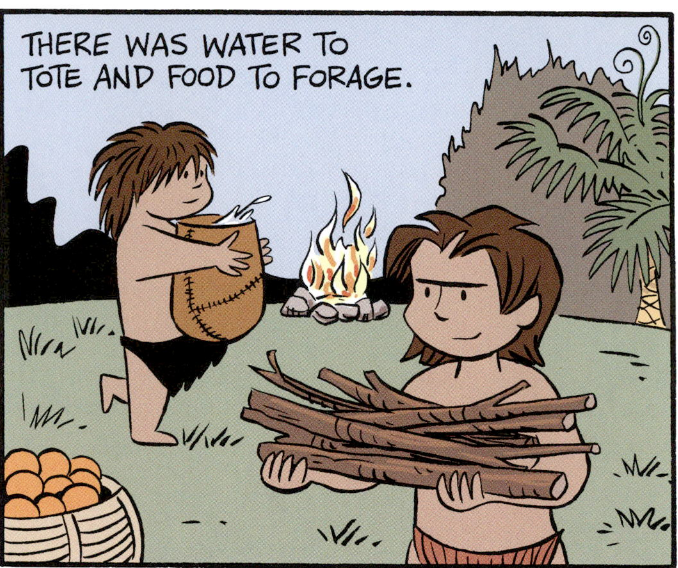
THERE WAS WATER TO TOTE AND FOOD TO FORAGE.

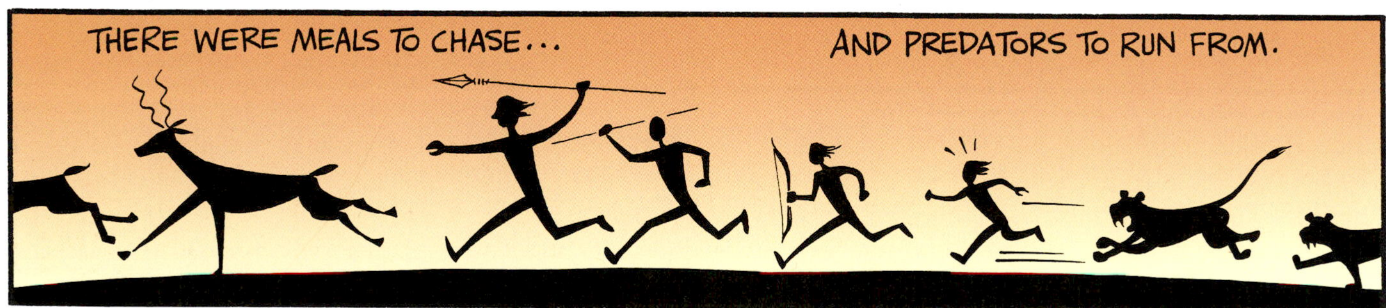
THERE WERE MEALS TO CHASE...
AND PREDATORS TO RUN FROM.

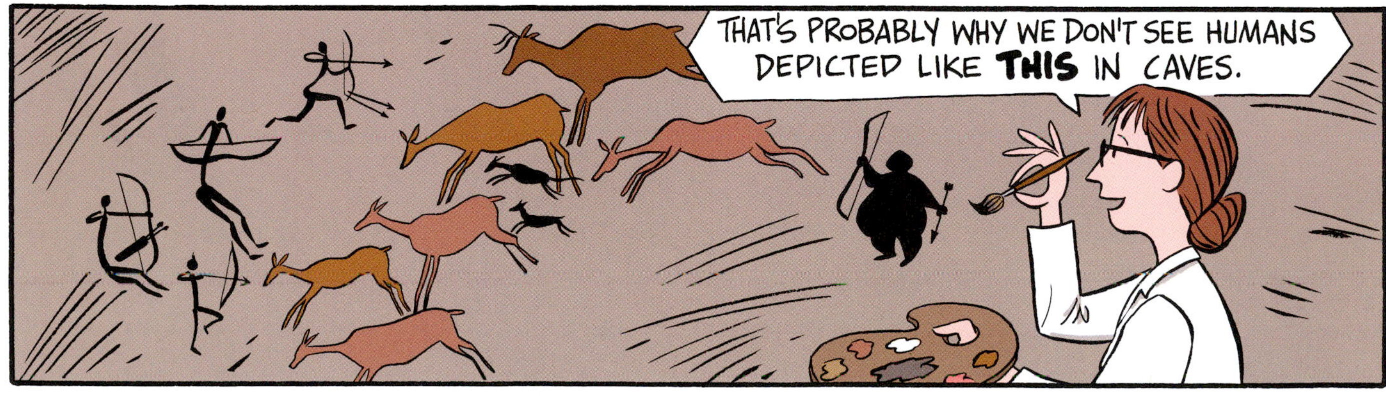
THAT'S PROBABLY WHY WE DON'T SEE HUMANS DEPICTED LIKE THIS IN CAVES.

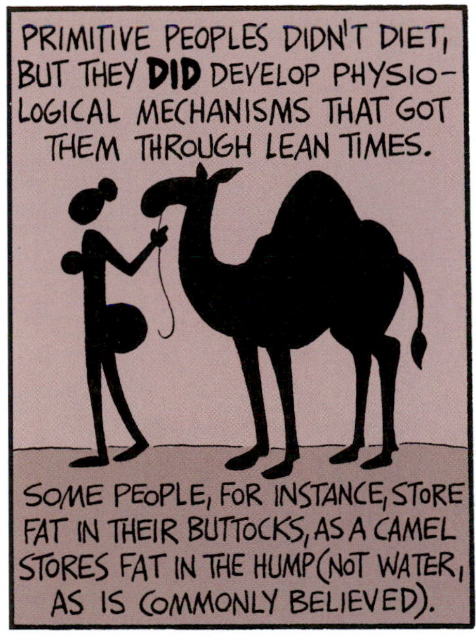
PRIMITIVE PEOPLES DIDN'T DIET, BUT THEY **DID** DEVELOP PHYSIOLOGICAL MECHANISMS THAT GOT THEM THROUGH LEAN TIMES.
SOME PEOPLE, FOR INSTANCE, STORE FAT IN THEIR BUTTOCKS, AS A CAMEL STORES FAT IN THE HUMP (NOT WATER, AS IS COMMONLY BELIEVED).

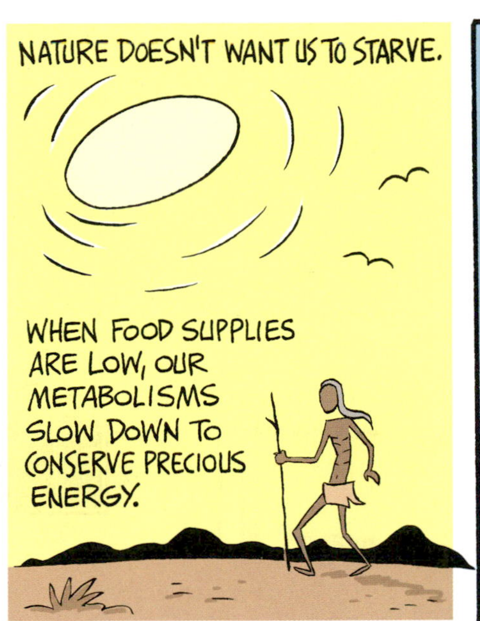
NATURE DOESN'T WANT US TO STARVE.
WHEN FOOD SUPPLIES ARE LOW, OUR METABOLISMS SLOW DOWN TO CONSERVE PRECIOUS ENERGY.

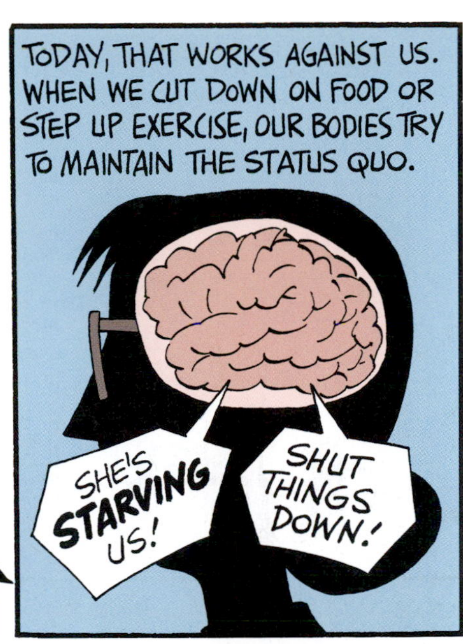
TODAY, THAT WORKS AGAINST US. WHEN WE CUT DOWN ON FOOD OR STEP UP EXERCISE, OUR BODIES TRY TO MAINTAIN THE STATUS QUO.
SHE'S **STARVING** US!
SHUT THINGS DOWN!

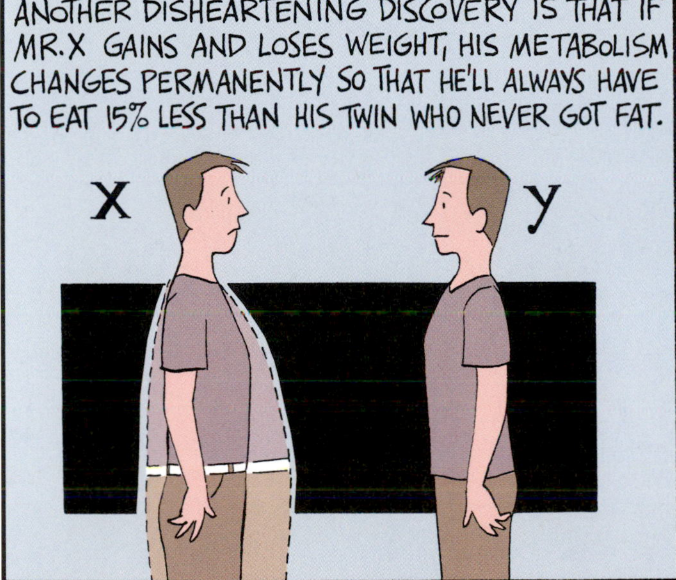
ANOTHER DISHEARTENING DISCOVERY IS THAT IF MR. X GAINS AND LOSES WEIGHT, HIS METABOLISM CHANGES PERMANENTLY SO THAT HE'LL ALWAYS HAVE TO EAT 15% LESS THAN HIS TWIN WHO NEVER GOT FAT.
X
Y

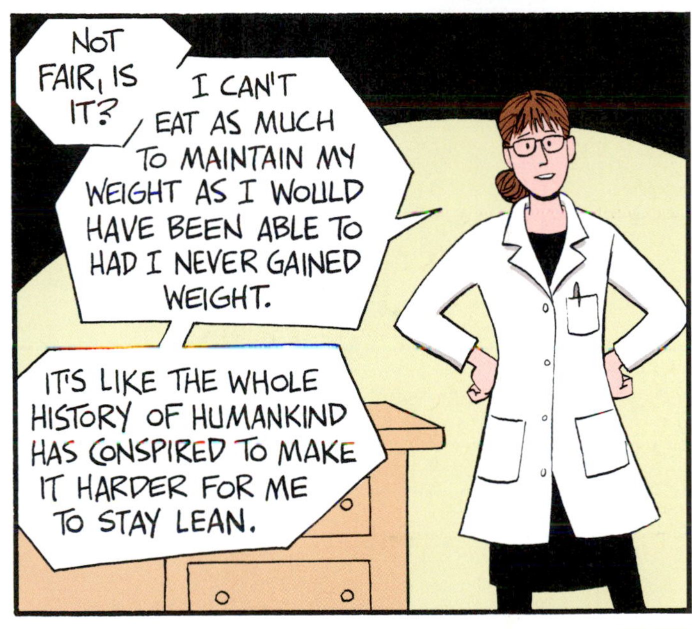
NOT FAIR, IS IT?
I CAN'T EAT AS MUCH TO MAINTAIN MY WEIGHT AS I WOULD HAVE BEEN ABLE TO HAD I NEVER GAINED WEIGHT.
IT'S LIKE THE WHOLE HISTORY OF HUMANKIND HAS CONSPIRED TO MAKE IT HARDER FOR ME TO STAY LEAN.

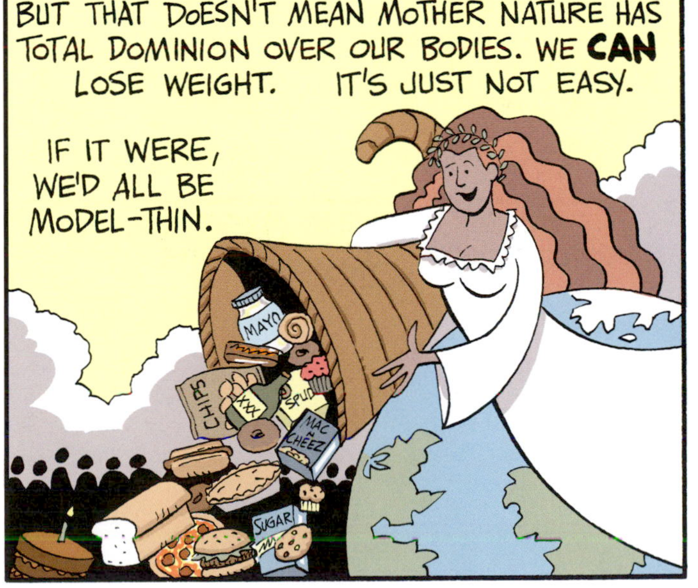
BUT THAT DOESN'T MEAN MOTHER NATURE HAS TOTAL DOMINION OVER OUR BODIES. WE **CAN** LOSE WEIGHT. IT'S JUST NOT EASY.
IF IT WERE, WE'D ALL BE MODEL-THIN.
MAYO
CHIPS
SPUD
MAC CHEEZ
SUGAR

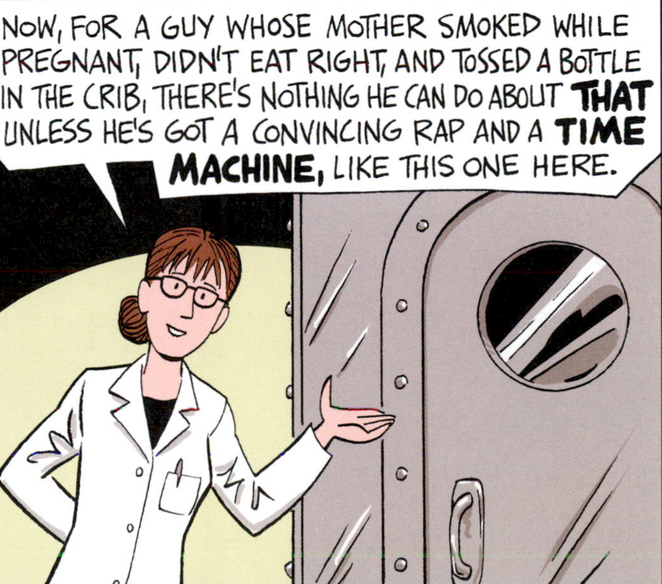
NOW, FOR A GUY WHOSE MOTHER SMOKED WHILE PREGNANT, DIDN'T EAT RIGHT, AND TOSSED A BOTTLE IN THE CRIB, THERE'S NOTHING HE CAN DO ABOUT **THAT** UNLESS HE'S GOT A CONVINCING RAP AND A **TIME MACHINE**, LIKE THIS ONE HERE.

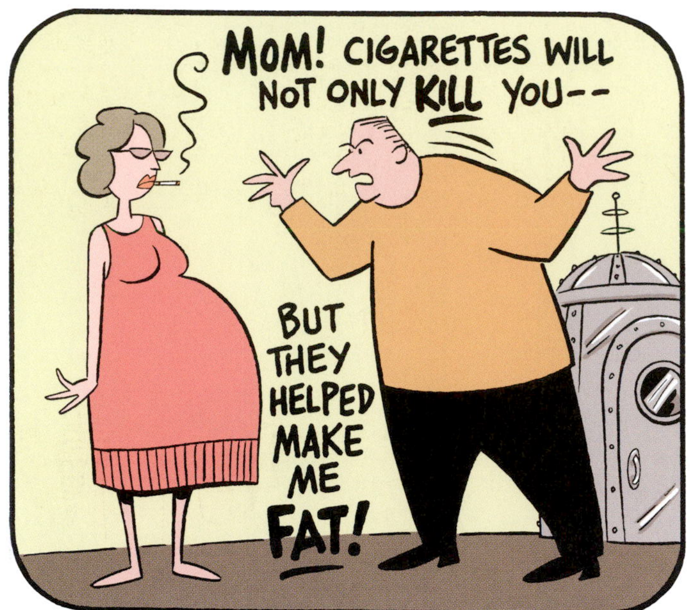
MOM! CIGARETTES WILL NOT ONLY KILL YOU--
BUT THEY HELPED MAKE ME FAT!

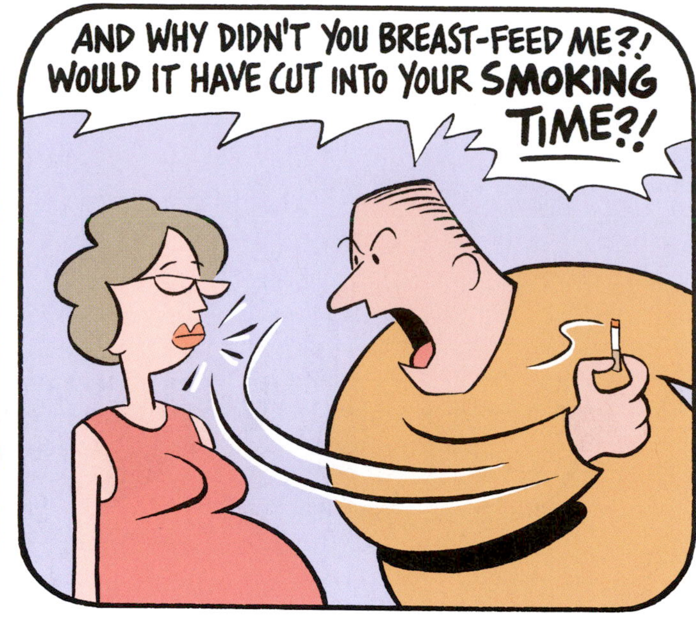
AND WHY DIDN'T YOU BREAST-FEED ME?! WOULD IT HAVE CUT INTO YOUR SMOKING TIME?!

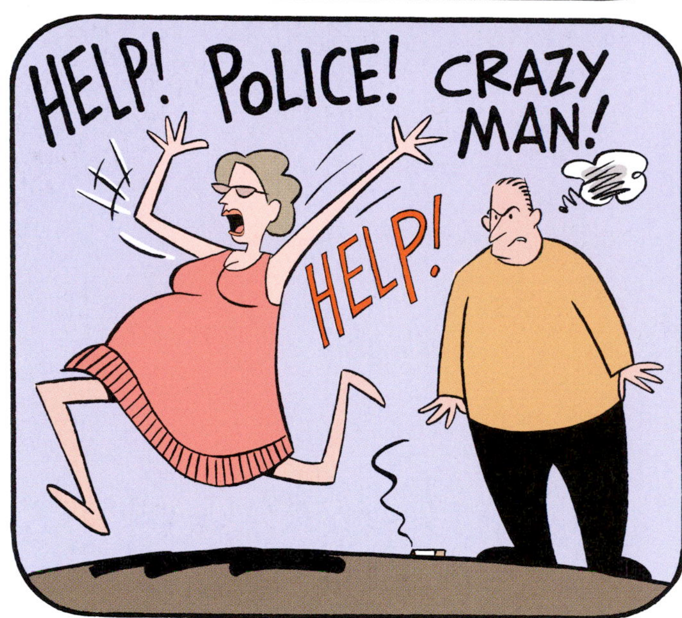
HELP! POLICE! CRAZY MAN!
HELP!

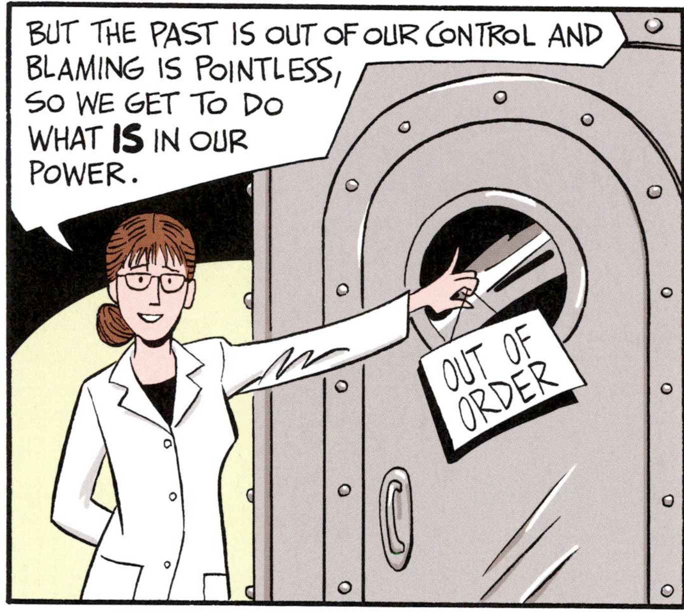
BUT THE PAST IS OUT OF OUR CONTROL AND BLAMING IS POINTLESS, SO WE GET TO DO WHAT IS IN OUR POWER.
OUT OF ORDER

ONE THING WE CAN DO IS BE AWARE. INFORMATION HAS COME TO LIGHT THAT OUR **FRIENDS** CAN INFLUENCE HOW MUCH WE WEIGH.

SOCIETAL STANDARDS HAVE A POWERFUL EFFECT.

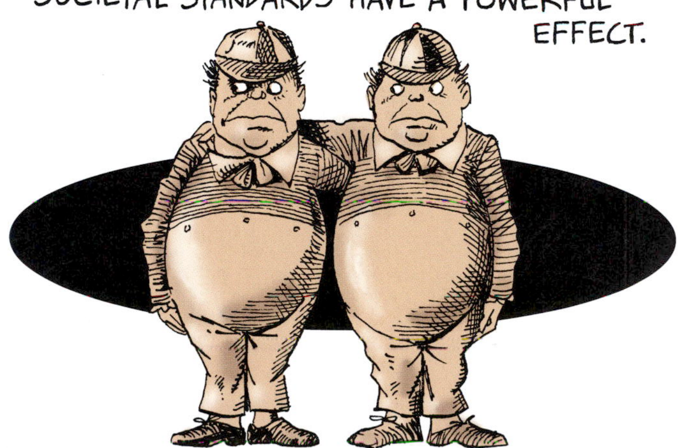

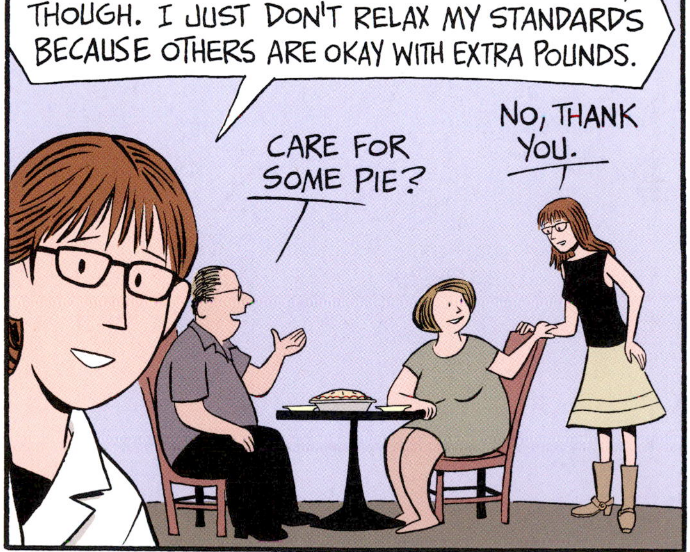
I DON'T HAVE TO AVOID MY HEFTY FRIENDS, THOUGH. I JUST DON'T RELAX MY STANDARDS BECAUSE OTHERS ARE OKAY WITH EXTRA POUNDS.
CARE FOR SOME PIE?
NO, THANK YOU.

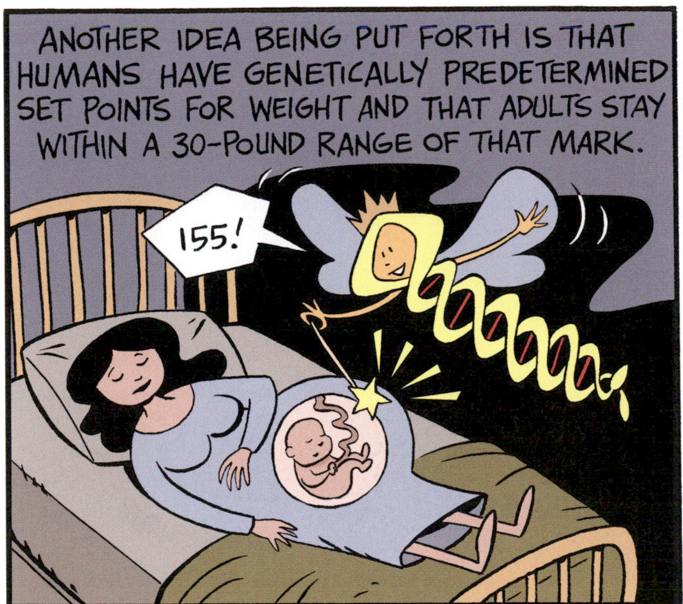
ANOTHER IDEA BEING PUT FORTH IS THAT HUMANS HAVE GENETICALLY PREDETERMINED SET POINTS FOR WEIGHT AND THAT ADULTS STAY WITHIN A 30-POUND RANGE OF THAT MARK.
155!

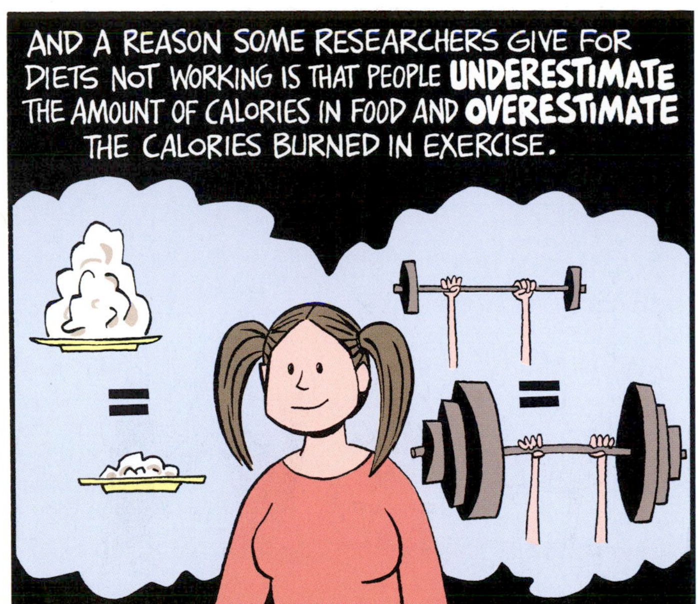
AND A REASON SOME RESEARCHERS GIVE FOR DIETS NOT WORKING IS THAT PEOPLE **UNDERESTIMATE** THE AMOUNT OF CALORIES IN FOOD AND **OVERESTIMATE** THE CALORIES BURNED IN EXERCISE.
=
=

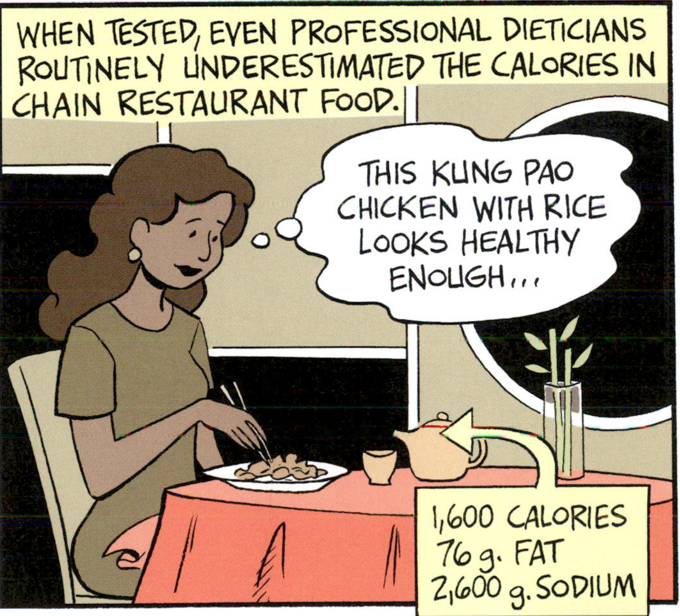
WHEN TESTED, EVEN PROFESSIONAL DIETICIANS ROUTINELY UNDERESTIMATED THE CALORIES IN CHAIN RESTAURANT FOOD.
THIS KUNG PAO CHICKEN WITH RICE LOOKS HEALTHY ENOUGH...
1,600 CALORIES
76 g. FAT
2,600 g. SODIUM

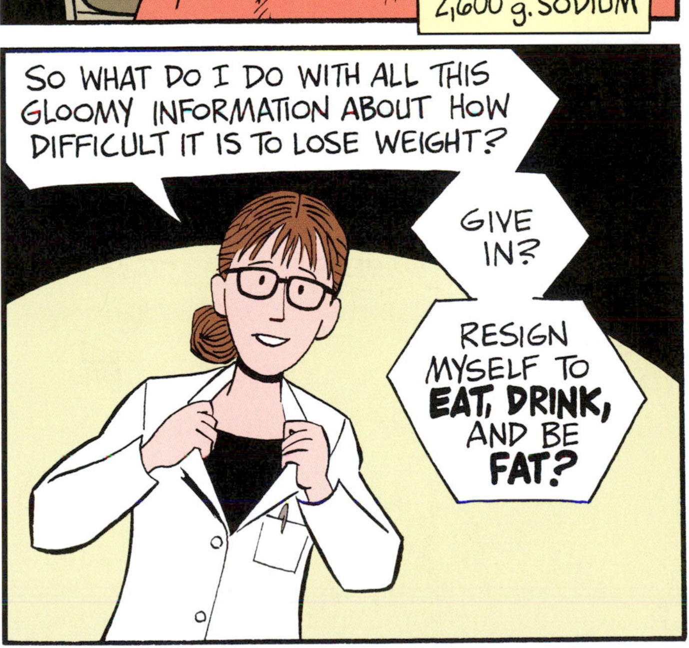
SO WHAT DO I DO WITH ALL THIS GLOOMY INFORMATION ABOUT HOW DIFFICULT IT IS TO LOSE WEIGHT?
GIVE IN?
RESIGN MYSELF TO **EAT, DRINK,** AND BE **FAT?**

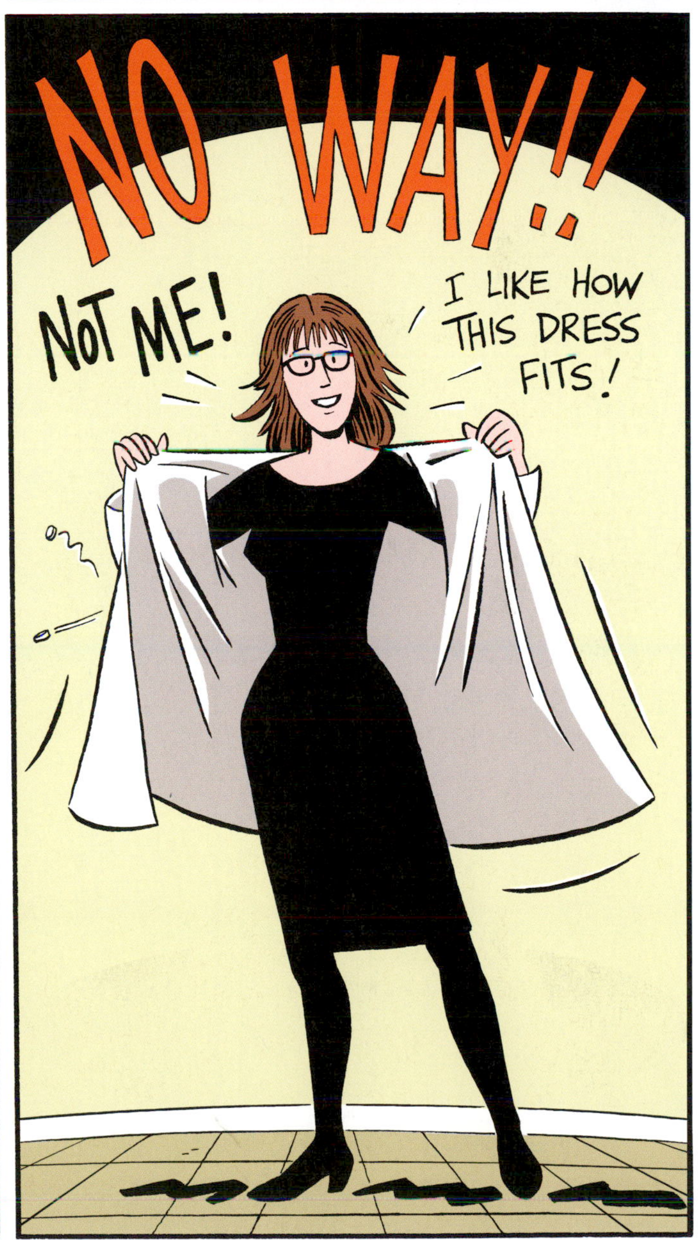
NO WAY!!
NOT ME!
I LIKE HOW THIS DRESS FITS!

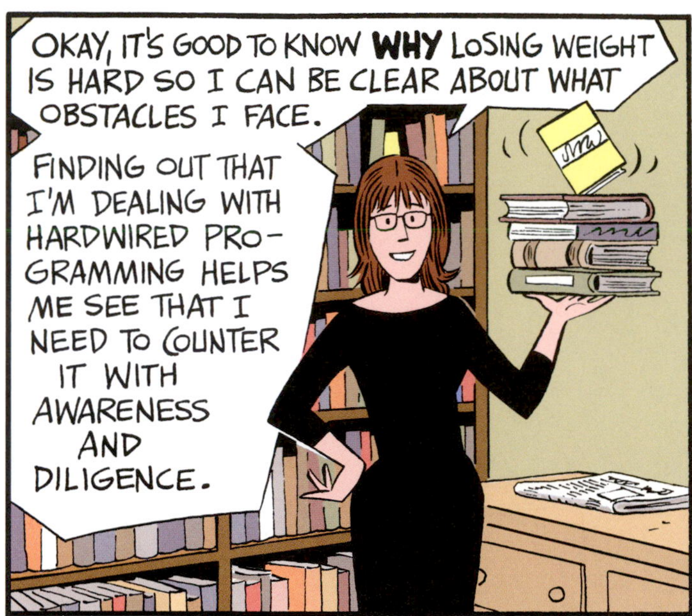
OKAY, IT'S GOOD TO KNOW **WHY** LOSING WEIGHT IS HARD SO I CAN BE CLEAR ABOUT WHAT OBSTACLES I FACE.
FINDING OUT THAT I'M DEALING WITH HARDWIRED PRO-GRAMMING HELPS ME SEE THAT I NEED TO COUNTER IT WITH AWARENESS AND DILIGENCE.

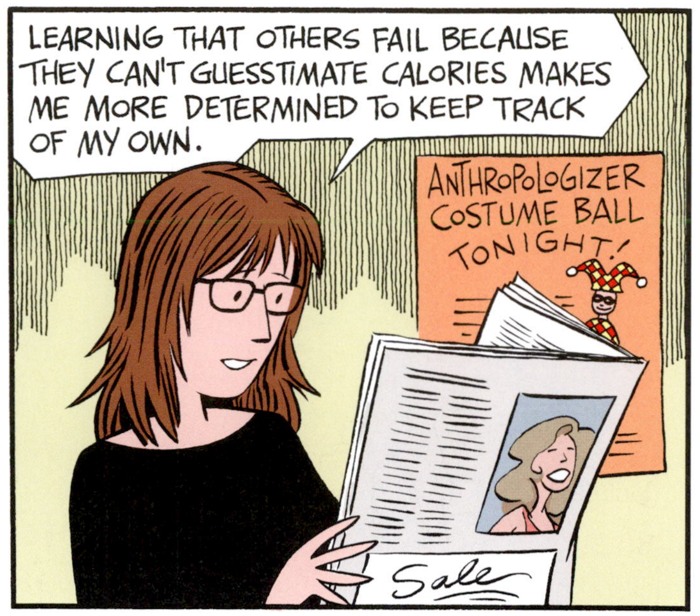
LEARNING THAT OTHERS FAIL BECAUSE THEY CAN'T GUESSTIMATE CALORIES MAKES ME MORE DETERMINED TO KEEP TRACK OF MY OWN.
ANTHROPOLOGIZER COSTUME BALL TONIGHT!
Sale

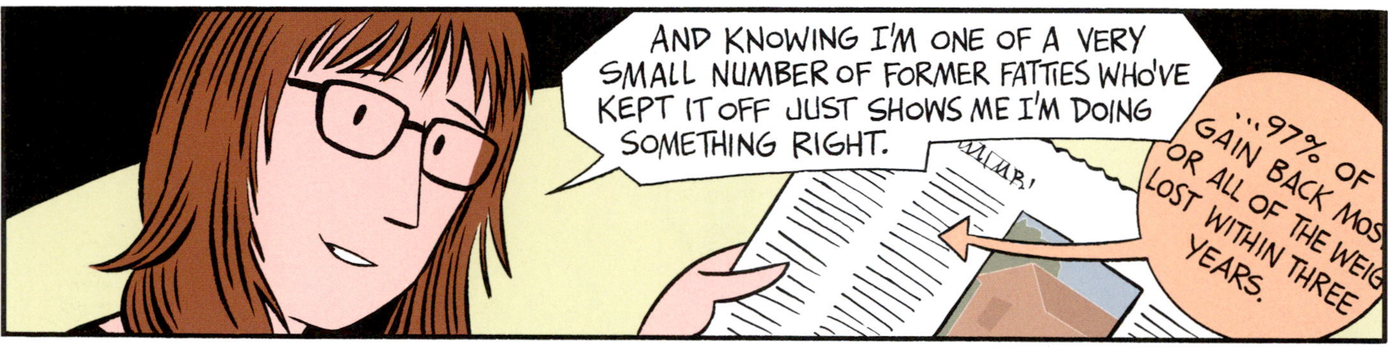
AND KNOWING I'M ONE OF A VERY SMALL NUMBER OF FORMER FATTIES WHO'VE KEPT IT OFF JUST SHOWS ME I'M DOING SOMETHING RIGHT.
...97% OF GAIN BACK MOS OR ALL OF THE WEIG LOST WITHIN THREE YEARS.

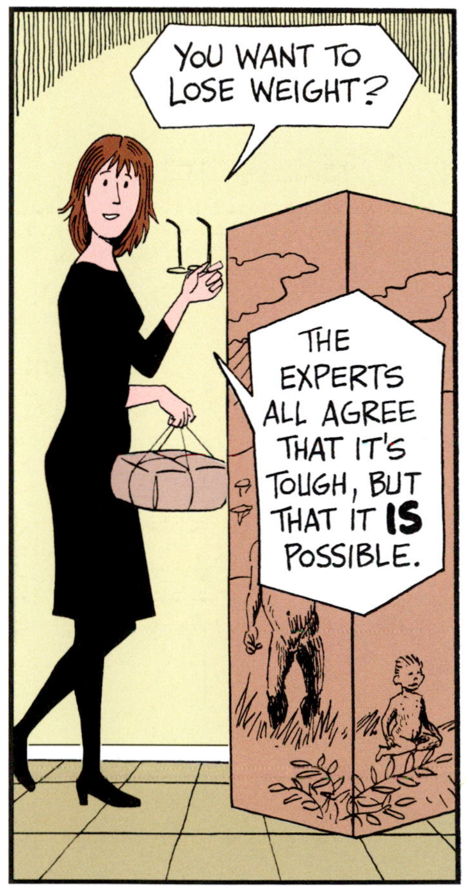
YOU WANT TO LOSE WEIGHT?
THE EXPERTS ALL AGREE THAT IT'S TOUGH, BUT THAT IT **IS** POSSIBLE.

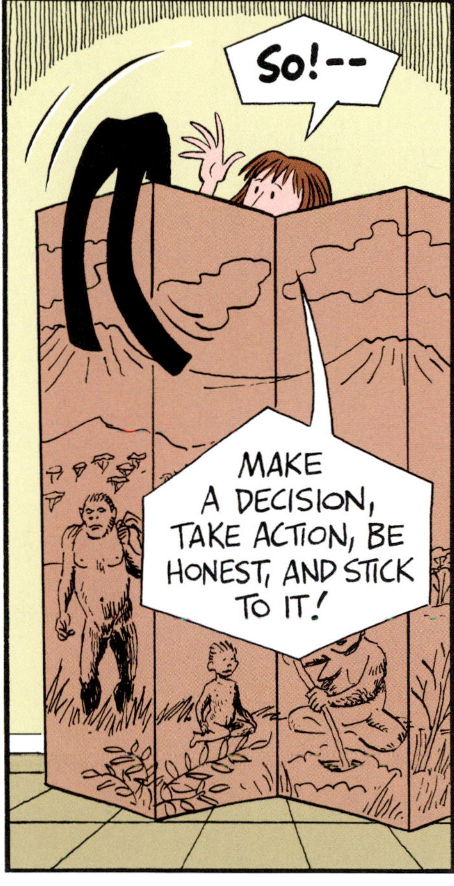
SO!--
MAKE A DECISION, TAKE ACTION, BE HONEST, AND STICK TO IT!

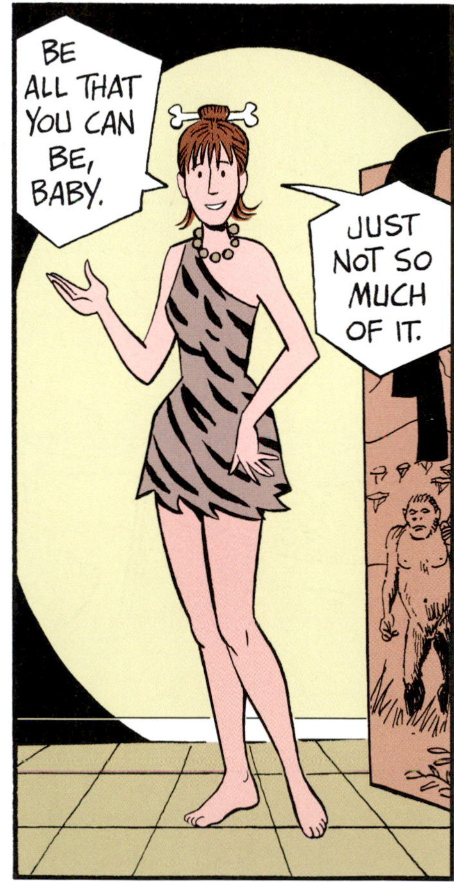
BE ALL THAT YOU CAN BE, BABY.
JUST NOT SO MUCH OF IT.

# What's in It for Me?

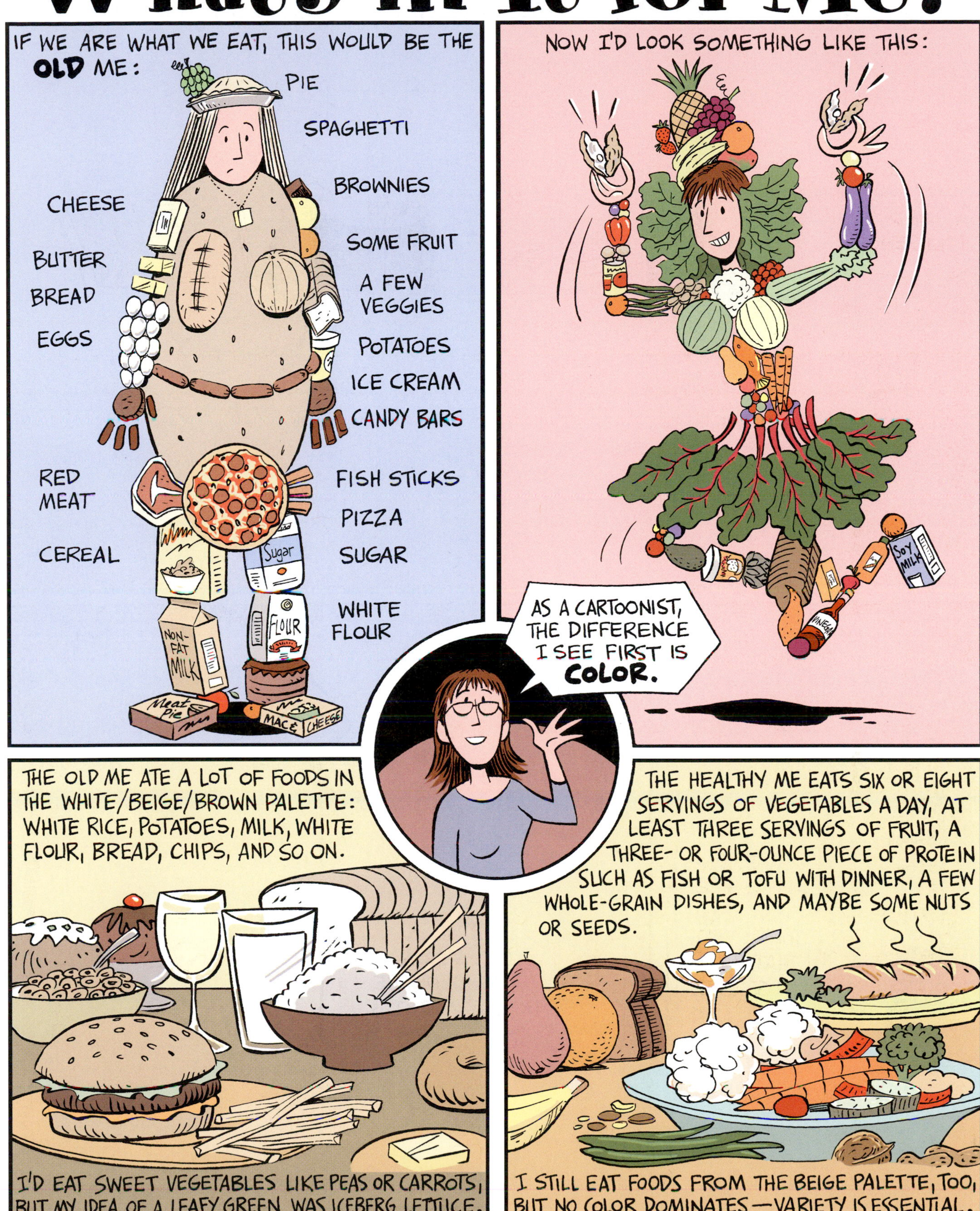

IF WE ARE WHAT WE EAT, THIS WOULD BE THE **OLD** ME:
PIE
SPAGHETTI
BROWNIES
CHEESE
SOME FRUIT
BUTTER
BREAD
A FEW VEGGIES
EGGS
POTATOES
ICE CREAM
CANDY BARS
RED MEAT
FISH STICKS
PIZZA
CEREAL
SUGAR
WHITE FLOUR
Sugar
FLOUR
NON-FAT MILK
Meat Pie
MAC & CHEESE
NOW I'D LOOK SOMETHING LIKE THIS:
SOY MILK
VINEGAR
AS A CARTOONIST, THE DIFFERENCE I SEE FIRST IS **COLOR.**
THE OLD ME ATE A LOT OF FOODS IN THE WHITE/BEIGE/BROWN PALETTE: WHITE RICE, POTATOES, MILK, WHITE FLOUR, BREAD, CHIPS, AND SO ON.
I'D EAT SWEET VEGETABLES LIKE PEAS OR CARROTS, BUT MY IDEA OF A LEAFY GREEN WAS ICEBERG LETTUCE.
THE HEALTHY ME EATS SIX OR EIGHT SERVINGS OF VEGETABLES A DAY, AT LEAST THREE SERVINGS OF FRUIT, A THREE- OR FOUR-OUNCE PIECE OF PROTEIN SUCH AS FISH OR TOFU WITH DINNER, A FEW WHOLE-GRAIN DISHES, AND MAYBE SOME NUTS OR SEEDS.
I STILL EAT FOODS FROM THE BEIGE PALETTE, TOO, BUT NO COLOR DOMINATES—VARIETY IS ESSENTIAL.

OUR BODIES EXTRACT THE VITAMINS AND NUTRIENTS WE NEED FOR GOOD HEALTH FROM OUR FOOD. THE WIDER THE VARIETY OF WHOLE FOODS WE EAT (NOT PROCESSED FOODS), THE MORE NUTRIENTS WE ABSORB THAT COMBINE FOR OPTIMUM HEALTH.

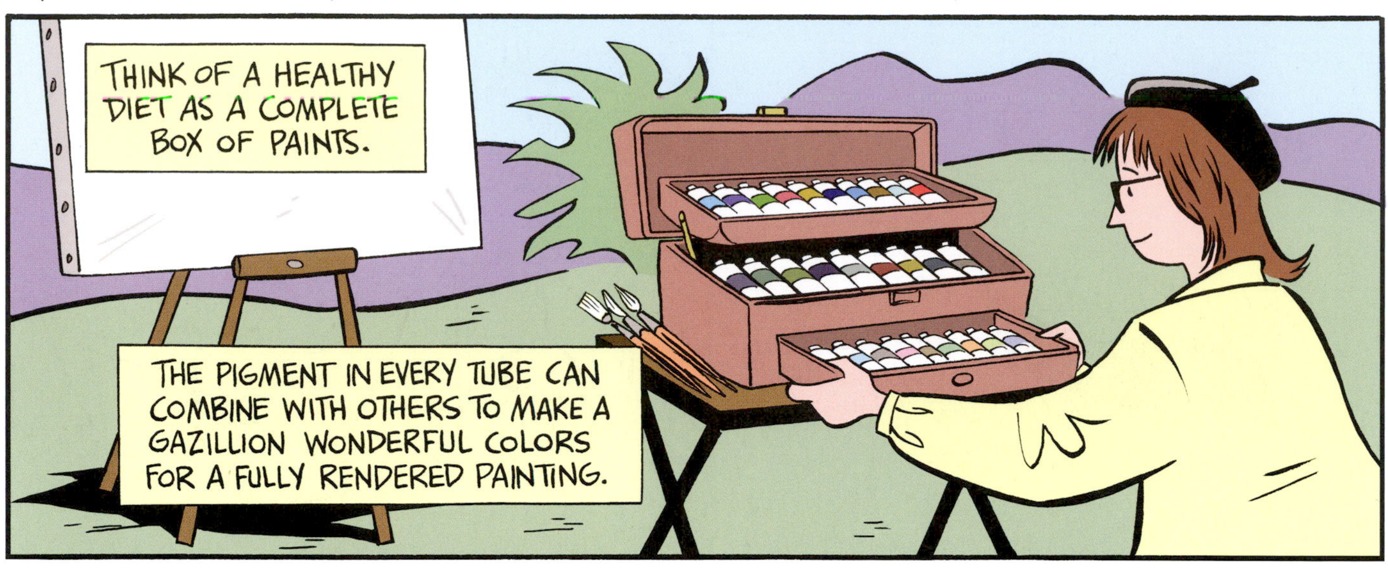

THINK OF A HEALTHY DIET AS A COMPLETE BOX OF PAINTS.
THE PIGMENT IN EVERY TUBE CAN COMBINE WITH OTHERS TO MAKE A GAZILLION WONDERFUL COLORS FOR A FULLY RENDERED PAINTING.

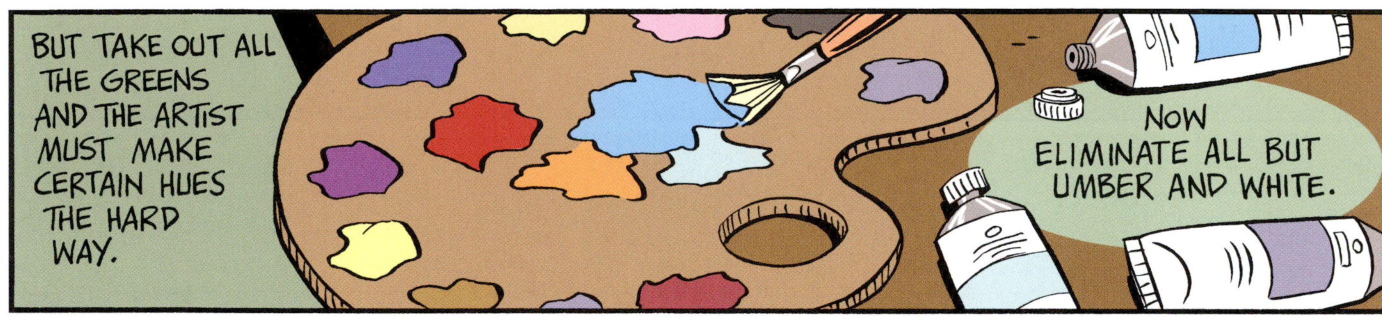

BUT TAKE OUT ALL THE GREENS AND THE ARTIST MUST MAKE CERTAIN HUES THE HARD WAY.
NOW ELIMINATE ALL BUT UMBER AND WHITE.

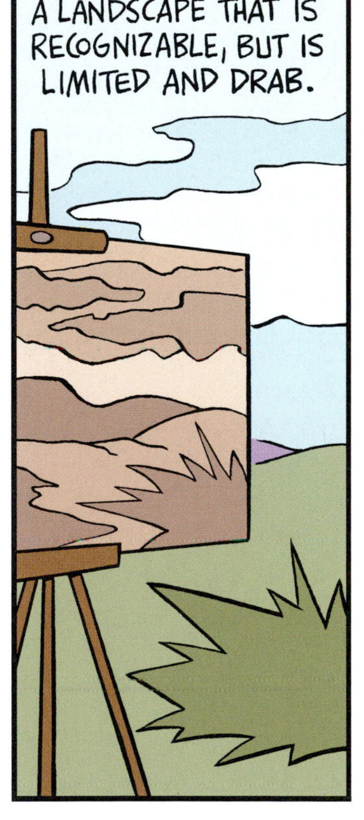

THE PAINTER CAN RENDER A LANDSCAPE THAT IS RECOGNIZABLE, BUT IS LIMITED AND DRAB.

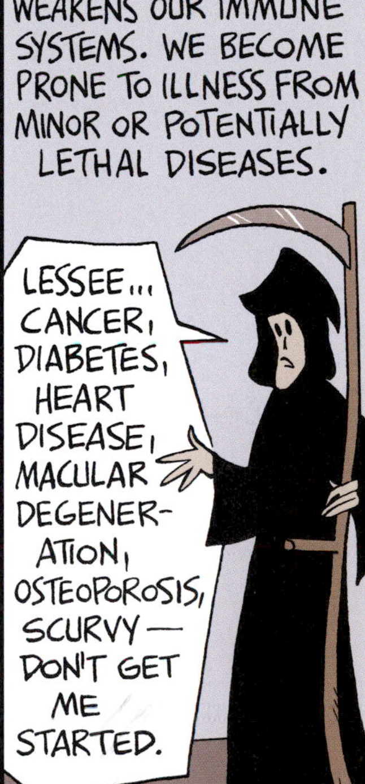

IN HUMAN TERMS, A DIET DEVOID OF WHOLE FOODS WEAKENS OUR IMMUNE SYSTEMS. WE BECOME PRONE TO ILLNESS FROM MINOR OR POTENTIALLY LETHAL DISEASES.
LESSEE... CANCER, DIABETES, HEART DISEASE, MACULAR DEGENER-ATION, OSTEOPOROSIS, SCURVY—DON'T GET ME STARTED.

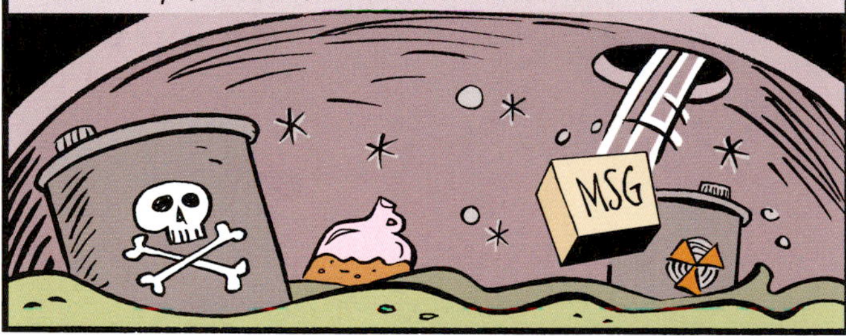

AND PROCESSED FOODS RIFE WITH CHEMICAL PRESERVATIVES AND ADDITIVES FURTHER IMPAIR OUR IMMUNE SYSTEMS BY OVERTAXING OUR FILTERS, MAINLY OUR LIVERS AND KIDNEYS.
MSG

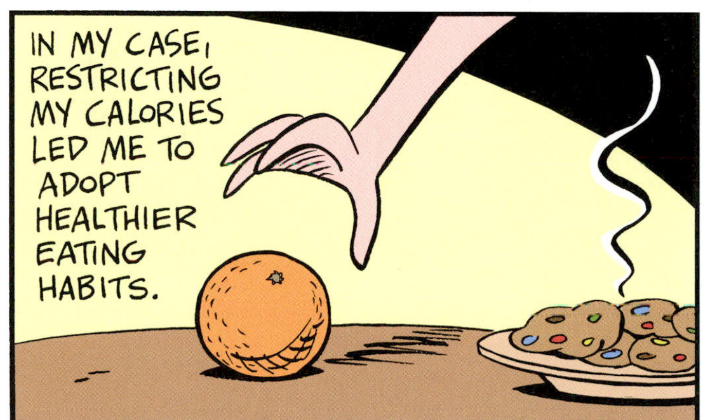

IN MY CASE, RESTRICTING MY CALORIES LED ME TO ADOPT HEALTHIER EATING HABITS.

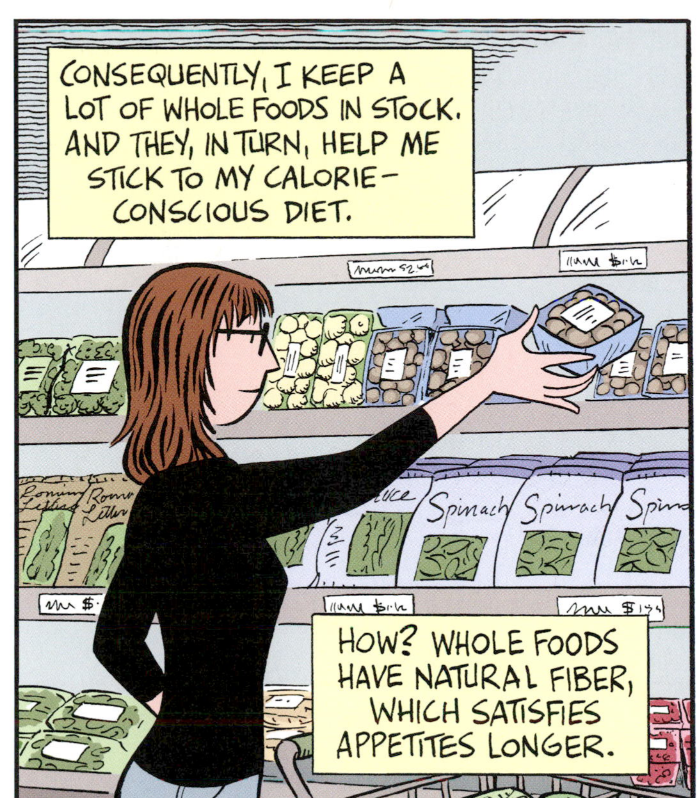
CONSEQUENTLY, I KEEP A LOT OF WHOLE FOODS IN STOCK. AND THEY, IN TURN, HELP ME STICK TO MY CALORIE-CONSCIOUS DIET.
Spinach
Spinach
HOW? WHOLE FOODS HAVE NATURAL FIBER, WHICH SATISFIES APPETITES LONGER.

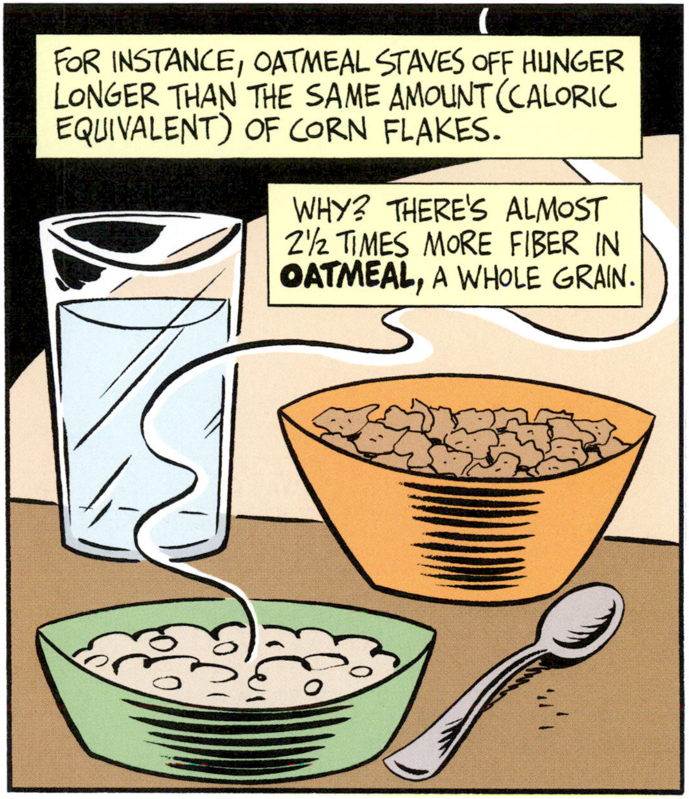
FOR INSTANCE, OATMEAL STAVES OFF HUNGER LONGER THAN THE SAME AMOUNT (CALORIC EQUIVALENT) OF CORN FLAKES.
WHY? THERE'S ALMOST 2½ TIMES MORE FIBER IN **OATMEAL**, A WHOLE GRAIN.

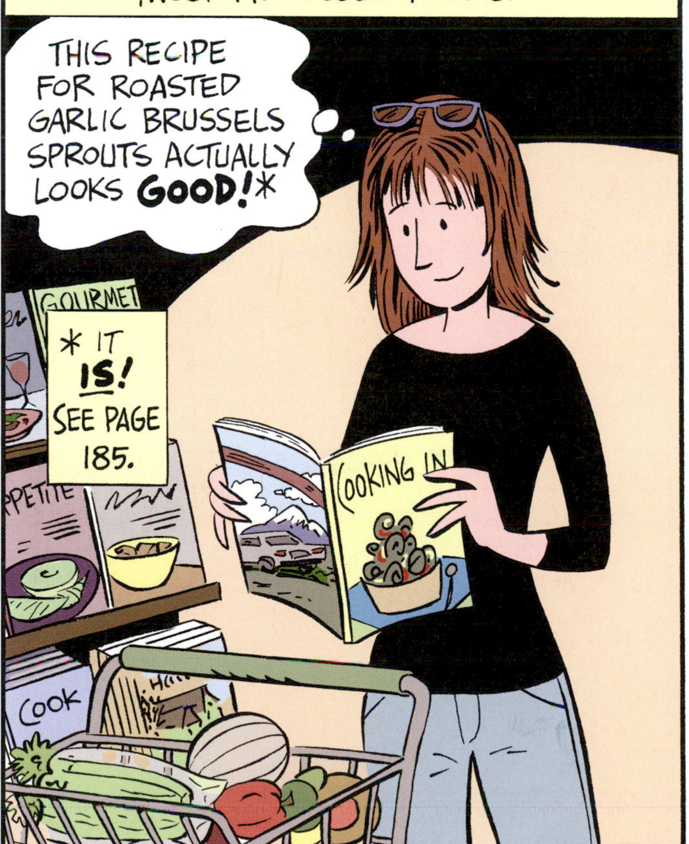
SO WHEN I STARTED RESTRICTING MY CALORIC INTAKE, THAT MEANT THAT TO STAY HAPPY (NOT HUNGRY) I NEEDED TO ADD MORE VEGETABLES AND WHOLE FOODS TO MY DIET AND ELIMINATE MOST PROCESSED FOODS.
THIS RECIPE FOR ROASTED GARLIC BRUSSELS SPROUTS ACTUALLY LOOKS **GOOD!***
GOURMET
* IT **IS!** SEE PAGE 185.
COOKING IN
COOK

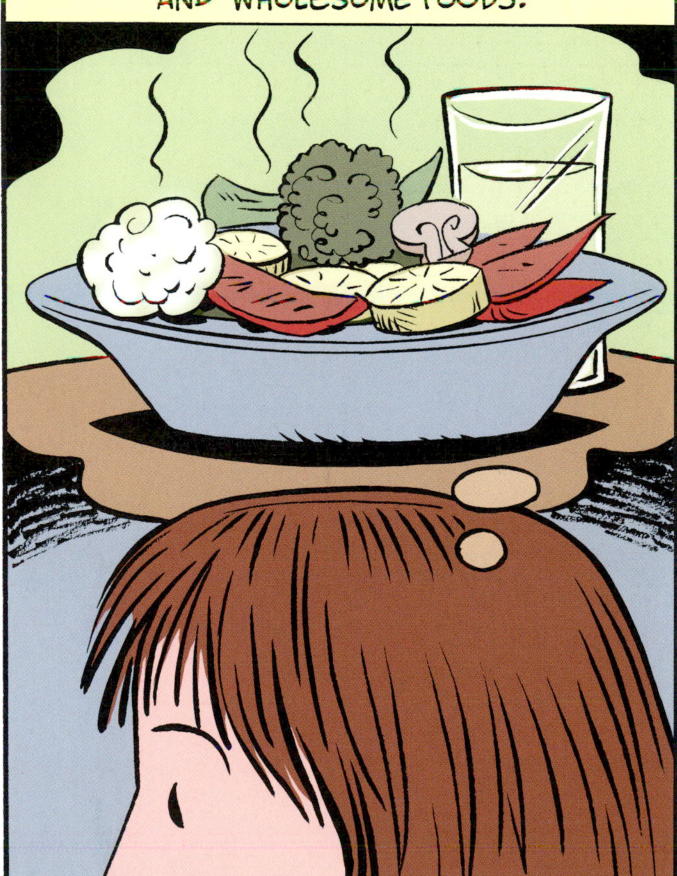
GRADUALLY, MY TASTES CHANGED SO THAT INSTEAD OF CRAVING SWEETS AND STARCHY THINGS, I NOW CRAVE FRESH VEGETABLES AND WHOLESOME FOODS.

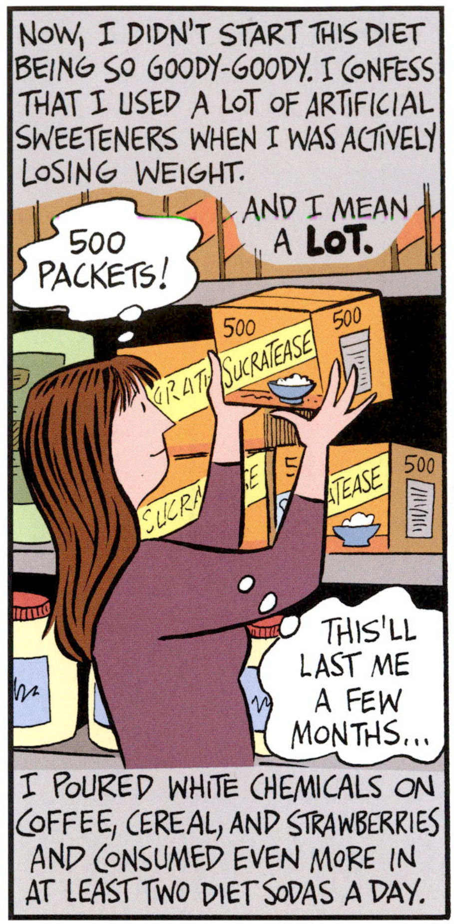
NOW, I DIDN'T START THIS DIET BEING SO GOODY-GOODY. I CONFESS THAT I USED A LOT OF ARTIFICIAL SWEETENERS WHEN I WAS ACTIVELY LOSING WEIGHT.
500 PACKETS!
AND I MEAN A **LOT.**
SUCRATEASE
THIS'LL LAST ME A FEW MONTHS...
I POURED WHITE CHEMICALS ON COFFEE, CEREAL, AND STRAWBERRIES AND CONSUMED EVEN MORE IN AT LEAST TWO DIET SODAS A DAY.

LATER I LEARNED THAT ONE PRODUCT I USED IS CHLORINATED SUCRALOSE—A CHLOROCARBON—AND IS IN THE SAME FAMILY AS **DDT** AND OTHER POISONS.
MM-MMM!
500 SUCRATEASE
A PERSISTENT RASH I'D HAD FOR YEARS MAGICALLY DISAPPEARED AS SOON AS I STOPPED USING THE SWEETENER IN THE LITTLE PAPER PACKETS.

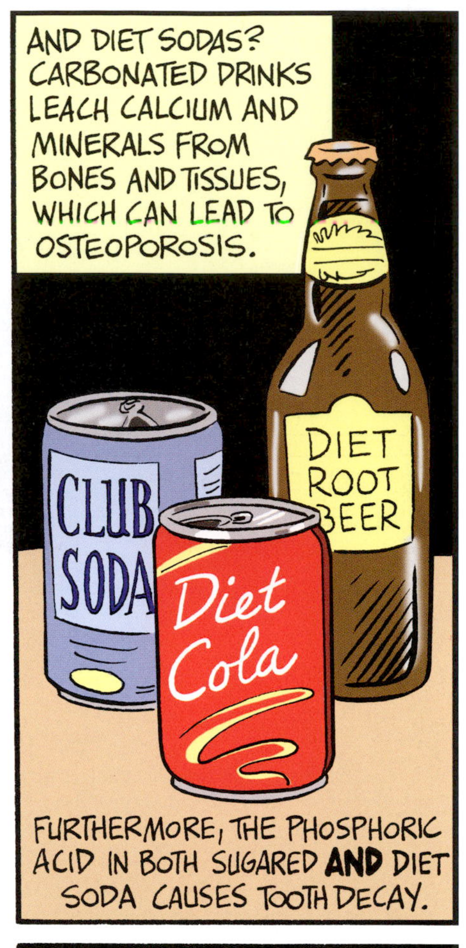
AND DIET SODAS? CARBONATED DRINKS LEACH CALCIUM AND MINERALS FROM BONES AND TISSUES, WHICH CAN LEAD TO OSTEOPOROSIS.
CLUB SODA
Diet Cola
DIET ROOT BEER
FURTHERMORE, THE PHOSPHORIC ACID IN BOTH SUGARED **AND** DIET SODA CAUSES TOOTH DECAY.

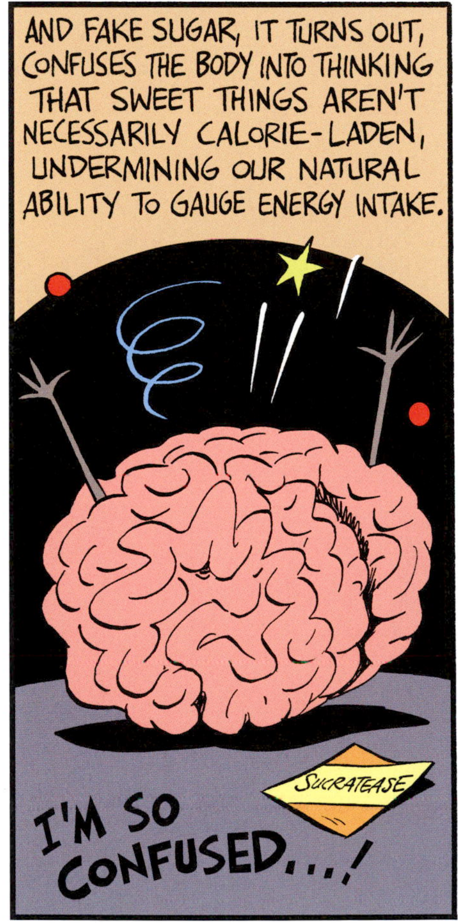
AND FAKE SUGAR, IT TURNS OUT, CONFUSES THE BODY INTO THINKING THAT SWEET THINGS AREN'T NECESSARILY CALORIE-LADEN, UNDERMINING OUR NATURAL ABILITY TO GAUGE ENERGY INTAKE.
SUCRATEASE
I'M SO CONFUSED...!

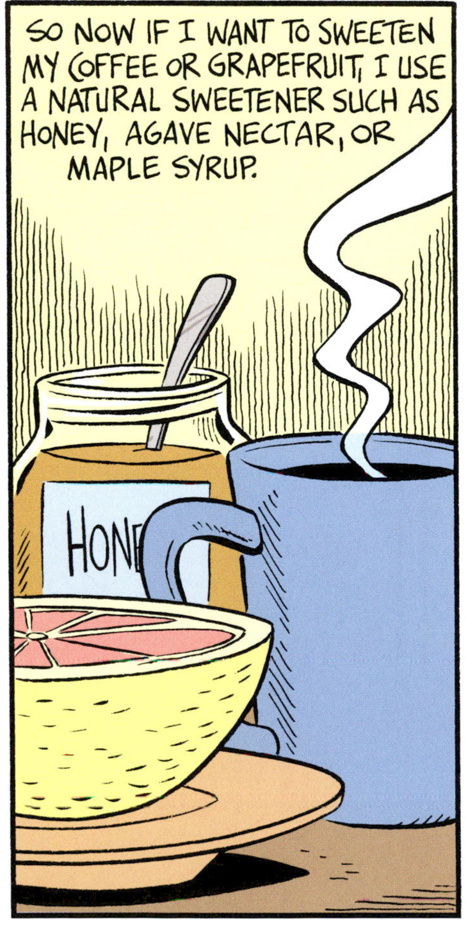
SO NOW IF I WANT TO SWEETEN MY COFFEE OR GRAPEFRUIT, I USE A NATURAL SWEETENER SUCH AS HONEY, AGAVE NECTAR, OR MAPLE SYRUP.
HONE

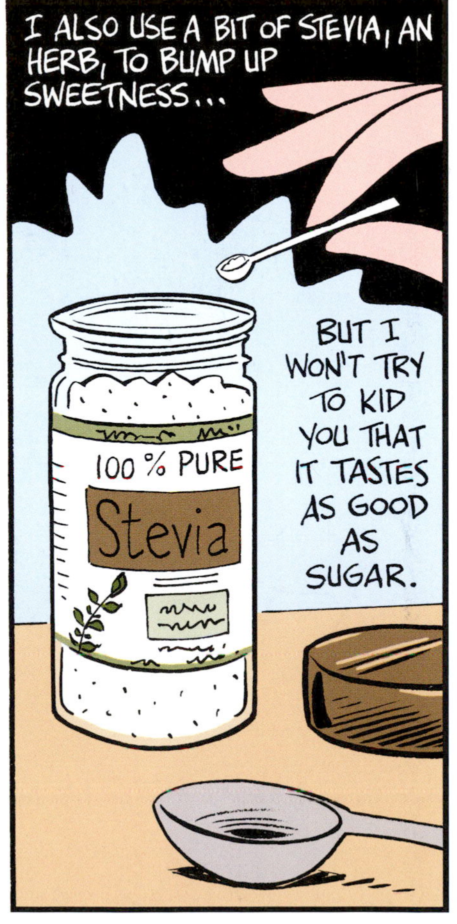
I ALSO USE A BIT OF STEVIA, AN HERB, TO BUMP UP SWEETNESS...
100 % PURE
Stevia
BUT I WON'T TRY TO KID YOU THAT IT TASTES AS GOOD AS SUGAR.

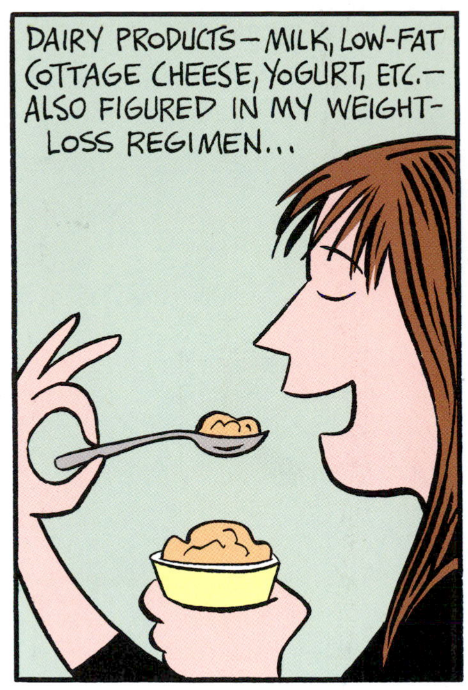
DAIRY PRODUCTS—MILK, LOW-FAT COTTAGE CHEESE, YOGURT, ETC.—ALSO FIGURED IN MY WEIGHT-LOSS REGIMEN...

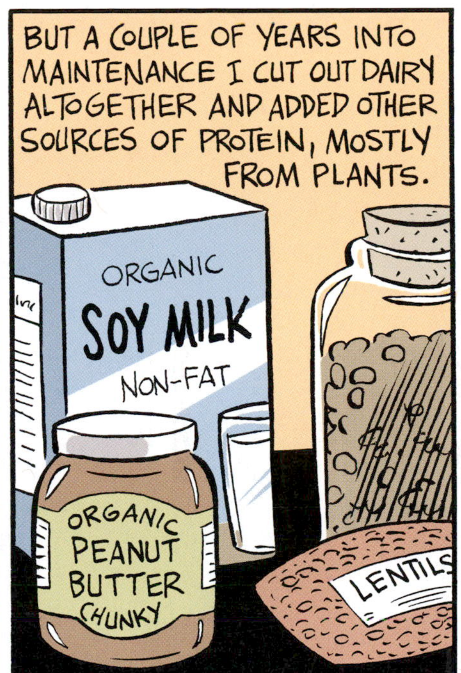
BUT A COUPLE OF YEARS INTO MAINTENANCE I CUT OUT DAIRY ALTOGETHER AND ADDED OTHER SOURCES OF PROTEIN, MOSTLY FROM PLANTS.
ORGANIC
SOY MILK
NON-FAT
ORGANIC
PEANUT
BUTTER
CHUNKY
LENTILS

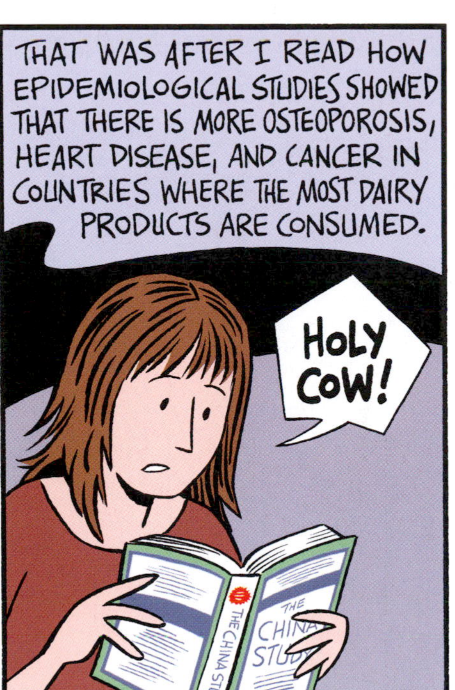
THAT WAS AFTER I READ HOW EPIDEMIOLOGICAL STUDIES SHOWED THAT THERE IS MORE OSTEOPOROSIS, HEART DISEASE, AND CANCER IN COUNTRIES WHERE THE MOST DAIRY PRODUCTS ARE CONSUMED.
HOLY COW!

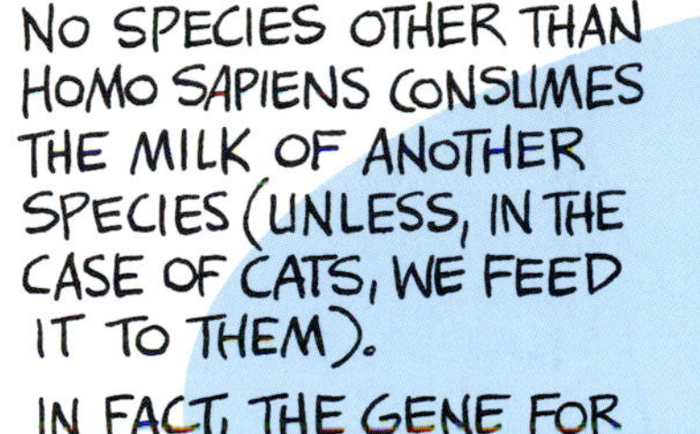
NO SPECIES OTHER THAN HOMO SAPIENS CONSUMES THE MILK OF ANOTHER SPECIES (UNLESS, IN THE CASE OF CATS, WE FEED IT TO THEM).
IN FACT, THE GENE FOR LACTOSE TOLERANCE APPEARED IN HUMANS ONLY 3,000 YEARS AGO, ONE OF OUR MOST RECENT MUTATIONS.

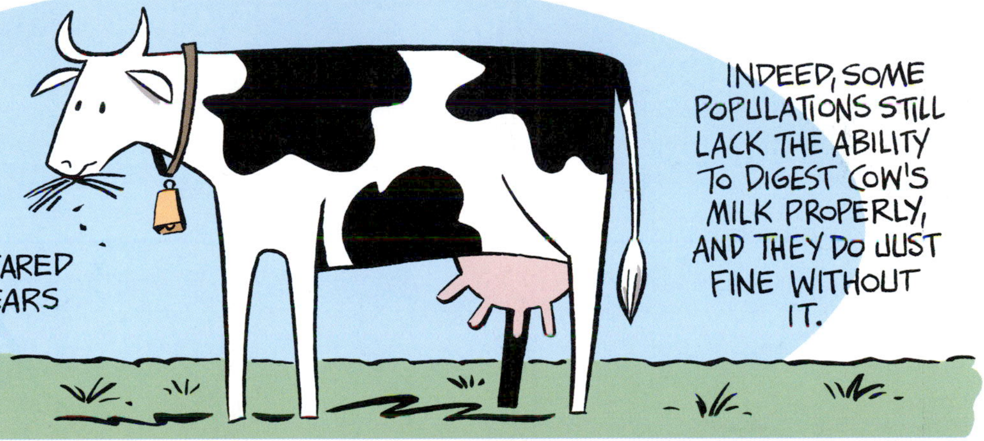
INDEED, SOME POPULATIONS STILL LACK THE ABILITY TO DIGEST COW'S MILK PROPERLY, AND THEY DO JUST FINE WITHOUT IT.

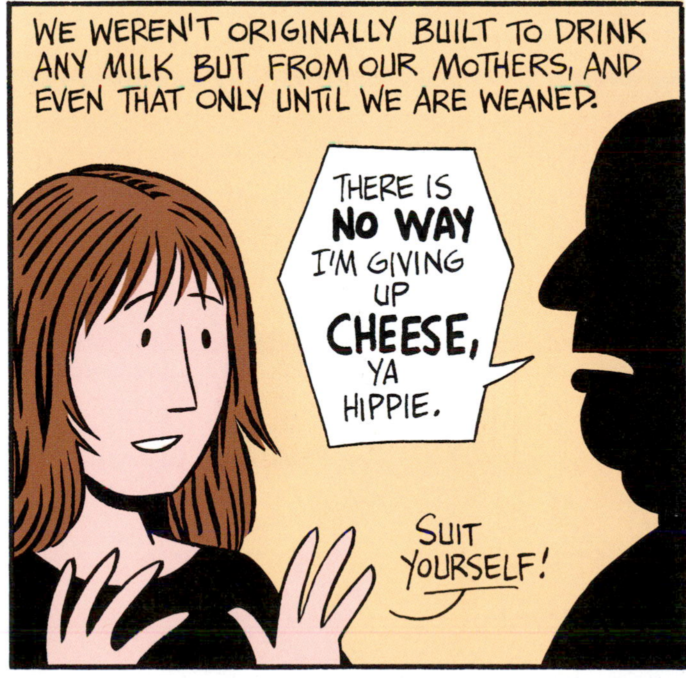
WE WEREN'T ORIGINALLY BUILT TO DRINK ANY MILK BUT FROM OUR MOTHERS, AND EVEN THAT ONLY UNTIL WE ARE WEANED.
THERE IS NO WAY I'M GIVING UP CHEESE, YA HIPPIE.
SUIT YOURSELF!

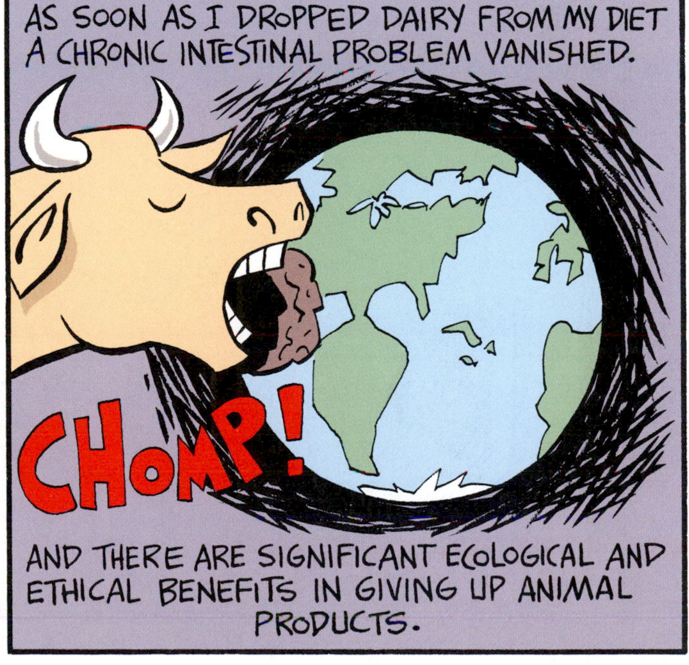
AS SOON AS I DROPPED DAIRY FROM MY DIET A CHRONIC INTESTINAL PROBLEM VANISHED.
CHOMP!
AND THERE ARE SIGNIFICANT ECOLOGICAL AND ETHICAL BENEFITS IN GIVING UP ANIMAL PRODUCTS.

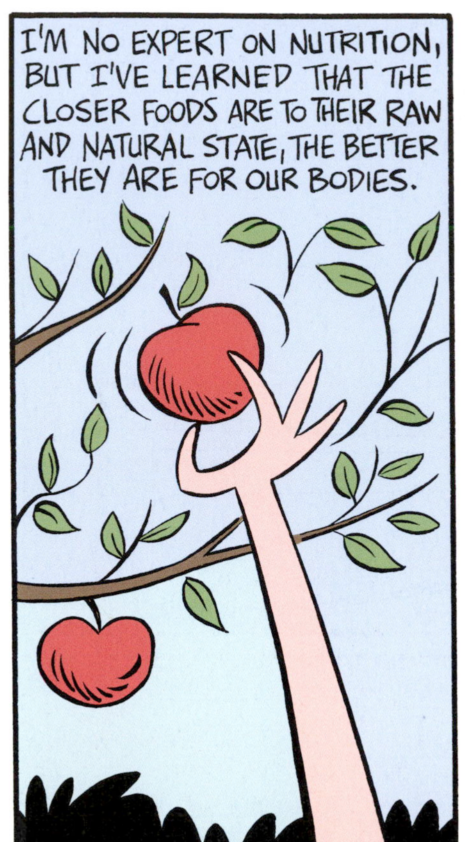
I'M NO EXPERT ON NUTRITION, BUT I'VE LEARNED THAT THE CLOSER FOODS ARE TO THEIR RAW AND NATURAL STATE, THE BETTER THEY ARE FOR OUR BODIES.

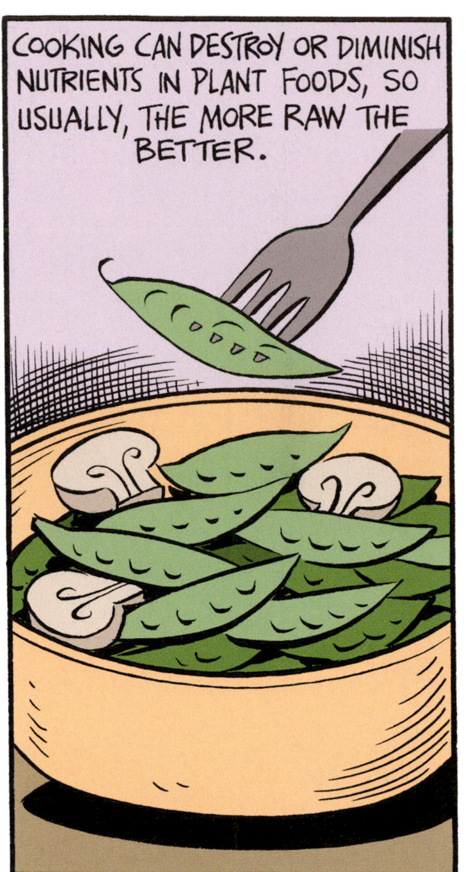
COOKING CAN DESTROY OR DIMINISH NUTRIENTS IN PLANT FOODS, SO USUALLY, THE MORE RAW THE BETTER.

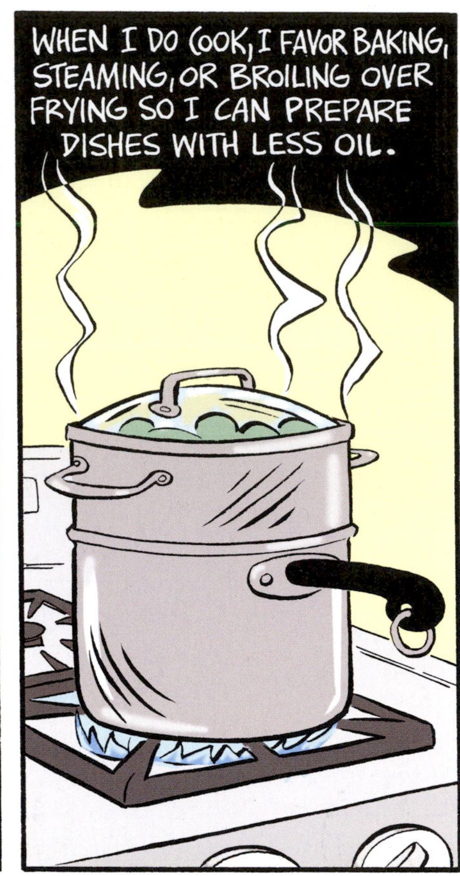
WHEN I DO COOK, I FAVOR BAKING, STEAMING, OR BROILING OVER FRYING SO I CAN PREPARE DISHES WITH LESS OIL.

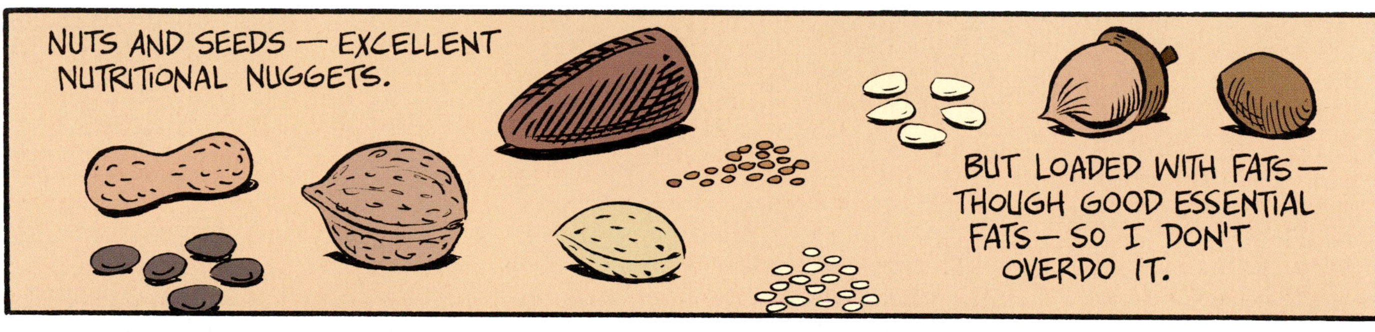
NUTS AND SEEDS — EXCELLENT NUTRITIONAL NUGGETS.
BUT LOADED WITH FATS — THOUGH GOOD ESSENTIAL FATS — SO I DON'T OVERDO IT.

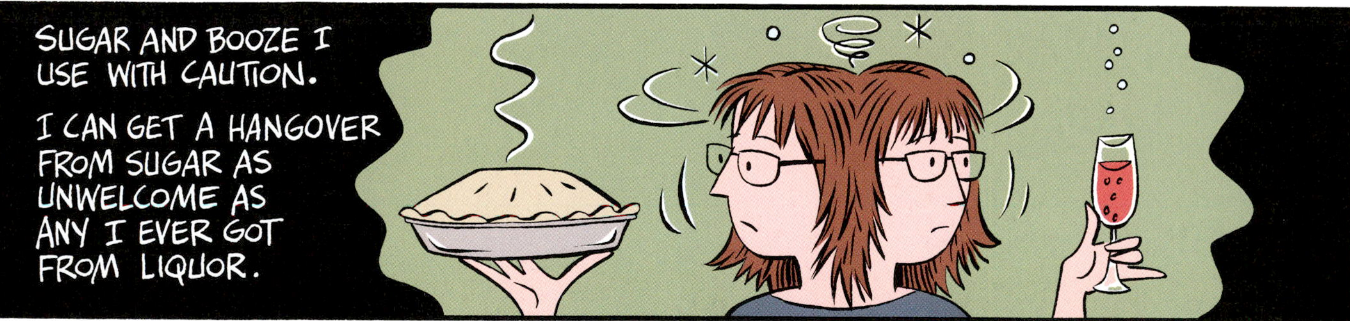
SUGAR AND BOOZE I USE WITH CAUTION.
I CAN GET A HANGOVER FROM SUGAR AS UNWELCOME AS ANY I EVER GOT FROM LIQUOR.

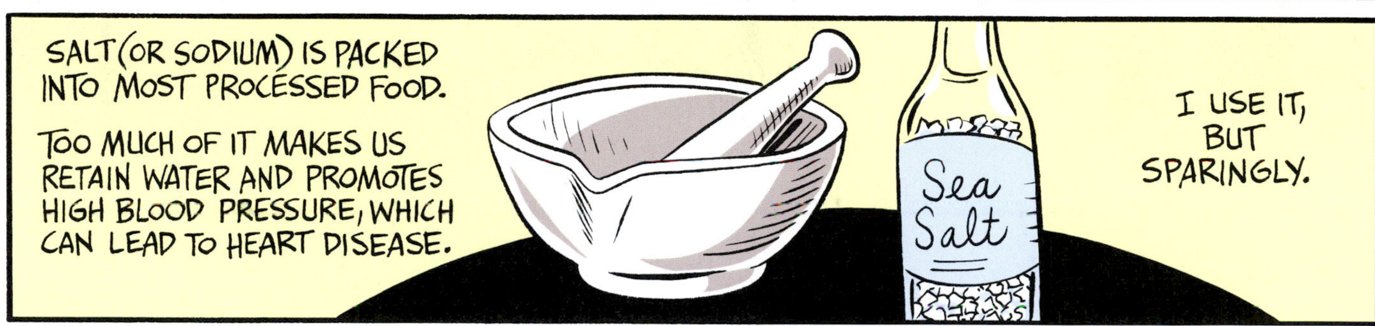
SALT (OR SODIUM) IS PACKED INTO MOST PROCESSED FOOD.
TOO MUCH OF IT MAKES US RETAIN WATER AND PROMOTES HIGH BLOOD PRESSURE, WHICH CAN LEAD TO HEART DISEASE.
Sea Salt
I USE IT, BUT SPARINGLY.

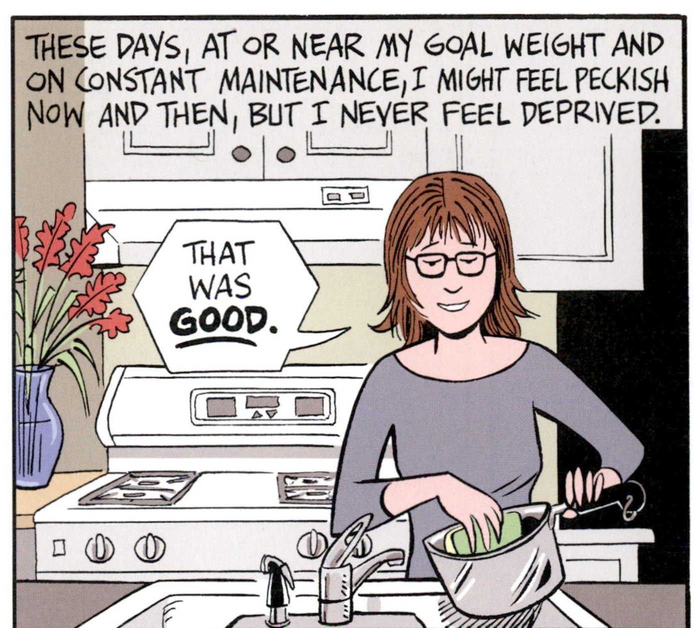
THESE DAYS, AT OR NEAR MY GOAL WEIGHT AND ON CONSTANT MAINTENANCE, I MIGHT FEEL PECKISH NOW AND THEN, BUT I NEVER FEEL DEPRIVED.
THAT WAS **GOOD**.

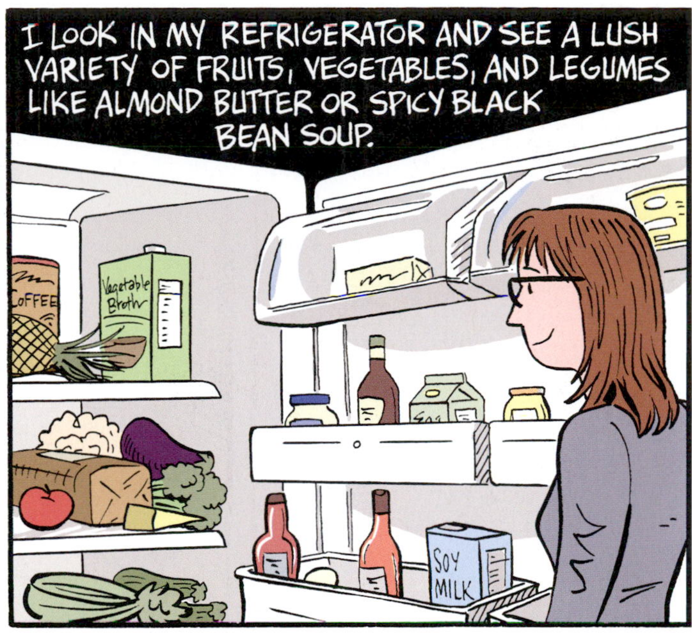
I LOOK IN MY REFRIGERATOR AND SEE A LUSH VARIETY OF FRUITS, VEGETABLES, AND LEGUMES LIKE ALMOND BUTTER OR SPICY BLACK BEAN SOUP.
COFFEE
Vegetable Broth
SOY MILK

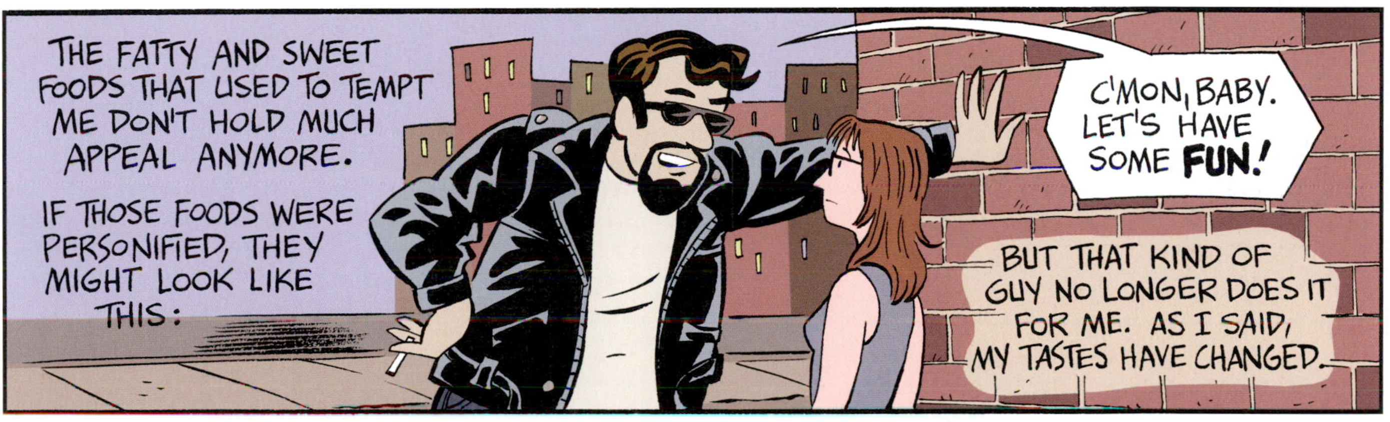
THE FATTY AND SWEET FOODS THAT USED TO TEMPT ME DON'T HOLD MUCH APPEAL ANYMORE.
IF THOSE FOODS WERE PERSONIFIED, THEY MIGHT LOOK LIKE THIS:
C'MON, BABY. LET'S HAVE SOME **FUN**!
BUT THAT KIND OF GUY NO LONGER DOES IT FOR ME. AS I SAID, MY TASTES HAVE CHANGED.

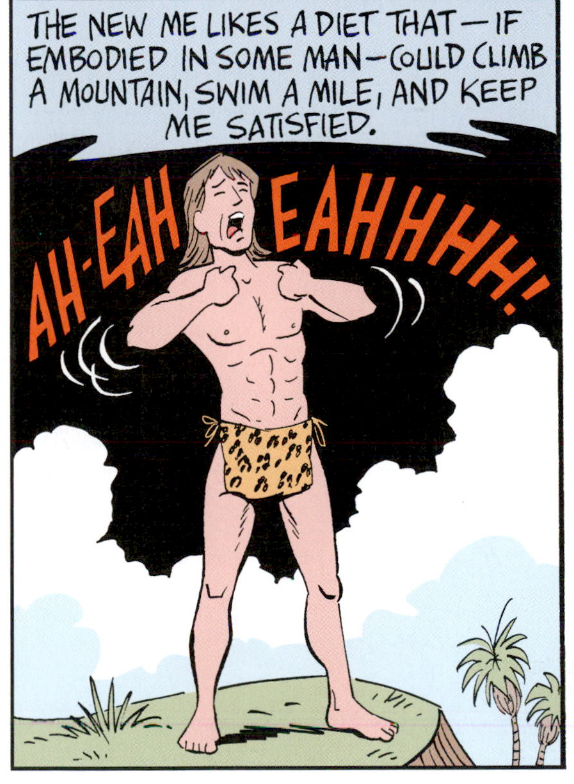
THE NEW ME LIKES A DIET THAT—IF EMBODIED IN SOME MAN—COULD CLIMB A MOUNTAIN, SWIM A MILE, AND KEEP ME SATISFIED.
AH-EAH EAHHHH!

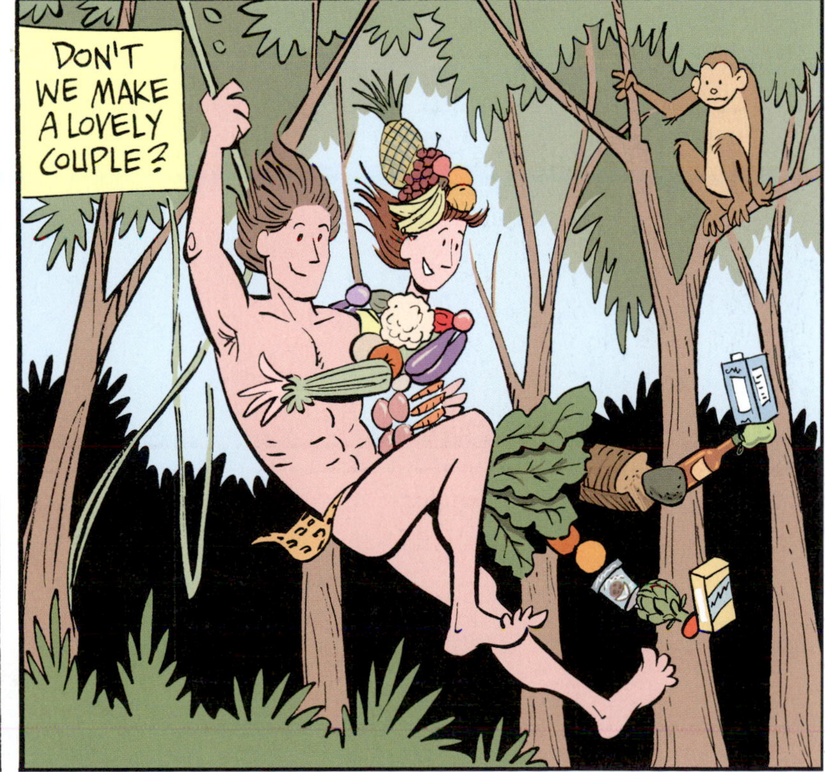
DON'T WE MAKE A LOVELY COUPLE?

# TIPS

AT THE BUFFET, CHOOSE A SMALL PLATE IF YOU CAN. A RESEARCHER FOUND THAT EVEN DIETICIANS UNCONSCIOUSLY LOADED UP ON MORE ICE CREAM WHEN THEY WERE GIVEN LARGER BOWLS AND SPOONS.

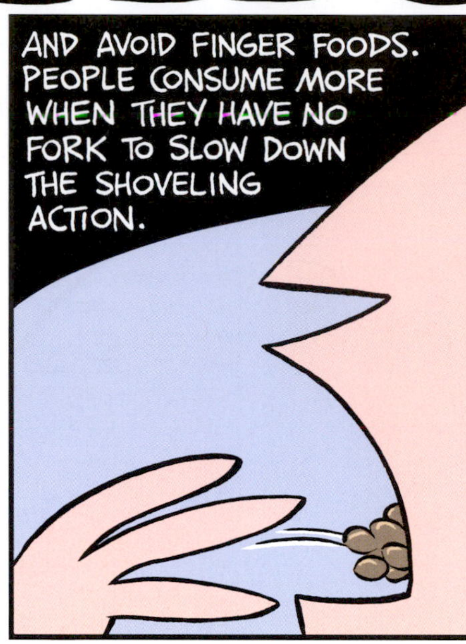

AND AVOID FINGER FOODS. PEOPLE CONSUME MORE WHEN THEY HAVE NO FORK TO SLOW DOWN THE SHOVELING ACTION.

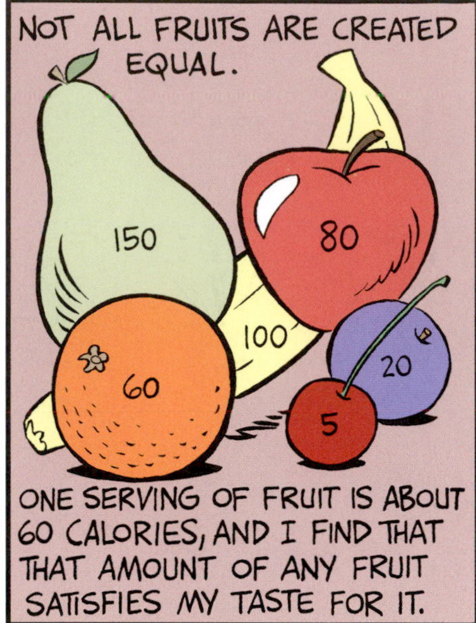

NOT ALL FRUITS ARE CREATED EQUAL.
150
80
100
20
60
5
ONE SERVING OF FRUIT IS ABOUT 60 CALORIES, AND I FIND THAT THAT AMOUNT OF ANY FRUIT SATISFIES MY TASTE FOR IT.

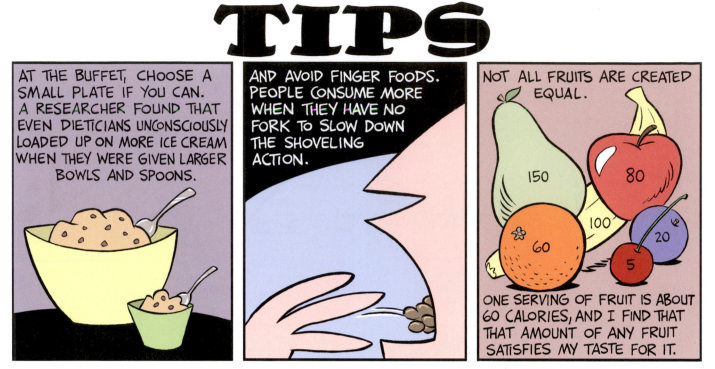

DON'T BELIEVE THE "NEGATIVE CALORIES" HYPE—BALONEY HAS CALORIES TOO. THE CALORIC BENEFIT FROM CHEWING/DIGESTING CELERY IS NEGLIGIBLE, ALTHOUGH EATING CELERY KEEPS ME FROM EATING THINGS THAT MAY BE MORE CALORIFIC.

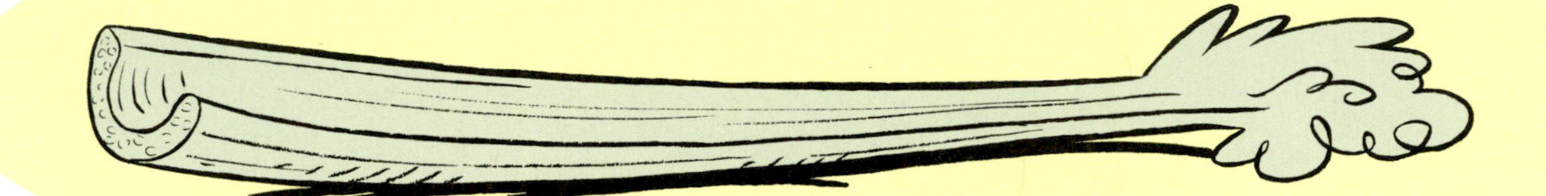

I'VE READ CLAIMS THAT AN APPLE (60-80 CALORIES) CAUSES THE BODY TO BURN MORE CALORIES DIGESTING IT THAN IT CONTAINS. IF YOU BELIEVE THAT, I HAVE A BRIDGE TO SELL YOU IN BROOKLYN.

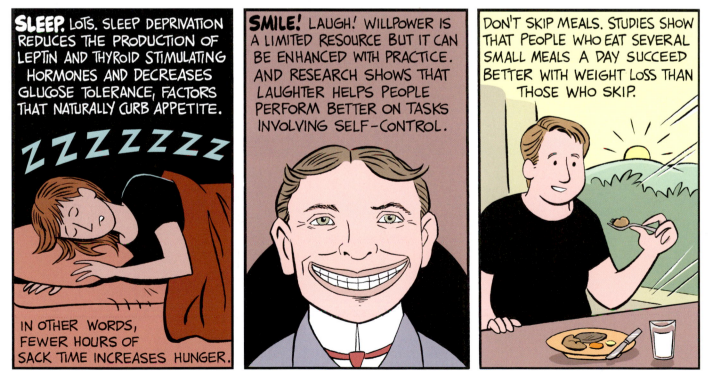

**SLEEP.** LOTS. SLEEP DEPRIVATION REDUCES THE PRODUCTION OF LEPTIN AND THYROID STIMULATING HORMONES AND DECREASES GLUCOSE TOLERANCE, FACTORS THAT NATURALLY CURB APPETITE.

ZZZZZZZ

IN OTHER WORDS, FEWER HOURS OF SACK TIME INCREASES HUNGER.

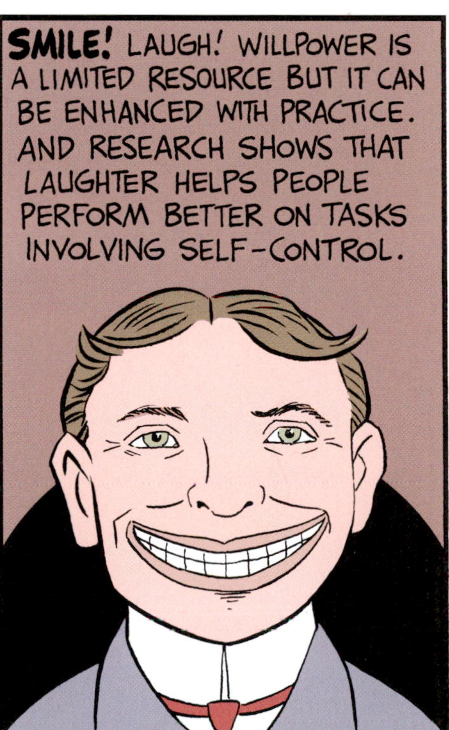

SMILE! LAUGH! WILLPOWER IS A LIMITED RESOURCE BUT IT CAN BE ENHANCED WITH PRACTICE. AND RESEARCH SHOWS THAT LAUGHTER HELPS PEOPLE PERFORM BETTER ON TASKS INVOLVING SELF-CONTROL.

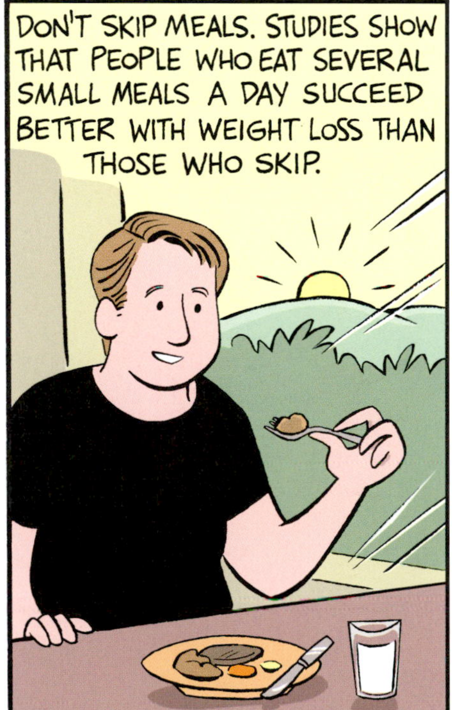

DON'T SKIP MEALS. STUDIES SHOW THAT PEOPLE WHO EAT SEVERAL SMALL MEALS A DAY SUCCEED BETTER WITH WEIGHT LOSS THAN THOSE WHO SKIP.

# At WORK or Play

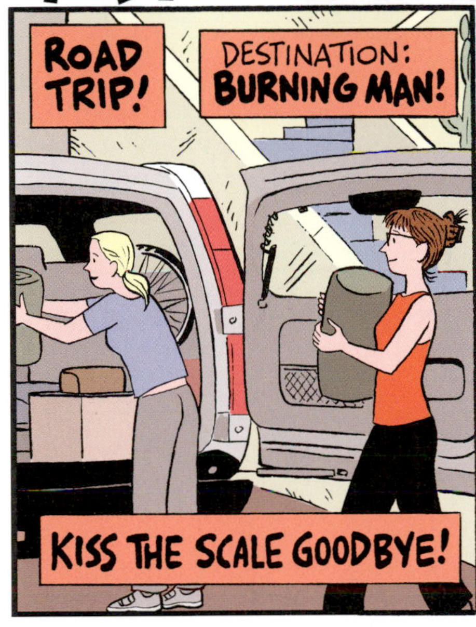
ROAD TRIP!
DESTINATION: BURNING MAN!
KISS THE SCALE GOODBYE!

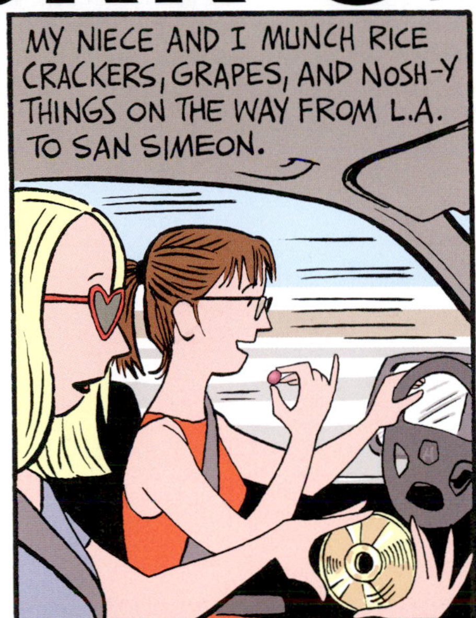
MY NIECE AND I MUNCH RICE CRACKERS, GRAPES, AND NOSH-Y THINGS ON THE WAY FROM L.A. TO SAN SIMEON.

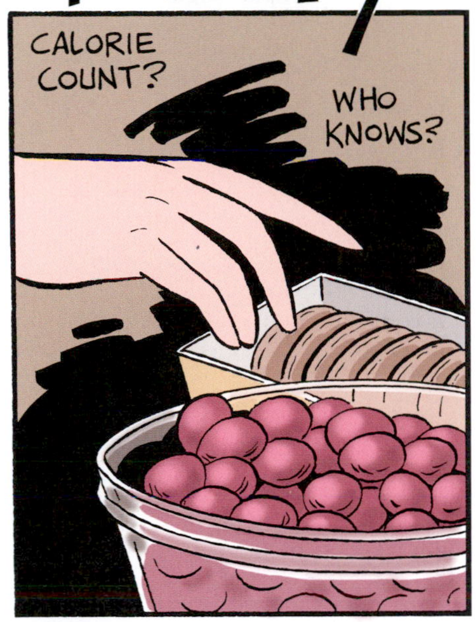
CALORIE COUNT?
WHO KNOWS?

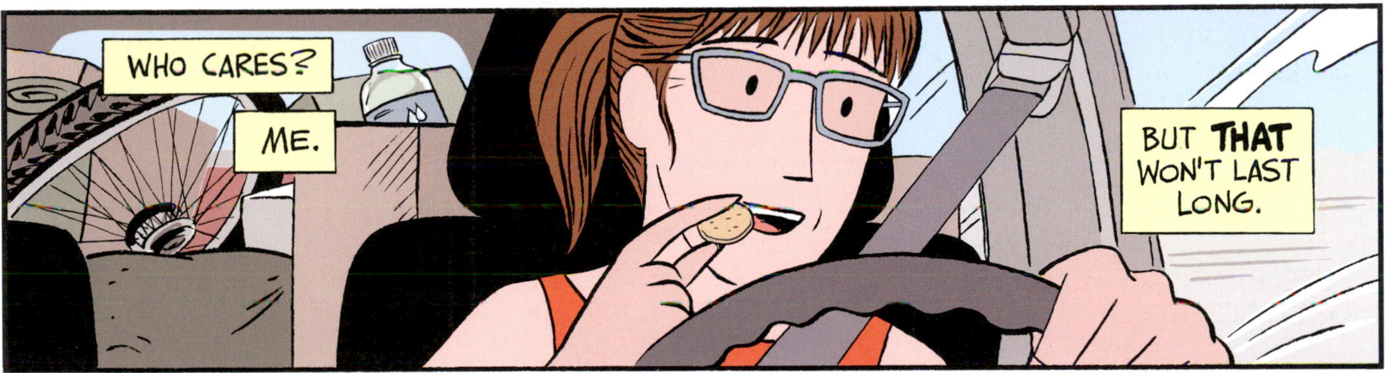
WHO CARES?
ME.
BUT THAT WON'T LAST LONG.

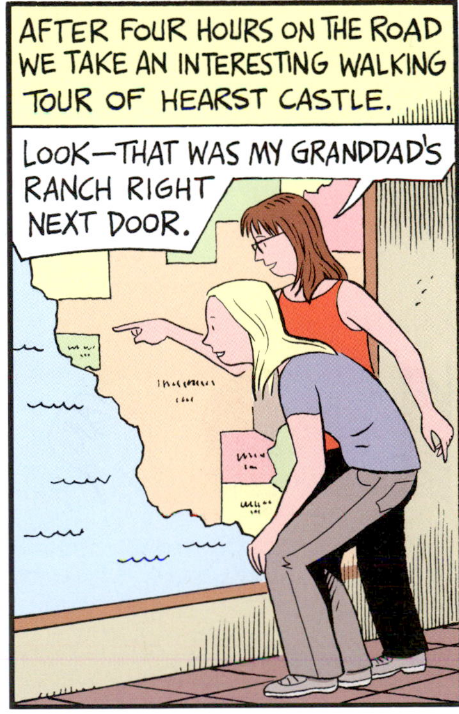
AFTER FOUR HOURS ON THE ROAD WE TAKE AN INTERESTING WALKING TOUR OF HEARST CASTLE.
LOOK—THAT WAS MY GRANDDAD'S RANCH RIGHT NEXT DOOR.

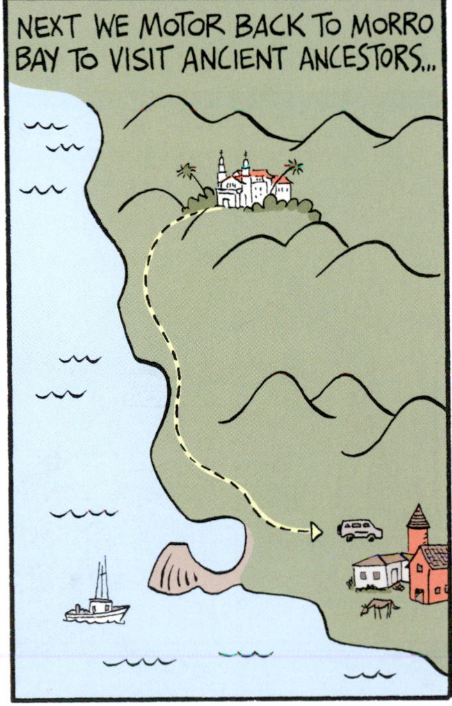
NEXT WE MOTOR BACK TO MORRO BAY TO VISIT ANCIENT ANCESTORS...

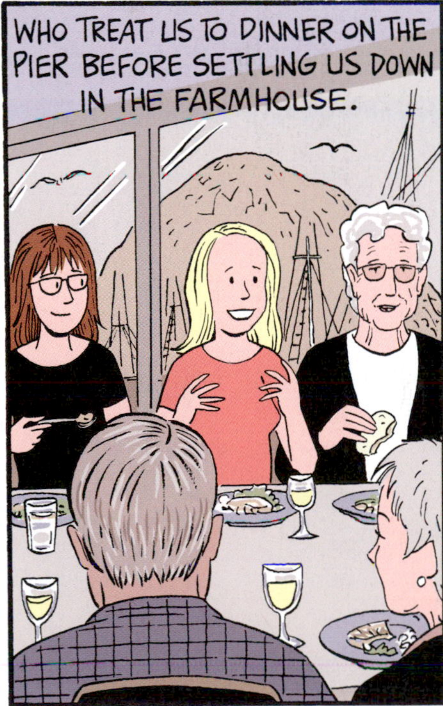
WHO TREAT US TO DINNER ON THE PIER BEFORE SETTLING US DOWN IN THE FARMHOUSE.

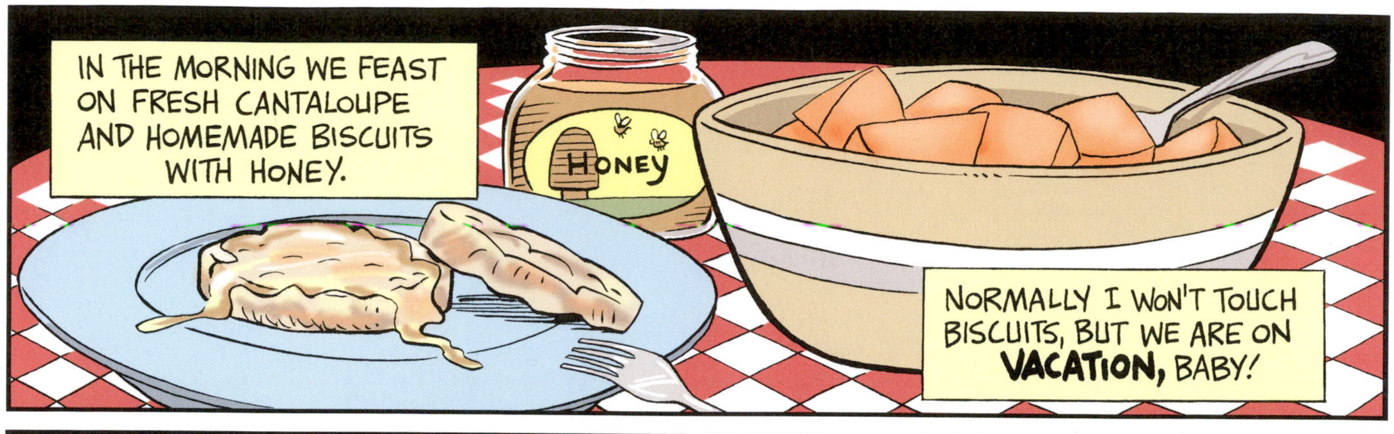
IN THE MORNING WE FEAST ON FRESH CANTALOUPE AND HOMEMADE BISCUITS WITH HONEY.
HONEY
NORMALLY I WON'T TOUCH BISCUITS, BUT WE ARE ON **VACATION**, BABY!

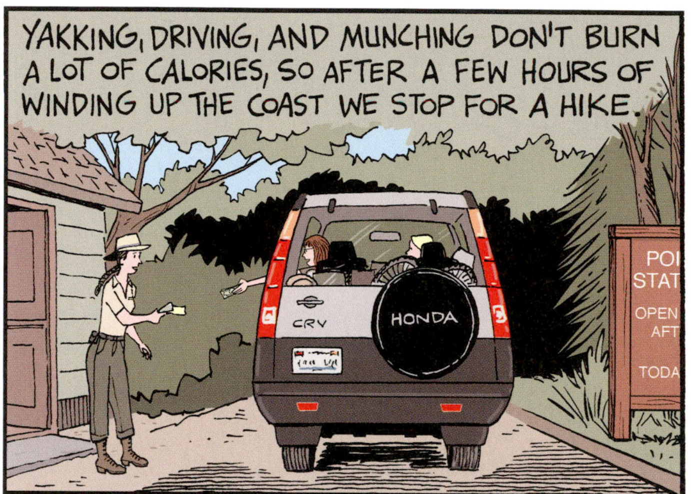
YAKKING, DRIVING, AND MUNCHING DON'T BURN A LOT OF CALORIES, SO AFTER A FEW HOURS OF WINDING UP THE COAST WE STOP FOR A HIKE.
CRV
HONDA

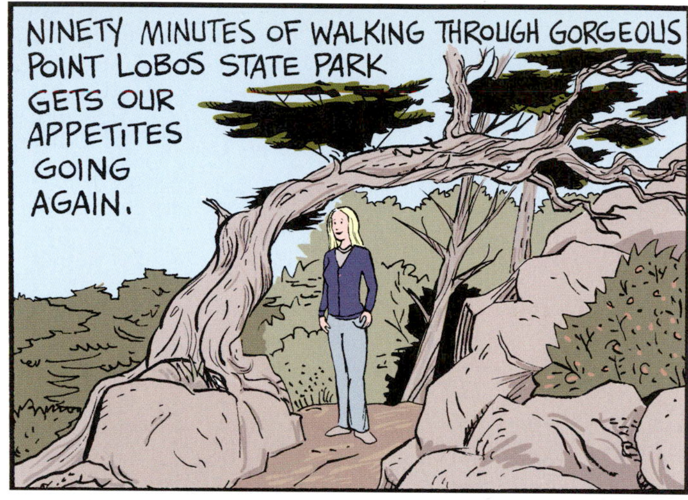
NINETY MINUTES OF WALKING THROUGH GORGEOUS POINT LOBOS STATE PARK GETS OUR APPETITES GOING AGAIN.

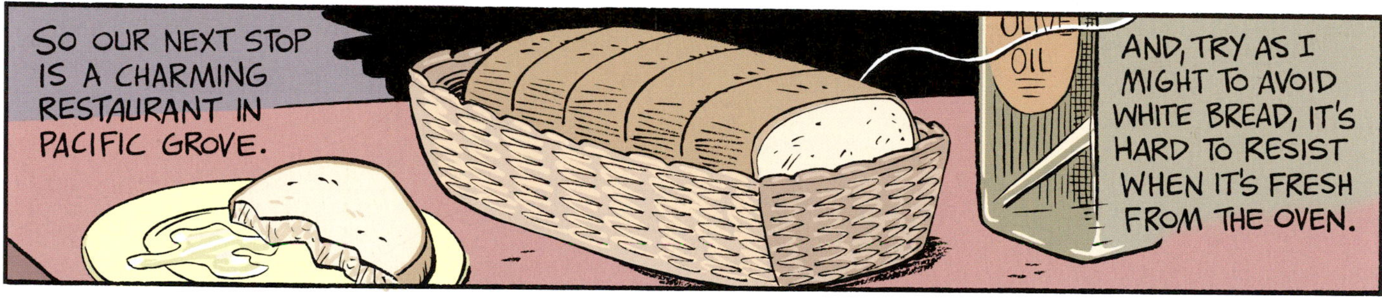
SO OUR NEXT STOP IS A CHARMING RESTAURANT IN PACIFIC GROVE.
OIL
AND, TRY AS I MIGHT TO AVOID WHITE BREAD, IT'S HARD TO RESIST WHEN IT'S FRESH FROM THE OVEN.

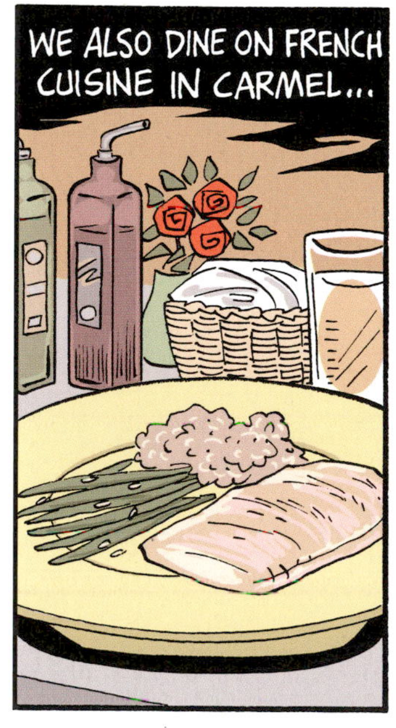
WE ALSO DINE ON FRENCH CUISINE IN CARMEL...

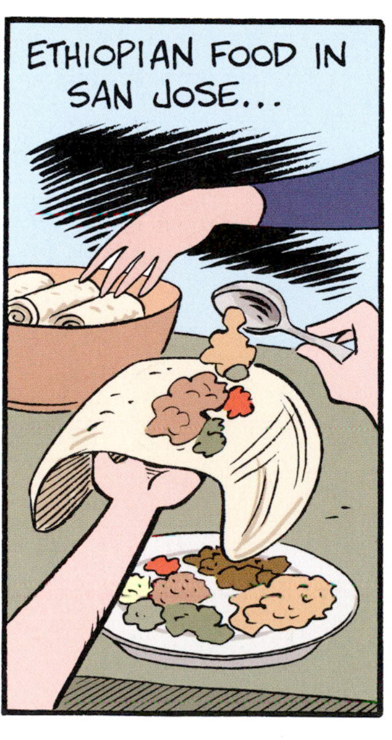
ETHIOPIAN FOOD IN SAN JOSE...

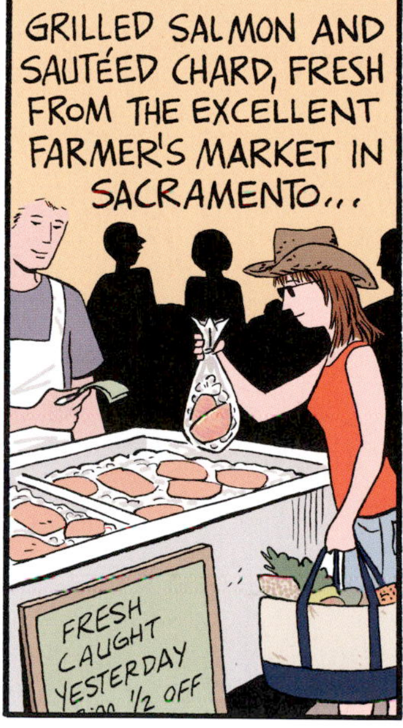
GRILLED SALMON AND SAUTÉED CHARD, FRESH FROM THE EXCELLENT FARMER'S MARKET IN SACRAMENTO...
FRESH CAUGHT YESTERDAY
1/2 OFF

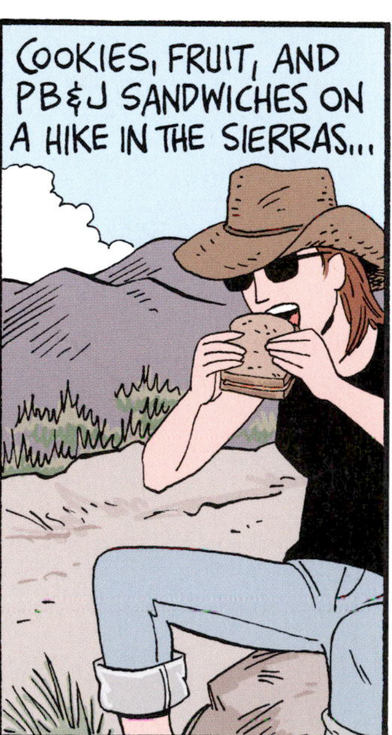
COOKIES, FRUIT, AND PB&J SANDWICHES ON A HIKE IN THE SIERRAS...

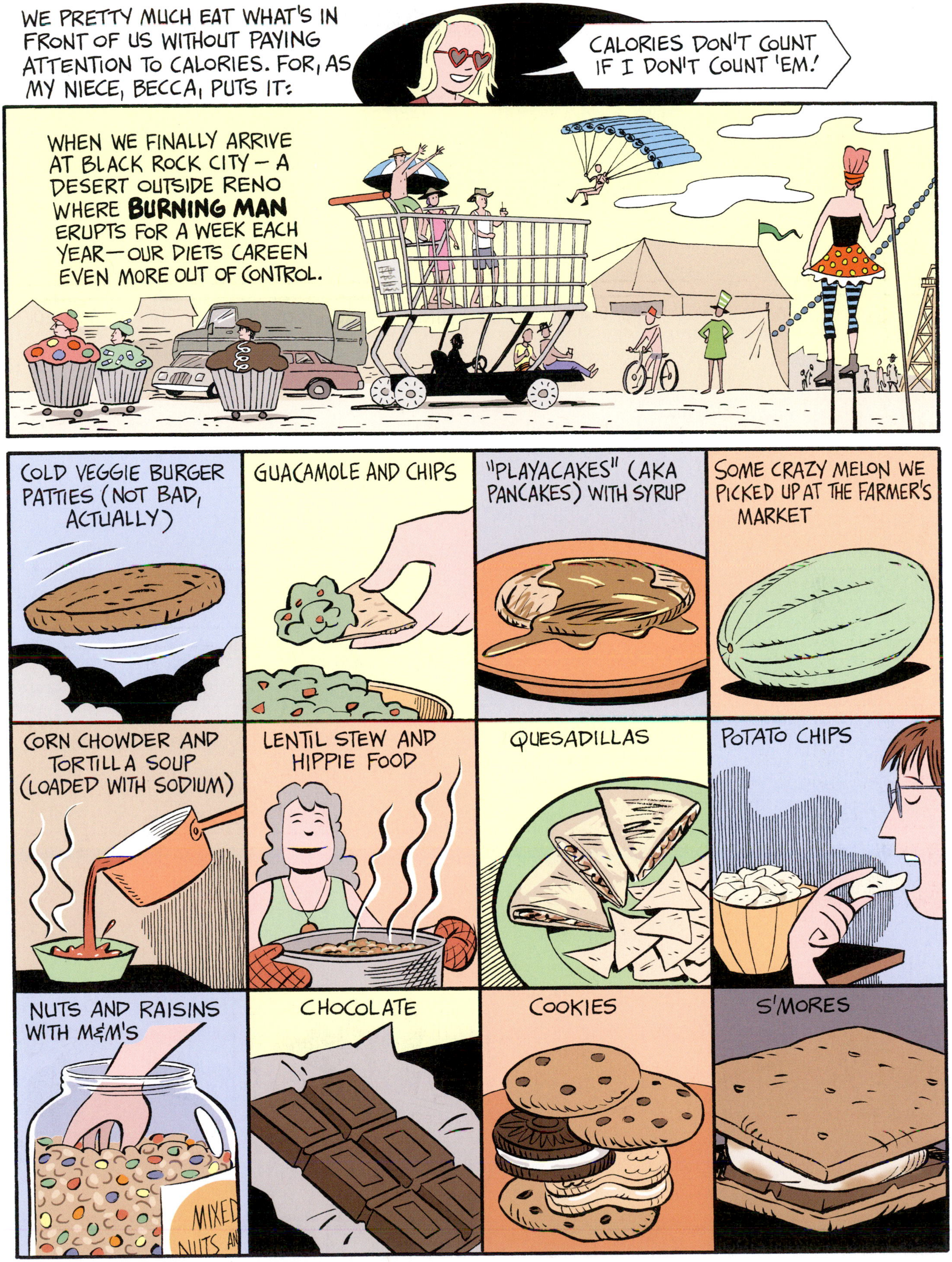

WE PRETTY MUCH EAT WHAT'S IN FRONT OF US WITHOUT PAYING ATTENTION TO CALORIES. FOR, AS MY NIECE, BECCA, PUTS IT:

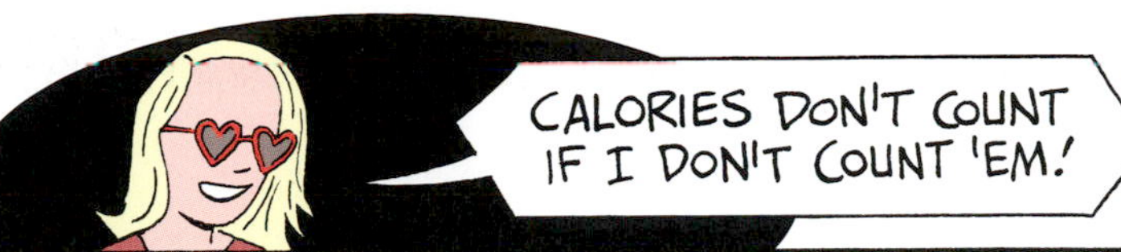

CALORIES DON'T COUNT IF I DON'T COUNT 'EM!

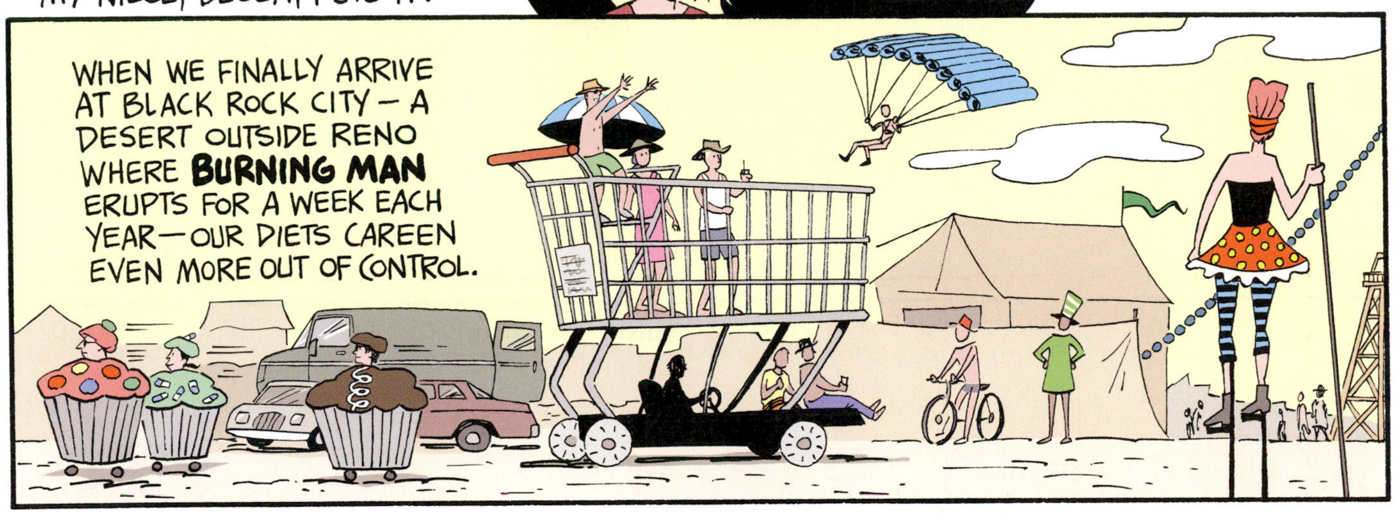

WHEN WE FINALLY ARRIVE AT BLACK ROCK CITY — A DESERT OUTSIDE RENO WHERE **BURNING MAN** ERUPTS FOR A WEEK EACH YEAR — OUR DIETS CAREEN EVEN MORE OUT OF CONTROL.

COLD VEGGIE BURGER PATTIES (NOT BAD, ACTUALLY)

GUACAMOLE AND CHIPS

"PLAYACAKES" (AKA PANCAKES) WITH SYRUP

SOME CRAZY MELON WE PICKED UP AT THE FARMER'S MARKET

CORN CHOWDER AND TORTILLA SOUP (LOADED WITH SODIUM)

LENTIL STEW AND HIPPIE FOOD

QUESADILLAS

POTATO CHIPS

NUTS AND RAISINS WITH M&M'S

MIXED NUTS AN

CHOCOLATE

COOKIES

S'MORES

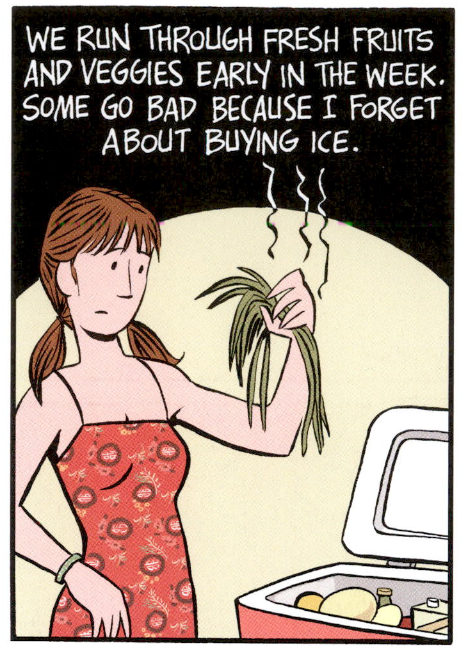
WE RUN THROUGH FRESH FRUITS AND VEGGIES EARLY IN THE WEEK. SOME GO BAD BECAUSE I FORGET ABOUT BUYING ICE.

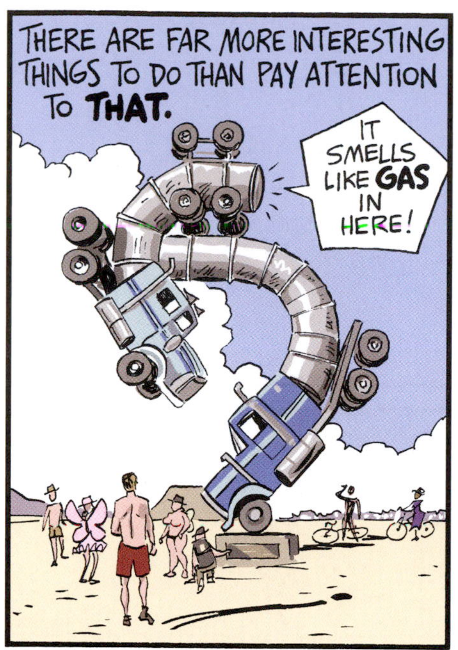
THERE ARE FAR MORE INTERESTING THINGS TO DO THAN PAY ATTENTION TO **THAT.**
IT SMELLS LIKE **GAS** IN HERE!

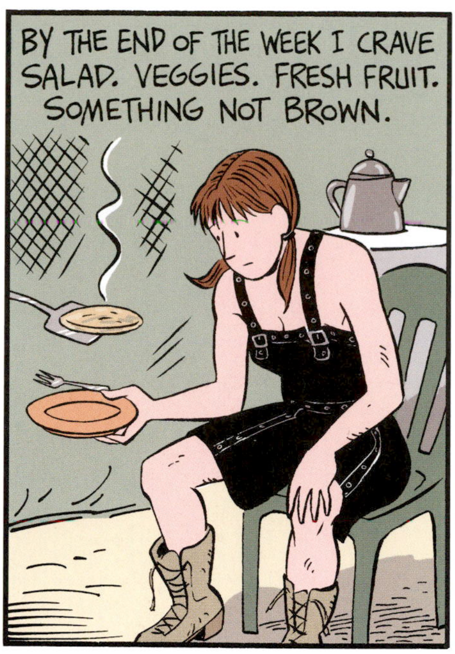
BY THE END OF THE WEEK I CRAVE SALAD. VEGGIES. FRESH FRUIT. SOMETHING NOT BROWN.

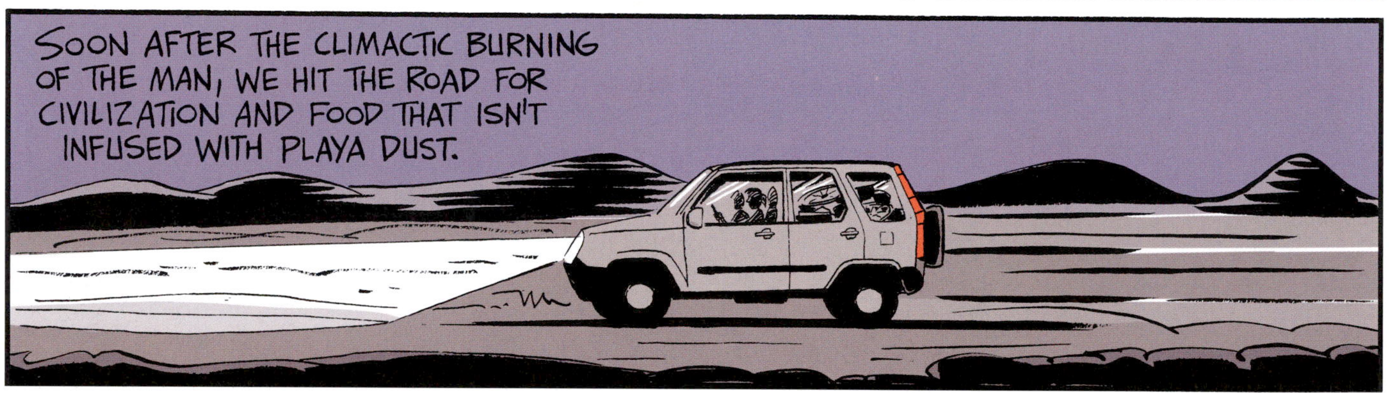
SOON AFTER THE CLIMACTIC BURNING OF THE MAN, WE HIT THE ROAD FOR CIVILIZATION AND FOOD THAT ISN'T INFUSED WITH PLAYA DUST.

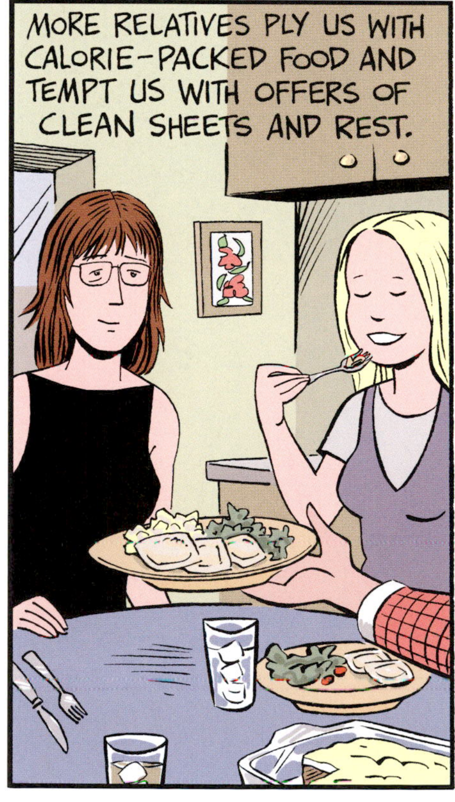
MORE RELATIVES PLY US WITH CALORIE-PACKED FOOD AND TEMPT US WITH OFFERS OF CLEAN SHEETS AND REST.

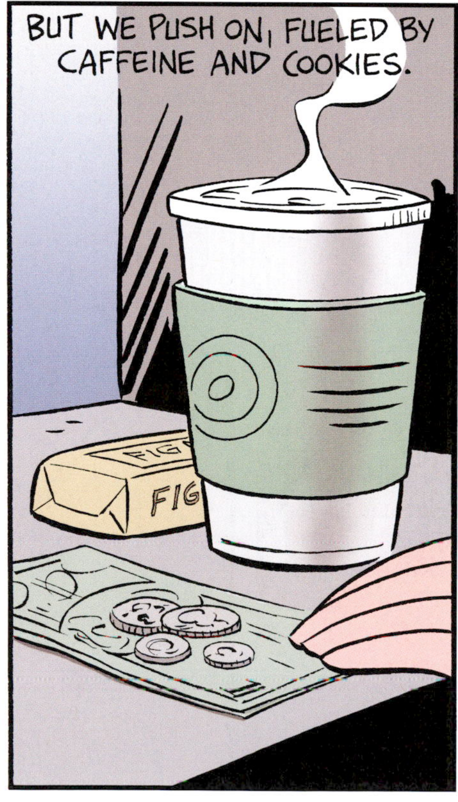
BUT WE PUSH ON, FUELED BY CAFFEINE AND COOKIES.
FIG

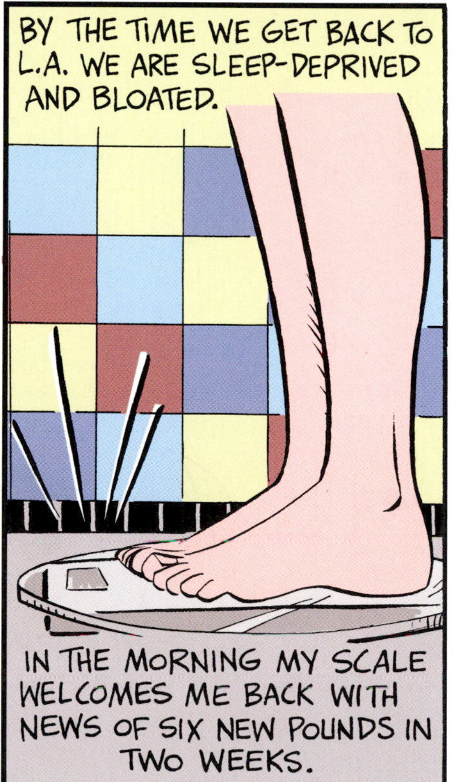
BY THE TIME WE GET BACK TO L.A. WE ARE SLEEP-DEPRIVED AND BLOATED.
IN THE MORNING MY SCALE WELCOMES ME BACK WITH NEWS OF SIX NEW POUNDS IN TWO WEEKS.

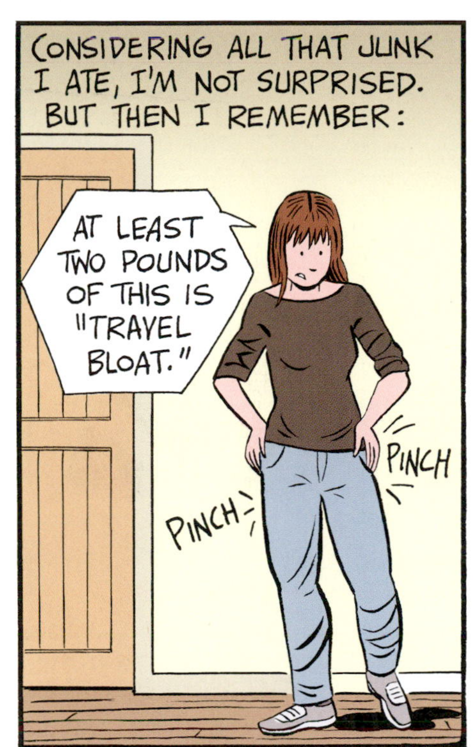
CONSIDERING ALL THAT JUNK I ATE, I'M NOT SURPRISED. BUT THEN I REMEMBER:
AT LEAST TWO POUNDS OF THIS IS "TRAVEL BLOAT."
PINCH
PINCH

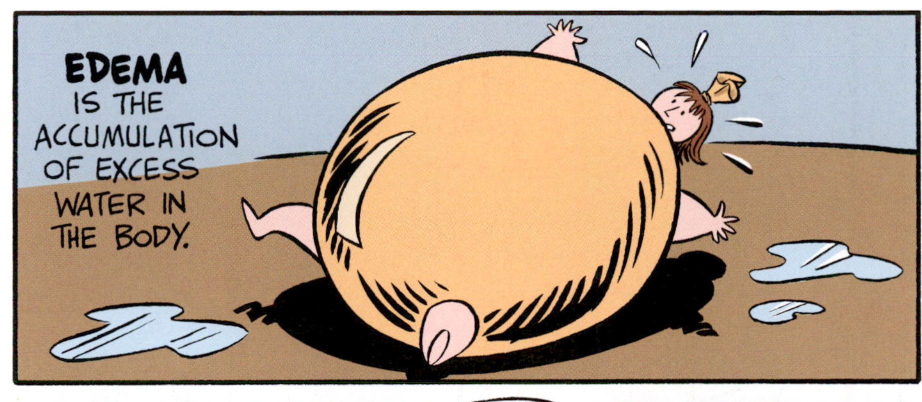
EDEMA IS THE ACCUMULATION OF EXCESS WATER IN THE BODY.

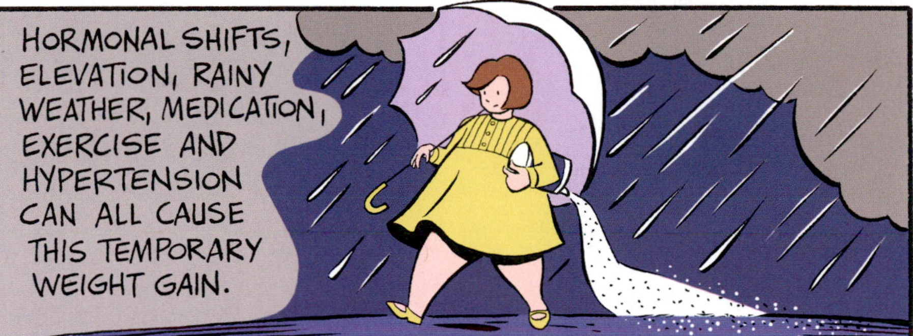
HORMONAL SHIFTS, ELEVATION, RAINY WEATHER, MEDICATION, EXERCISE AND HYPERTENSION CAN ALL CAUSE THIS TEMPORARY WEIGHT GAIN.

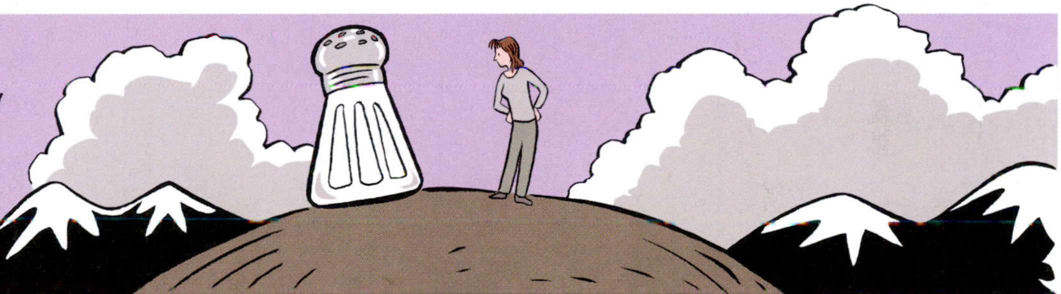
TRAVEL ALWAYS KICKS IT IN FOR ME, ESPECIALLY IF I FLY OR, IN THIS CASE, CONSUME A LOT OF SALTY FOODS AT A HIGH ELEVATION.

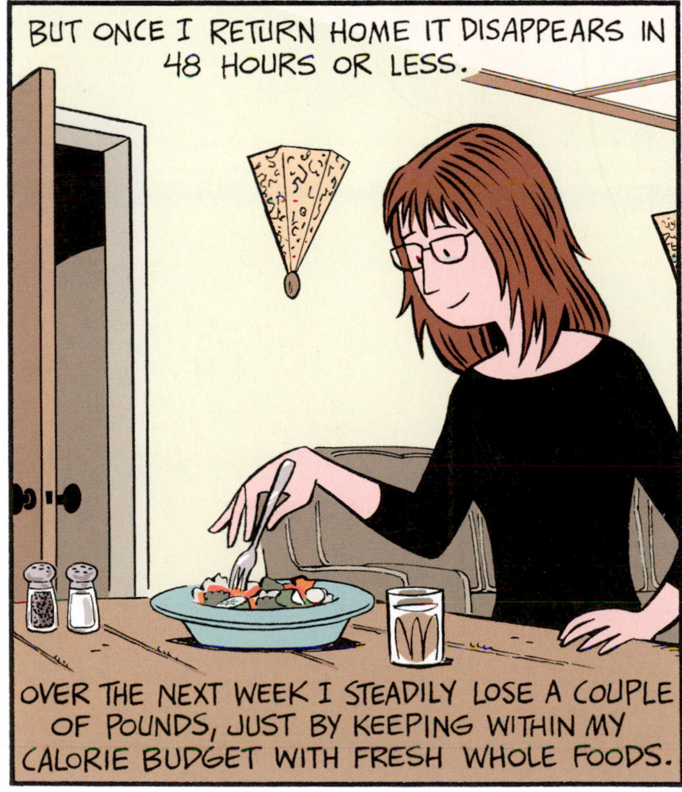
BUT ONCE I RETURN HOME IT DISAPPEARS IN 48 HOURS OR LESS.
OVER THE NEXT WEEK I STEADILY LOSE A COUPLE OF POUNDS, JUST BY KEEPING WITHIN MY CALORIE BUDGET WITH FRESH WHOLE FOODS.

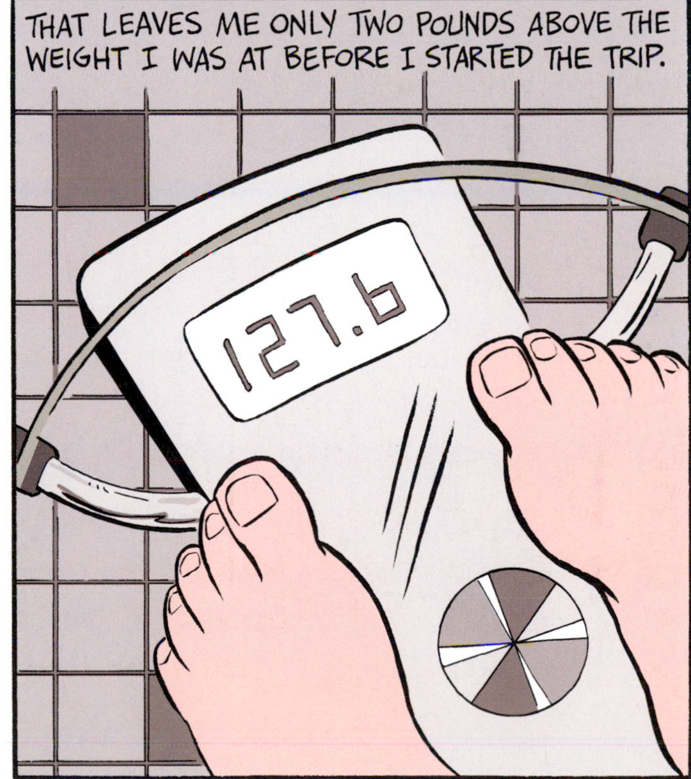
THAT LEAVES ME ONLY TWO POUNDS ABOVE THE WEIGHT I WAS AT BEFORE I STARTED THE TRIP.
127.6

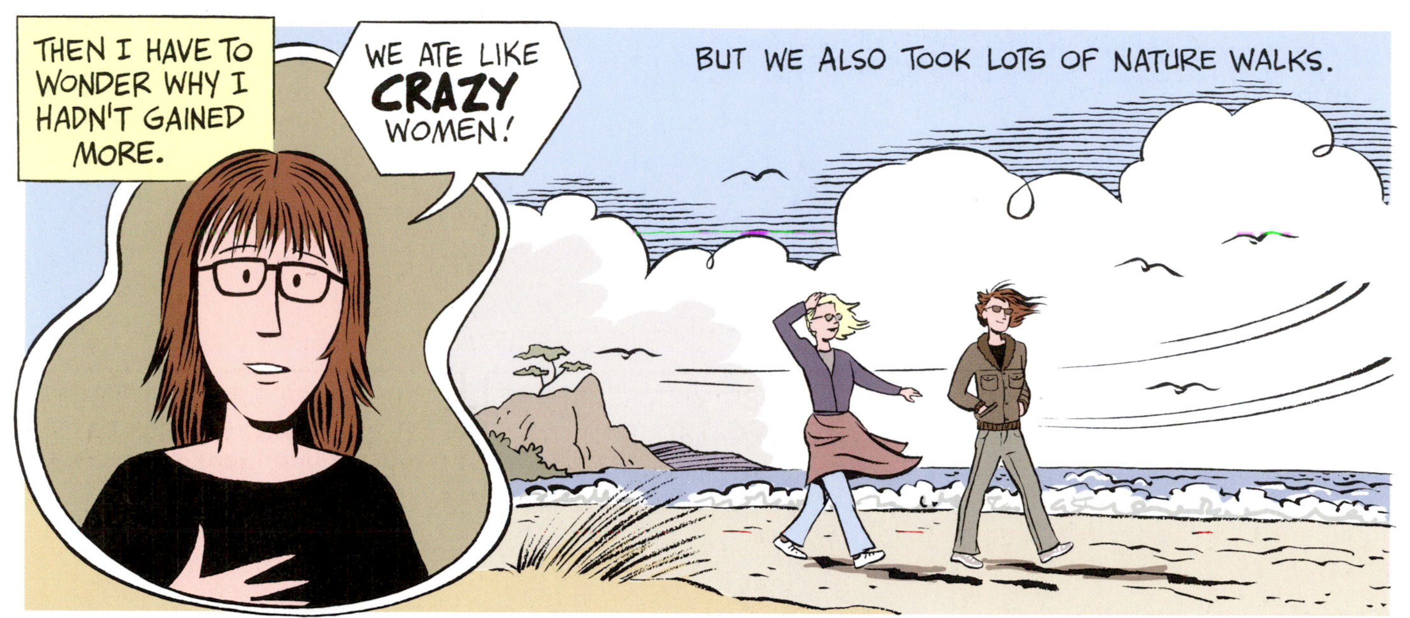
THEN I HAVE TO WONDER WHY I HADN'T GAINED MORE.
WE ATE LIKE CRAZY WOMEN!
BUT WE ALSO TOOK LOTS OF NATURE WALKS.

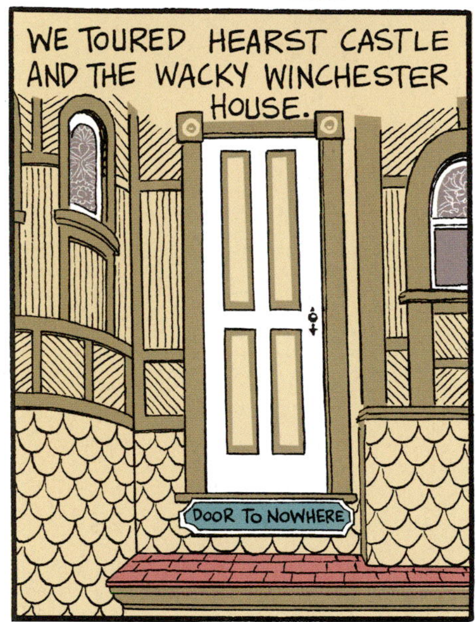
WE TOURED HEARST CASTLE AND THE WACKY WINCHESTER HOUSE.
DOOR TO NOWHERE

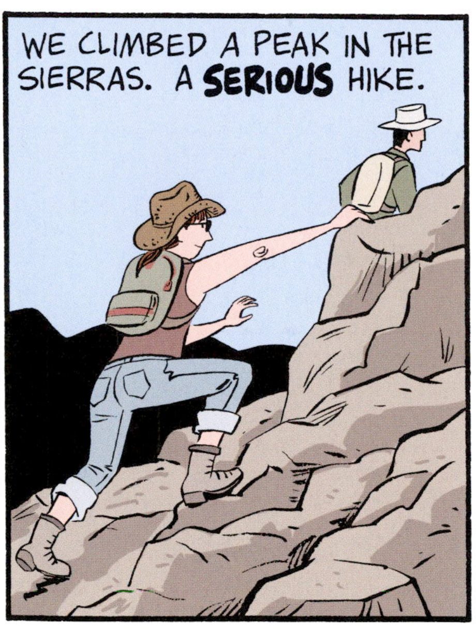
WE CLIMBED A PEAK IN THE SIERRAS. A SERIOUS HIKE.

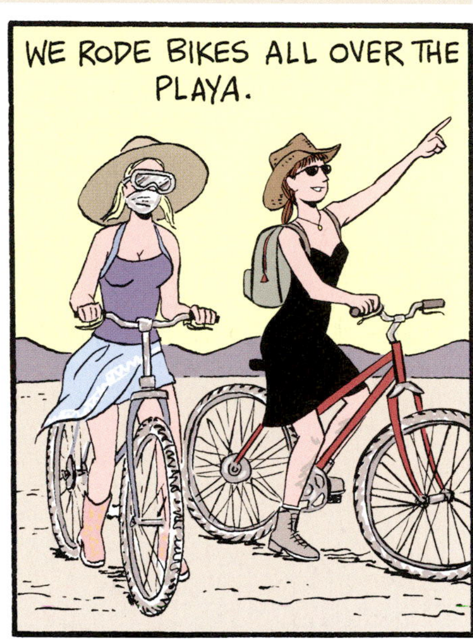
WE RODE BIKES ALL OVER THE PLAYA.

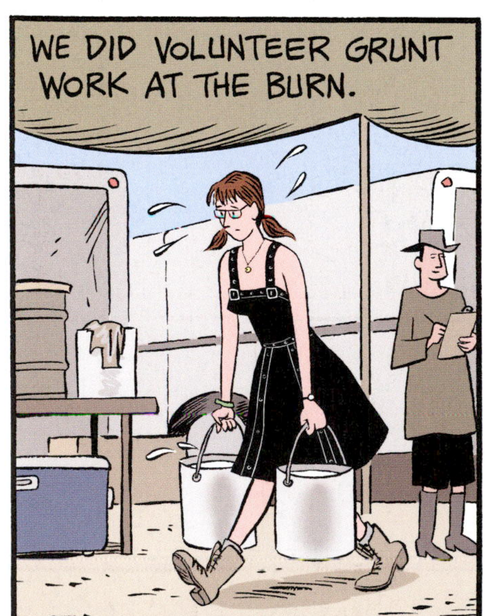
WE DID VOLUNTEER GRUNT WORK AT THE BURN.

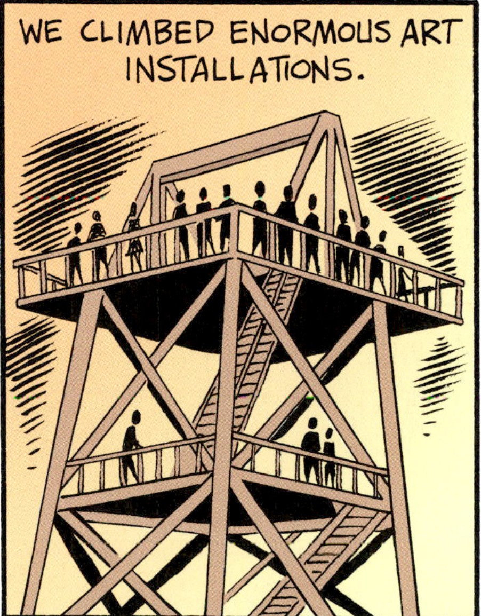
WE CLIMBED ENORMOUS ART INSTALLATIONS.

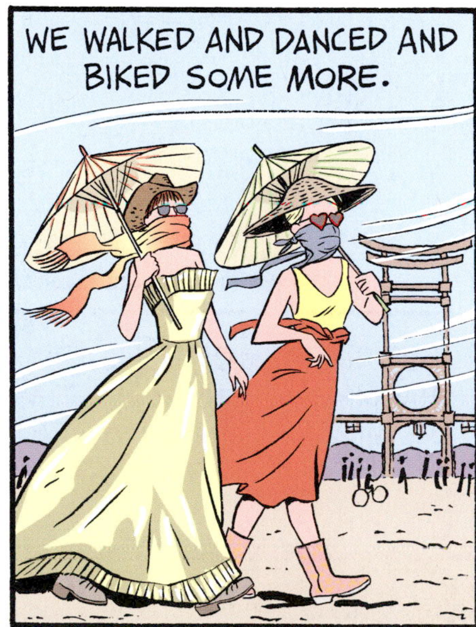
WE WALKED AND DANCED AND BIKED SOME MORE.

IN SHORT, LOTS OF ACTIVITY BURNED OFF MANY UNKNOWN EXCESS CALORIES.

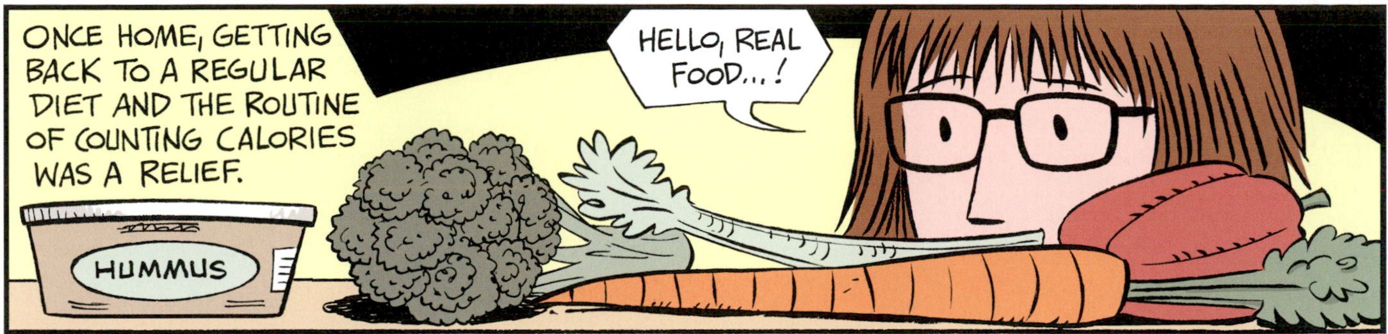
ONCE HOME, GETTING BACK TO A REGULAR DIET AND THE ROUTINE OF COUNTING CALORIES WAS A RELIEF.
HELLO, REAL FOOD...!
HUMMUS

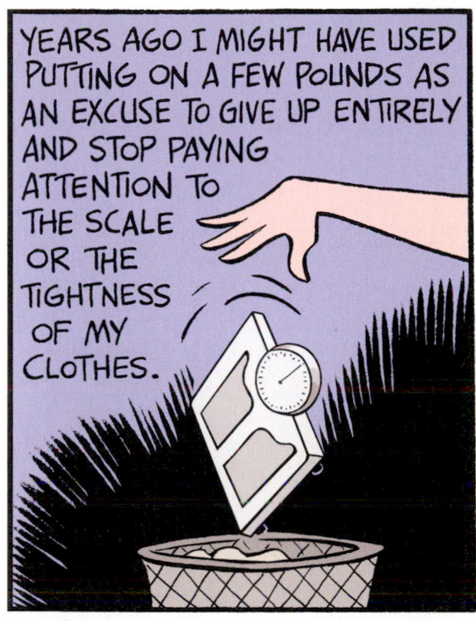
YEARS AGO I MIGHT HAVE USED PUTTING ON A FEW POUNDS AS AN EXCUSE TO GIVE UP ENTIRELY AND STOP PAYING ATTENTION TO THE SCALE OR THE TIGHTNESS OF MY CLOTHES.

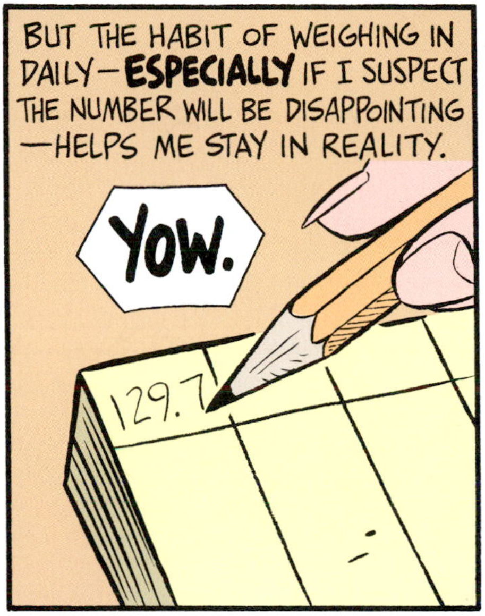
BUT THE HABIT OF WEIGHING IN DAILY—ESPECIALLY IF I SUSPECT THE NUMBER WILL BE DISAPPOINTING—HELPS ME STAY IN REALITY.
YOW.
129.7

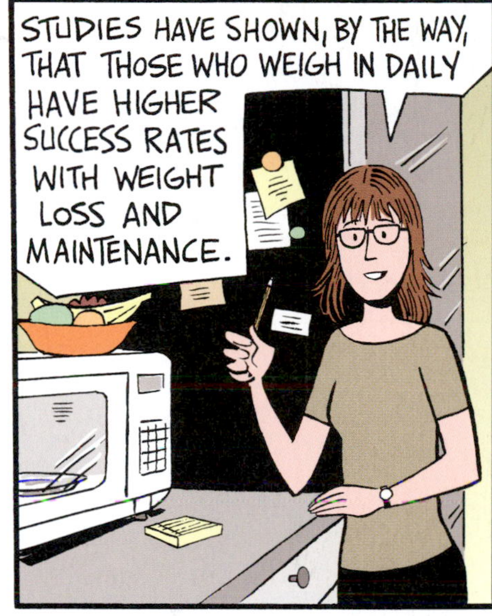
STUDIES HAVE SHOWN, BY THE WAY, THAT THOSE WHO WEIGH IN DAILY HAVE HIGHER SUCCESS RATES WITH WEIGHT LOSS AND MAINTENANCE.

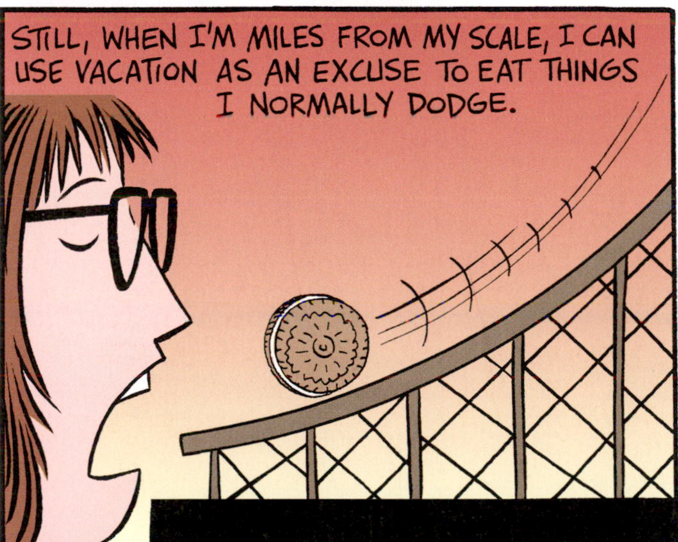
STILL, WHEN I'M MILES FROM MY SCALE, I CAN USE VACATION AS AN EXCUSE TO EAT THINGS I NORMALLY DODGE.

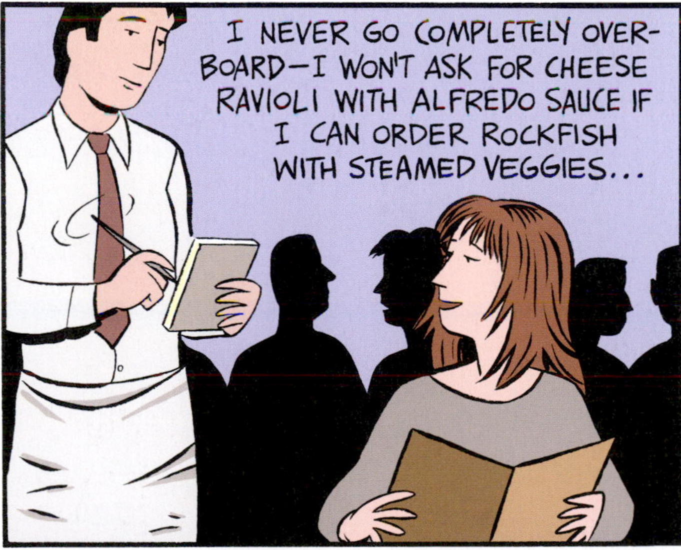
I NEVER GO COMPLETELY OVERBOARD—I WON'T ASK FOR CHEESE RAVIOLI WITH ALFREDO SAUCE IF I CAN ORDER ROCKFISH WITH STEAMED VEGGIES...

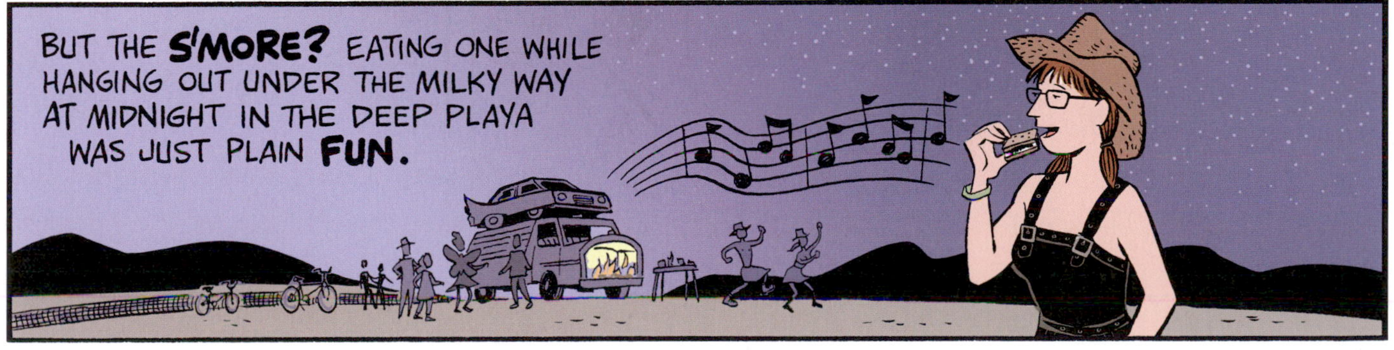
BUT THE S'MORE? EATING ONE WHILE HANGING OUT UNDER THE MILKY WAY AT MIDNIGHT IN THE DEEP PLAYA WAS JUST PLAIN FUN.

# WHICH BRINGS US TO THE OPPOSITE OF FUN... WORK!

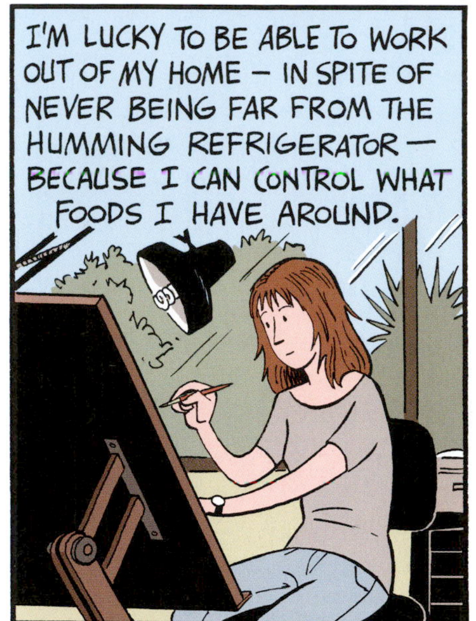
I'M LUCKY TO BE ABLE TO WORK OUT OF MY HOME – IN SPITE OF NEVER BEING FAR FROM THE HUMMING REFRIGERATOR – BECAUSE I CAN CONTROL WHAT FOODS I HAVE AROUND.

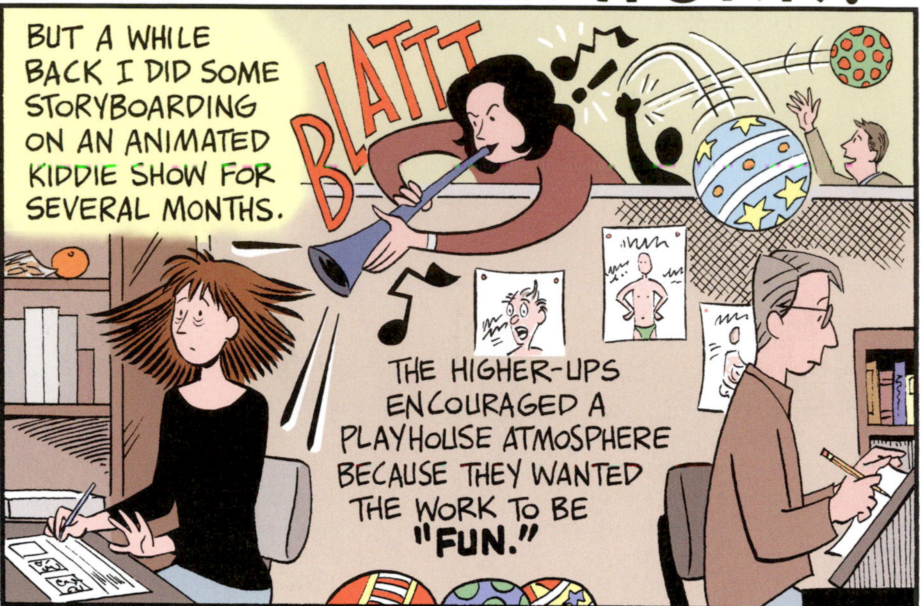
BUT A WHILE BACK I DID SOME STORYBOARDING ON AN ANIMATED KIDDIE SHOW FOR SEVERAL MONTHS.
BLATT
THE HIGHER-UPS ENCOURAGED A PLAYHOUSE ATMOSPHERE BECAUSE THEY WANTED THE WORK TO BE "FUN."

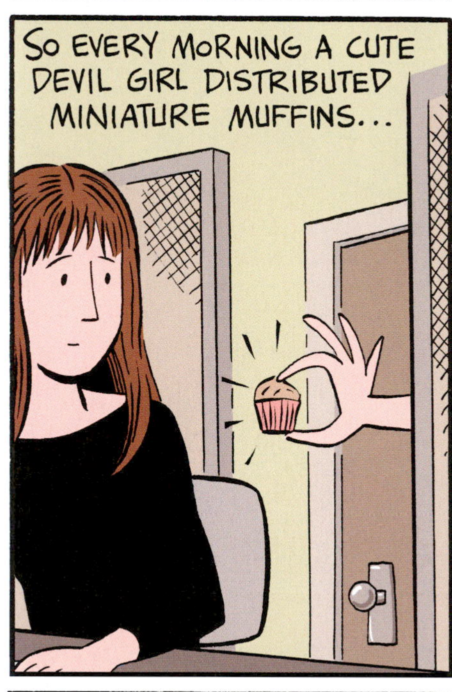
SO EVERY MORNING A CUTE DEVIL GIRL DISTRIBUTED MINIATURE MUFFINS...

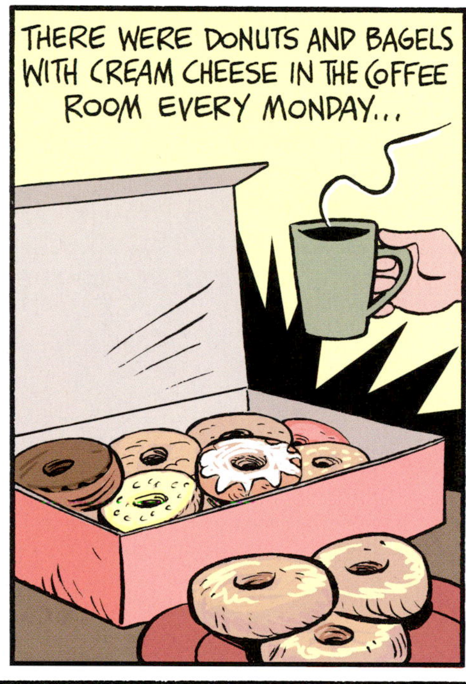
THERE WERE DONUTS AND BAGELS WITH CREAM CHEESE IN THE COFFEE ROOM EVERY MONDAY...

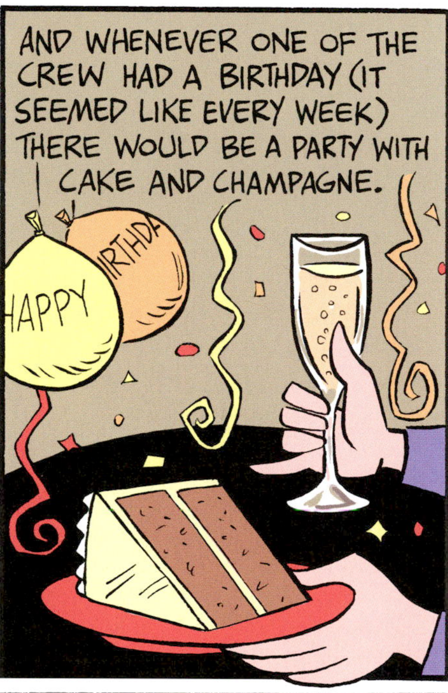
AND WHENEVER ONE OF THE CREW HAD A BIRTHDAY (IT SEEMED LIKE EVERY WEEK) THERE WOULD BE A PARTY WITH CAKE AND CHAMPAGNE.

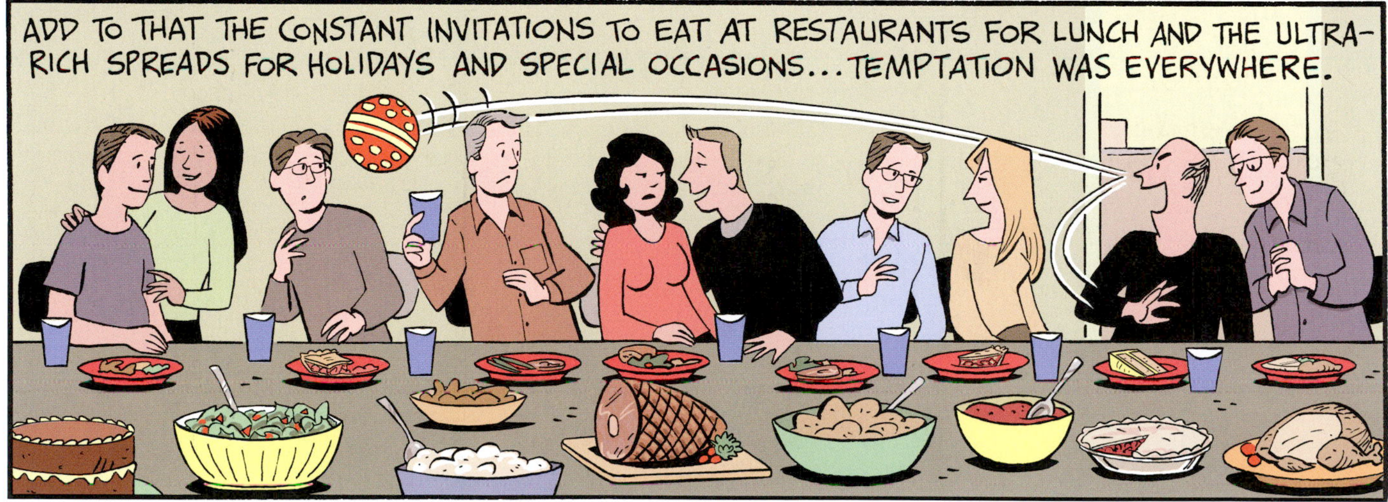
ADD TO THAT THE CONSTANT INVITATIONS TO EAT AT RESTAURANTS FOR LUNCH AND THE ULTRA-RICH SPREADS FOR HOLIDAYS AND SPECIAL OCCASIONS... TEMPTATION WAS EVERYWHERE.

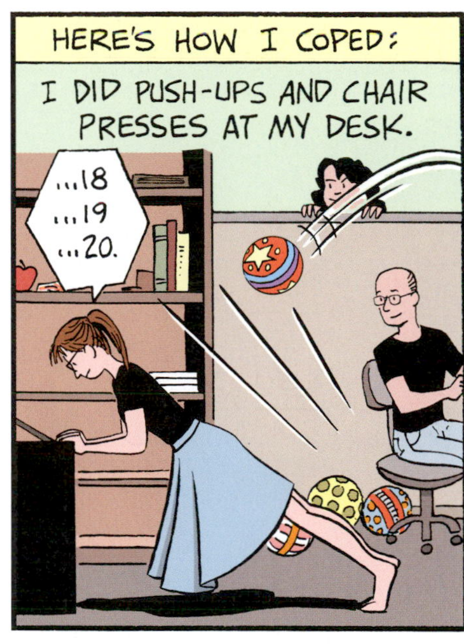
HERE'S HOW I COPED:
I DID PUSH-UPS AND CHAIR PRESSES AT MY DESK.
...18
...19
...20.

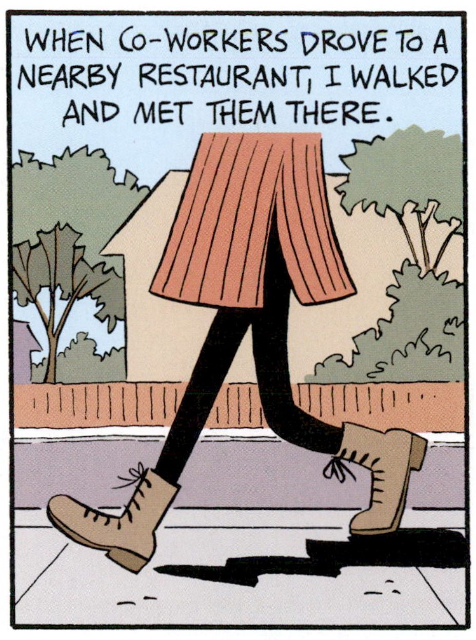
WHEN CO-WORKERS DROVE TO A NEARBY RESTAURANT, I WALKED AND MET THEM THERE.

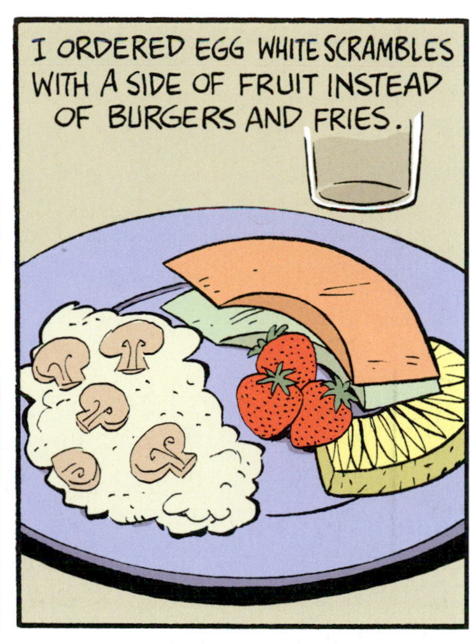
I ORDERED EGG WHITE SCRAMBLES WITH A SIDE OF FRUIT INSTEAD OF BURGERS AND FRIES.

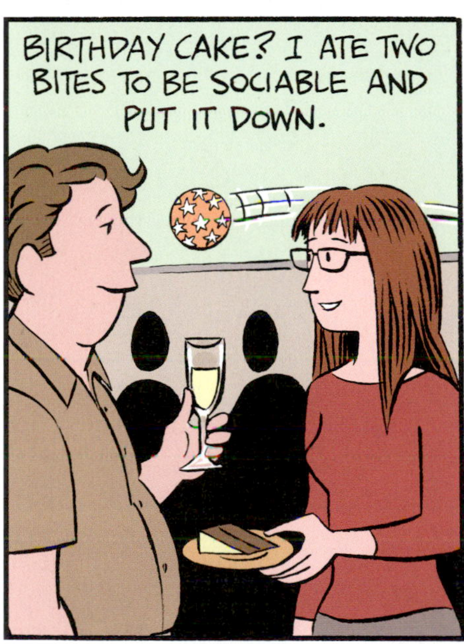
BIRTHDAY CAKE? I ATE TWO BITES TO BE SOCIABLE AND PUT IT DOWN.

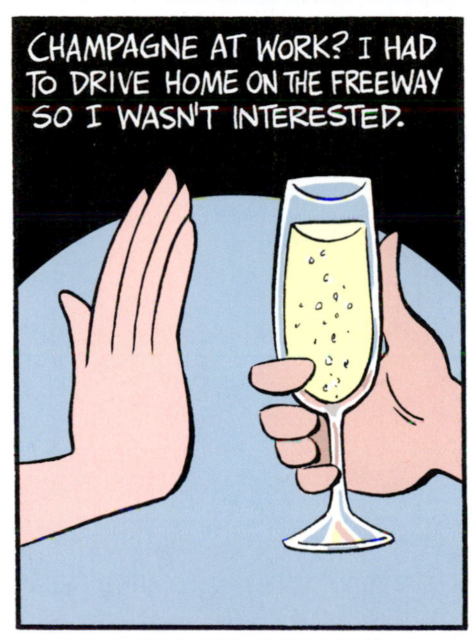
CHAMPAGNE AT WORK? I HAD TO DRIVE HOME ON THE FREEWAY SO I WASN'T INTERESTED.

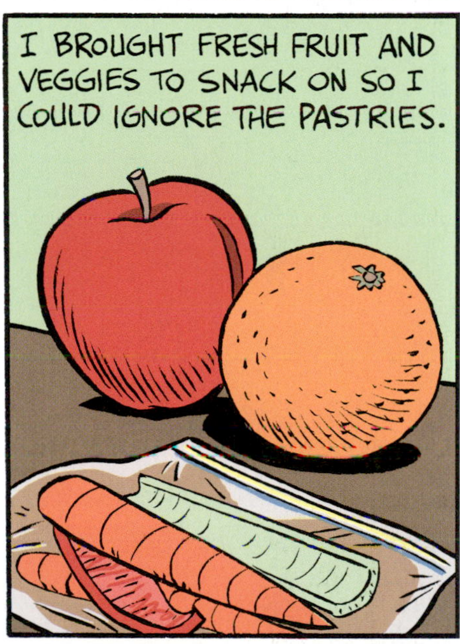
I BROUGHT FRESH FRUIT AND VEGGIES TO SNACK ON SO I COULD IGNORE THE PASTRIES.

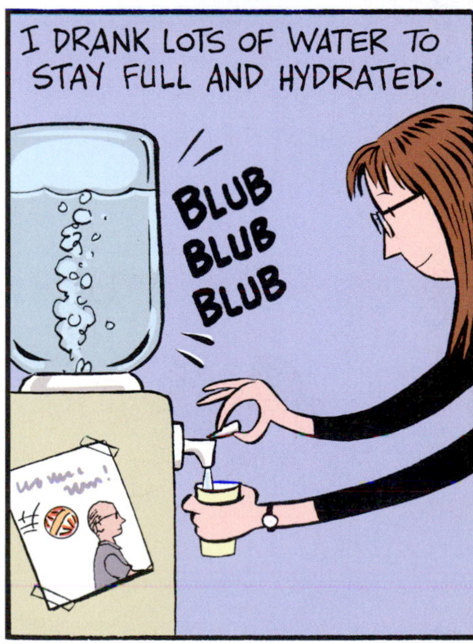
I DRANK LOTS OF WATER TO STAY FULL AND HYDRATED.
BLUB
BLUB
BLUB

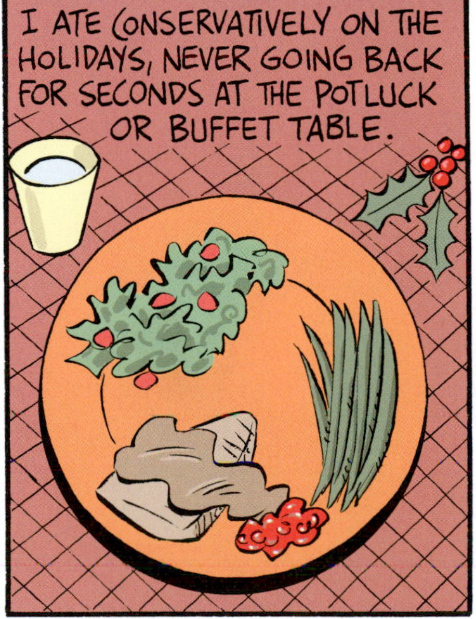
I ATE CONSERVATIVELY ON THE HOLIDAYS, NEVER GOING BACK FOR SECONDS AT THE POTLUCK OR BUFFET TABLE.

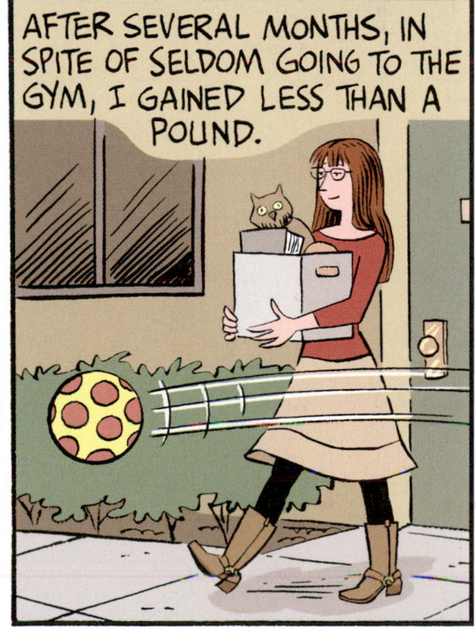
AFTER SEVERAL MONTHS, IN SPITE OF SELDOM GOING TO THE GYM, I GAINED LESS THAN A POUND.

OTHER WORK-AROUNDS AT WORK INCLUDE:

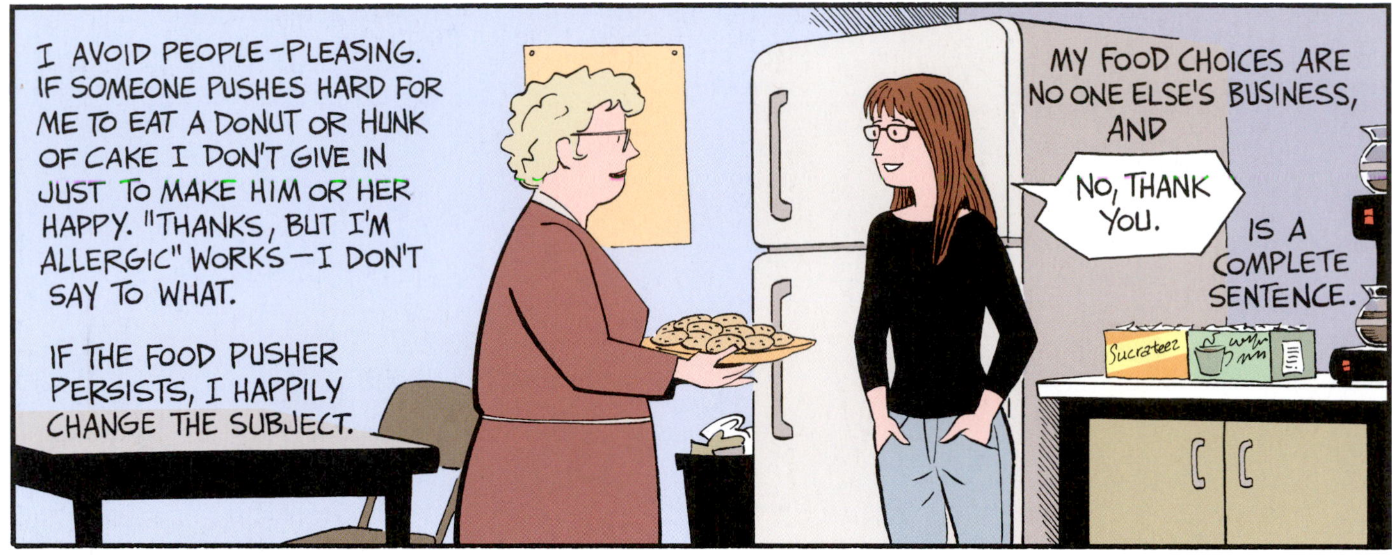

I AVOID PEOPLE-PLEASING. IF SOMEONE PUSHES HARD FOR ME TO EAT A DONUT OR HUNK OF CAKE I DON'T GIVE IN JUST TO MAKE HIM OR HER HAPPY. "THANKS, BUT I'M ALLERGIC" WORKS—I DON'T SAY TO WHAT.
IF THE FOOD PUSHER PERSISTS, I HAPPILY CHANGE THE SUBJECT.
MY FOOD CHOICES ARE NO ONE ELSE'S BUSINESS, AND
NO, THANK YOU.
IS A COMPLETE SENTENCE.
Sucrateez


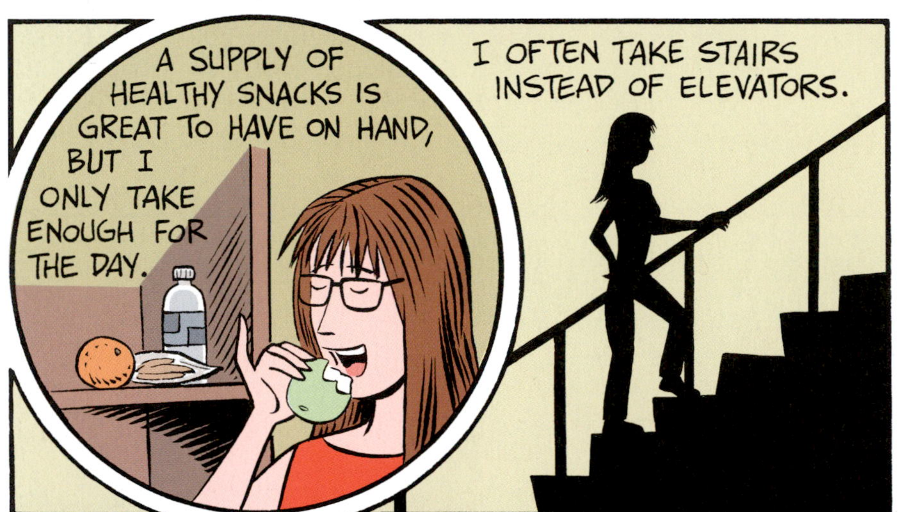

A SUPPLY OF HEALTHY SNACKS IS GREAT TO HAVE ON HAND, BUT I ONLY TAKE ENOUGH FOR THE DAY.
I OFTEN TAKE STAIRS INSTEAD OF ELEVATORS.


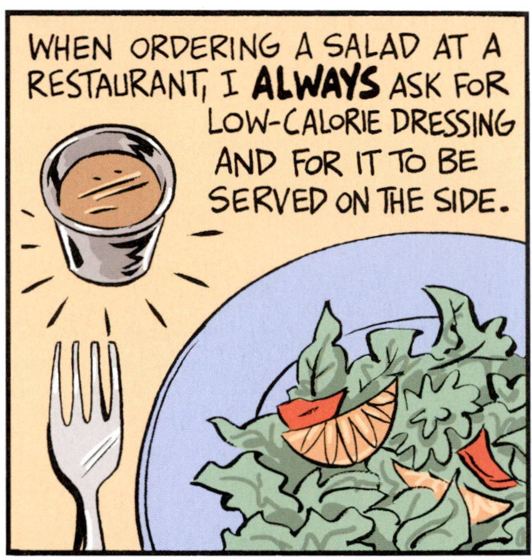

WHEN ORDERING A SALAD AT A RESTAURANT, I **ALWAYS** ASK FOR LOW-CALORIE DRESSING AND FOR IT TO BE SERVED ON THE SIDE.


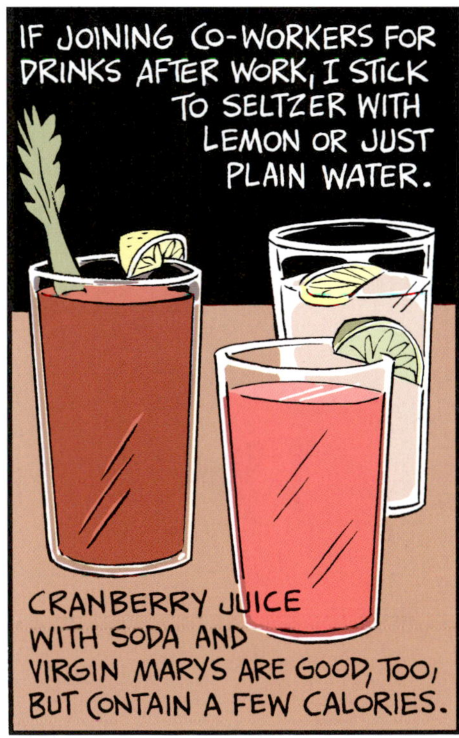

IF JOINING CO-WORKERS FOR DRINKS AFTER WORK, I STICK TO SELTZER WITH LEMON OR JUST PLAIN WATER.
CRANBERRY JUICE WITH SODA AND VIRGIN MARYS ARE GOOD, TOO, BUT CONTAIN A FEW CALORIES.


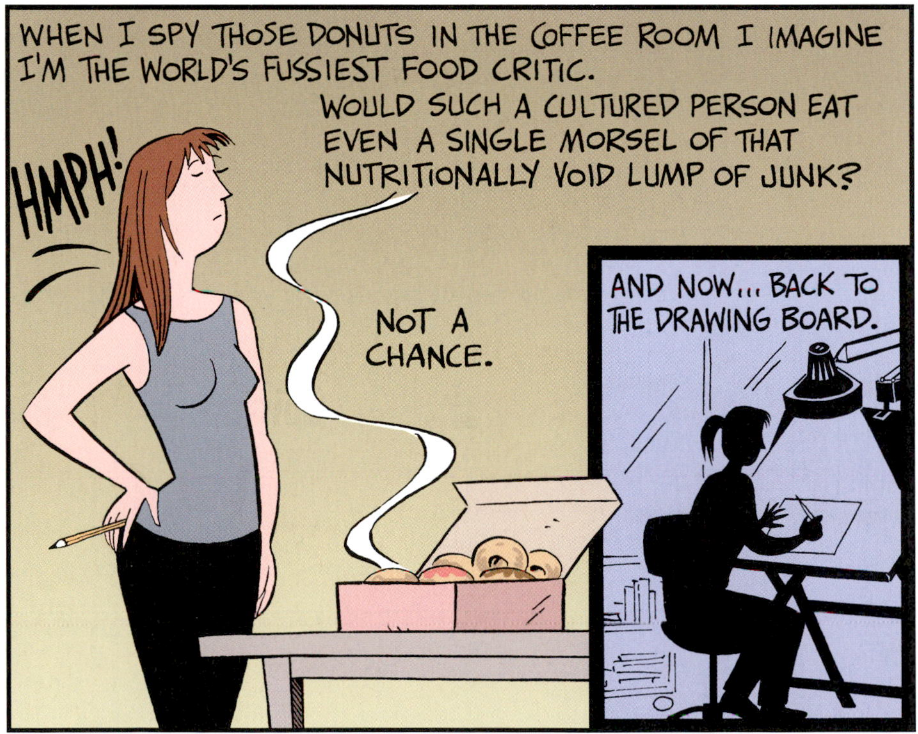

WHEN I SPY THOSE DONUTS IN THE COFFEE ROOM I IMAGINE I'M THE WORLD'S FUSSIEST FOOD CRITIC.
WOULD SUCH A CULTURED PERSON EAT EVEN A SINGLE MORSEL OF THAT NUTRITIONALLY VOID LUMP OF JUNK?
HMPH!
NOT A CHANCE.
AND NOW... BACK TO THE DRAWING BOARD.

# FLIPPING THE SWITCH

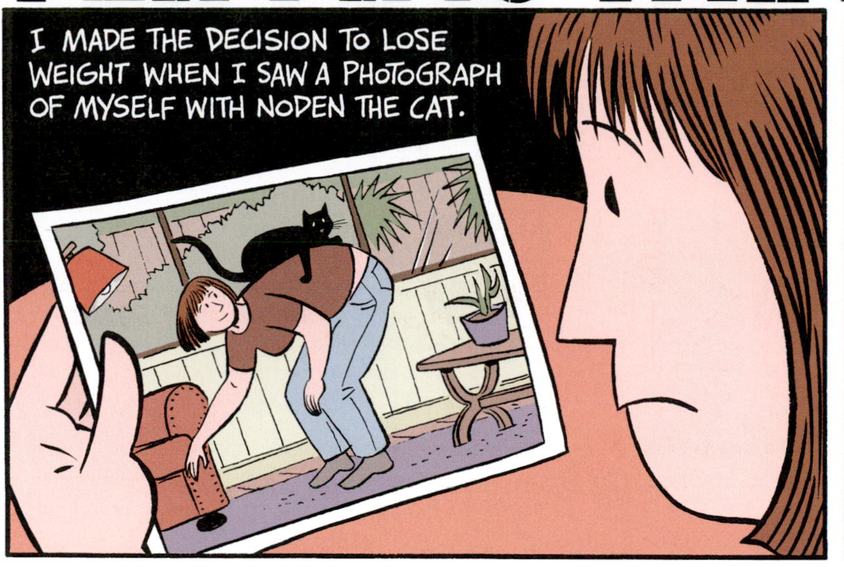
I MADE THE DECISION TO LOSE WEIGHT WHEN I SAW A PHOTOGRAPH OF MYSELF WITH NODEN THE CAT.

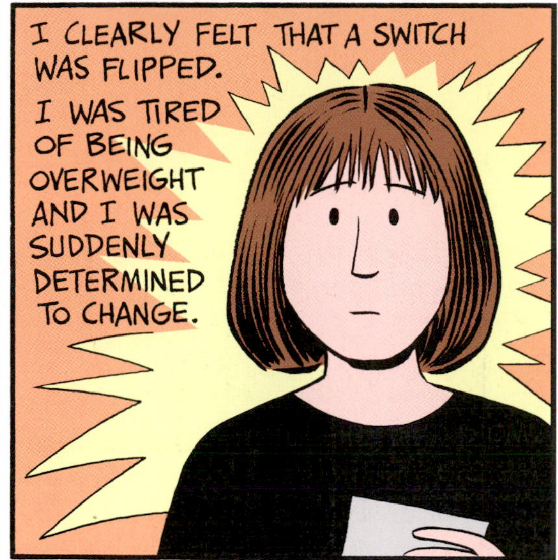
I CLEARLY FELT THAT A SWITCH WAS FLIPPED.
I WAS TIRED OF BEING OVERWEIGHT AND I WAS SUDDENLY DETERMINED TO CHANGE.

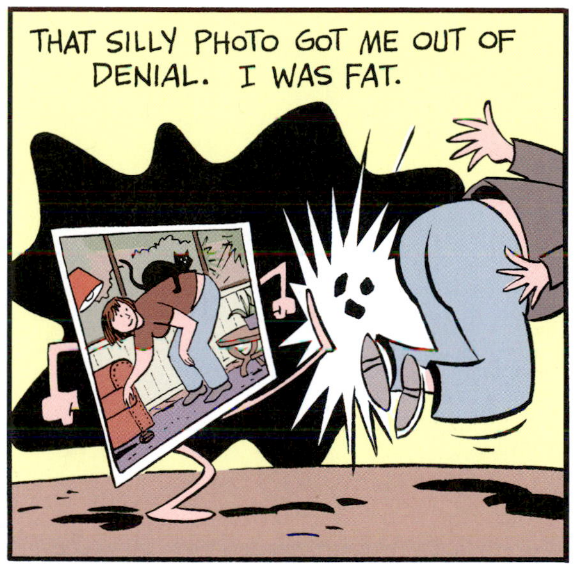
THAT SILLY PHOTO GOT ME OUT OF DENIAL. I WAS FAT.

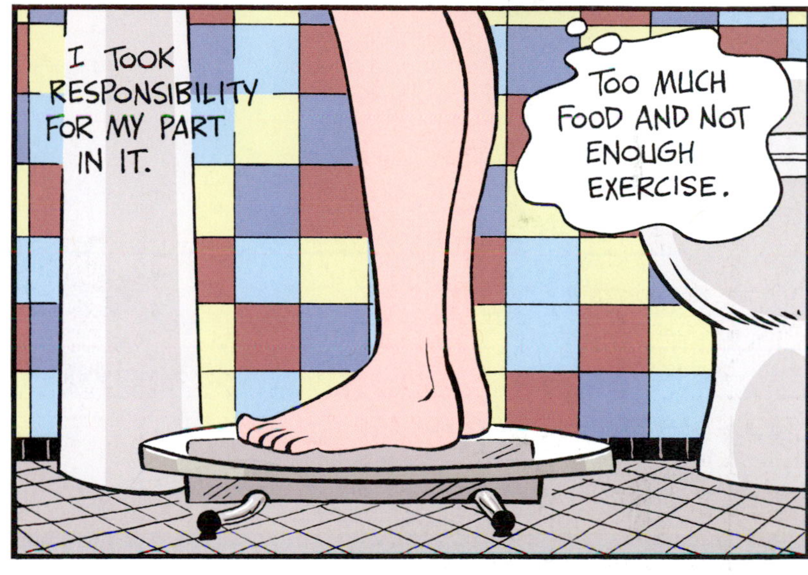
I TOOK RESPONSIBILITY FOR MY PART IN IT.
TOO MUCH FOOD AND NOT ENOUGH EXERCISE.

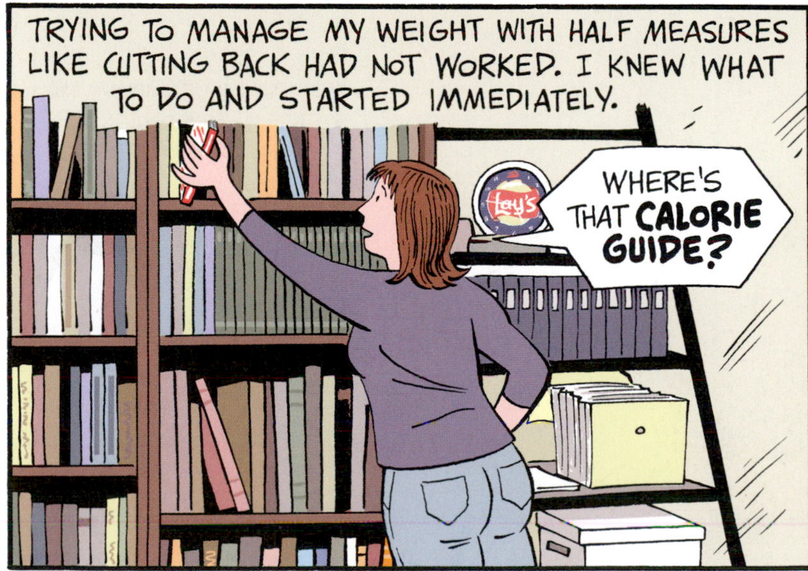
TRYING TO MANAGE MY WEIGHT WITH HALF MEASURES LIKE CUTTING BACK HAD NOT WORKED. I KNEW WHAT TO DO AND STARTED IMMEDIATELY.
WHERE'S THAT CALORIE GUIDE?

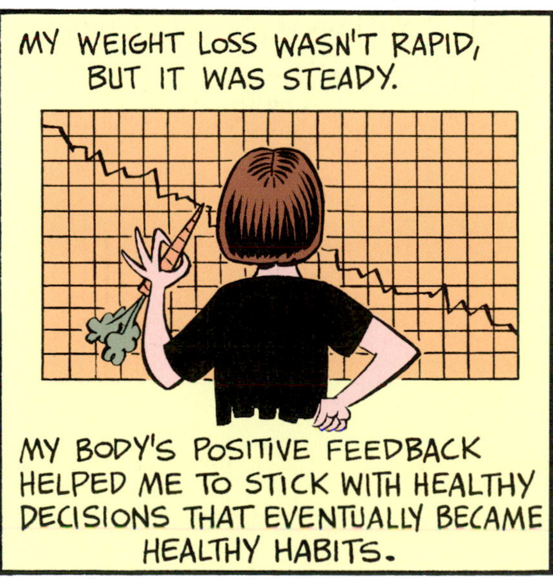
MY WEIGHT LOSS WASN'T RAPID, BUT IT WAS STEADY.
MY BODY'S POSITIVE FEEDBACK HELPED ME TO STICK WITH HEALTHY DECISIONS THAT EVENTUALLY BECAME HEALTHY HABITS.

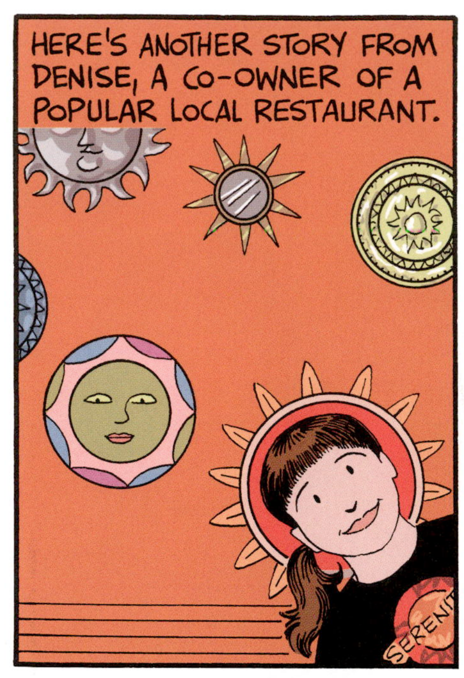
HERE'S ANOTHER STORY FROM DENISE, A CO-OWNER OF A POPULAR LOCAL RESTAURANT.

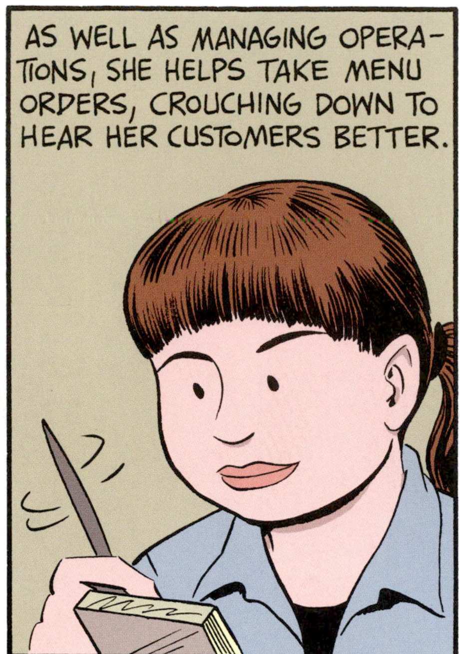
AS WELL AS MANAGING OPERATIONS, SHE HELPS TAKE MENU ORDERS, CROUCHING DOWN TO HEAR HER CUSTOMERS BETTER.

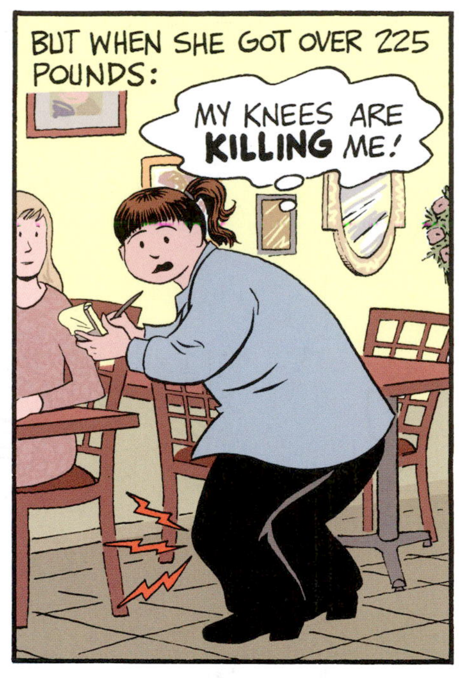
BUT WHEN SHE GOT OVER 225 POUNDS:
MY KNEES ARE **KILLING** ME!

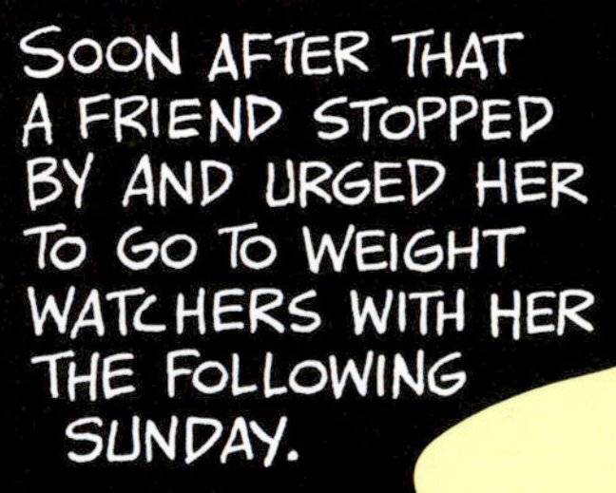
SOON AFTER THAT A FRIEND STOPPED BY AND URGED HER TO GO TO WEIGHT WATCHERS WITH HER THE FOLLOWING SUNDAY.

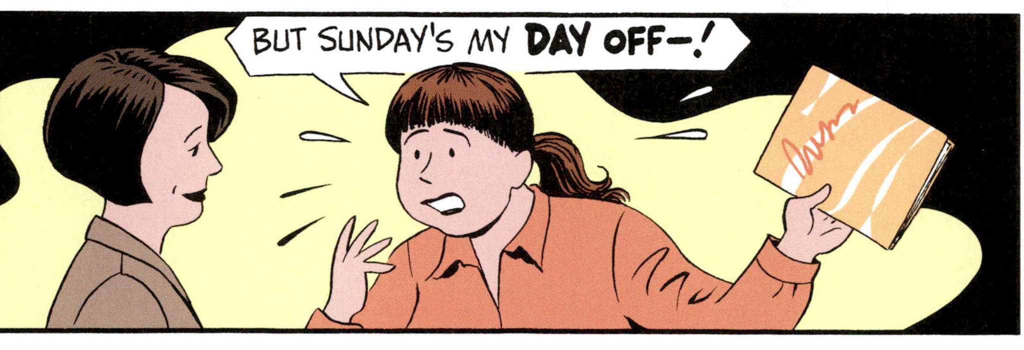
BUT SUNDAY'S MY **DAY OFF**—!

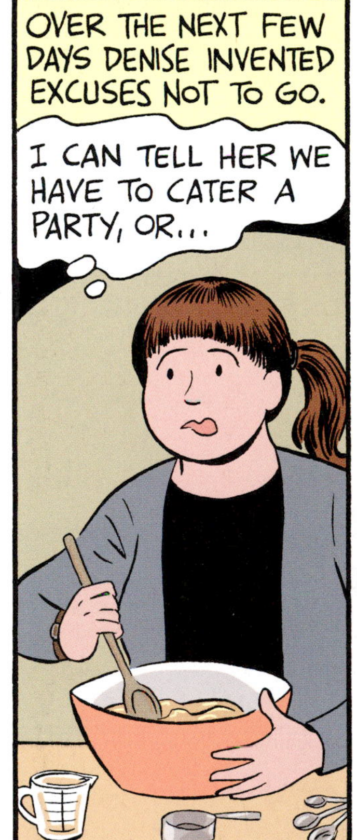
OVER THE NEXT FEW DAYS DENISE INVENTED EXCUSES NOT TO GO.
I CAN TELL HER WE HAVE TO CATER A PARTY, OR...

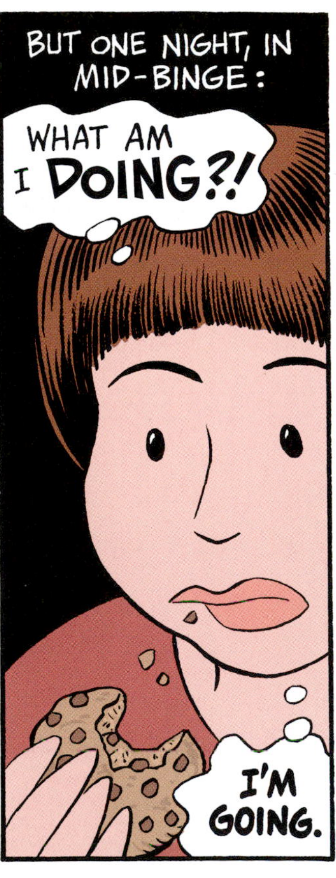
BUT ONE NIGHT, IN MID-BINGE:
WHAT AM I **DOING?!**
I'M GOING.

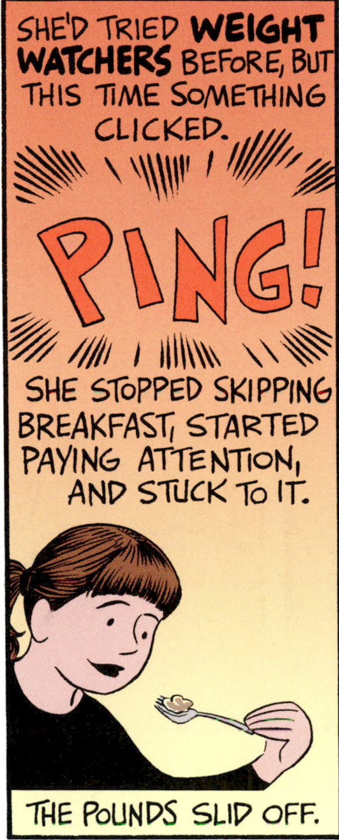
SHE'D TRIED **WEIGHT WATCHERS** BEFORE, BUT THIS TIME SOMETHING CLICKED.
PING!
SHE STOPPED SKIPPING BREAKFAST, STARTED PAYING ATTENTION, AND STUCK TO IT.
THE POUNDS SLID OFF.

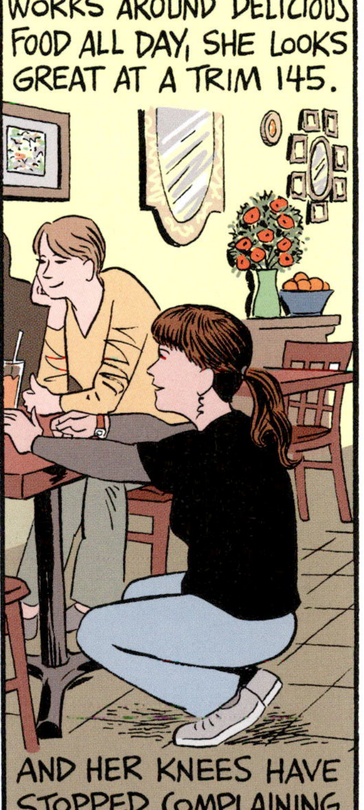
NOW, EVEN THOUGH SHE WORKS AROUND DELICIOUS FOOD ALL DAY, SHE LOOKS GREAT AT A TRIM 145.
AND HER KNEES HAVE STOPPED COMPLAINING.

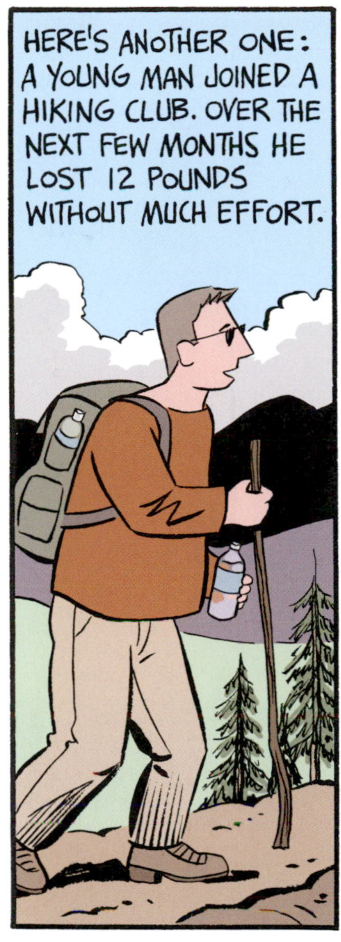
HERE'S ANOTHER ONE: A YOUNG MAN JOINED A HIKING CLUB. OVER THE NEXT FEW MONTHS HE LOST 12 POUNDS WITHOUT MUCH EFFORT.

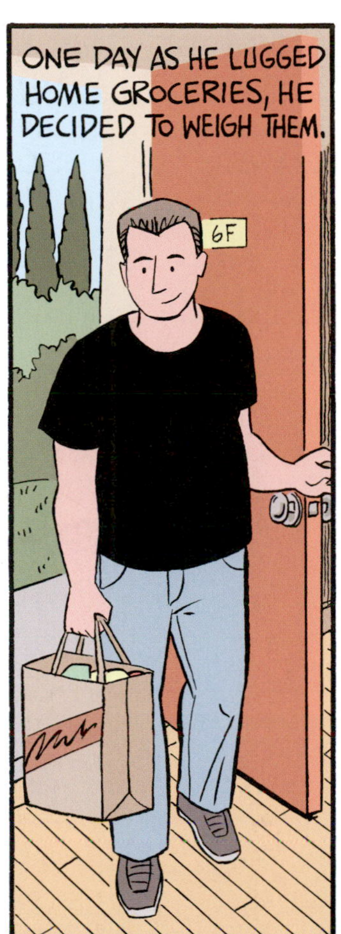
ONE DAY AS HE LUGGED HOME GROCERIES, HE DECIDED TO WEIGH THEM.
6F

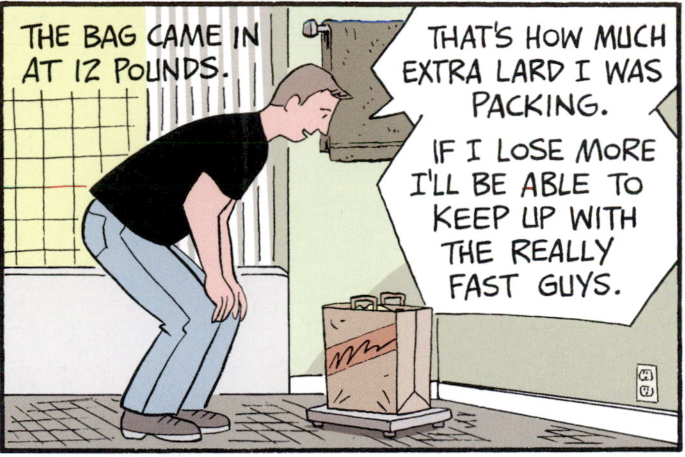
THE BAG CAME IN AT 12 POUNDS.
THAT'S HOW MUCH EXTRA LARD I WAS PACKING.
IF I LOSE MORE I'LL BE ABLE TO KEEP UP WITH THE REALLY FAST GUYS.

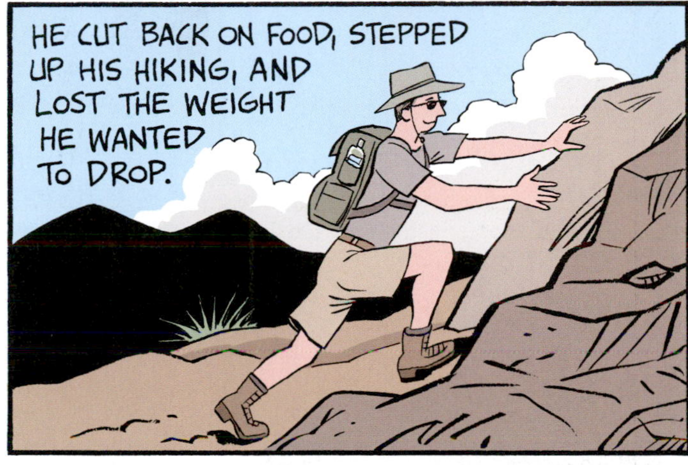
HE CUT BACK ON FOOD, STEPPED UP HIS HIKING, AND LOST THE WEIGHT HE WANTED TO DROP.

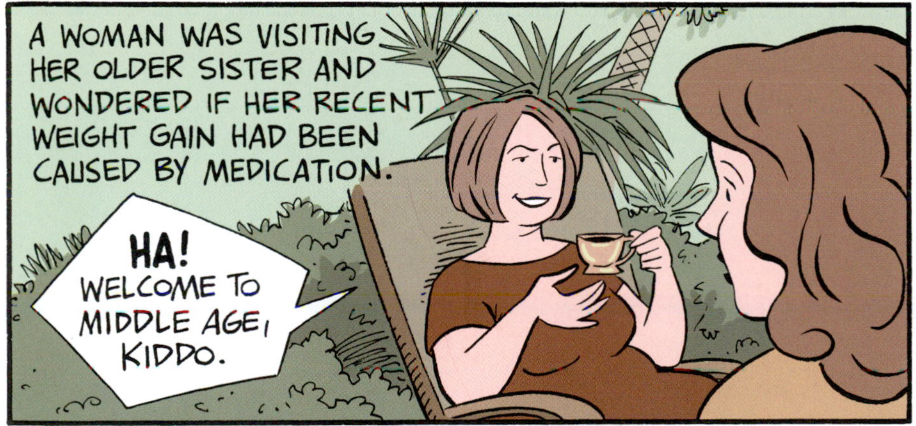
A WOMAN WAS VISITING HER OLDER SISTER AND WONDERED IF HER RECENT WEIGHT GAIN HAD BEEN CAUSED BY MEDICATION.
HA! WELCOME TO MIDDLE AGE, KIDDO.

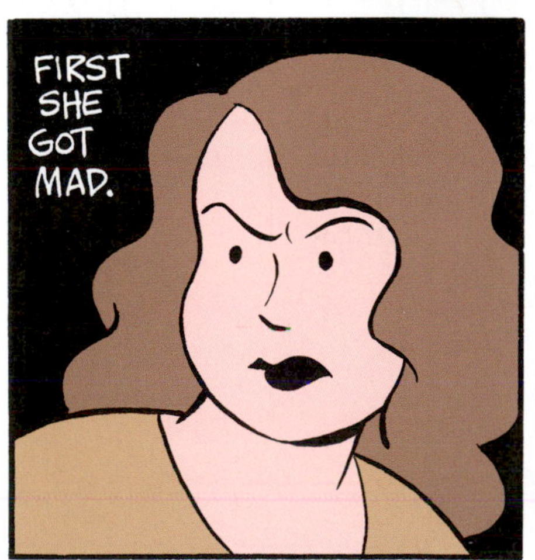
FIRST SHE GOT MAD.

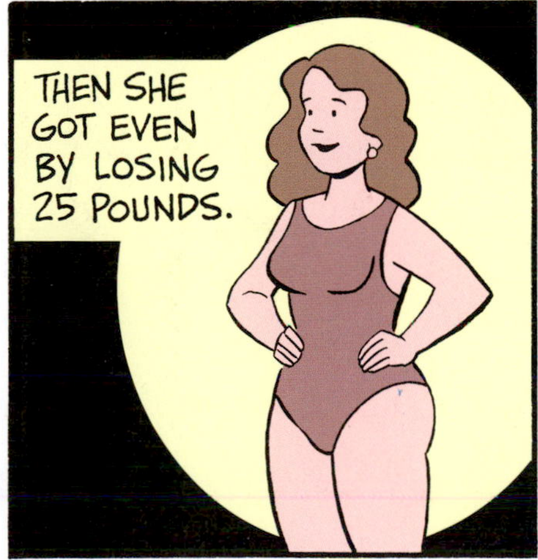
THEN SHE GOT EVEN BY LOSING 25 POUNDS.

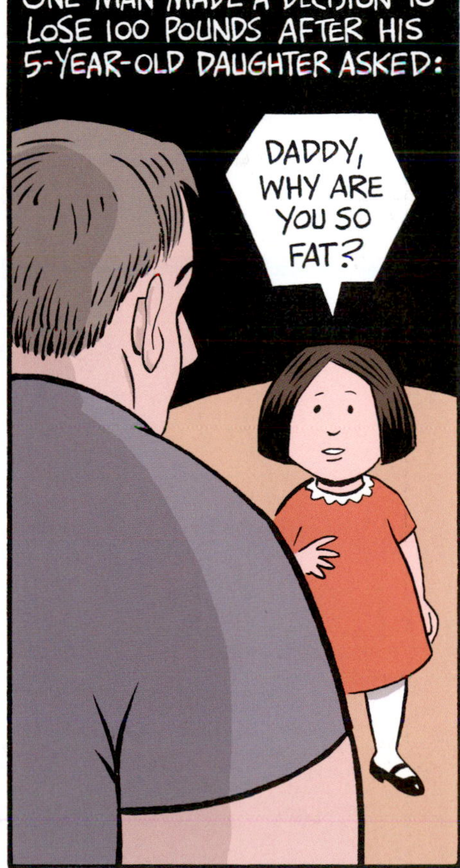
ONE MAN MADE A DECISION TO LOSE 100 POUNDS AFTER HIS 5-YEAR-OLD DAUGHTER ASKED:
DADDY, WHY ARE YOU SO FAT?

THERE ARE TONS OF STORIES LIKE THESE. USUALLY, SOME EXTERNAL INFORMATION PULLS THE TRIGGER THAT PROMPTS CHANGE.

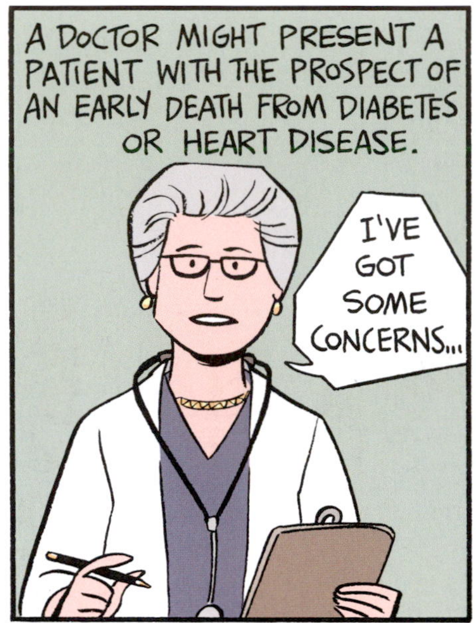
A DOCTOR MIGHT PRESENT A PATIENT WITH THE PROSPECT OF AN EARLY DEATH FROM DIABETES OR HEART DISEASE.
I'VE GOT SOME CONCERNS...

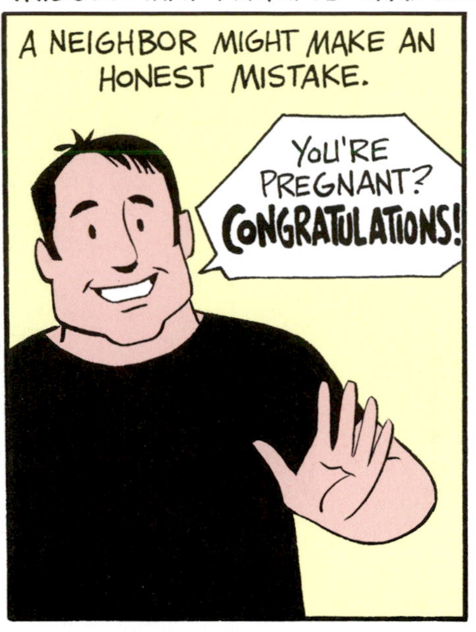
A NEIGHBOR MIGHT MAKE AN HONEST MISTAKE.
YOU'RE PREGNANT? CONGRATULATIONS!

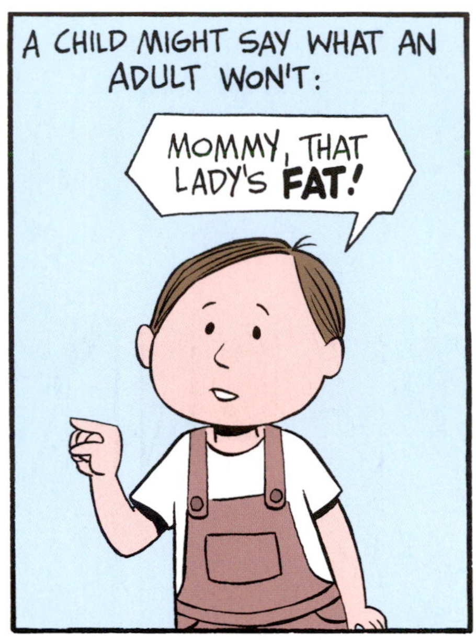
A CHILD MIGHT SAY WHAT AN ADULT WON'T:
MOMMY, THAT LADY'S FAT!

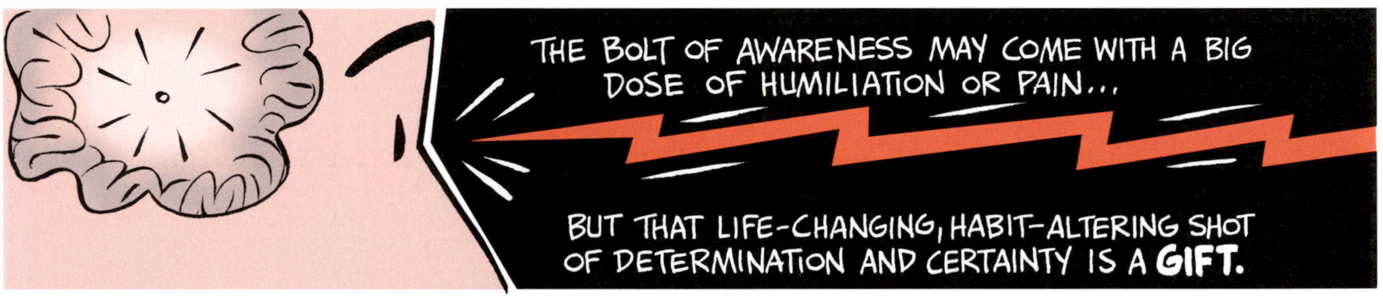
THE BOLT OF AWARENESS MAY COME WITH A BIG DOSE OF HUMILIATION OR PAIN...
BUT THAT LIFE-CHANGING, HABIT-ALTERING SHOT OF DETERMINATION AND CERTAINTY IS A GIFT.

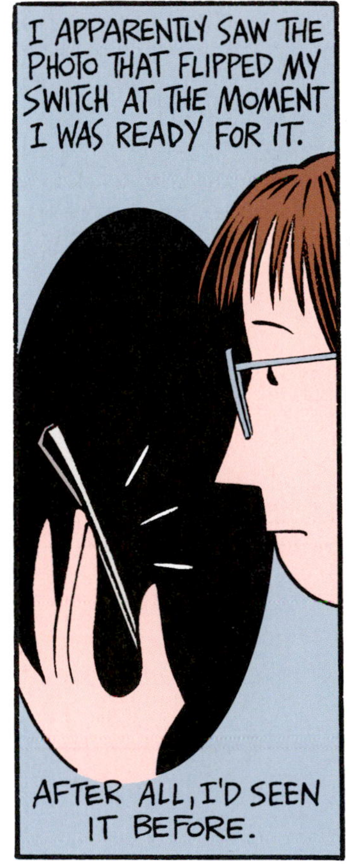
I APPARENTLY SAW THE PHOTO THAT FLIPPED MY SWITCH AT THE MOMENT I WAS READY FOR IT.
AFTER ALL, I'D SEEN IT BEFORE.

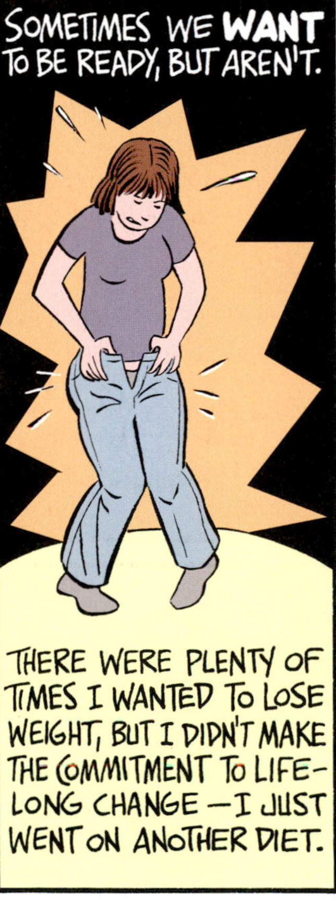
SOMETIMES WE WANT TO BE READY, BUT AREN'T.
THERE WERE PLENTY OF TIMES I WANTED TO LOSE WEIGHT, BUT I DIDN'T MAKE THE COMMITMENT TO LIFE-LONG CHANGE—I JUST WENT ON ANOTHER DIET.

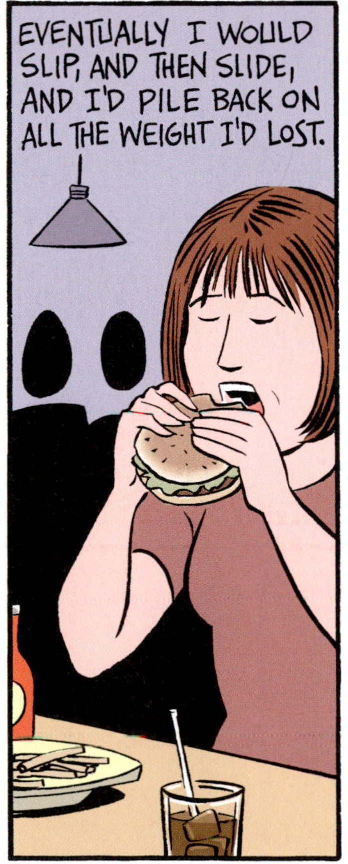
EVENTUALLY I WOULD SLIP, AND THEN SLIDE, AND I'D PILE BACK ON ALL THE WEIGHT I'D LOST.

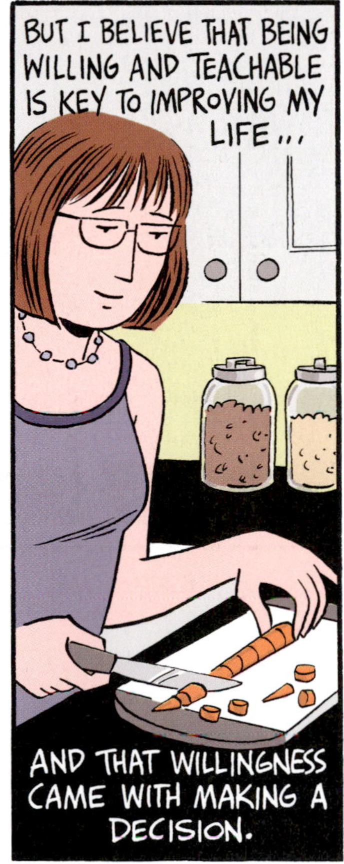
BUT I BELIEVE THAT BEING WILLING AND TEACHABLE IS KEY TO IMPROVING MY LIFE...
AND THAT WILLINGNESS CAME WITH MAKING A DECISION.

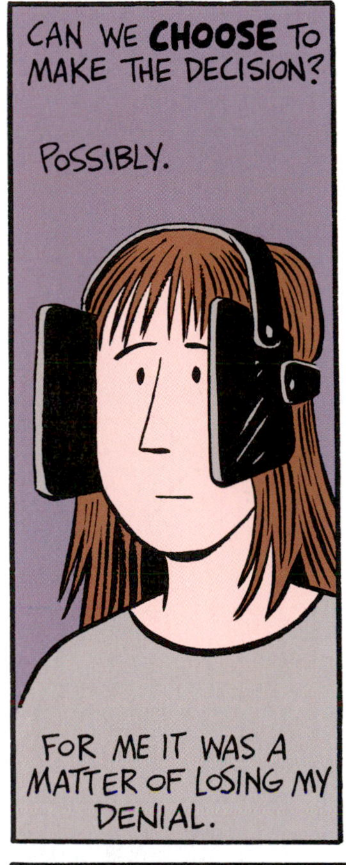
CAN WE **CHOOSE** TO MAKE THE DECISION?
POSSIBLY.
FOR ME IT WAS A MATTER OF LOSING MY DENIAL.

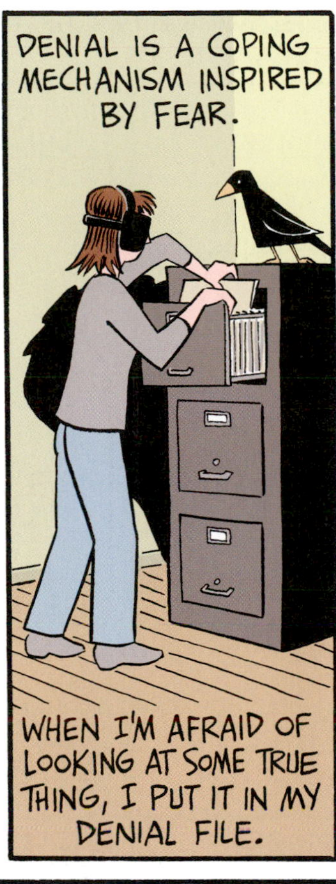
DENIAL IS A COPING MECHANISM INSPIRED BY FEAR.
WHEN I'M AFRAID OF LOOKING AT SOME TRUE THING, I PUT IT IN MY DENIAL FILE.

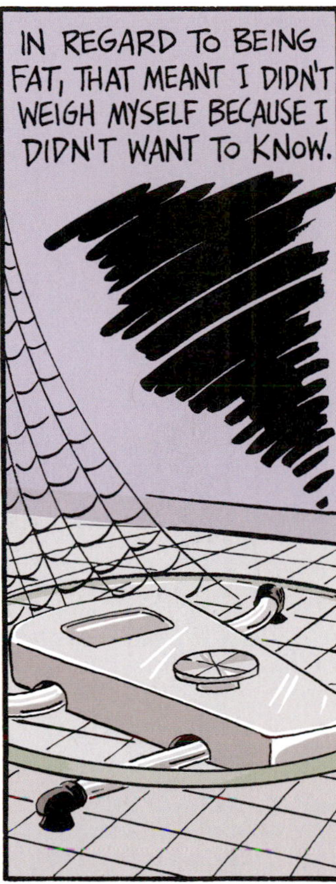
IN REGARD TO BEING FAT, THAT MEANT I DIDN'T WEIGH MYSELF BECAUSE I DIDN'T WANT TO KNOW.

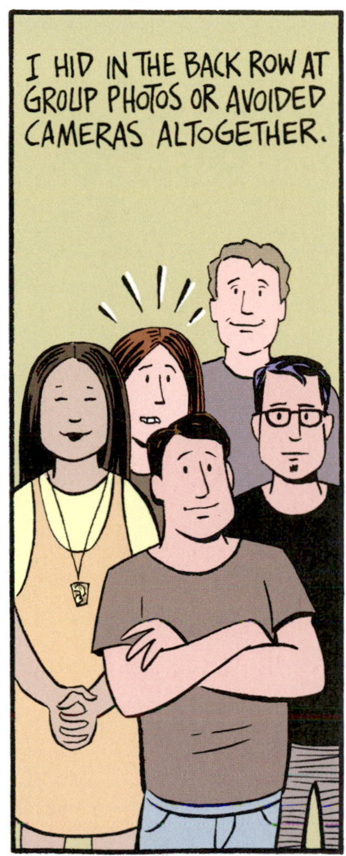
I HID IN THE BACK ROW AT GROUP PHOTOS OR AVOIDED CAMERAS ALTOGETHER.

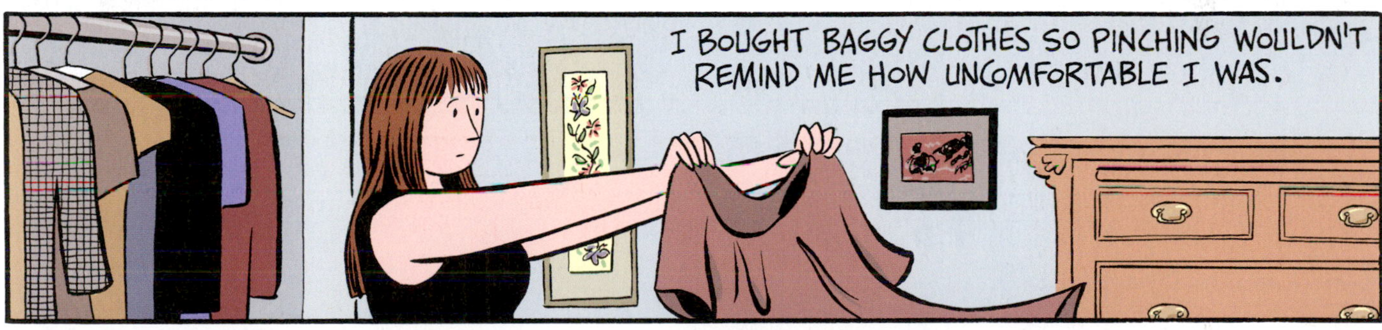
I BOUGHT BAGGY CLOTHES SO PINCHING WOULDN'T REMIND ME HOW UNCOMFORTABLE I WAS.

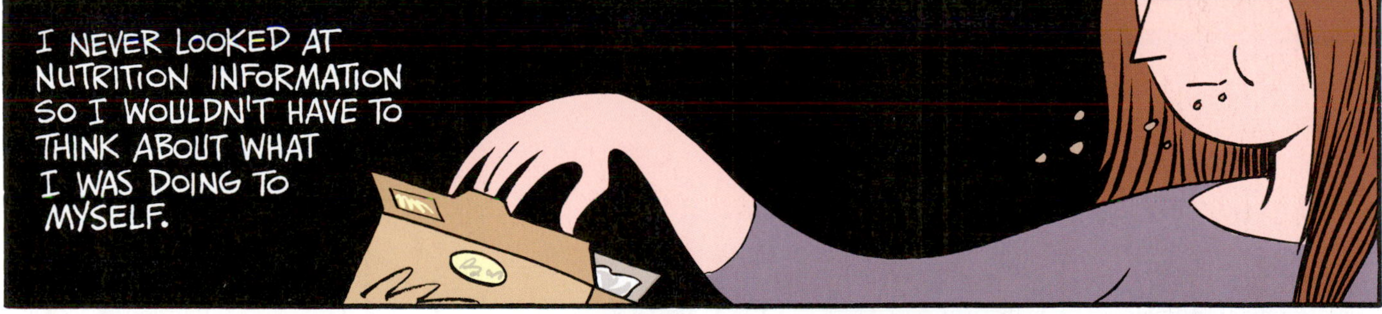
I NEVER LOOKED AT NUTRITION INFORMATION SO I WOULDN'T HAVE TO THINK ABOUT WHAT I WAS DOING TO MYSELF.

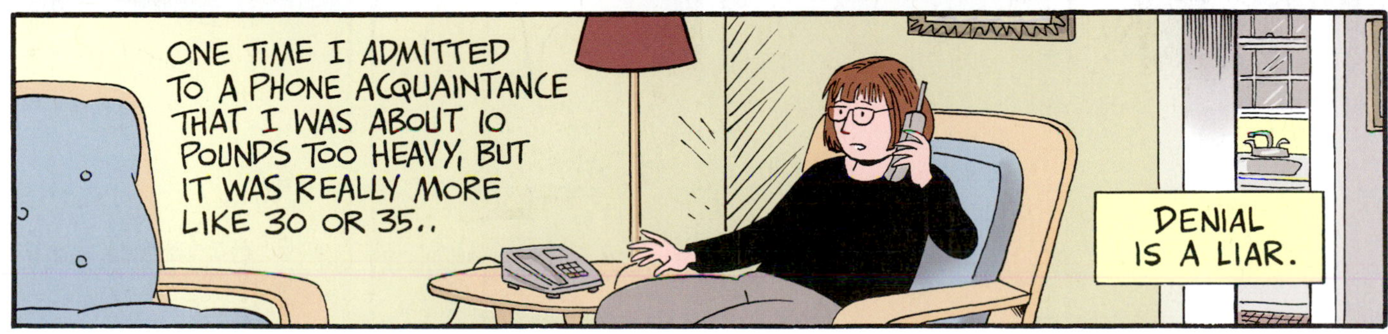
ONE TIME I ADMITTED TO A PHONE ACQUAINTANCE THAT I WAS ABOUT 10 POUNDS TOO HEAVY, BUT IT WAS REALLY MORE LIKE 30 OR 35..
DENIAL IS A LIAR.

HERE ARE SUGGESTIONS ON HOW TO GET OUT OF DENIAL SO THAT YOU MIGHT BE ABLE TO MAKE THAT BIG DECISION.

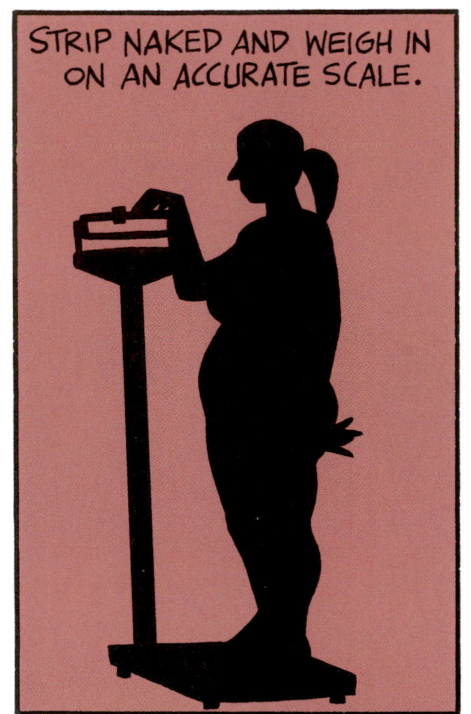

STRIP NAKED AND WEIGH IN ON AN ACCURATE SCALE.

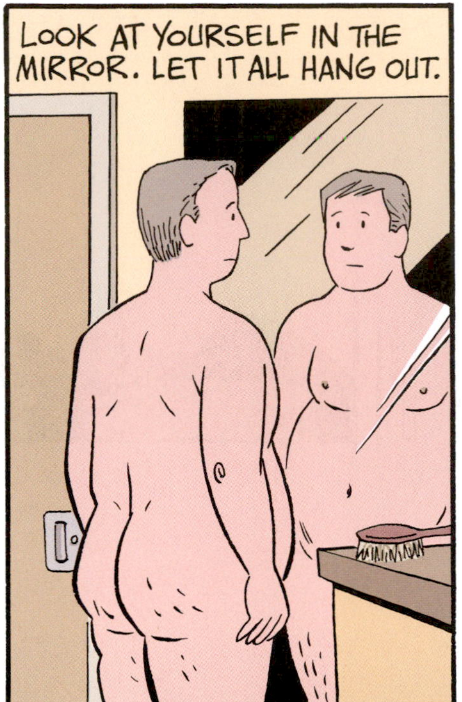

LOOK AT YOURSELF IN THE MIRROR. LET IT ALL HANG OUT.

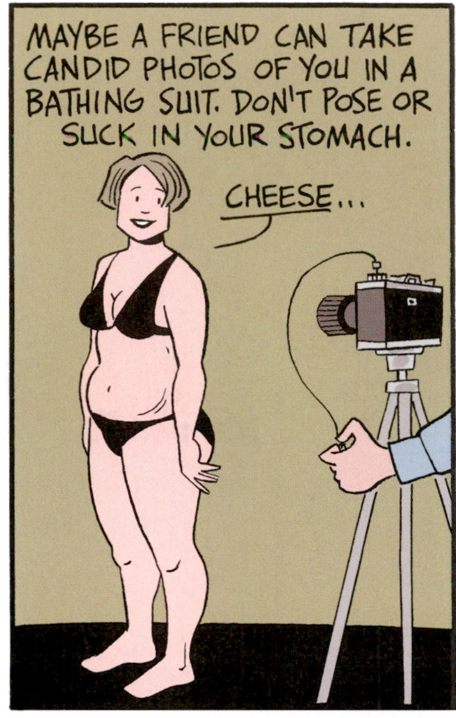

MAYBE A FRIEND CAN TAKE CANDID PHOTOS OF YOU IN A BATHING SUIT. DON'T POSE OR SUCK IN YOUR STOMACH.
CHEESE...

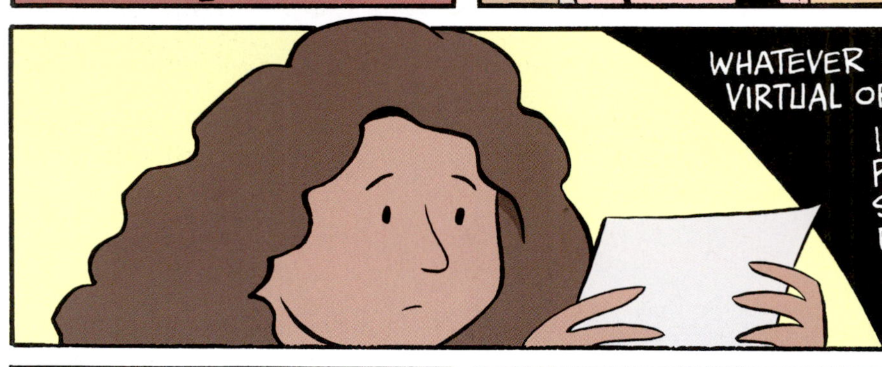

WHATEVER INFORMATION YOU GET, VIRTUAL OR ACTUAL, IS REALITY.
IF IT HURTS, THAT'S OK. PAIN MOTIVATES CHANGE SO WE CAN GET RELIEF FROM PAIN.

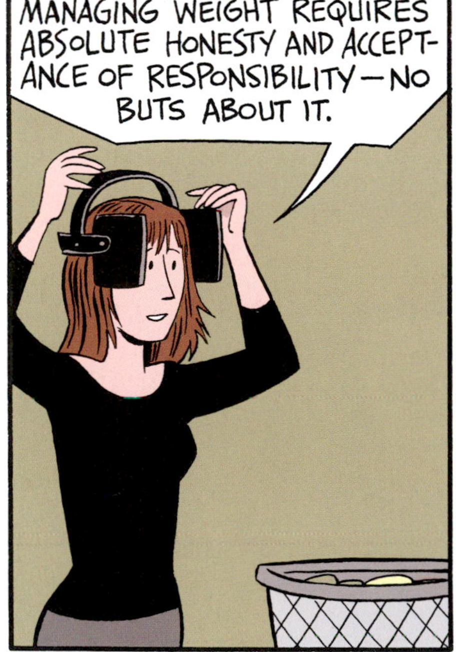

FOR OVEREATERS LIKE MYSELF, MANAGING WEIGHT REQUIRES ABSOLUTE HONESTY AND ACCEPTANCE OF RESPONSIBILITY—NO BUTS ABOUT IT.

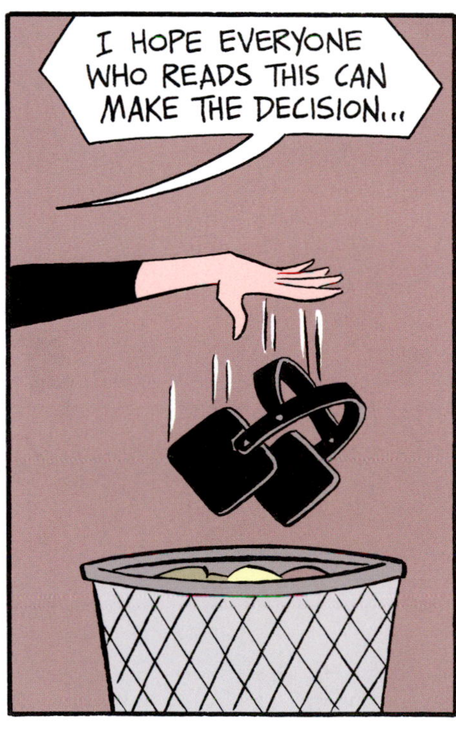

I HOPE EVERYONE WHO READS THIS CAN MAKE THE DECISION...

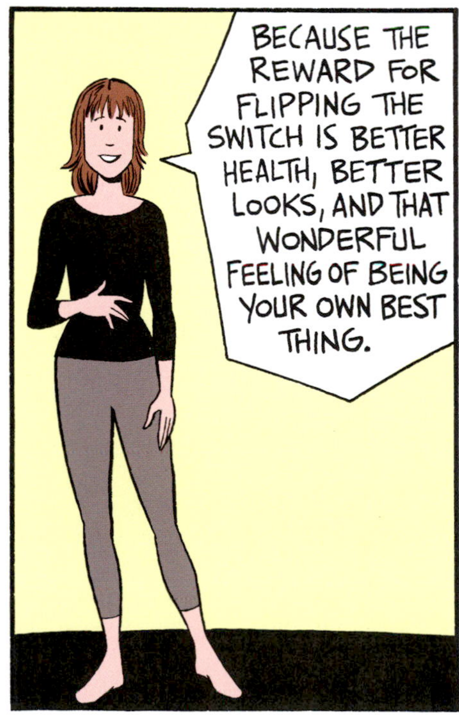

BECAUSE THE REWARD FOR FLIPPING THE SWITCH IS BETTER HEALTH, BETTER LOOKS, AND THAT WONDERFUL FEELING OF BEING YOUR OWN BEST THING.

# GETTING GOOD to GO

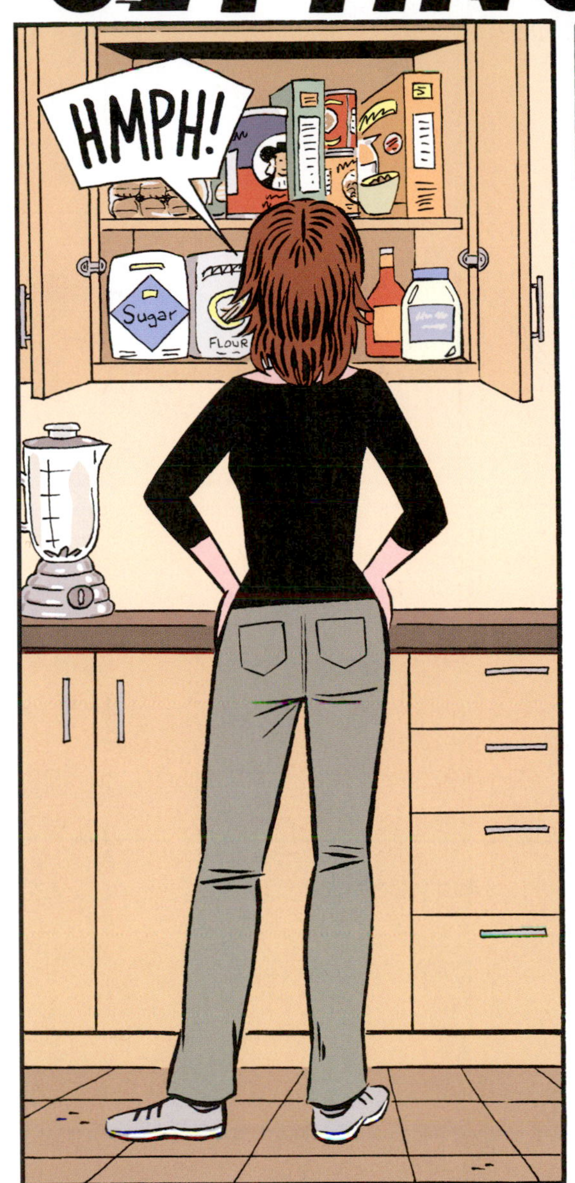

HMPH!
Sugar
FLOUR


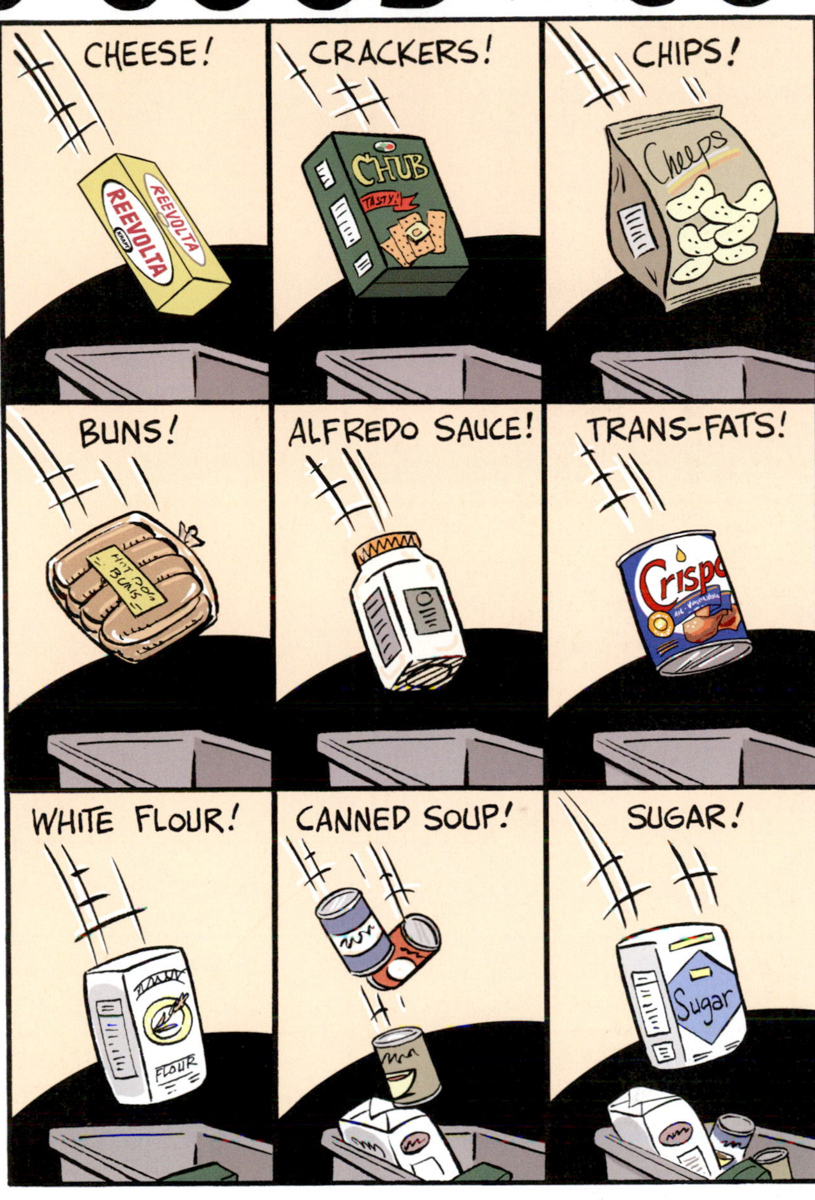

CHEESE!
REEVOLTA
CRACKERS!
CHUB
TASTY
CHIPS!
Cheeps
BUNS!
HOT DOG BUNS
ALFREDO SAUCE!
TRANS-FATS!
Crispo
WHITE FLOUR!
FLOUR
CANNED SOUP!
SUGAR!
Sugar


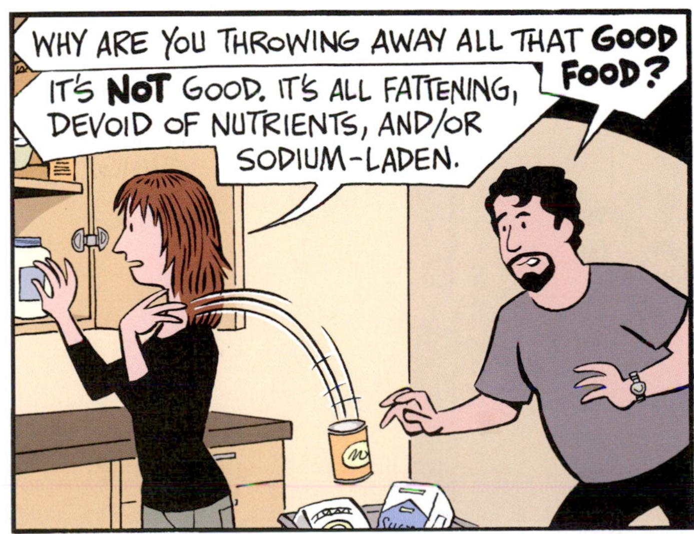

WHY ARE YOU THROWING AWAY ALL THAT **GOOD FOOD?**
IT'S **NOT** GOOD. IT'S ALL FATTENING, DEVOID OF NUTRIENTS, AND/OR SODIUM-LADEN.


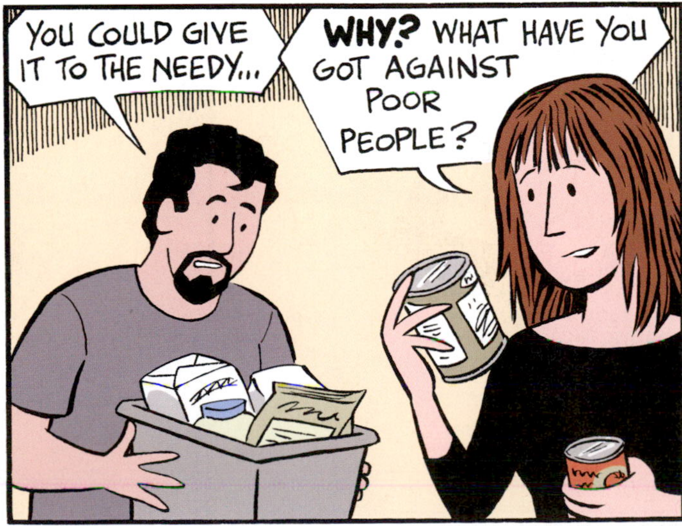

YOU COULD GIVE IT TO THE NEEDY...
**WHY?** WHAT HAVE YOU GOT AGAINST POOR PEOPLE?

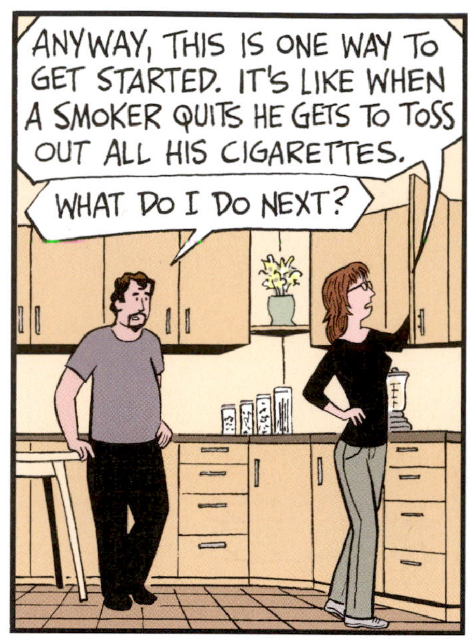
ANYWAY, THIS IS ONE WAY TO GET STARTED. IT'S LIKE WHEN A SMOKER QUITS HE GETS TO TOSS OUT ALL HIS CIGARETTES.
WHAT DO I DO NEXT?
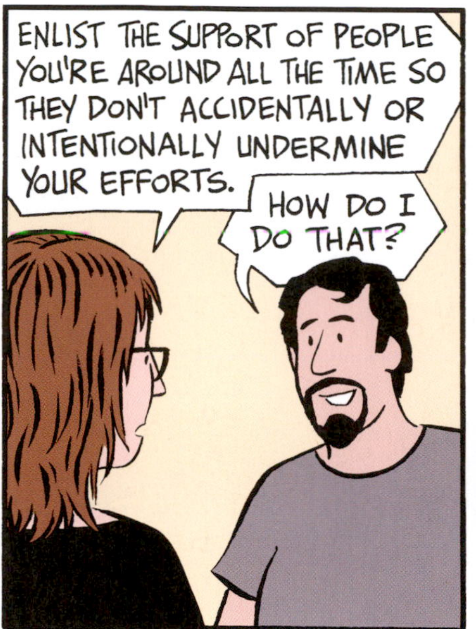
ENLIST THE SUPPORT OF PEOPLE YOU'RE AROUND ALL THE TIME SO THEY DON'T ACCIDENTALLY OR INTENTIONALLY UNDERMINE YOUR EFFORTS.
HOW DO I DO THAT?
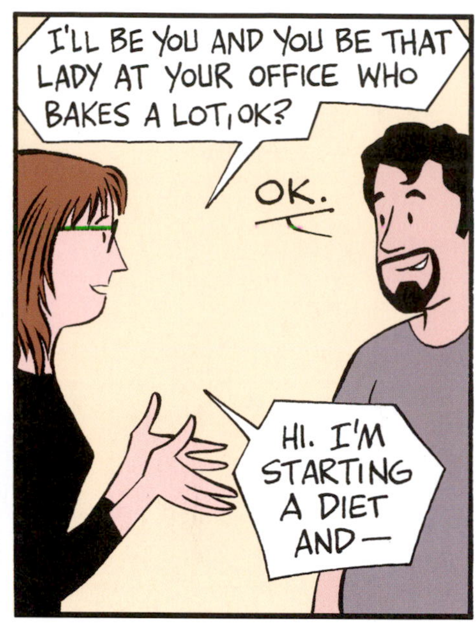
I'LL BE YOU AND YOU BE THAT LADY AT YOUR OFFICE WHO BAKES A LOT, OK?
OK.
HI. I'M STARTING A DIET AND—
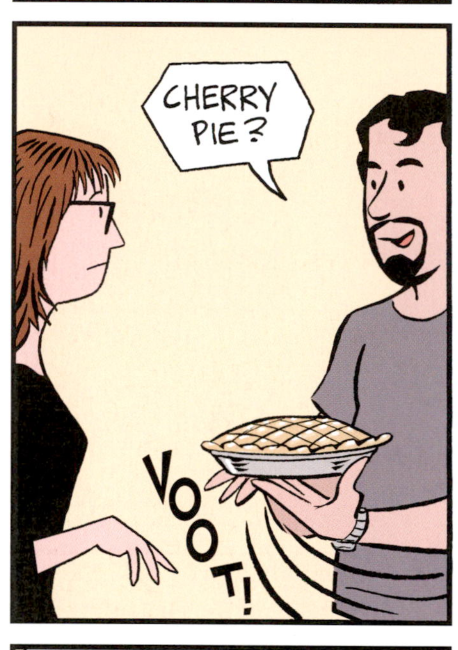
CHERRY PIE?
VOOT!
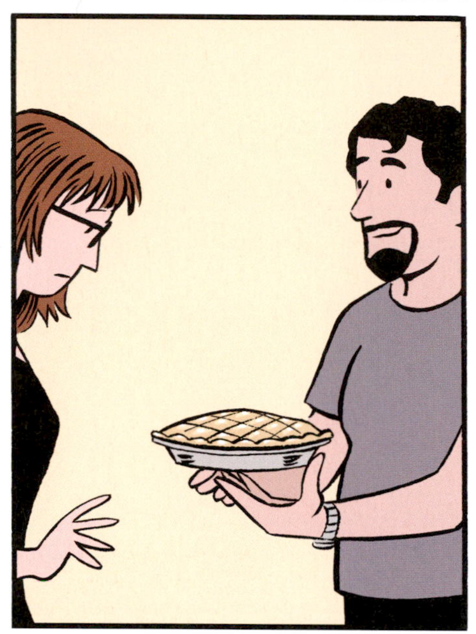
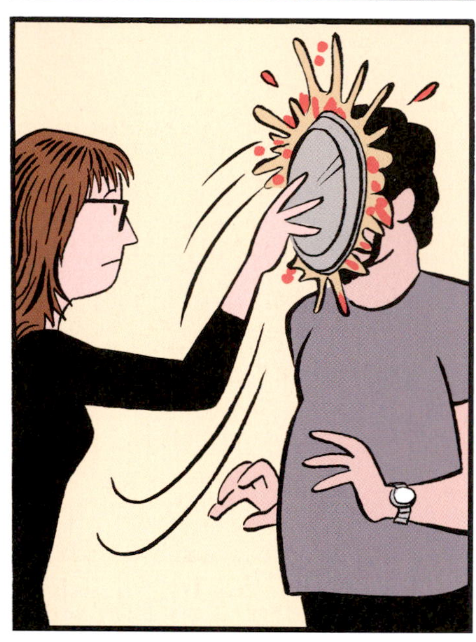
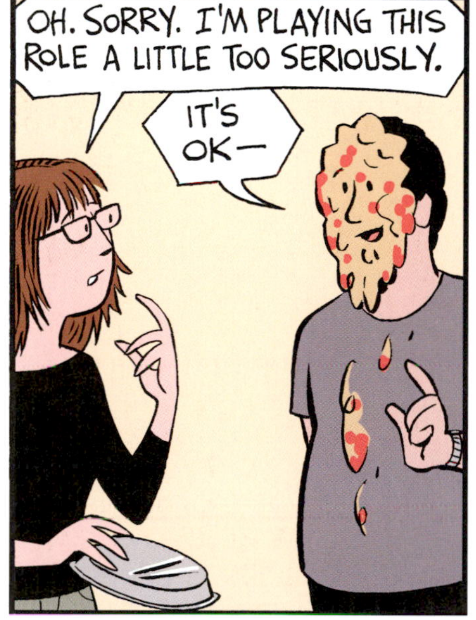
OH. SORRY. I'M PLAYING THIS ROLE A LITTLE TOO SERIOUSLY.
IT'S OK—
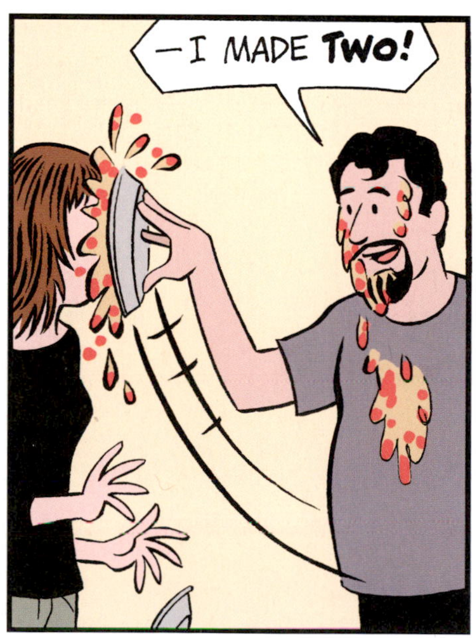
—I MADE **TWO!**
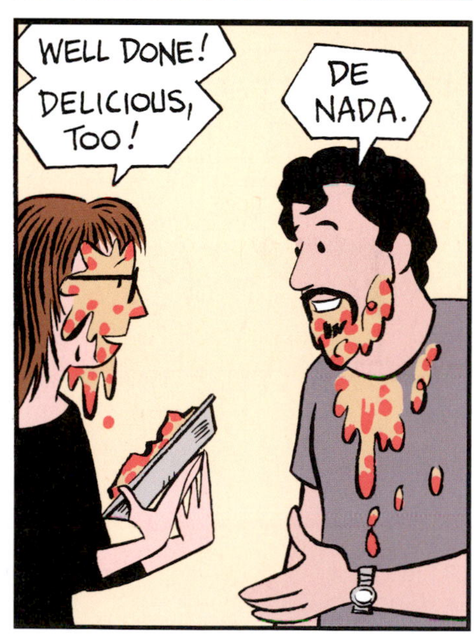
WELL DONE!
DELICIOUS, TOO!
DE NADA.

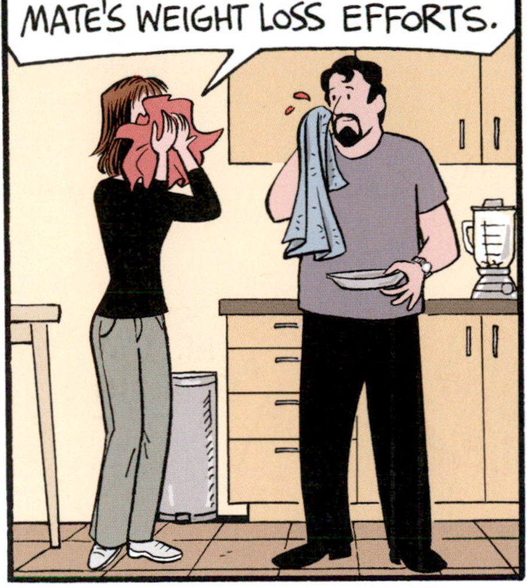
YOU KNOW, THERE **ARE** PEOPLE WHO—CONSCIOUSLY OR NOT—SABOTAGE THEIR FRIENDS' OR MATE'S WEIGHT LOSS EFFORTS.

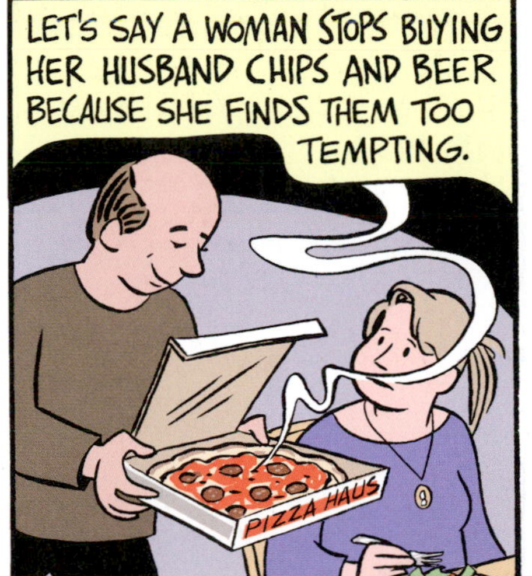
LET'S SAY A WOMAN STOPS BUYING HER HUSBAND CHIPS AND BEER BECAUSE SHE FINDS THEM TOO TEMPTING.
PIZZA HAUS
HE MIGHT COAX HER OFF HER DIET SO HE CAN GET WHAT HE WANTS.

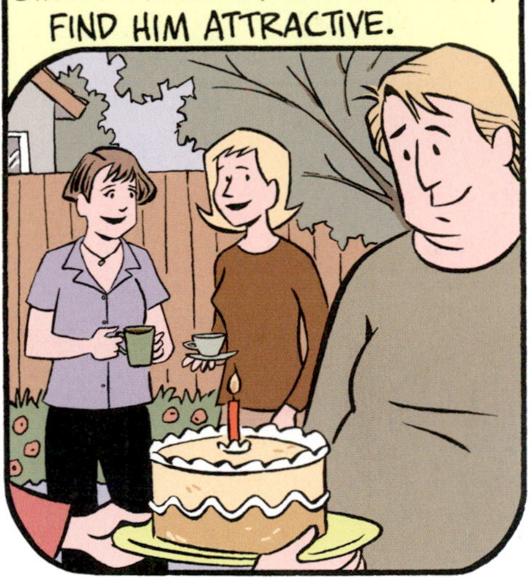
OR A WIFE MAY NOT WANT HER MAN TO LOSE HIS BIG GUT BECAUSE HER SINGLE FRIENDS MIGHT SUDDENLY FIND HIM ATTRACTIVE.

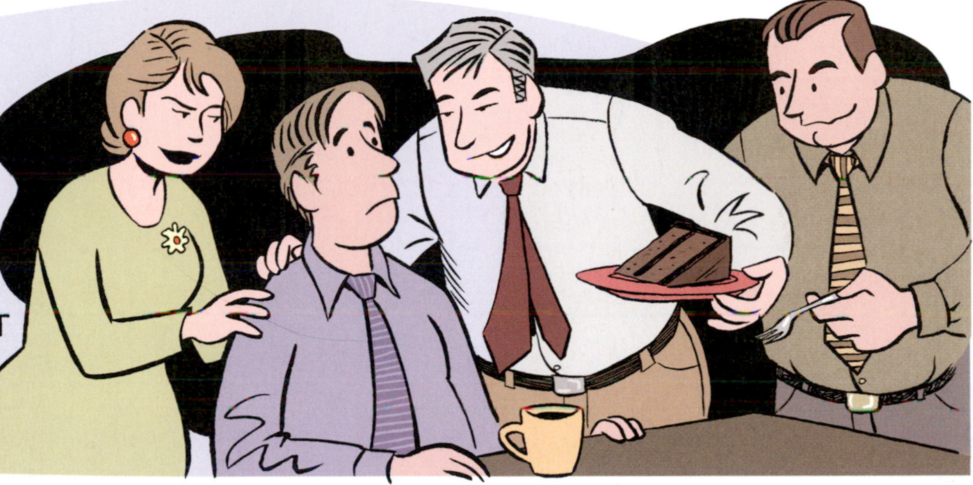
OR LET'S SAY AN OFFICE WORKER SUCCESSFULLY LOSES WEIGHT. SINCE SLIMMER EMPLOYEES GET MORE PROMOTIONS AND PAY (UNFAIR, BUT TRUE), HIS CO-WORKERS MAY BECOME COMPETITIVE AND ATTEMPT TO SABOTAGE HIS EFFORTS.

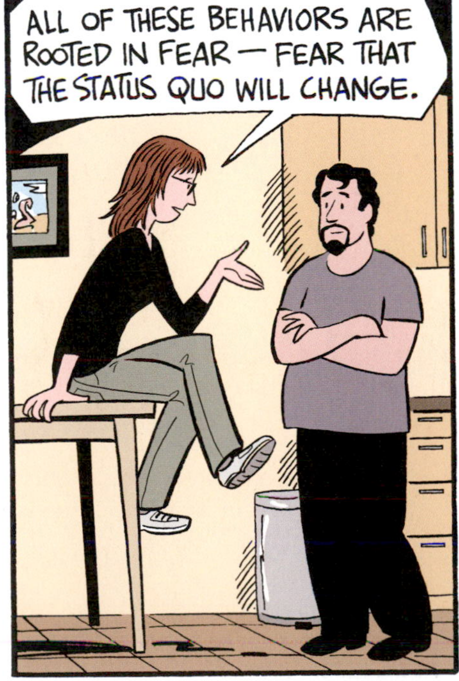
ALL OF THESE BEHAVIORS ARE ROOTED IN FEAR—FEAR THAT THE STATUS QUO WILL CHANGE.

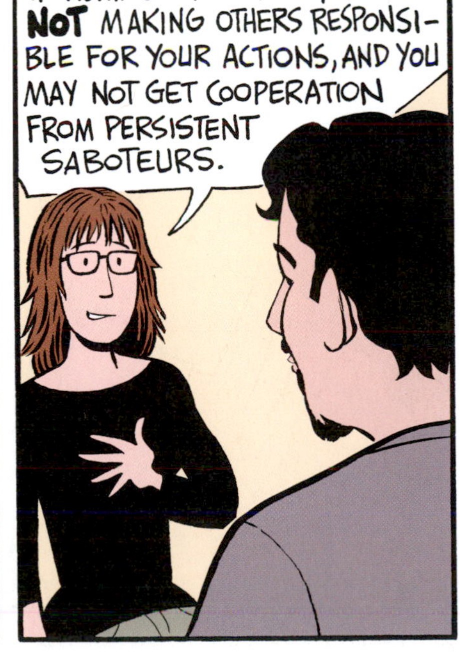
IN ASKING FOR SUPPORT, YOU'RE **NOT** MAKING OTHERS RESPONSIBLE FOR YOUR ACTIONS, AND YOU MAY NOT GET COOPERATION FROM PERSISTENT SABOTEURS.

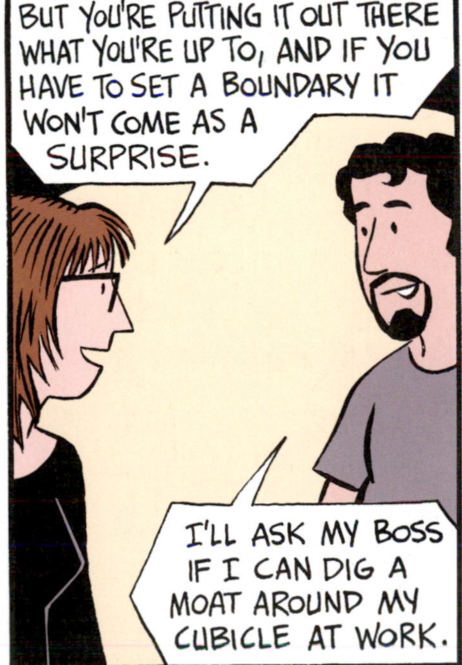
BUT YOU'RE PUTTING IT OUT THERE WHAT YOU'RE UP TO, AND IF YOU HAVE TO SET A BOUNDARY IT WON'T COME AS A SURPRISE.
I'LL ASK MY BOSS IF I CAN DIG A MOAT AROUND MY CUBICLE AT WORK.

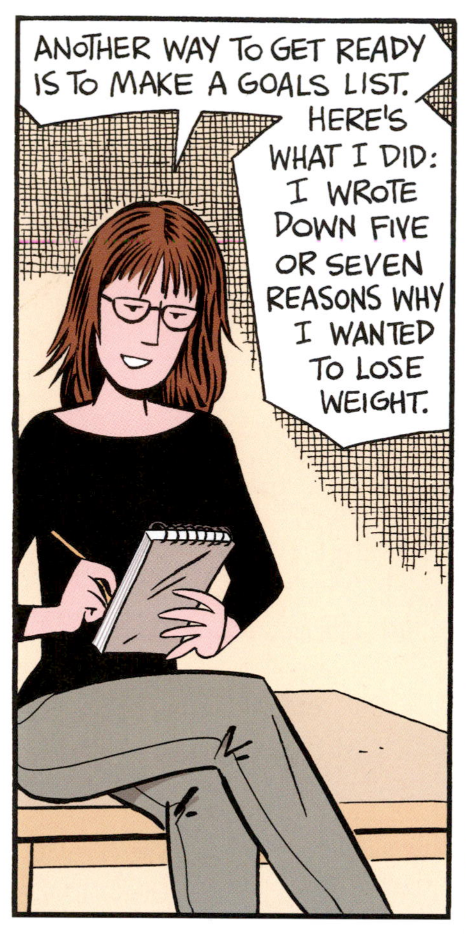
ANOTHER WAY TO GET READY IS TO MAKE A GOALS LIST.
HERE'S WHAT I DID: I WROTE DOWN FIVE OR SEVEN REASONS WHY I WANTED TO LOSE WEIGHT.

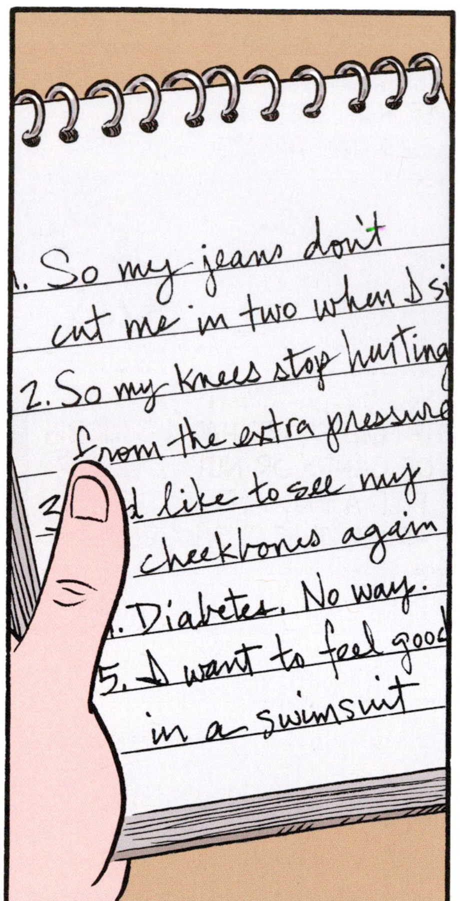
1. So my jeans don't cut me in two when I si
2. So my knees stop hurting from the extra pressure
3. I'd like to see my cheekbones again
4. Diabetes. No way.
5. I want to feel good in a swimsuit

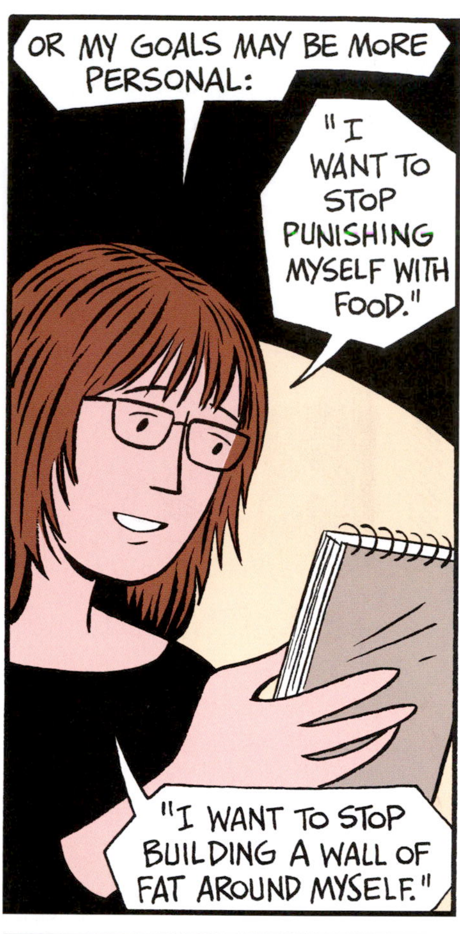
OR MY GOALS MAY BE MORE PERSONAL:
"I WANT TO STOP PUNISHING MYSELF WITH FOOD."
"I WANT TO STOP BUILDING A WALL OF FAT AROUND MYSELF."

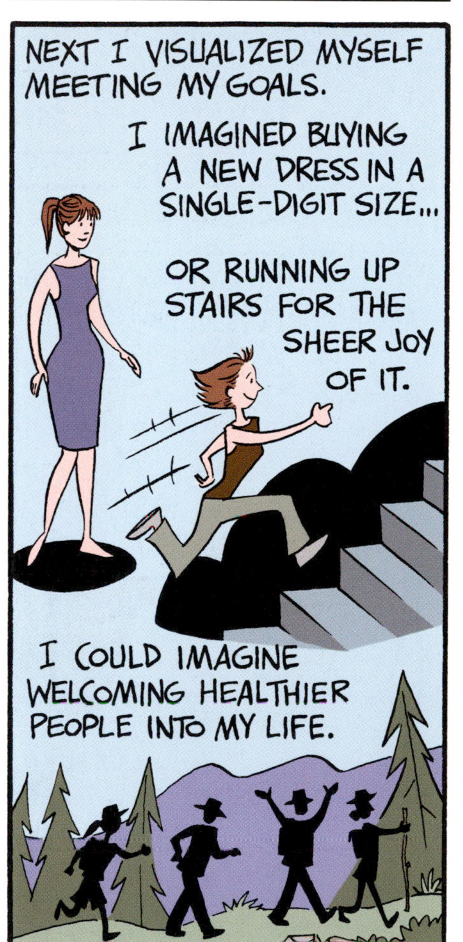
NEXT I VISUALIZED MYSELF MEETING MY GOALS.
I IMAGINED BUYING A NEW DRESS IN A SINGLE-DIGIT SIZE...
OR RUNNING UP STAIRS FOR THE SHEER JOY OF IT.
I COULD IMAGINE WELCOMING HEALTHIER PEOPLE INTO MY LIFE.

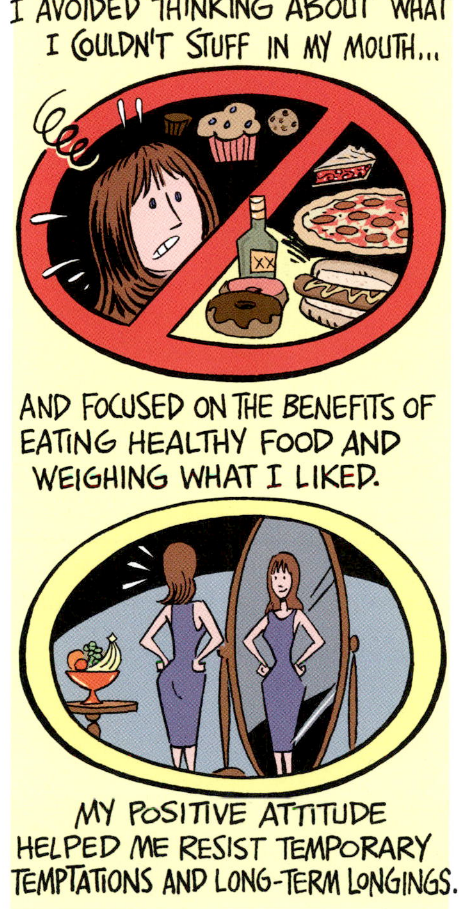
I AVOIDED THINKING ABOUT WHAT I COULDN'T STUFF IN MY MOUTH...
AND FOCUSED ON THE BENEFITS OF EATING HEALTHY FOOD AND WEIGHING WHAT I LIKED.
MY POSITIVE ATTITUDE HELPED ME RESIST TEMPORARY TEMPTATIONS AND LONG-TERM LONGINGS.

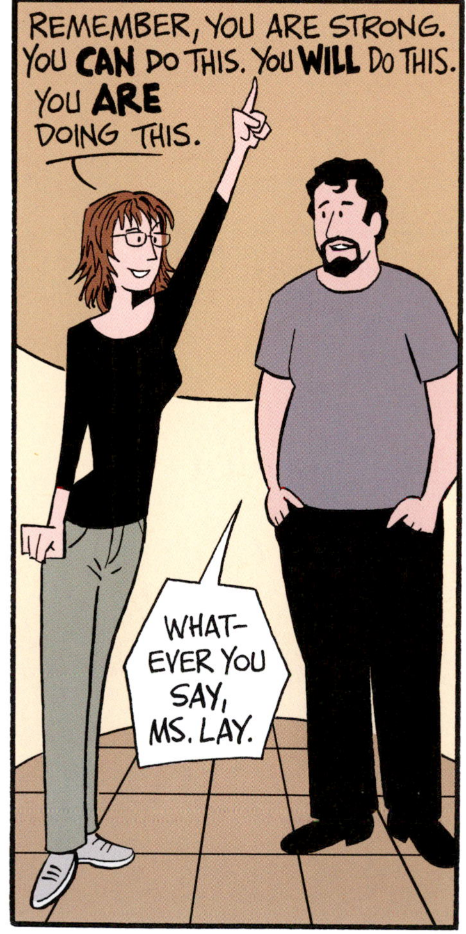
REMEMBER, YOU ARE STRONG. YOU **CAN** DO THIS. YOU **WILL** DO THIS. YOU **ARE** DOING THIS.
WHAT-EVER YOU SAY, MS. LAY.

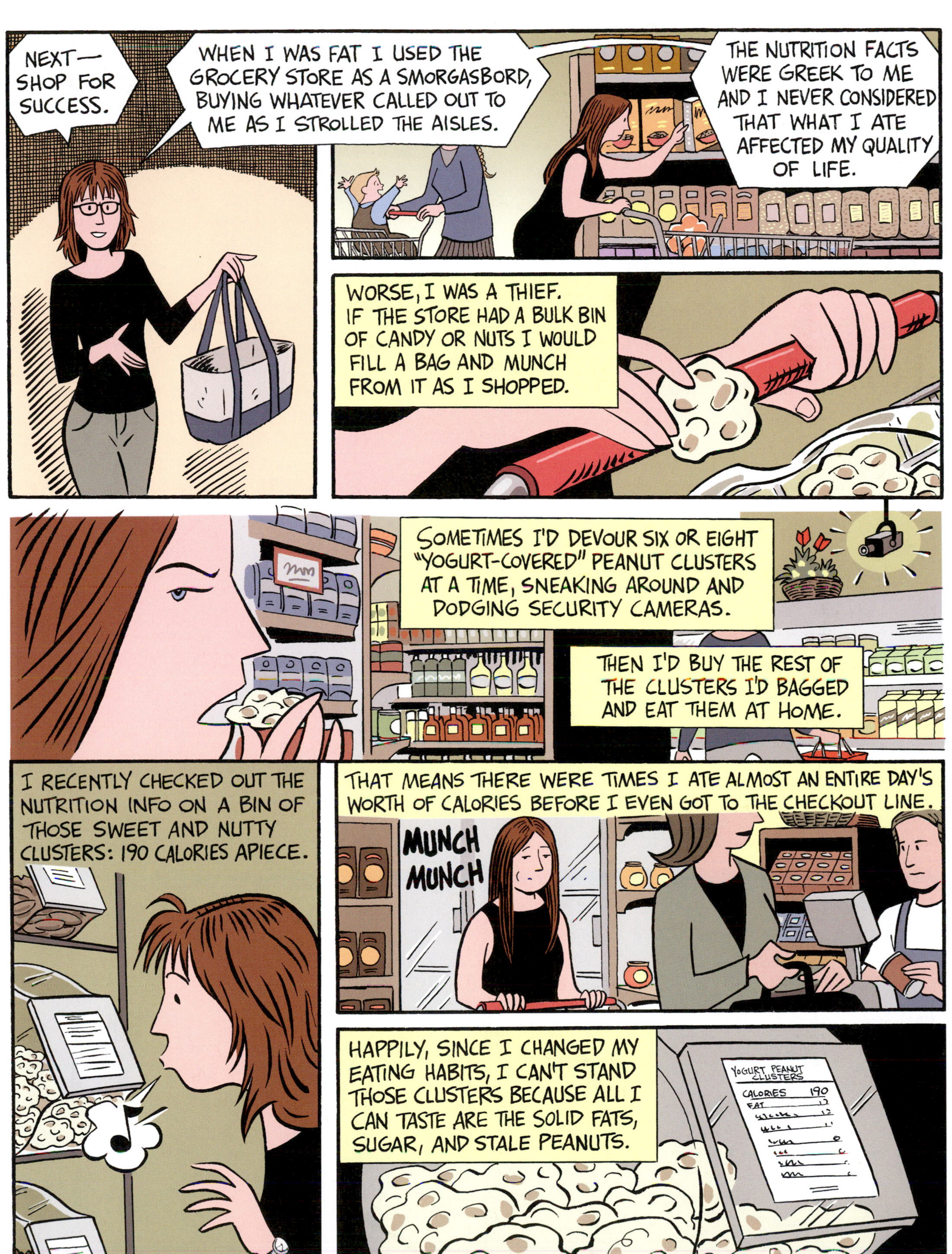
NEXT—
SHOP FOR SUCCESS.
WHEN I WAS FAT I USED THE GROCERY STORE AS A SMORGASBORD, BUYING WHATEVER CALLED OUT TO ME AS I STROLLED THE AISLES.
THE NUTRITION FACTS WERE GREEK TO ME AND I NEVER CONSIDERED THAT WHAT I ATE AFFECTED MY QUALITY OF LIFE.
WORSE, I WAS A THIEF. IF THE STORE HAD A BULK BIN OF CANDY OR NUTS I WOULD FILL A BAG AND MUNCH FROM IT AS I SHOPPED.
SOMETIMES I'D DEVOUR SIX OR EIGHT "YOGURT-COVERED" PEANUT CLUSTERS AT A TIME, SNEAKING AROUND AND DODGING SECURITY CAMERAS.
THEN I'D BUY THE REST OF THE CLUSTERS I'D BAGGED AND EAT THEM AT HOME.
I RECENTLY CHECKED OUT THE NUTRITION INFO ON A BIN OF THOSE SWEET AND NUTTY CLUSTERS: 190 CALORIES APIECE.
THAT MEANS THERE WERE TIMES I ATE ALMOST AN ENTIRE DAY'S WORTH OF CALORIES BEFORE I EVEN GOT TO THE CHECKOUT LINE.
MUNCH
MUNCH
HAPPILY, SINCE I CHANGED MY EATING HABITS, I CAN'T STAND THOSE CLUSTERS BECAUSE ALL I CAN TASTE ARE THE SOLID FATS, SUGAR, AND STALE PEANUTS.
YOGURT PEANUT CLUSTERS
CALORIES 190

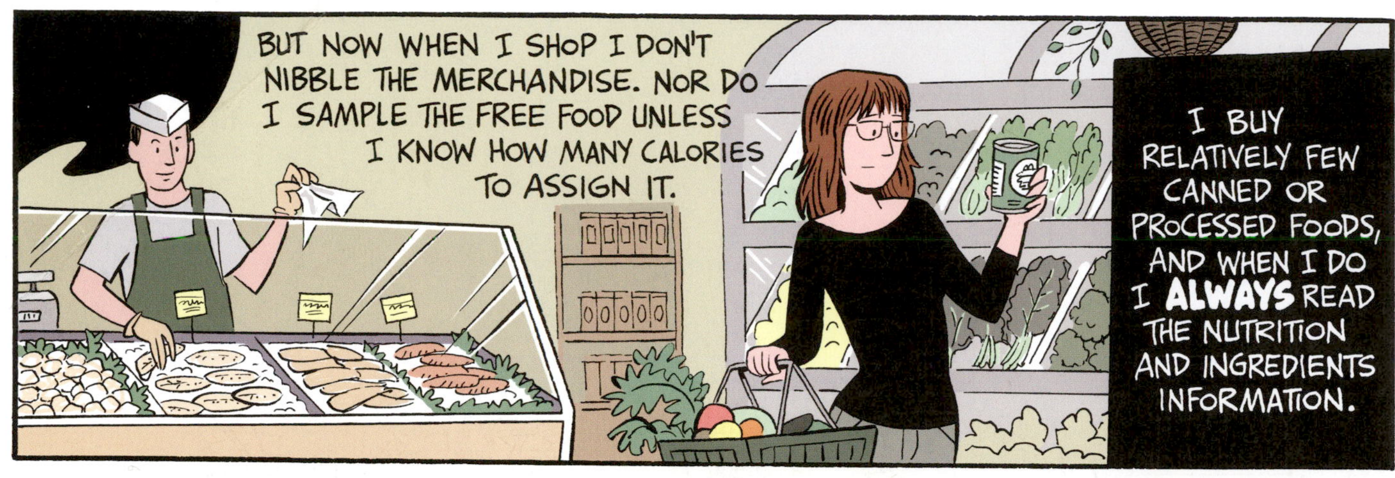

BUT NOW WHEN I SHOP I DON'T NIBBLE THE MERCHANDISE. NOR DO I SAMPLE THE FREE FOOD UNLESS I KNOW HOW MANY CALORIES TO ASSIGN IT.
I BUY RELATIVELY FEW CANNED OR PROCESSED FOODS, AND WHEN I DO I **ALWAYS** READ THE NUTRITION AND INGREDIENTS INFORMATION.

IF GRAPES ARE ON SALE BUT COME IN 3-POUND BAGS, I'M NOT SHY ABOUT MAKING UP A SMALLER BAG. THERE'S NO SENSE BUYING MORE THAN I CAN EAT BEFORE THE FOOD LOSES FRESHNESS.

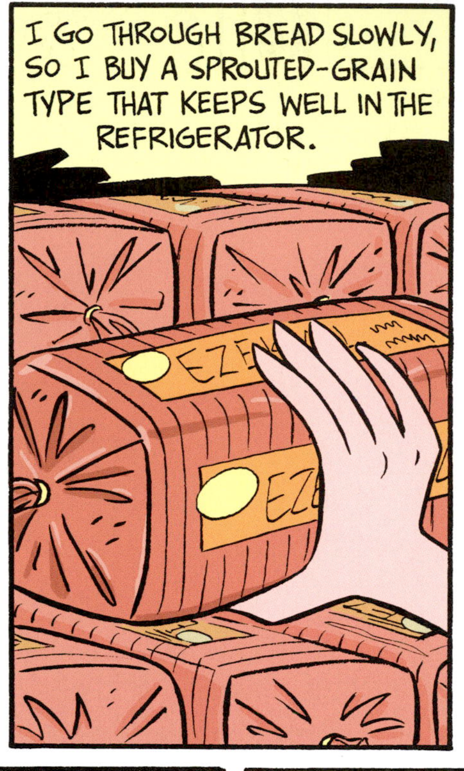

I GO THROUGH BREAD SLOWLY, SO I BUY A SPROUTED-GRAIN TYPE THAT KEEPS WELL IN THE REFRIGERATOR.

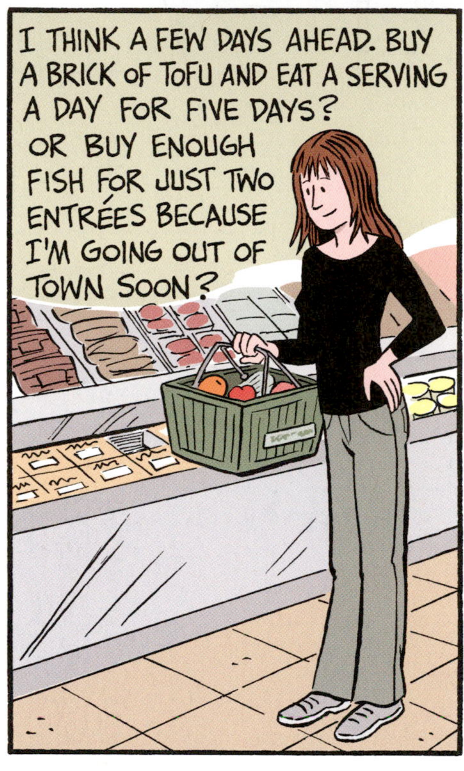

I THINK A FEW DAYS AHEAD. BUY A BRICK OF TOFU AND EAT A SERVING A DAY FOR FIVE DAYS?
OR BUY ENOUGH FISH FOR JUST TWO ENTRÉES BECAUSE I'M GOING OUT OF TOWN SOON?

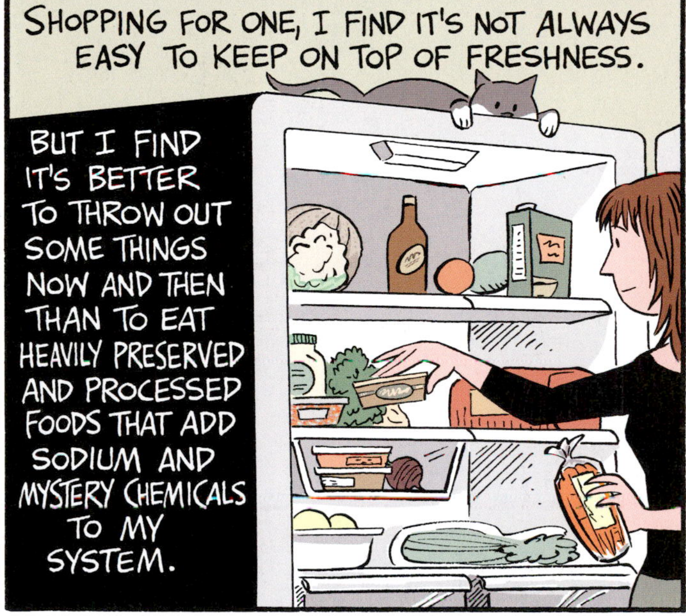

SHOPPING FOR ONE, I FIND IT'S NOT ALWAYS EASY TO KEEP ON TOP OF FRESHNESS.
BUT I FIND IT'S BETTER TO THROW OUT SOME THINGS NOW AND THEN THAN TO EAT HEAVILY PRESERVED AND PROCESSED FOODS THAT ADD SODIUM AND MYSTERY CHEMICALS TO MY SYSTEM.

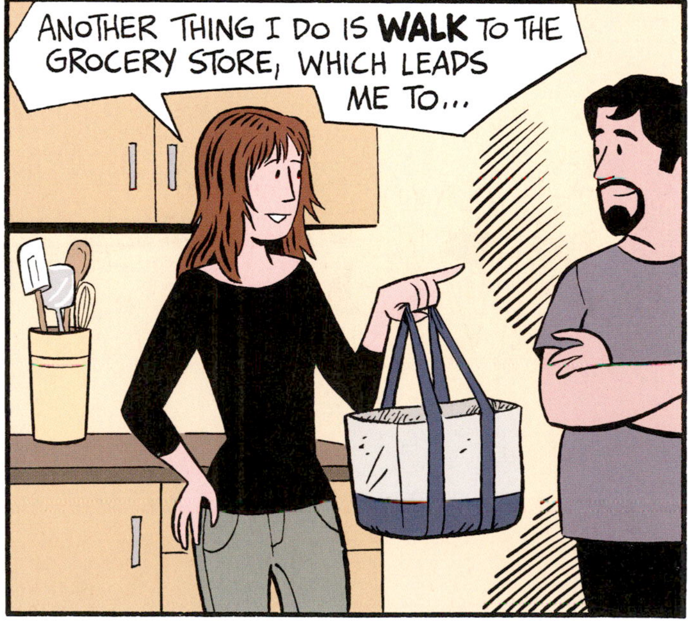

ANOTHER THING I DO IS **WALK** TO THE GROCERY STORE, WHICH LEADS ME TO...

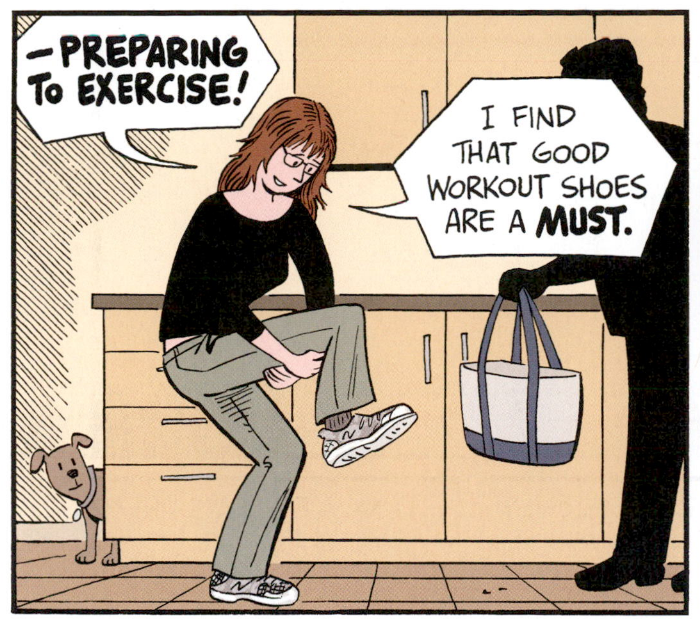
—PREPARING TO EXERCISE!
I FIND THAT GOOD WORKOUT SHOES ARE A MUST.

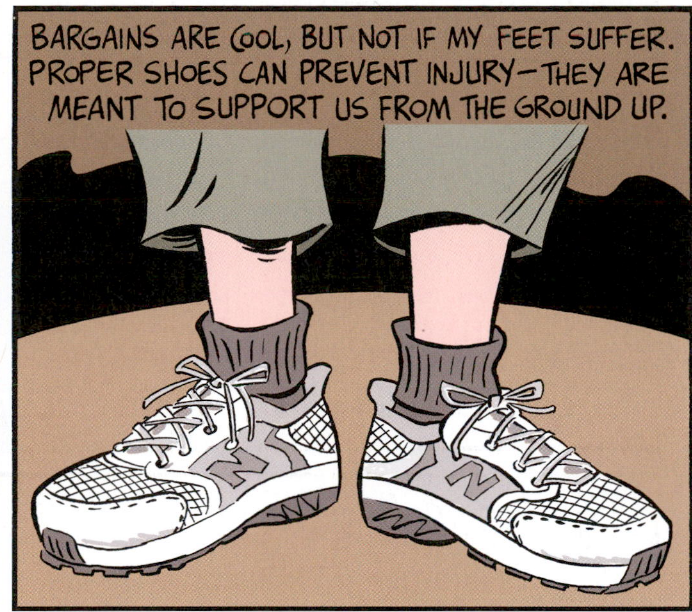
BARGAINS ARE COOL, BUT NOT IF MY FEET SUFFER. PROPER SHOES CAN PREVENT INJURY—THEY ARE MEANT TO SUPPORT US FROM THE GROUND UP.

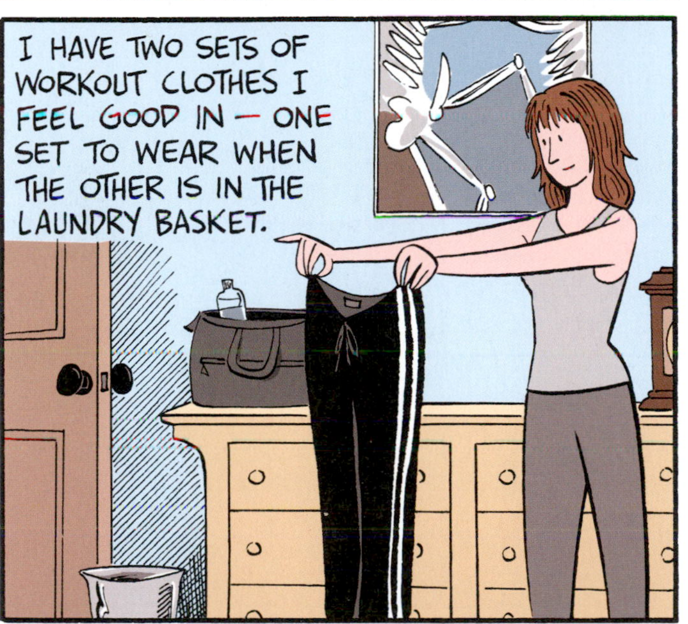
I HAVE TWO SETS OF WORKOUT CLOTHES I FEEL GOOD IN — ONE SET TO WEAR WHEN THE OTHER IS IN THE LAUNDRY BASKET.

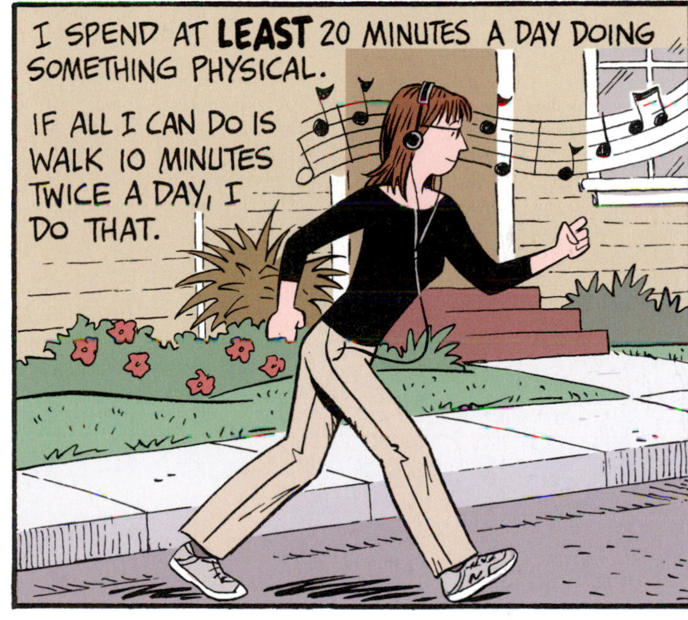
I SPEND AT LEAST 20 MINUTES A DAY DOING SOMETHING PHYSICAL.
IF ALL I CAN DO IS WALK 10 MINUTES TWICE A DAY, I DO THAT.

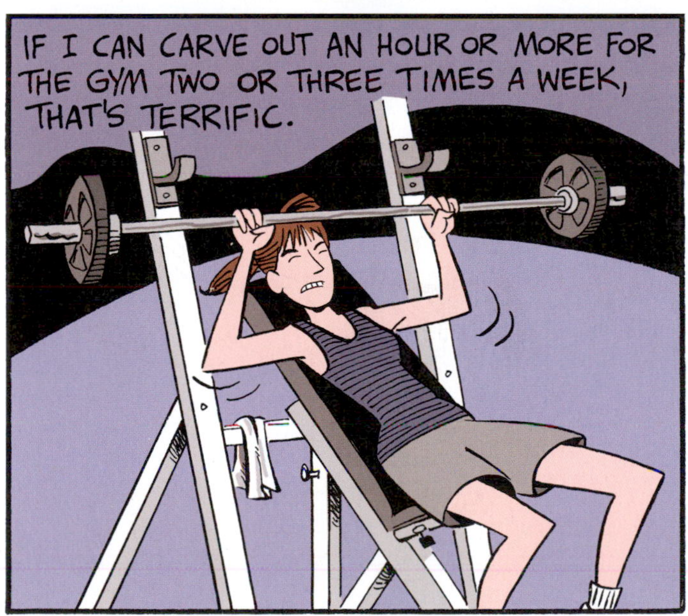
IF I CAN CARVE OUT AN HOUR OR MORE FOR THE GYM TWO OR THREE TIMES A WEEK, THAT'S TERRIFIC.

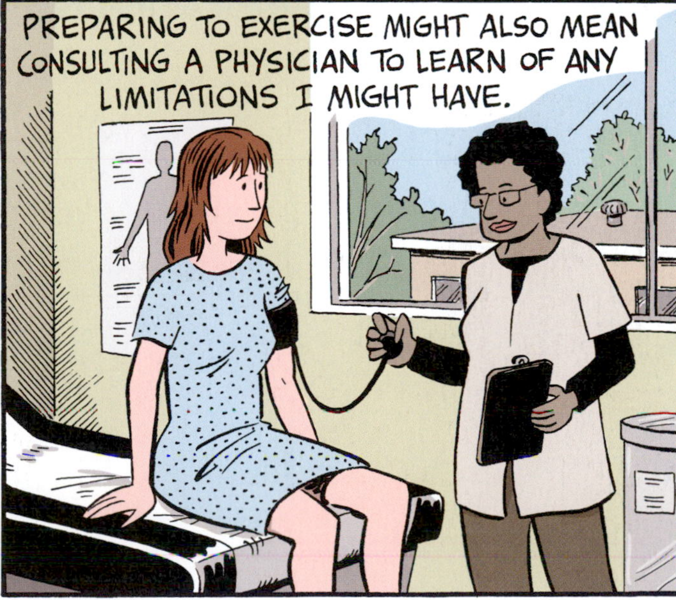
PREPARING TO EXERCISE MIGHT ALSO MEAN CONSULTING A PHYSICIAN TO LEARN OF ANY LIMITATIONS I MIGHT HAVE.

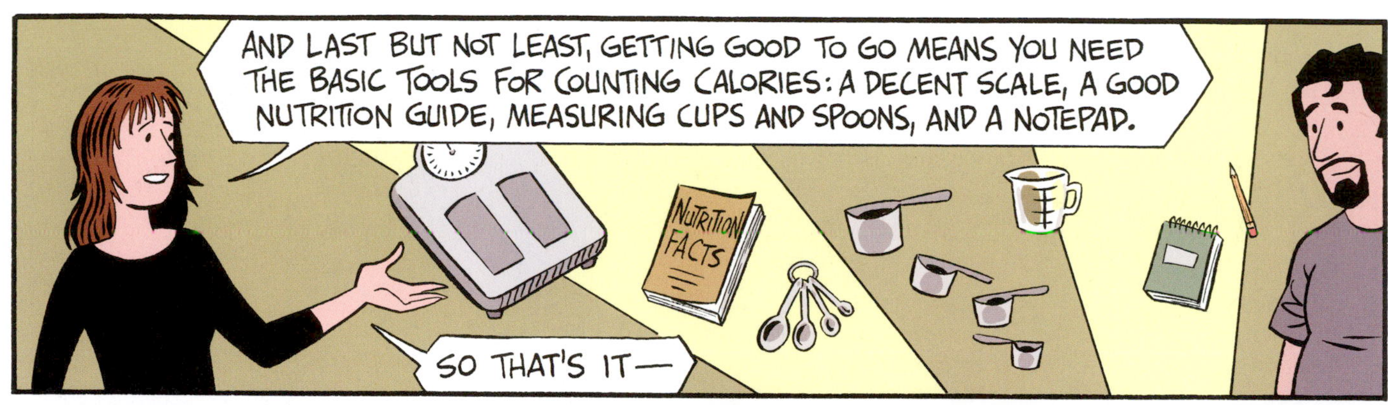
AND LAST BUT NOT LEAST, GETTING GOOD TO GO MEANS YOU NEED THE BASIC TOOLS FOR COUNTING CALORIES: A DECENT SCALE, A GOOD NUTRITION GUIDE, MEASURING CUPS AND SPOONS, AND A NOTEPAD.
NUTRITION FACTS
SO THAT'S IT—

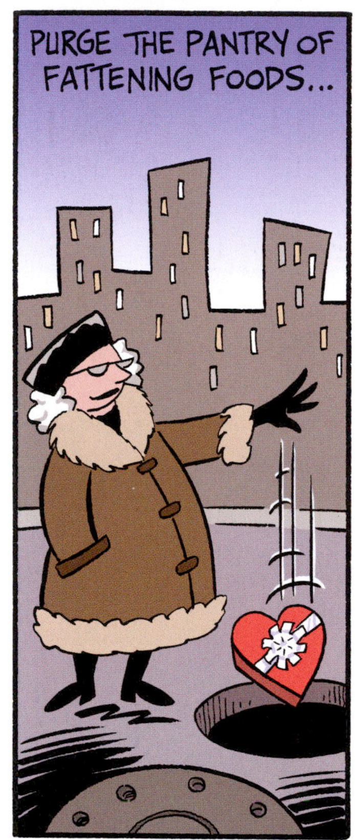
PURGE THE PANTRY OF FATTENING FOODS...

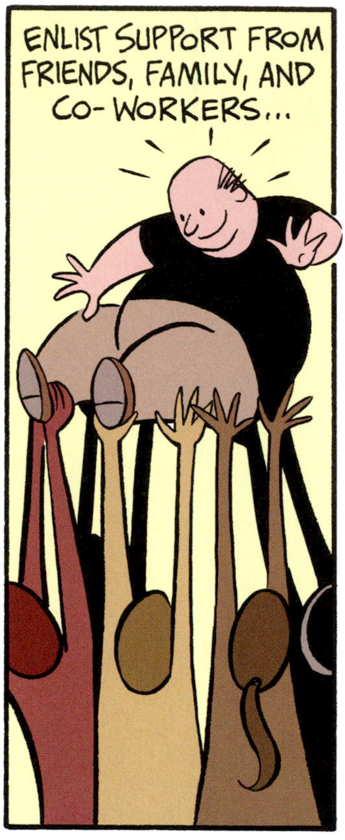
ENLIST SUPPORT FROM FRIENDS, FAMILY, AND CO-WORKERS...

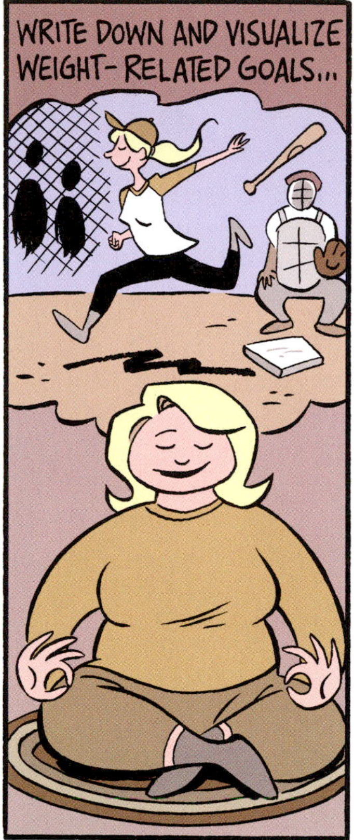
WRITE DOWN AND VISUALIZE WEIGHT-RELATED GOALS...

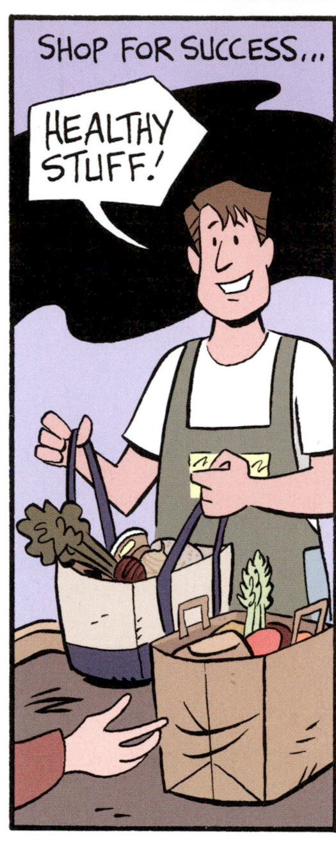
SHOP FOR SUCCESS...
HEALTHY STUFF!

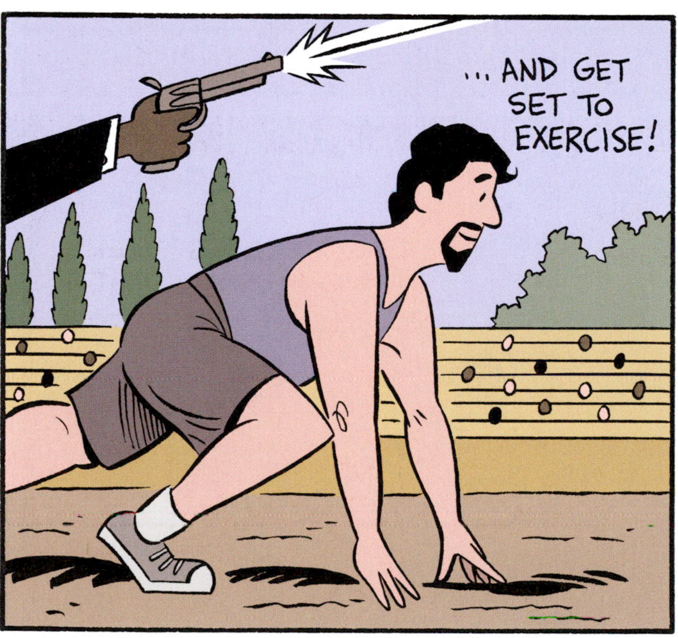
...AND GET SET TO EXERCISE!

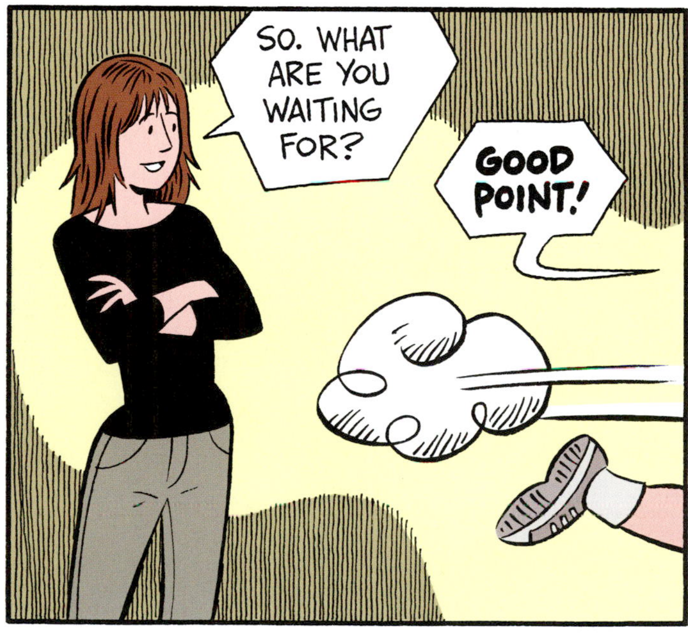
SO. WHAT ARE YOU WAITING FOR?
GOOD POINT!

# The Gymless Workout

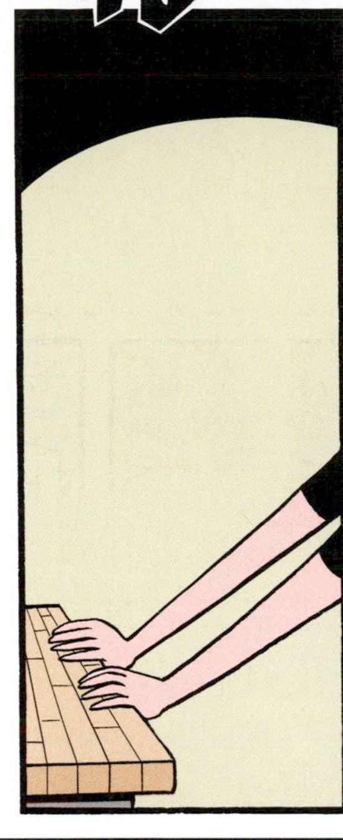
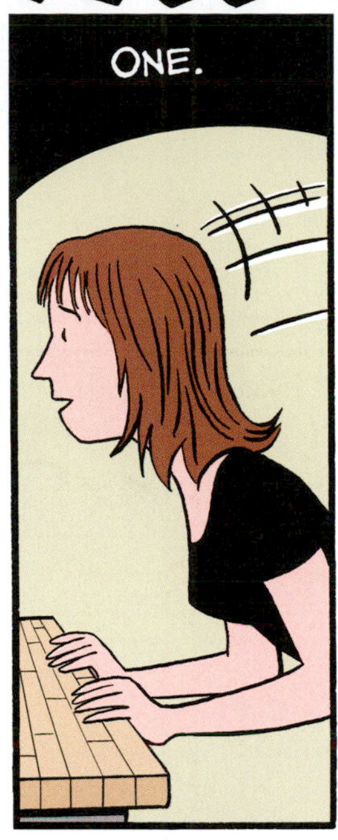

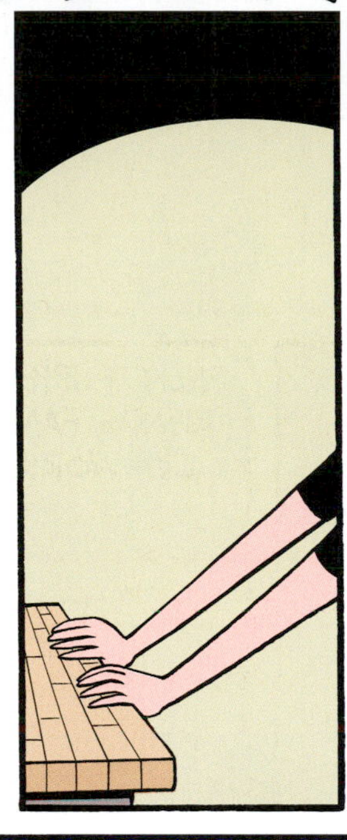
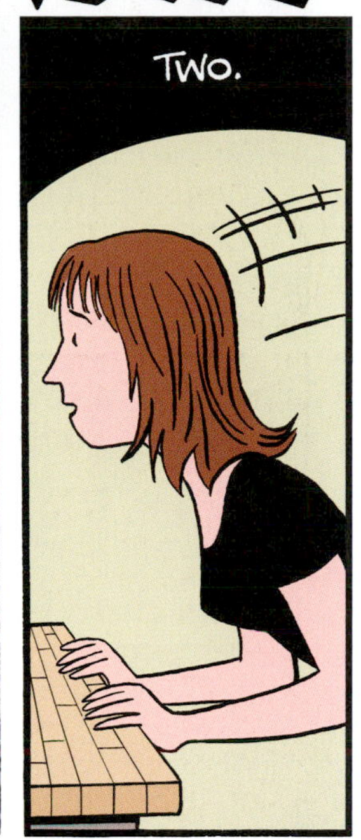

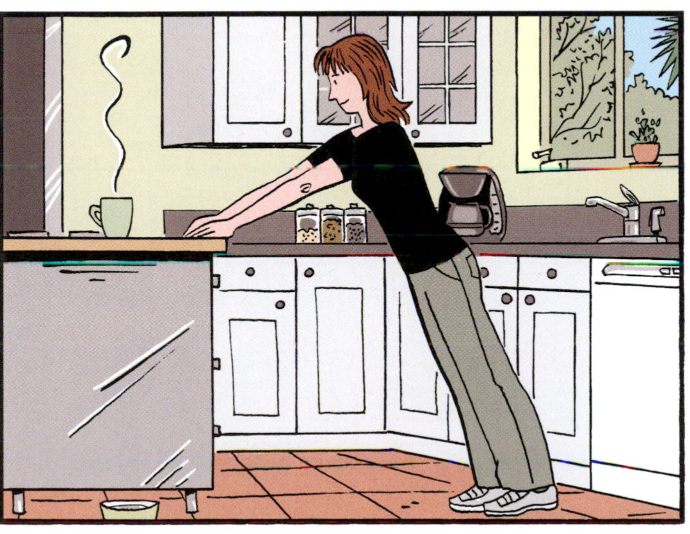
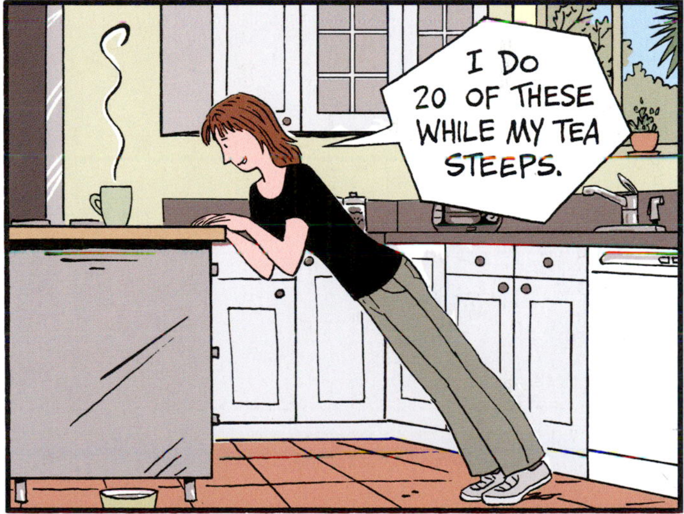

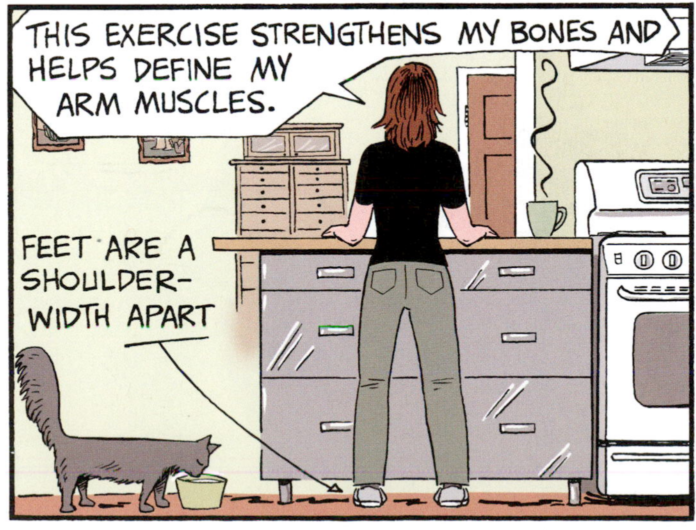

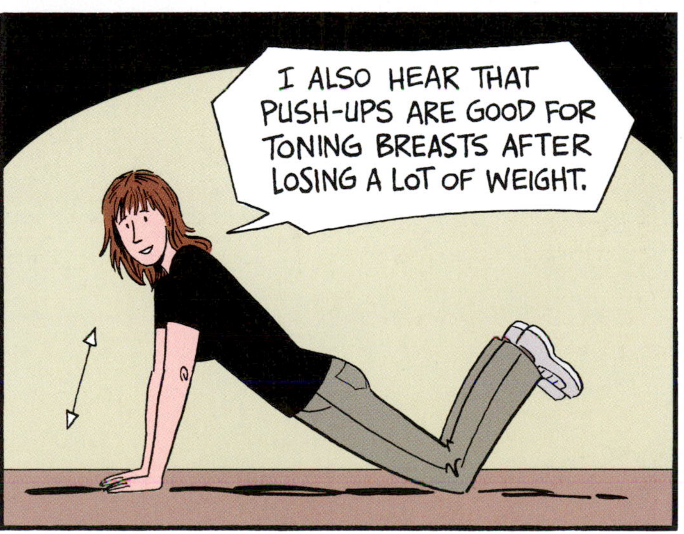

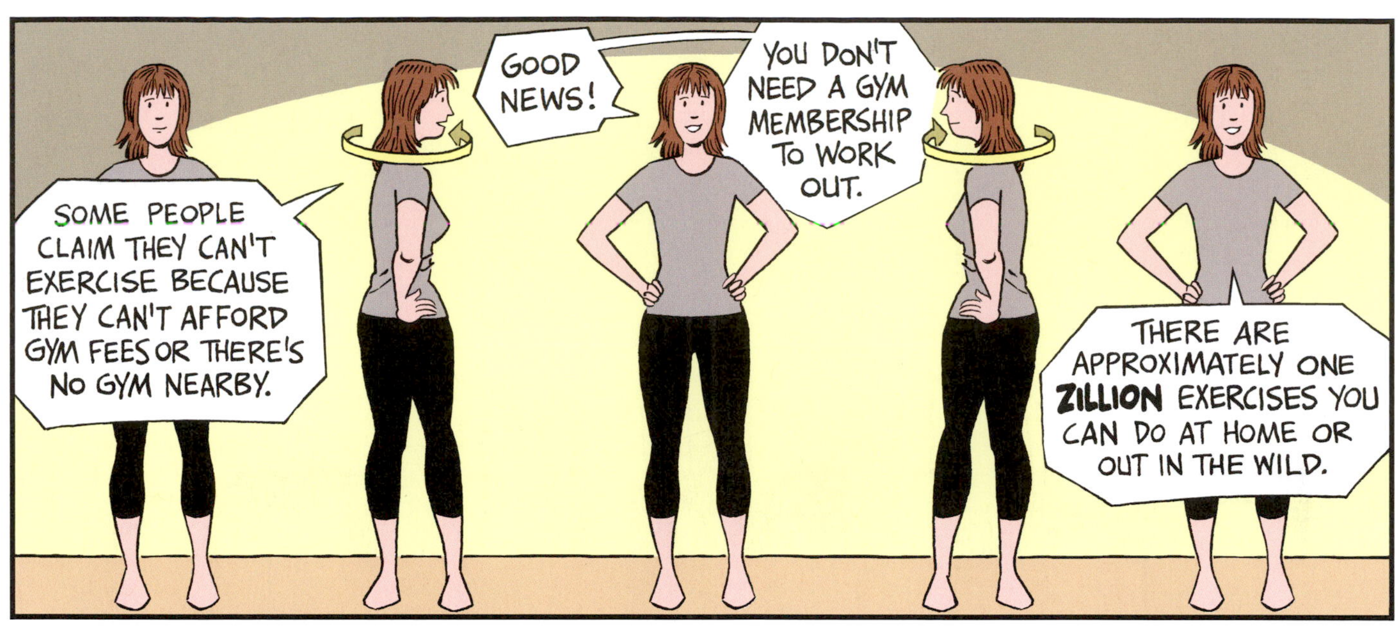
SOME PEOPLE CLAIM THEY CAN'T EXERCISE BECAUSE THEY CAN'T AFFORD GYM FEES OR THERE'S NO GYM NEARBY.
GOOD NEWS!
YOU DON'T NEED A GYM MEMBERSHIP TO WORK OUT.
THERE ARE APPROXIMATELY ONE **ZILLION** EXERCISES YOU CAN DO AT HOME OR OUT IN THE WILD.

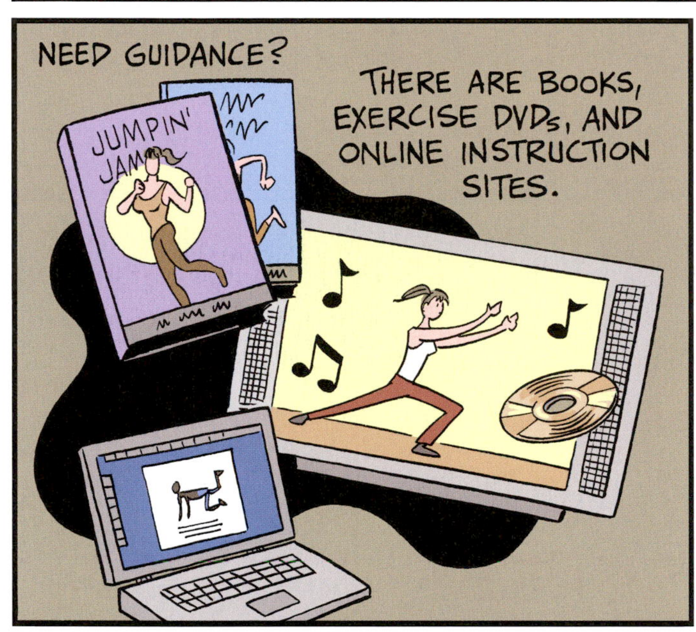
NEED GUIDANCE?
THERE ARE BOOKS, EXERCISE DVDs, AND ONLINE INSTRUCTION SITES.
JUMPIN' JAM

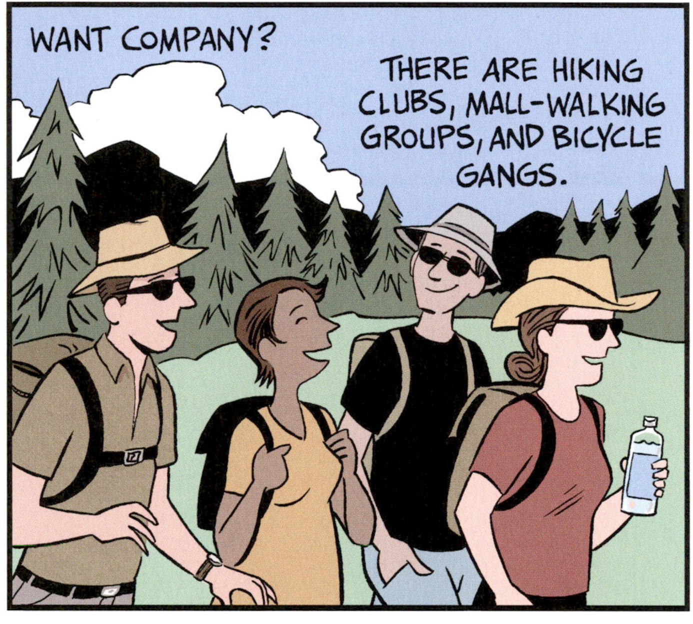
WANT COMPANY?
THERE ARE HIKING CLUBS, MALL-WALKING GROUPS, AND BICYCLE GANGS.

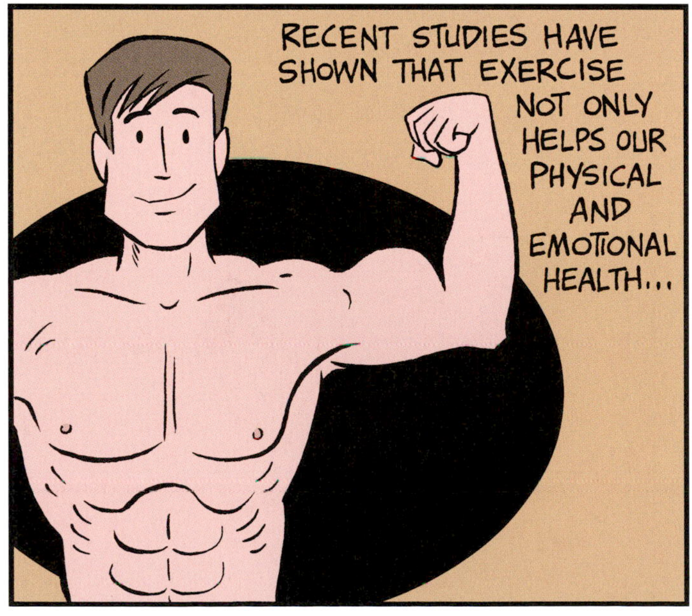
RECENT STUDIES HAVE SHOWN THAT EXERCISE NOT ONLY HELPS OUR PHYSICAL AND EMOTIONAL HEALTH...

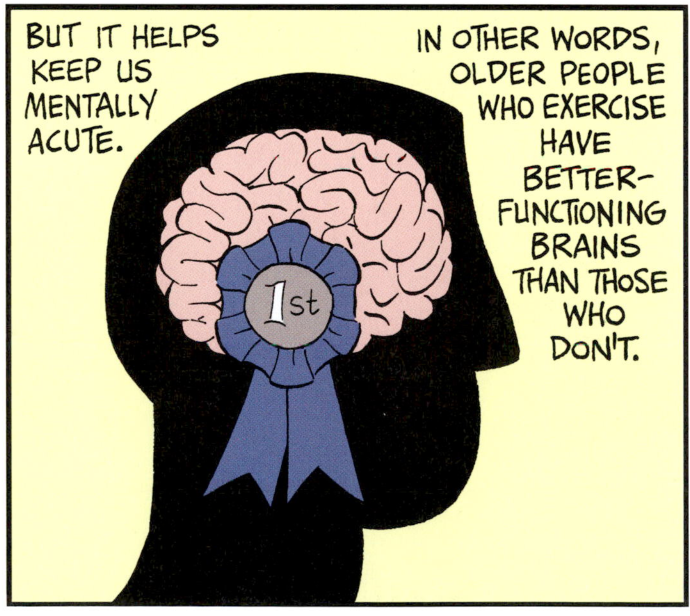
BUT IT HELPS KEEP US MENTALLY ACUTE.
IN OTHER WORDS, OLDER PEOPLE WHO EXERCISE HAVE BETTER-FUNCTIONING BRAINS THAN THOSE WHO DON'T.
1st

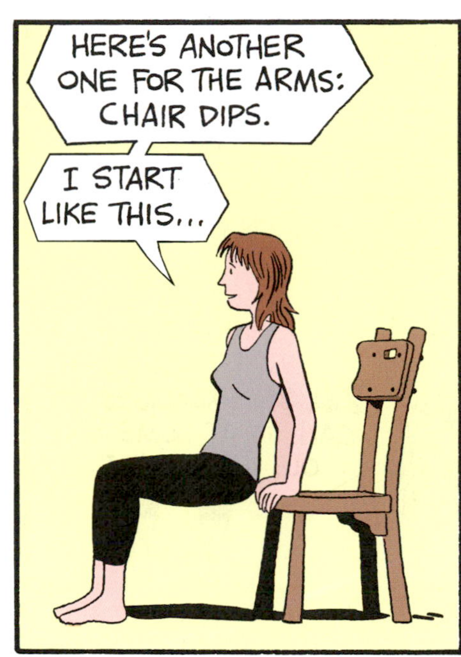
HERE'S ANOTHER ONE FOR THE ARMS: CHAIR DIPS.
I START LIKE THIS...

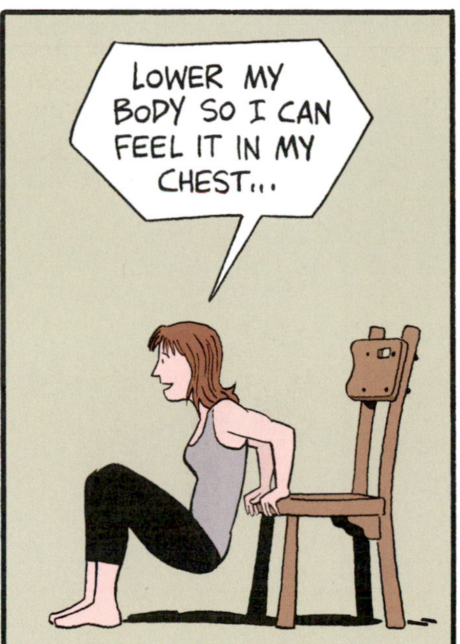
LOWER MY BODY SO I CAN FEEL IT IN MY CHEST...

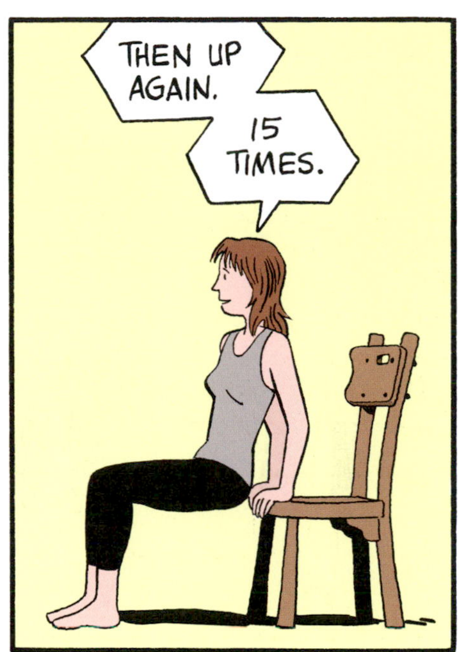
THEN UP AGAIN.
15 TIMES.

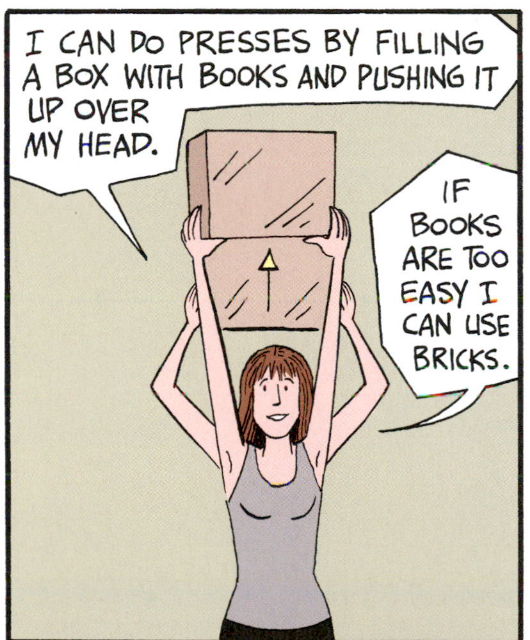
I CAN DO PRESSES BY FILLING A BOX WITH BOOKS AND PUSHING IT UP OVER MY HEAD.
IF BOOKS ARE TOO EASY I CAN USE BRICKS.

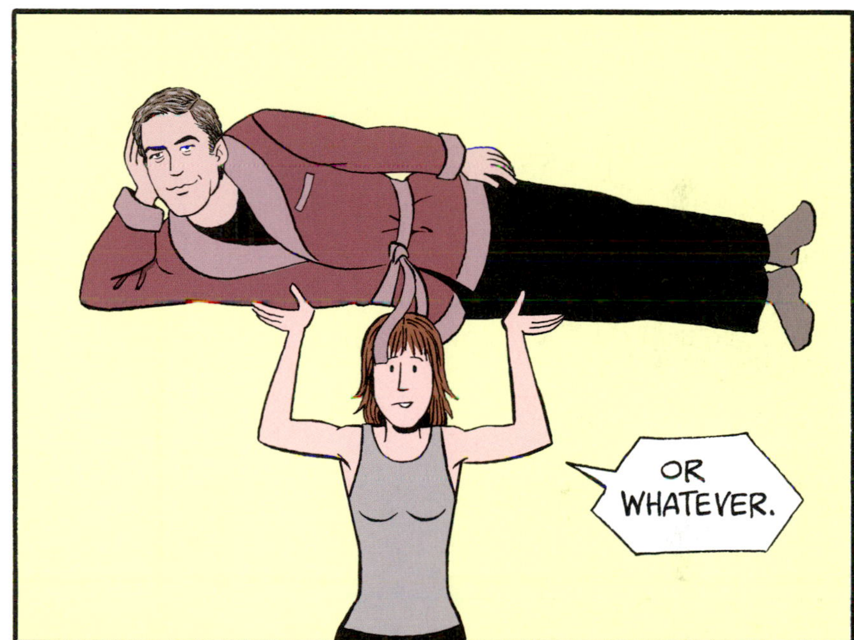
OR WHATEVER.

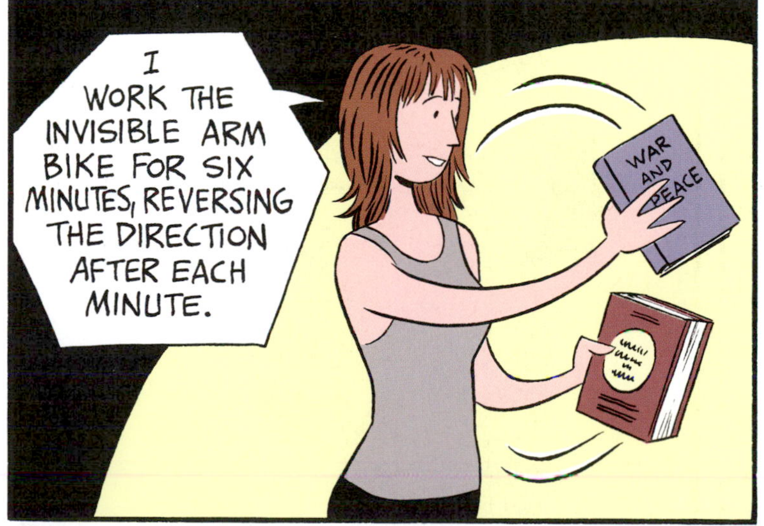
I WORK THE INVISIBLE ARM BIKE FOR SIX MINUTES, REVERSING THE DIRECTION AFTER EACH MINUTE.
WAR AND PEACE

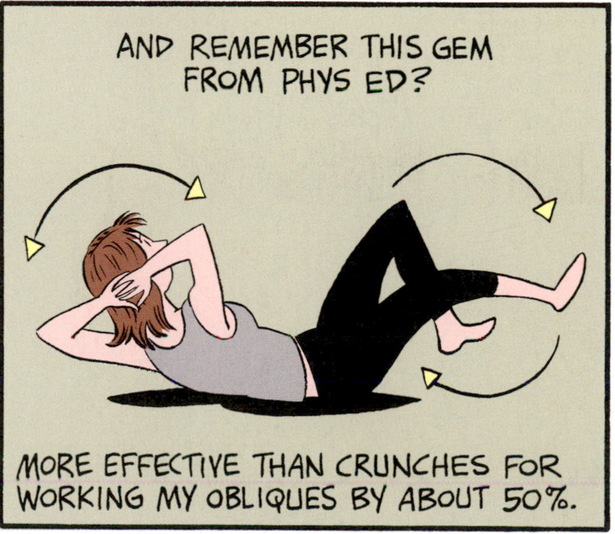
AND REMEMBER THIS GEM FROM PHYS ED?
MORE EFFECTIVE THAN CRUNCHES FOR WORKING MY OBLIQUES BY ABOUT 50%.

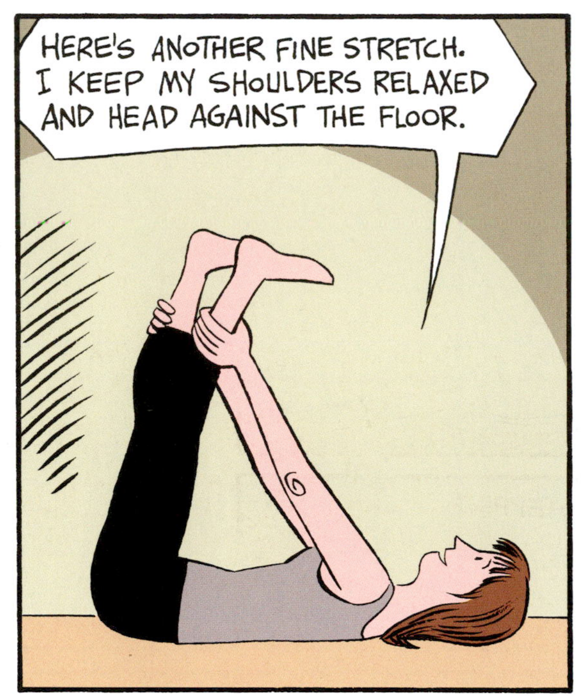
HERE'S ANOTHER FINE STRETCH. I KEEP MY SHOULDERS RELAXED AND HEAD AGAINST THE FLOOR.

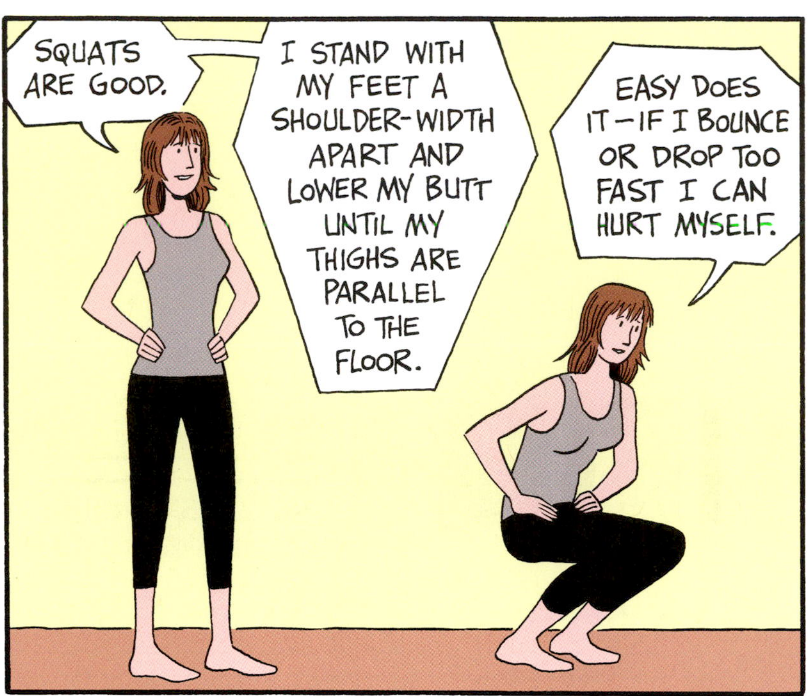
SQUATS ARE GOOD.
I STAND WITH MY FEET A SHOULDER-WIDTH APART AND LOWER MY BUTT UNTIL MY THIGHS ARE PARALLEL TO THE FLOOR.
EASY DOES IT—IF I BOUNCE OR DROP TOO FAST I CAN HURT MYSELF.

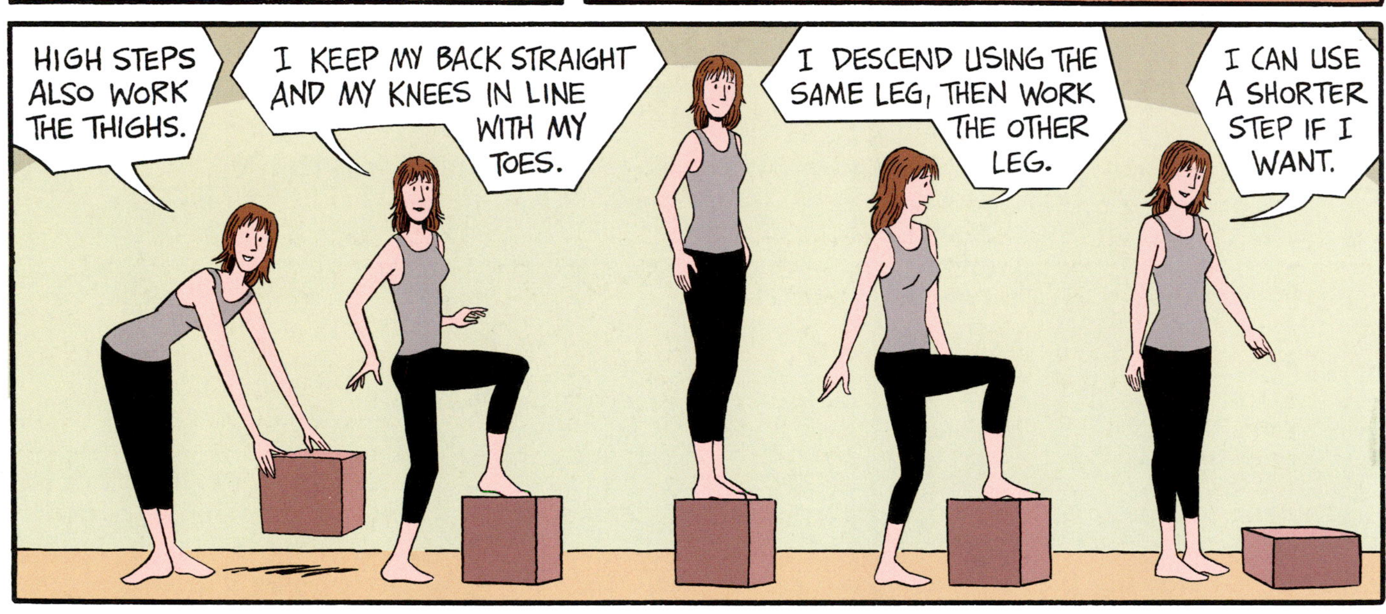
HIGH STEPS ALSO WORK THE THIGHS.
I KEEP MY BACK STRAIGHT AND MY KNEES IN LINE WITH MY TOES.
I DESCEND USING THE SAME LEG, THEN WORK THE OTHER LEG.
I CAN USE A SHORTER STEP IF I WANT.

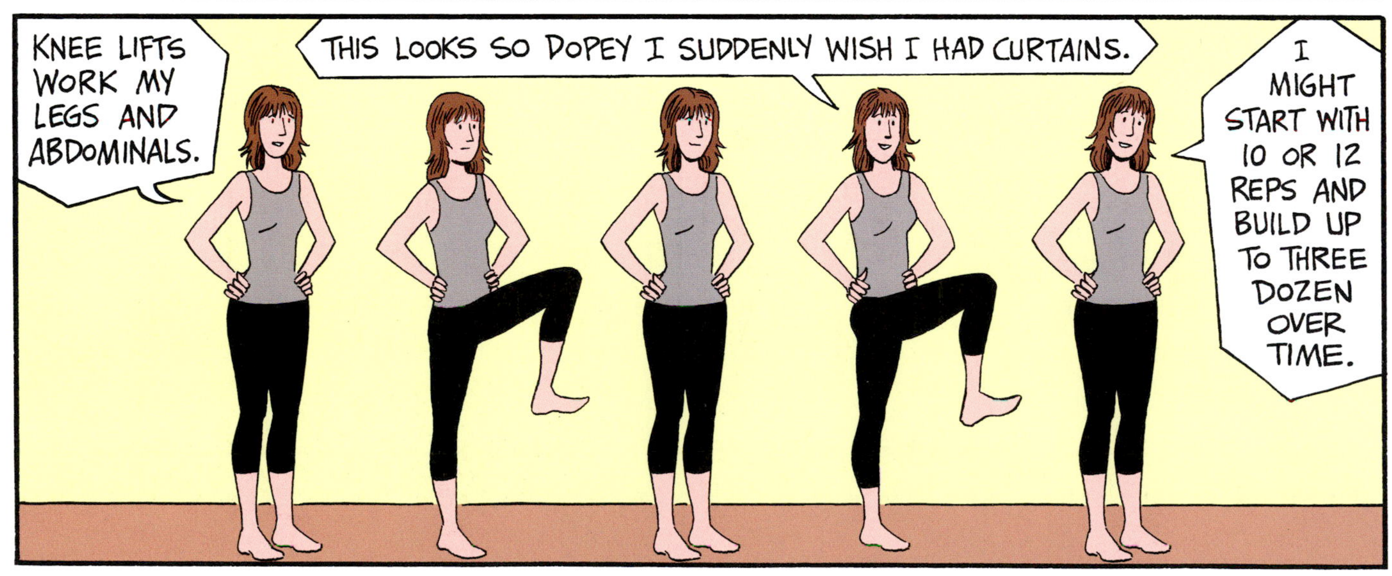
KNEE LIFTS WORK MY LEGS AND ABDOMINALS.
THIS LOOKS SO DOPEY I SUDDENLY WISH I HAD CURTAINS.
I MIGHT START WITH 10 OR 12 REPS AND BUILD UP TO THREE DOZEN OVER TIME.

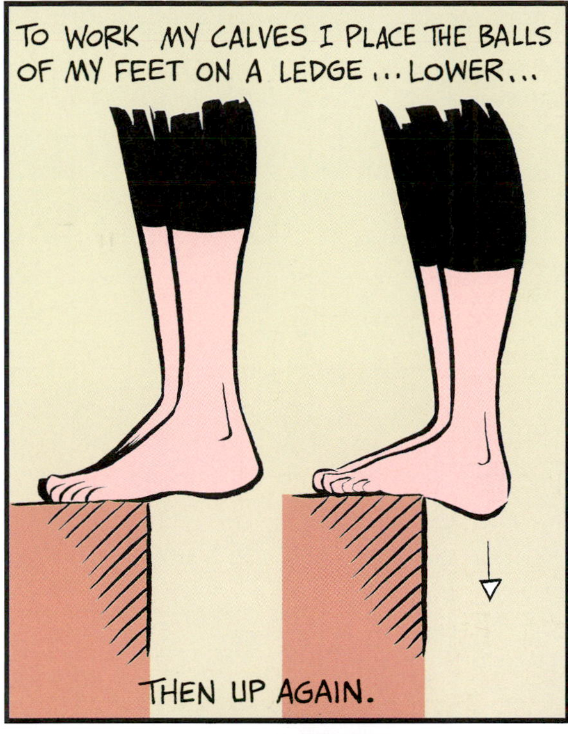
TO WORK MY CALVES I PLACE THE BALLS OF MY FEET ON A LEDGE... LOWER...
THEN UP AGAIN.

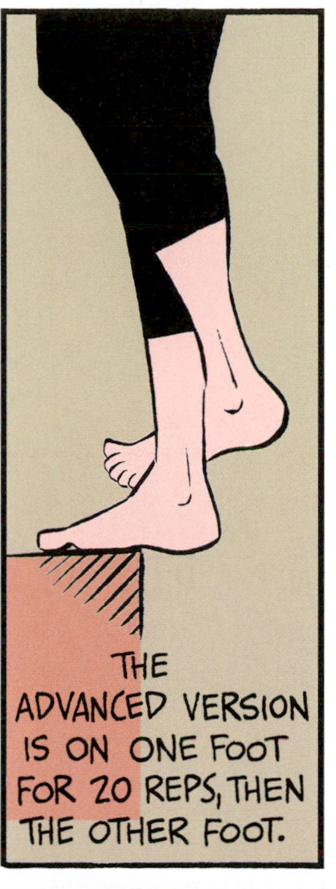
THE ADVANCED VERSION IS ON ONE FOOT FOR 20 REPS, THEN THE OTHER FOOT.

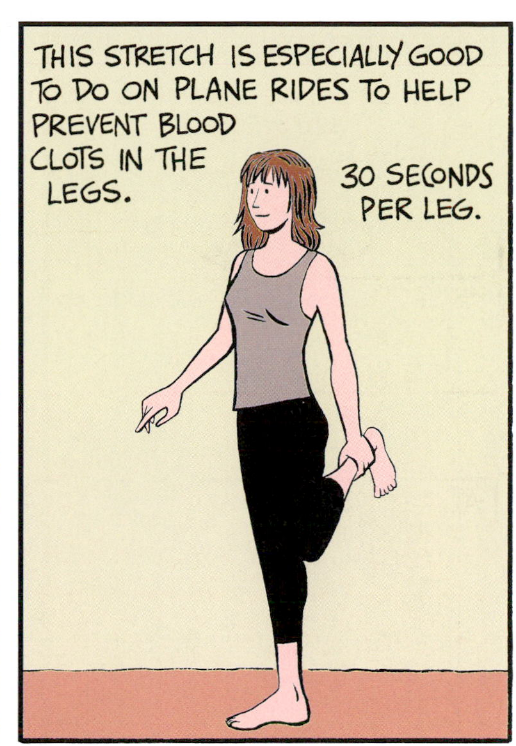
THIS STRETCH IS ESPECIALLY GOOD TO DO ON PLANE RIDES TO HELP PREVENT BLOOD CLOTS IN THE LEGS.
30 SECONDS PER LEG.

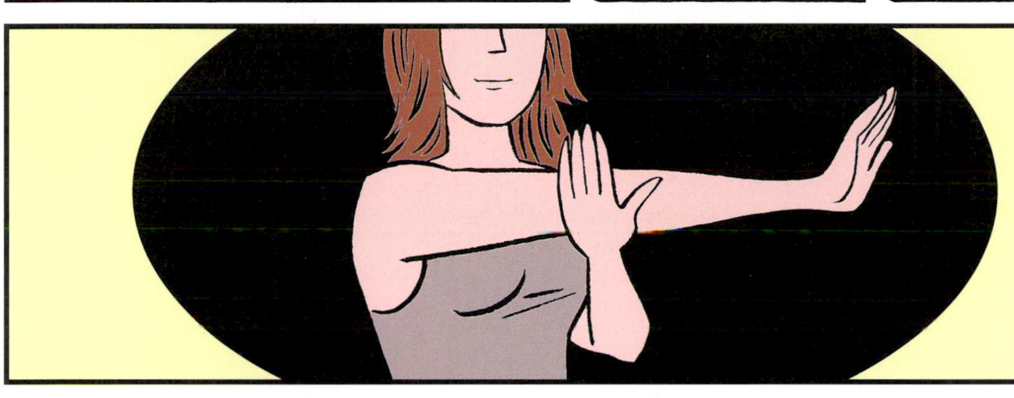
A SHOULDER STRETCH — 15 SECONDS FOR EACH SIDE...

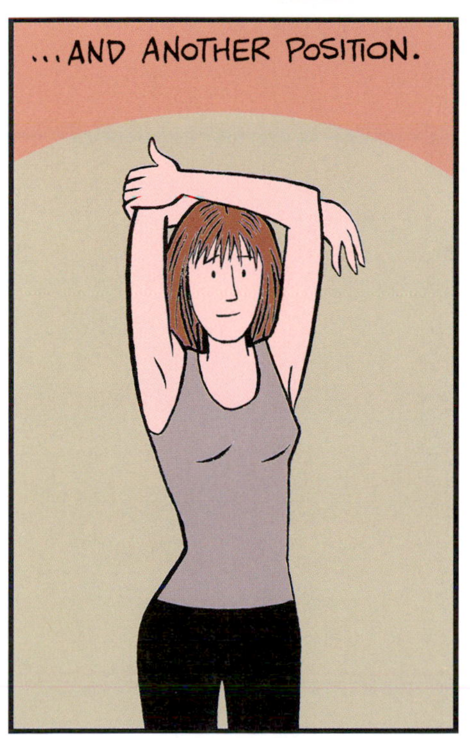
...AND ANOTHER POSITION.

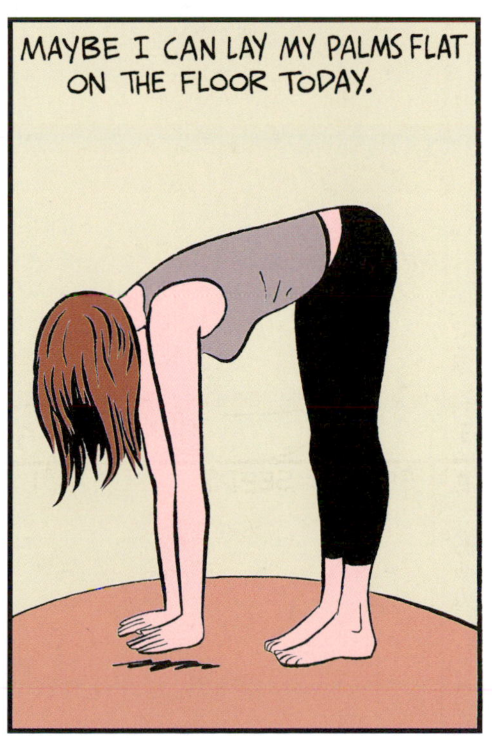
MAYBE I CAN LAY MY PALMS FLAT ON THE FLOOR TODAY.

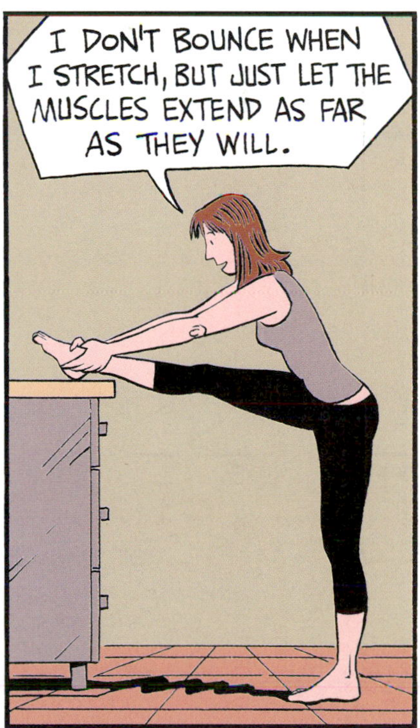
I DON'T BOUNCE WHEN I STRETCH, BUT JUST LET THE MUSCLES EXTEND AS FAR AS THEY WILL.

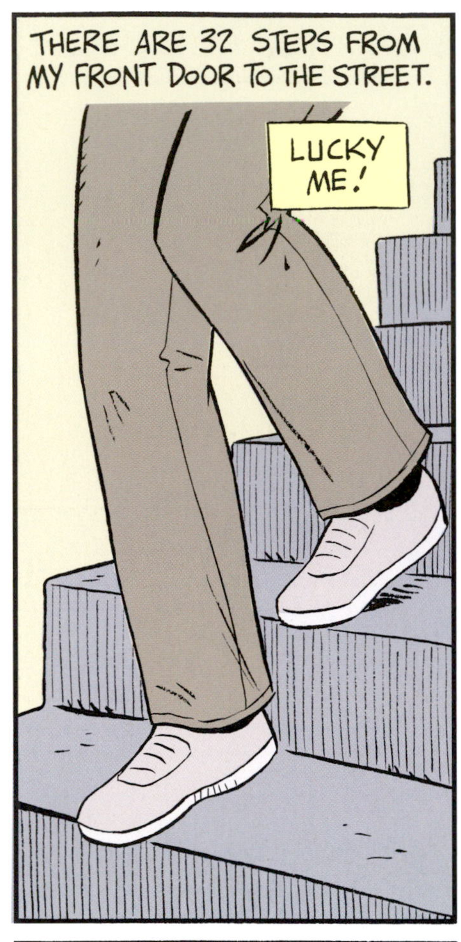
THERE ARE 32 STEPS FROM MY FRONT DOOR TO THE STREET.
LUCKY ME!

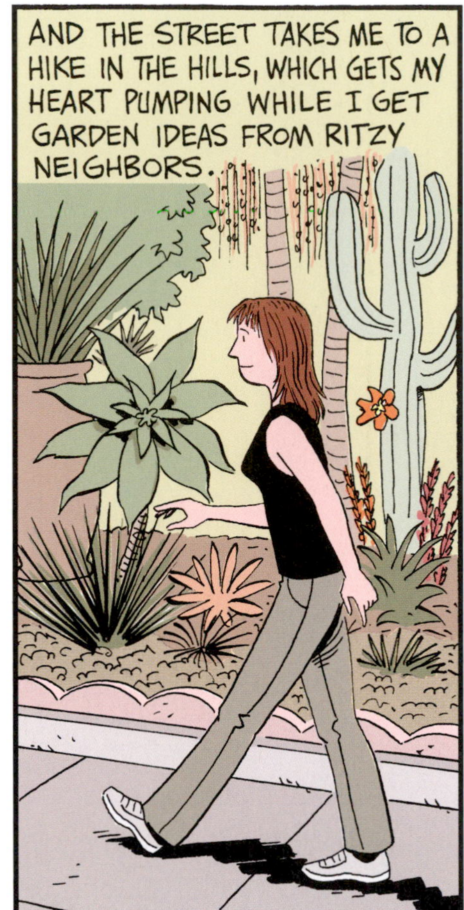
AND THE STREET TAKES ME TO A HIKE IN THE HILLS, WHICH GETS MY HEART PUMPING WHILE I GET GARDEN IDEAS FROM RITZY NEIGHBORS.

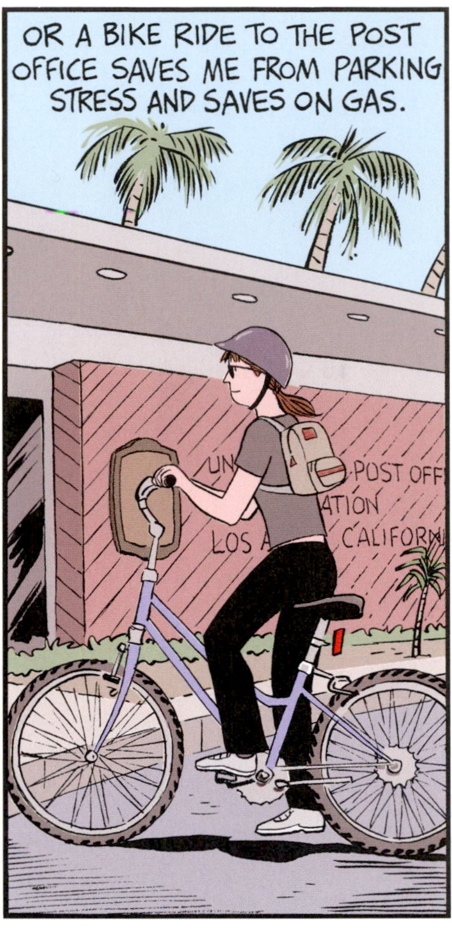
OR A BIKE RIDE TO THE POST OFFICE SAVES ME FROM PARKING STRESS AND SAVES ON GAS.

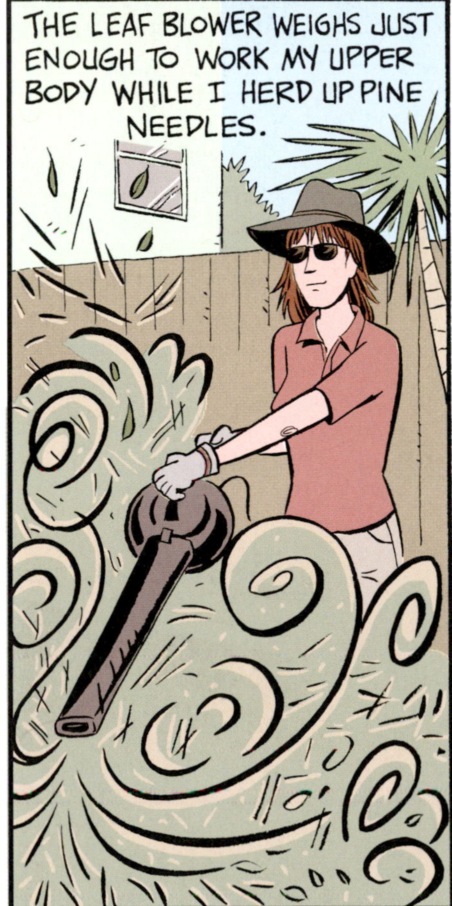
THE LEAF BLOWER WEIGHS JUST ENOUGH TO WORK MY UPPER BODY WHILE I HERD UP PINE NEEDLES.

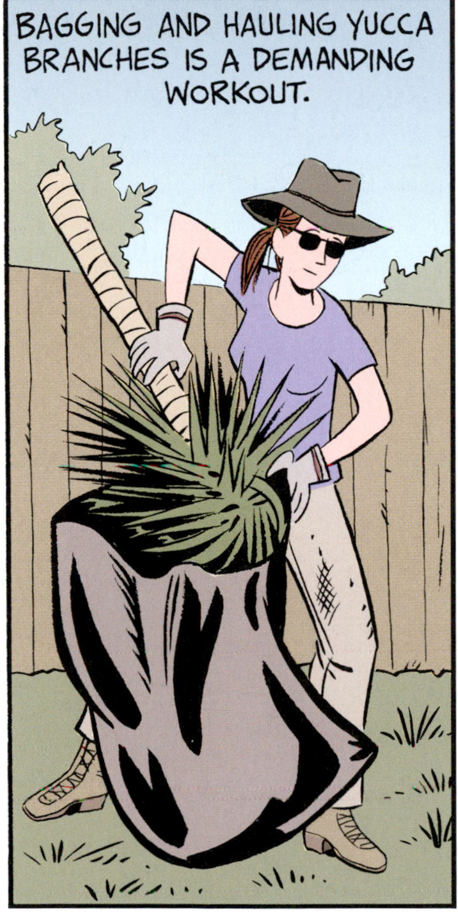
BAGGING AND HAULING YUCCA BRANCHES IS A DEMANDING WORKOUT.

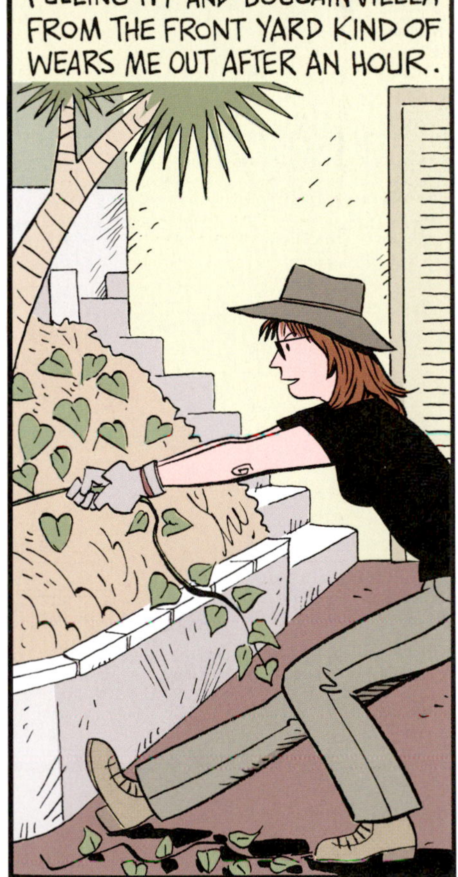
PULLING IVY AND BOUGAINVILLEA FROM THE FRONT YARD KIND OF WEARS ME OUT AFTER AN HOUR.

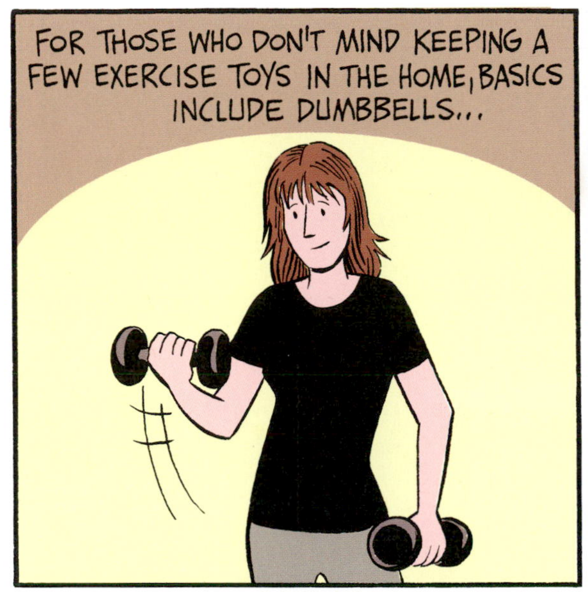

FOR THOSE WHO DON'T MIND KEEPING A FEW EXERCISE TOYS IN THE HOME, BASICS INCLUDE DUMBBELLS...

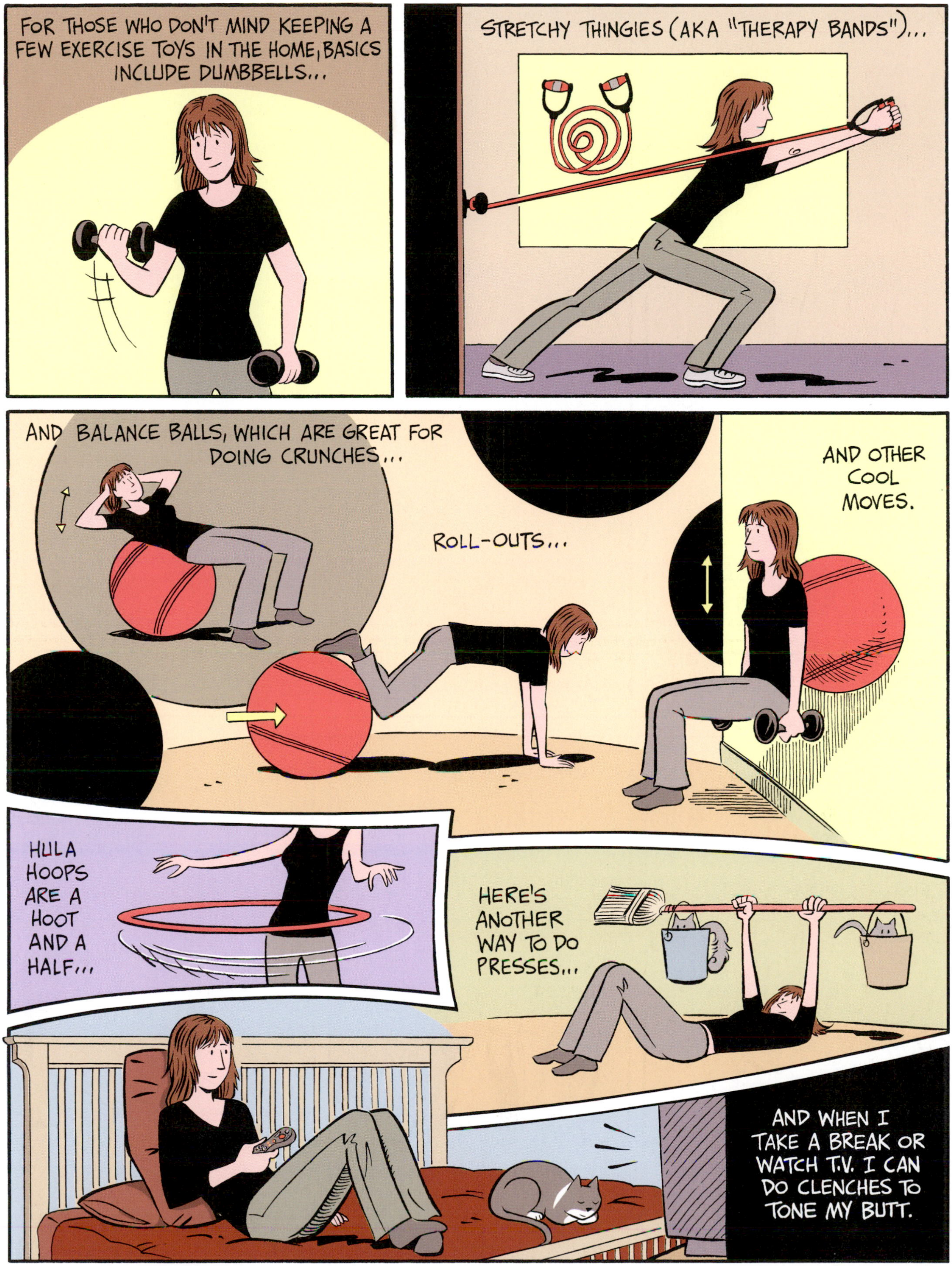

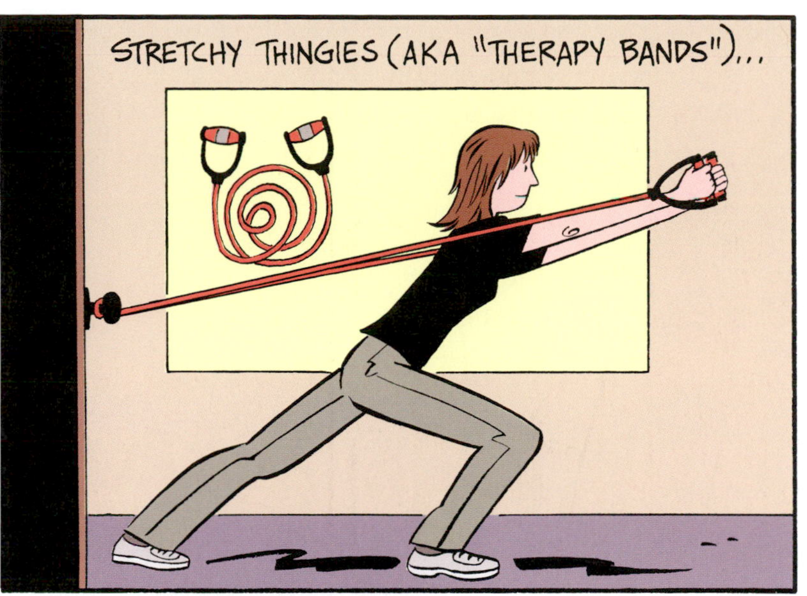

STRETCHY THINGIES (AKA "THERAPY BANDS")...

AND BALANCE BALLS, WHICH ARE GREAT FOR DOING CRUNCHES...

ROLL-OUTS...

AND OTHER COOL MOVES.

HULA HOOPS ARE A HOOT AND A HALF...

HERE'S ANOTHER WAY TO DO PRESSES...

AND WHEN I TAKE A BREAK OR WATCH T.V. I CAN DO CLENCHES TO TONE MY BUTT.

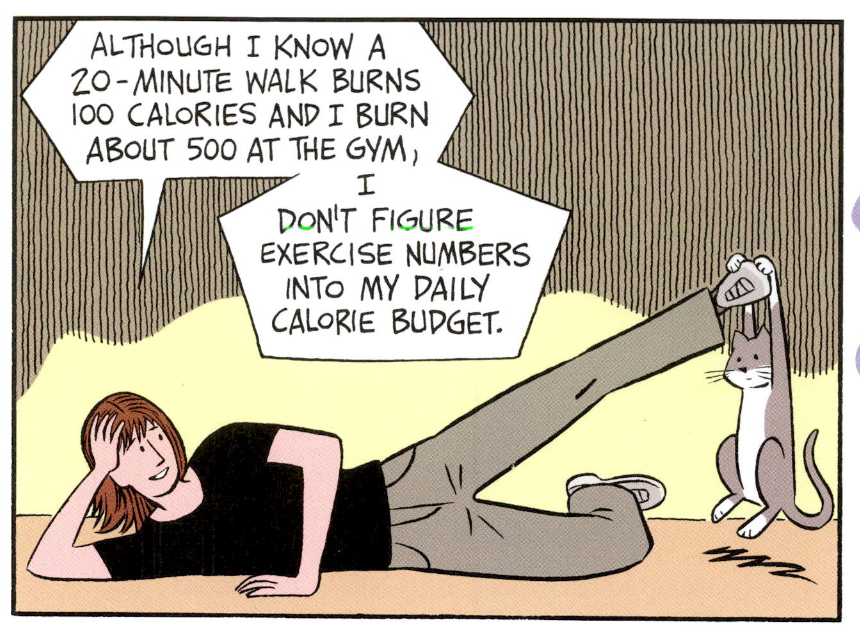
ALTHOUGH I KNOW A 20-MINUTE WALK BURNS 100 CALORIES AND I BURN ABOUT 500 AT THE GYM,
I DON'T FIGURE EXERCISE NUMBERS INTO MY DAILY CALORIE BUDGET.

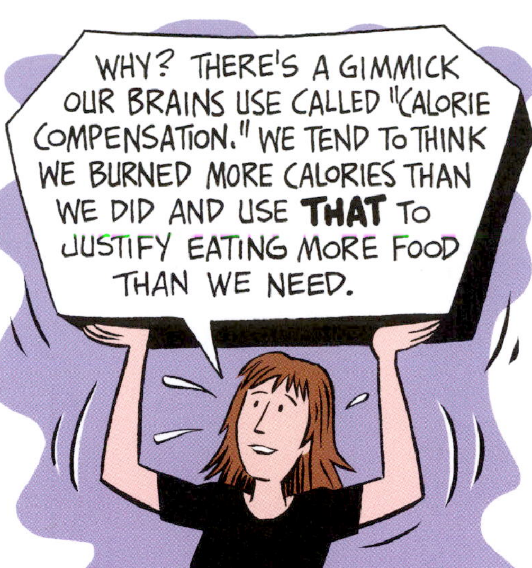
WHY? THERE'S A GIMMICK OUR BRAINS USE CALLED "CALORIE COMPENSATION." WE TEND TO THINK WE BURNED MORE CALORIES THAN WE DID AND USE **THAT** TO JUSTIFY EATING MORE FOOD THAN WE NEED.

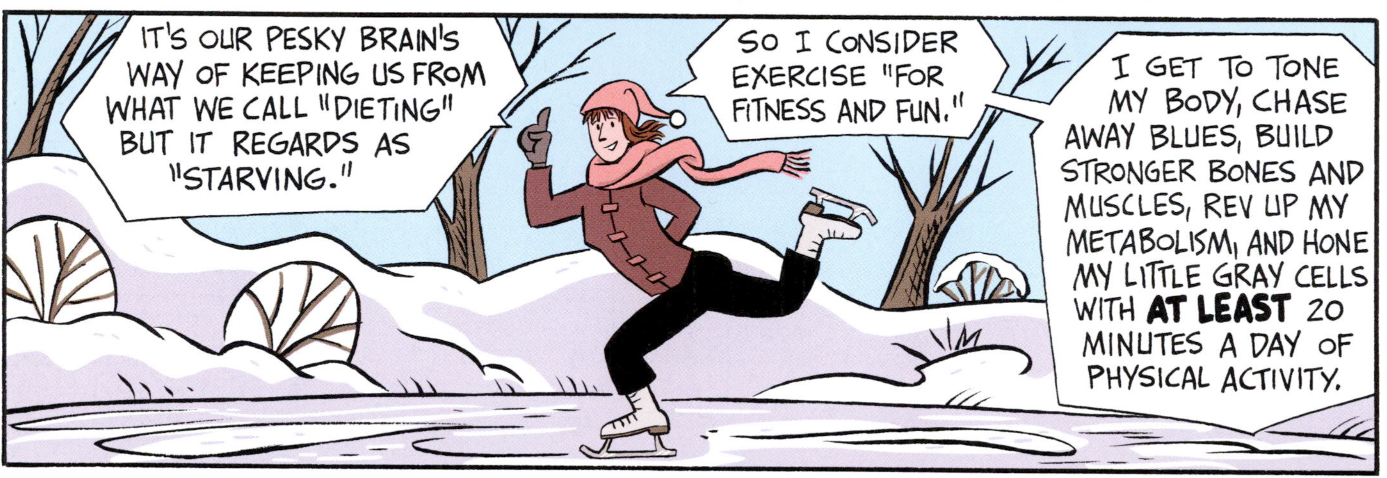
IT'S OUR PESKY BRAIN'S WAY OF KEEPING US FROM WHAT WE CALL "DIETING" BUT IT REGARDS AS "STARVING."
SO I CONSIDER EXERCISE "FOR FITNESS AND FUN."
I GET TO TONE MY BODY, CHASE AWAY BLUES, BUILD STRONGER BONES AND MUSCLES, REV UP MY METABOLISM, AND HONE MY LITTLE GRAY CELLS WITH **AT LEAST** 20 MINUTES A DAY OF PHYSICAL ACTIVITY.

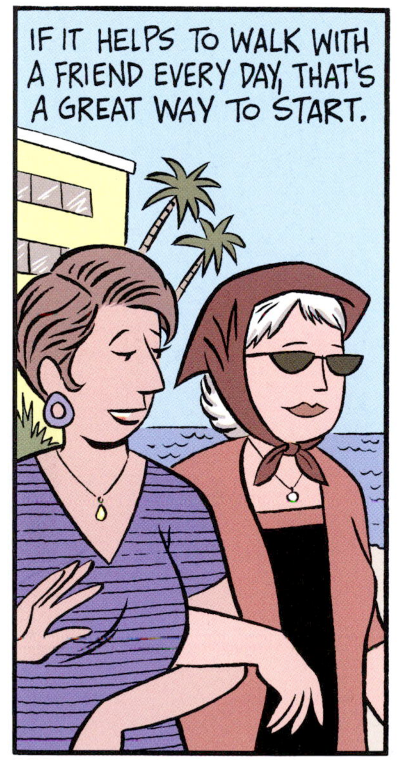
IF IT HELPS TO WALK WITH A FRIEND EVERY DAY, THAT'S A GREAT WAY TO START.

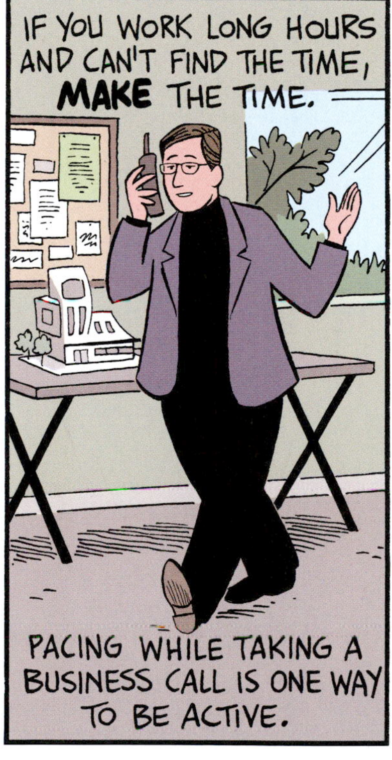
IF YOU WORK LONG HOURS AND CAN'T FIND THE TIME, **MAKE** THE TIME.
PACING WHILE TAKING A BUSINESS CALL IS ONE WAY TO BE ACTIVE.

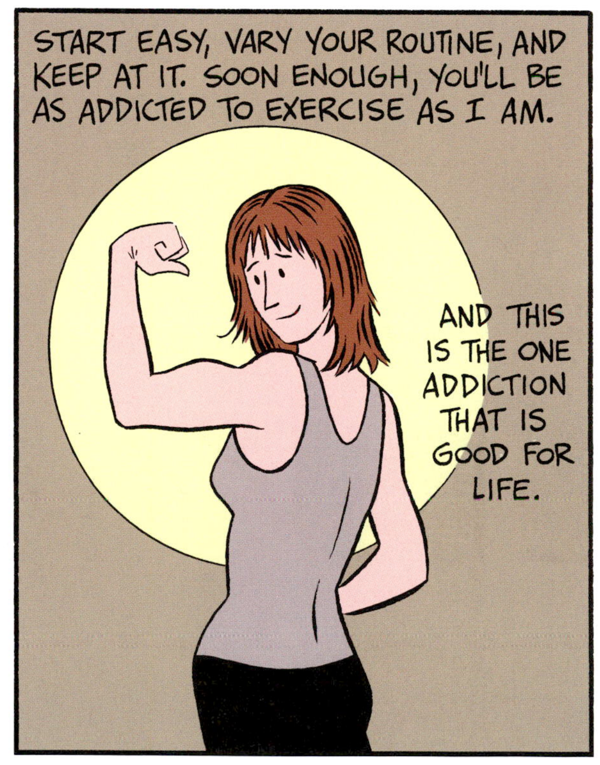
START EASY, VARY YOUR ROUTINE, AND KEEP AT IT. SOON ENOUGH, YOU'LL BE AS ADDICTED TO EXERCISE AS I AM.
AND THIS IS THE ONE ADDICTION THAT IS GOOD FOR LIFE.

# At the Gym

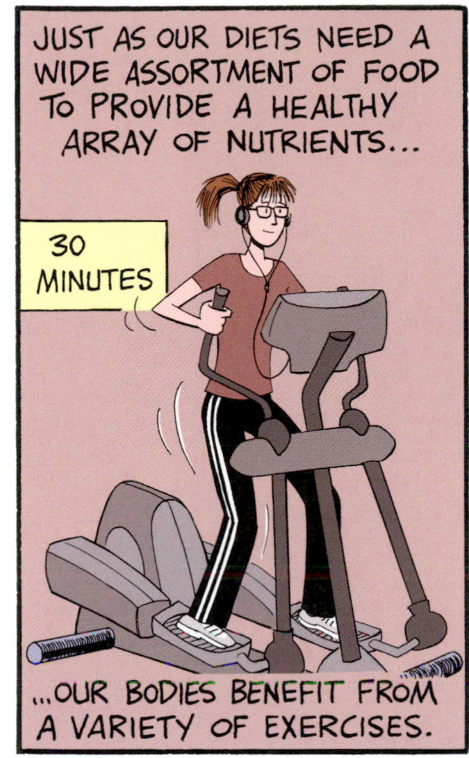
JUST AS OUR DIETS NEED A WIDE ASSORTMENT OF FOOD TO PROVIDE A HEALTHY ARRAY OF NUTRIENTS...
30 MINUTES
...OUR BODIES BENEFIT FROM A VARIETY OF EXERCISES.

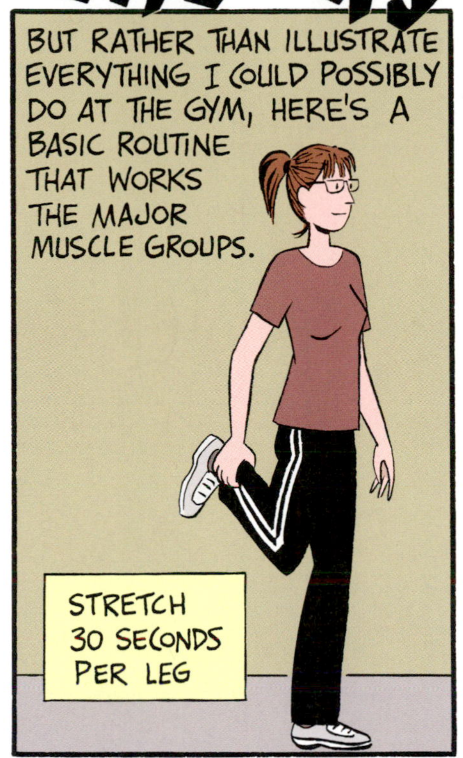
BUT RATHER THAN ILLUSTRATE EVERYTHING I COULD POSSIBLY DO AT THE GYM, HERE'S A BASIC ROUTINE THAT WORKS THE MAJOR MUSCLE GROUPS.
STRETCH 30 SECONDS PER LEG

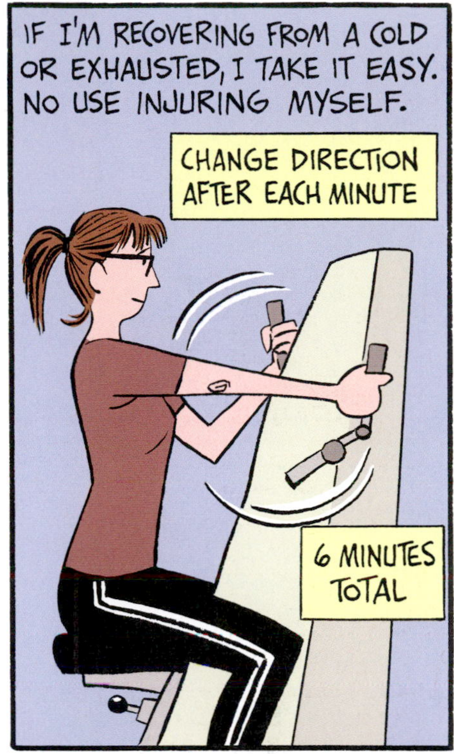
IF I'M RECOVERING FROM A COLD OR EXHAUSTED, I TAKE IT EASY. NO USE INJURING MYSELF.
CHANGE DIRECTION AFTER EACH MINUTE
6 MINUTES TOTAL

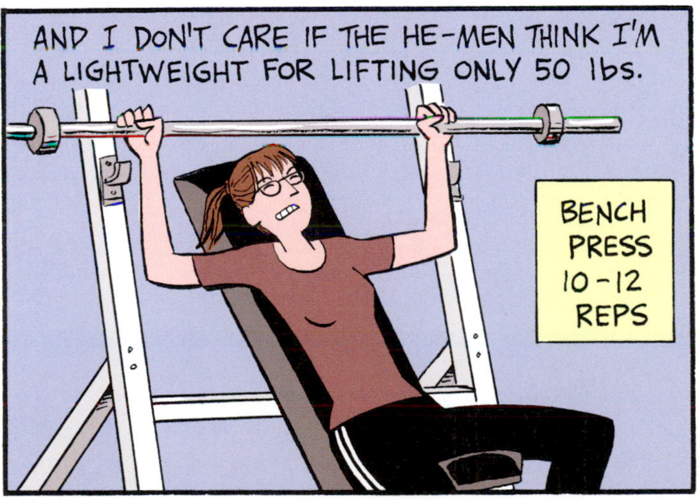
AND I DON'T CARE IF THE HE-MEN THINK I'M A LIGHTWEIGHT FOR LIFTING ONLY 50 lbs.
BENCH PRESS 10-12 REPS

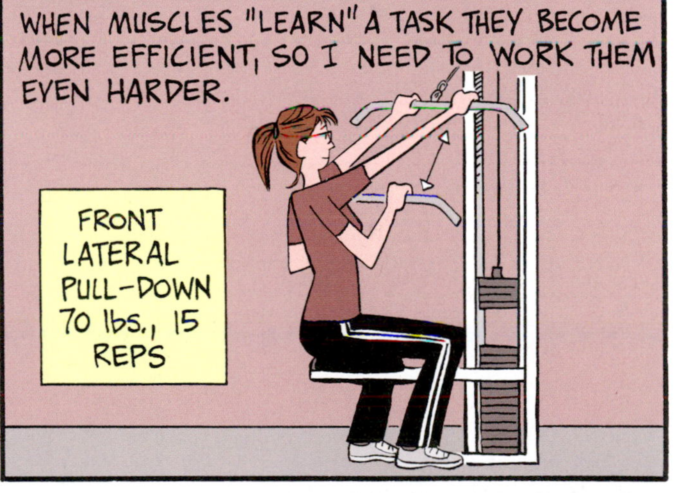
WHEN MUSCLES "LEARN" A TASK THEY BECOME MORE EFFICIENT, SO I NEED TO WORK THEM EVEN HARDER.
FRONT LATERAL PULL-DOWN 70 lbs., 15 REPS

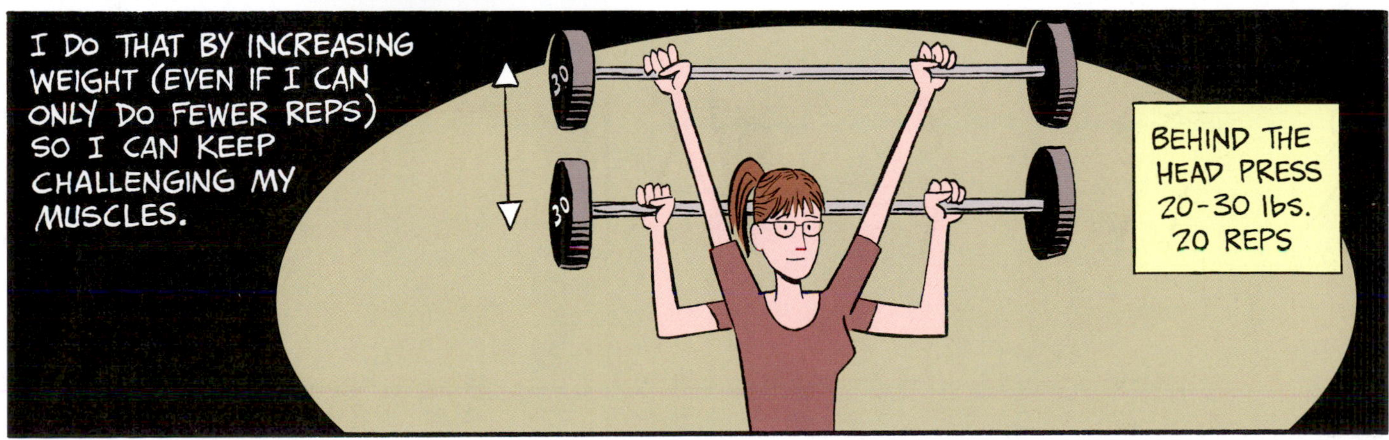
I DO THAT BY INCREASING WEIGHT (EVEN IF I CAN ONLY DO FEWER REPS) SO I CAN KEEP CHALLENGING MY MUSCLES.
30
30
BEHIND THE HEAD PRESS 20-30 lbs. 20 REPS

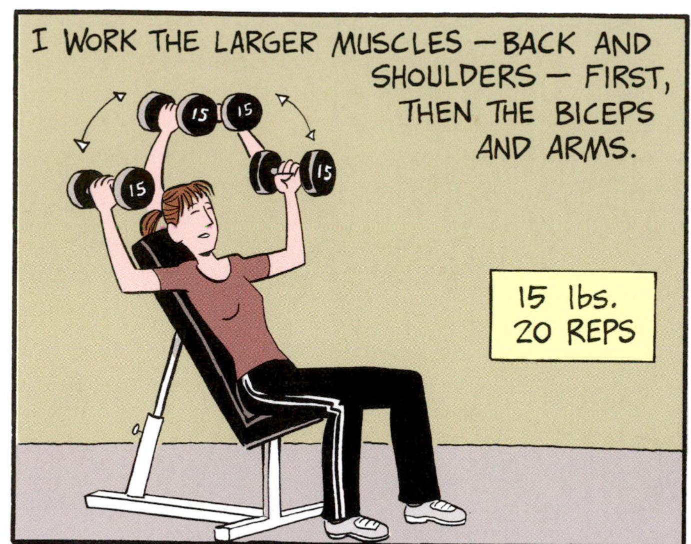
I WORK THE LARGER MUSCLES — BACK AND SHOULDERS — FIRST, THEN THE BICEPS AND ARMS.
15 15 15 15
15 lbs. 20 REPS

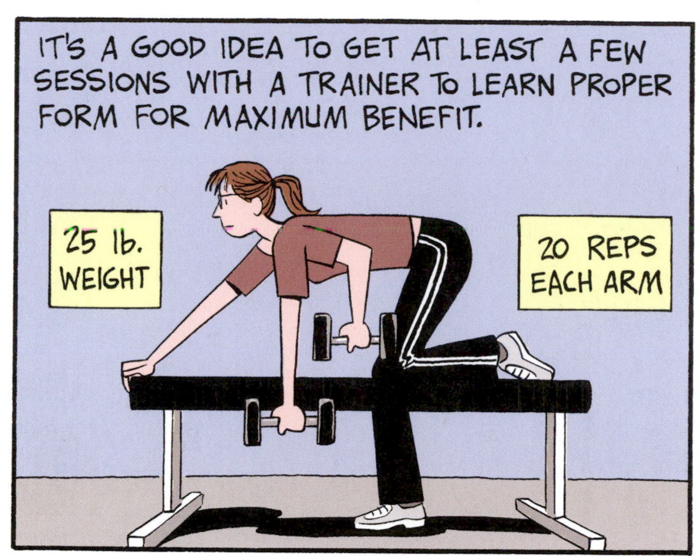
IT'S A GOOD IDEA TO GET AT LEAST A FEW SESSIONS WITH A TRAINER TO LEARN PROPER FORM FOR MAXIMUM BENEFIT.
25 lb. WEIGHT
20 REPS EACH ARM

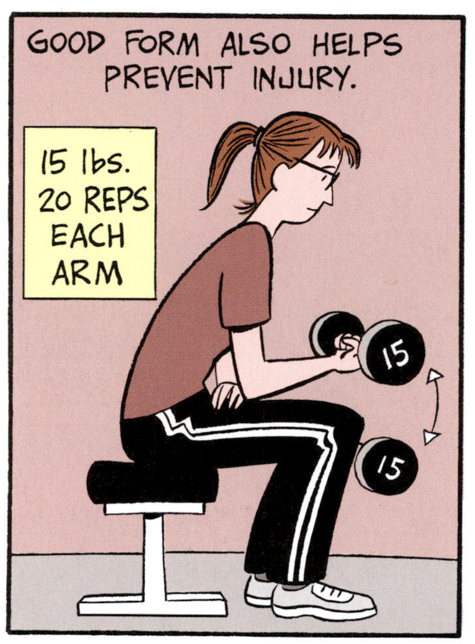
GOOD FORM ALSO HELPS PREVENT INJURY.
15 lbs. 20 REPS EACH ARM
15
15

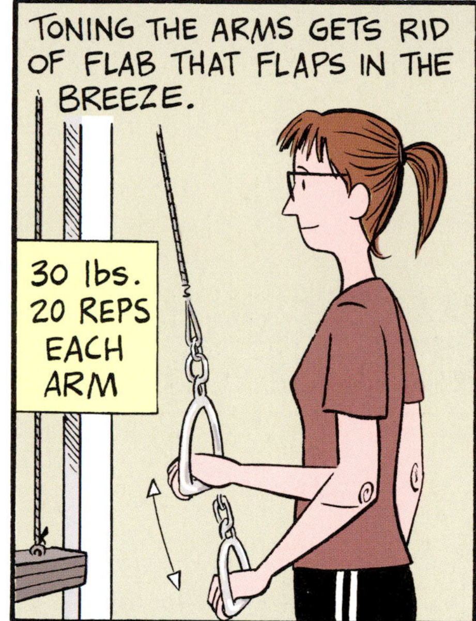
TONING THE ARMS GETS RID OF FLAB THAT FLAPS IN THE BREEZE.
30 lbs. 20 REPS EACH ARM

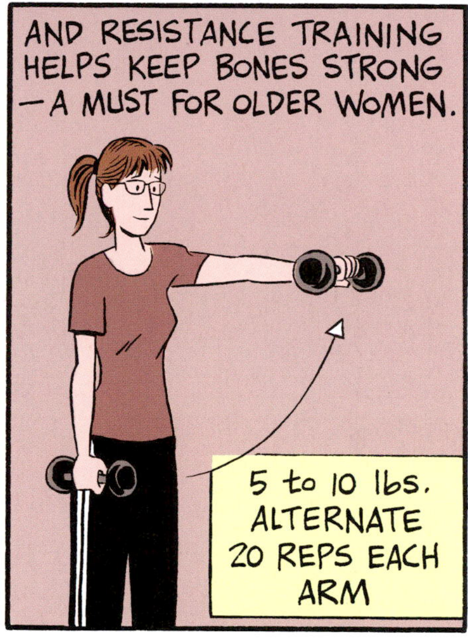
AND RESISTANCE TRAINING HELPS KEEP BONES STRONG — A MUST FOR OLDER WOMEN.
5 to 10 lbs. ALTERNATE 20 REPS EACH ARM

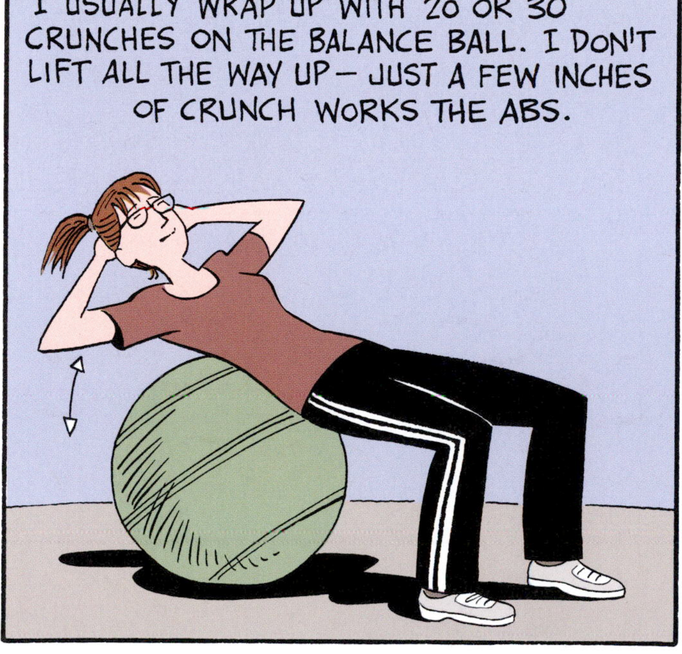
I USUALLY WRAP UP WITH 20 OR 30 CRUNCHES ON THE BALANCE BALL. I DON'T LIFT ALL THE WAY UP — JUST A FEW INCHES OF CRUNCH WORKS THE ABS.

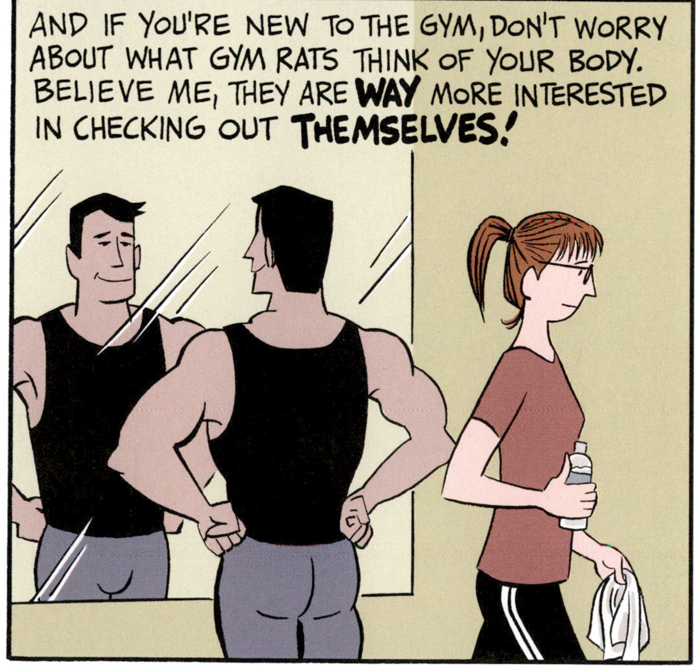
AND IF YOU'RE NEW TO THE GYM, DON'T WORRY ABOUT WHAT GYM RATS THINK OF YOUR BODY. BELIEVE ME, THEY ARE WAY MORE INTERESTED IN CHECKING OUT THEMSELVES!

# A LIFELONG CHANGE

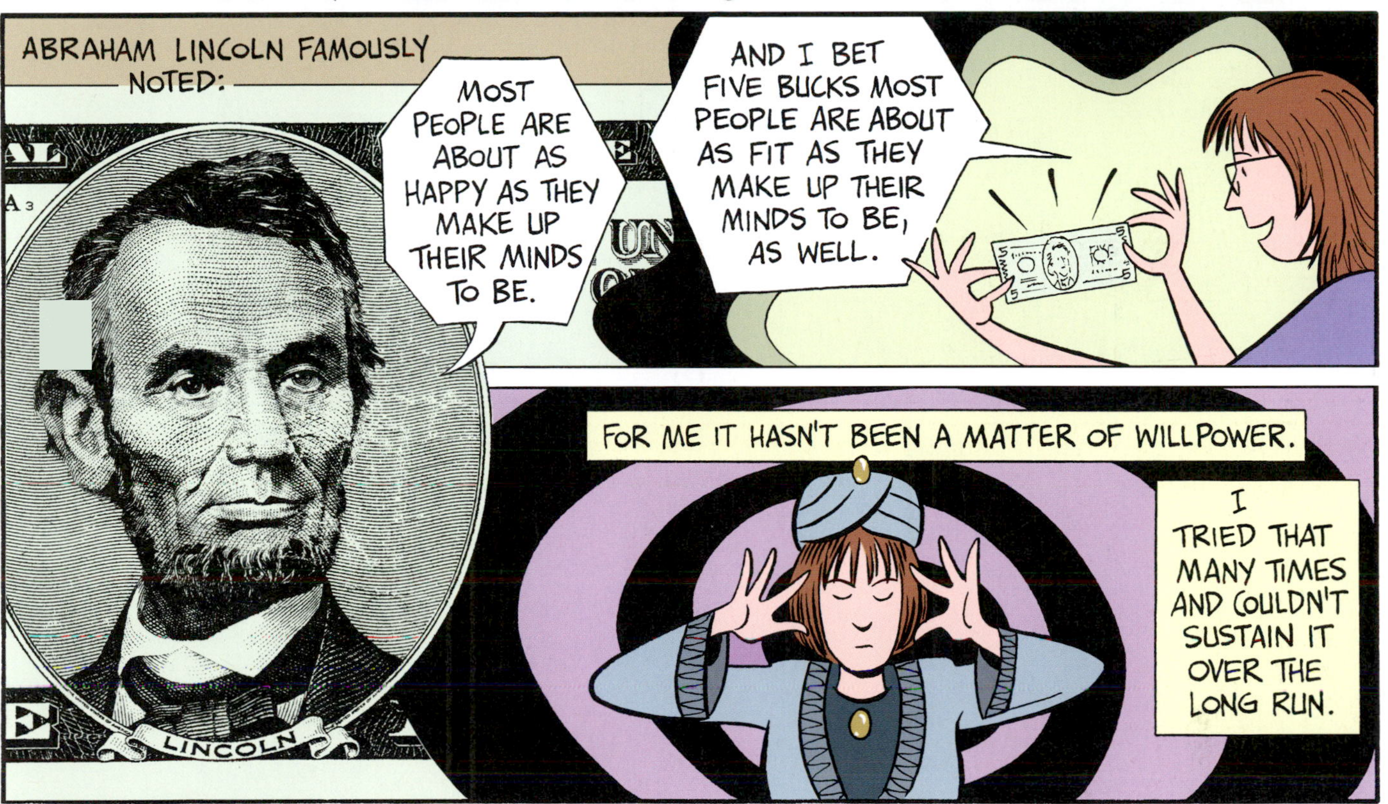
ABRAHAM LINCOLN FAMOUSLY NOTED:
MOST PEOPLE ARE ABOUT AS HAPPY AS THEY MAKE UP THEIR MINDS TO BE.
AND I BET FIVE BUCKS MOST PEOPLE ARE ABOUT AS FIT AS THEY MAKE UP THEIR MINDS TO BE, AS WELL.
LINCOLN
FOR ME IT HASN'T BEEN A MATTER OF WILLPOWER.
I TRIED THAT MANY TIMES AND COULDN'T SUSTAIN IT OVER THE LONG RUN.

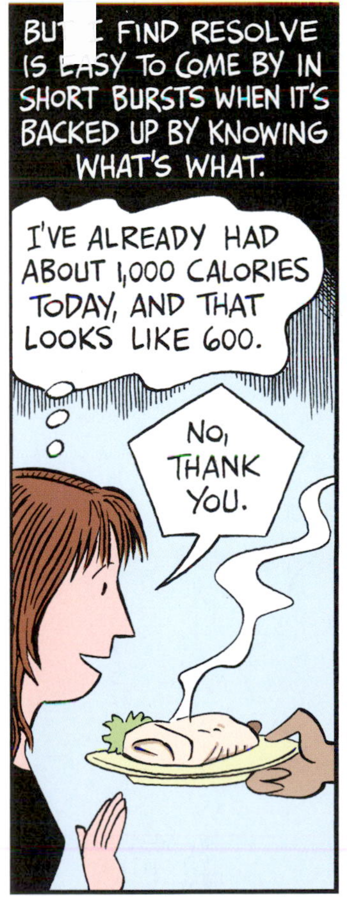
BUT I FIND RESOLVE IS EASY TO COME BY IN SHORT BURSTS WHEN IT'S BACKED UP BY KNOWING WHAT'S WHAT.
I'VE ALREADY HAD ABOUT 1,000 CALORIES TODAY, AND THAT LOOKS LIKE 600.
NO, THANK YOU.

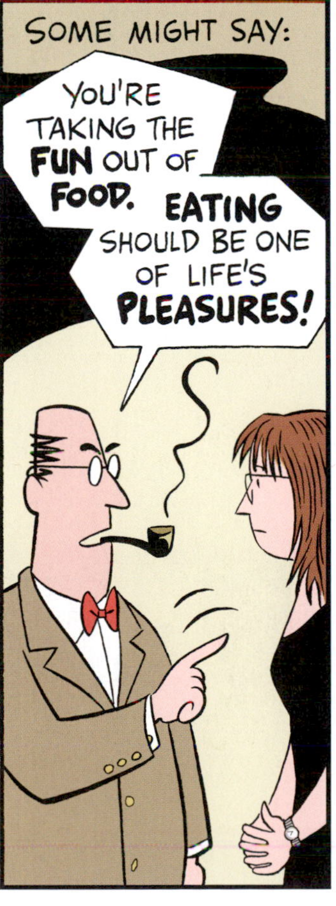
SOME MIGHT SAY:
YOU'RE TAKING THE **FUN** OUT OF **FOOD. EATING** SHOULD BE ONE OF LIFE'S **PLEASURES!**

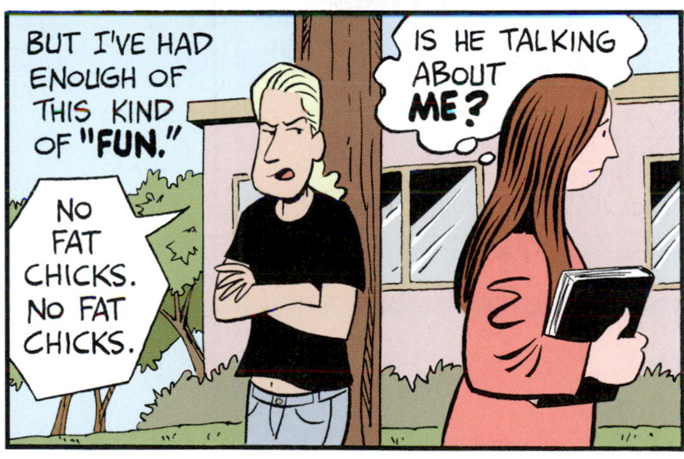
BUT I'VE HAD ENOUGH OF THIS KIND OF **"FUN."**
IS HE TALKING ABOUT **ME?**
NO FAT CHICKS. NO FAT CHICKS.

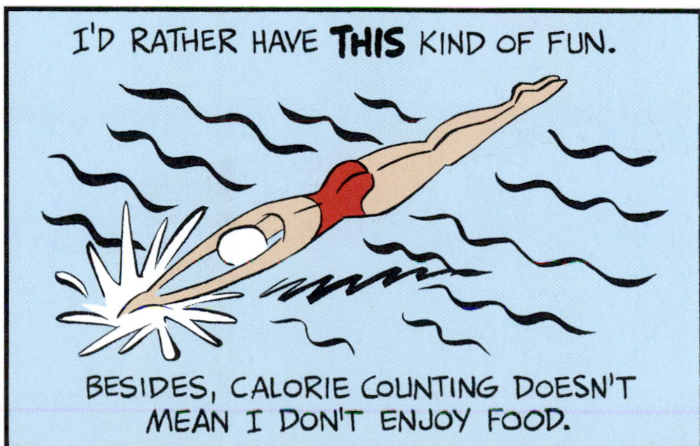
I'D RATHER HAVE **THIS** KIND OF FUN.
BESIDES, CALORIE COUNTING DOESN'T MEAN I DON'T ENJOY FOOD.

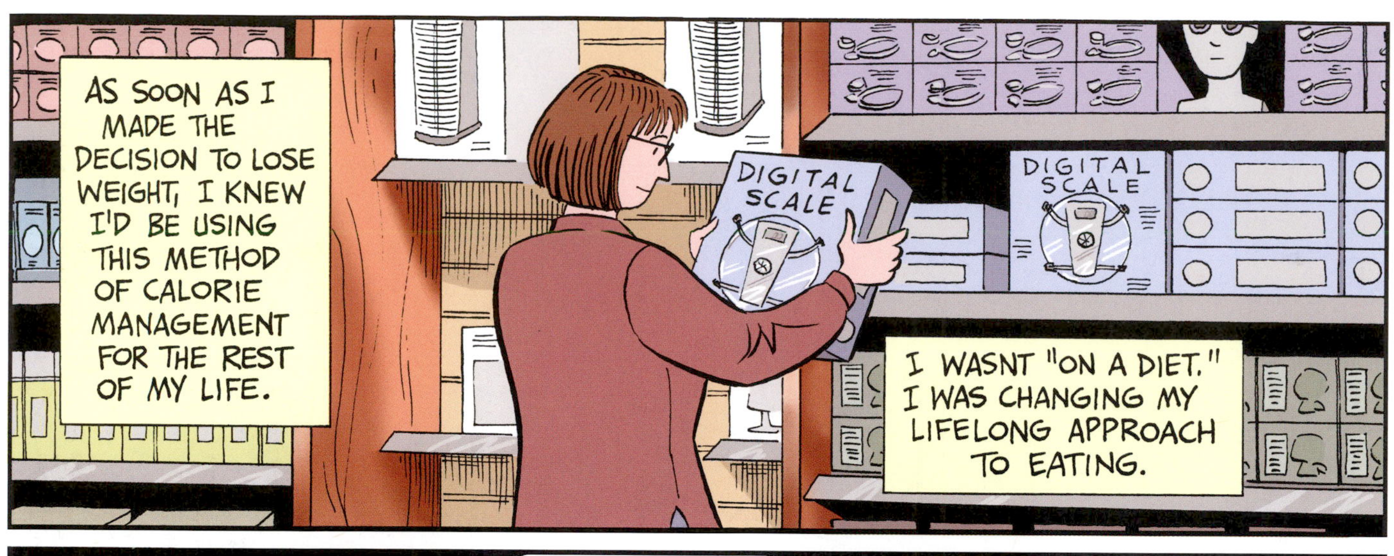
AS SOON AS I MADE THE DECISION TO LOSE WEIGHT, I KNEW I'D BE USING THIS METHOD OF CALORIE MANAGEMENT FOR THE REST OF MY LIFE.
DIGITAL SCALE
DIGITAL SCALE
I WASNT "ON A DIET." I WAS CHANGING MY LIFELONG APPROACH TO EATING.

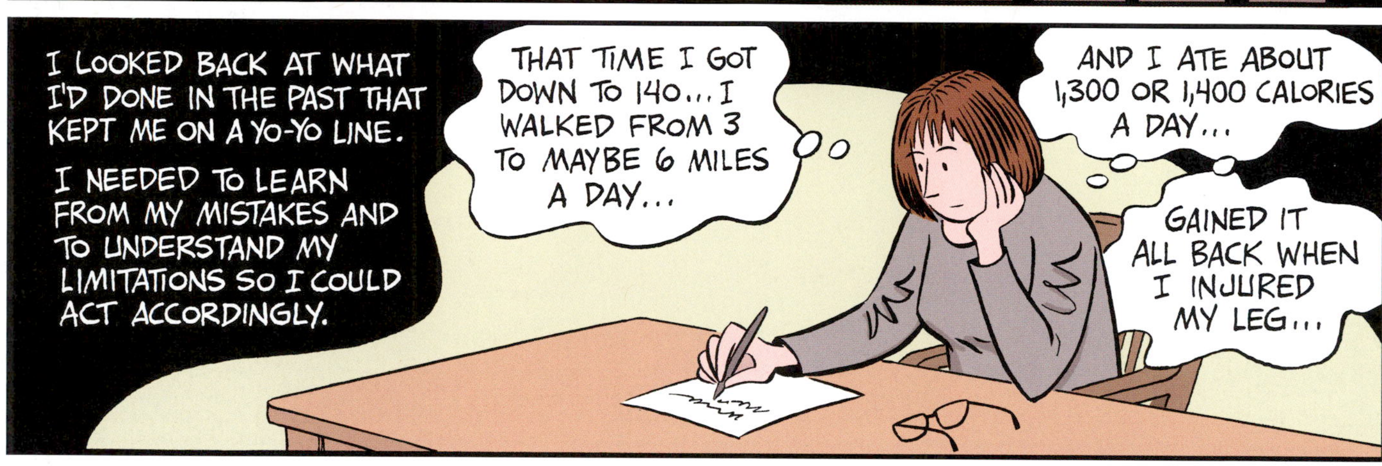
I LOOKED BACK AT WHAT I'D DONE IN THE PAST THAT KEPT ME ON A YO-YO LINE.
I NEEDED TO LEARN FROM MY MISTAKES AND TO UNDERSTAND MY LIMITATIONS SO I COULD ACT ACCORDINGLY.
THAT TIME I GOT DOWN TO 140... I WALKED FROM 3 TO MAYBE 6 MILES A DAY...
AND I ATE ABOUT 1,300 OR 1,400 CALORIES A DAY...
GAINED IT ALL BACK WHEN I INJURED MY LEG...

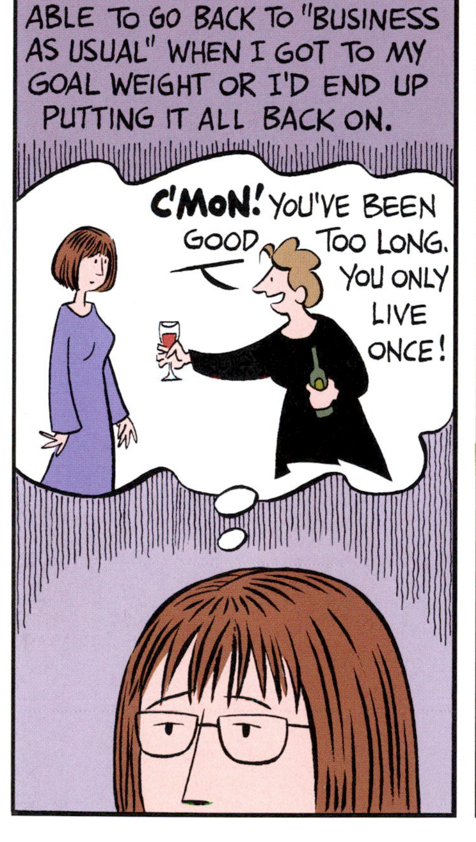
I SAW THAT I WOULDN'T BE ABLE TO GO BACK TO "BUSINESS AS USUAL" WHEN I GOT TO MY GOAL WEIGHT OR I'D END UP PUTTING IT ALL BACK ON.
C'MON! YOU'VE BEEN GOOD TOO LONG. YOU ONLY LIVE ONCE!

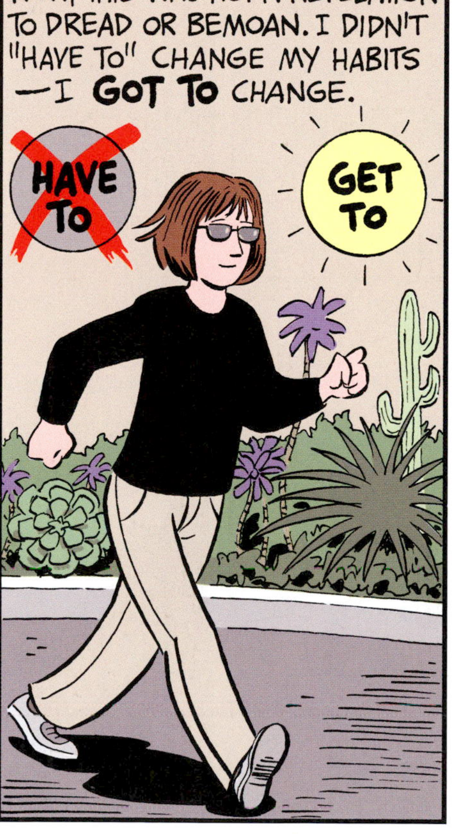
NOW, THIS WAS NOT A REVELATION TO DREAD OR BEMOAN. I DIDN'T "HAVE TO" CHANGE MY HABITS —I GOT TO CHANGE.
HAVE TO
GET TO

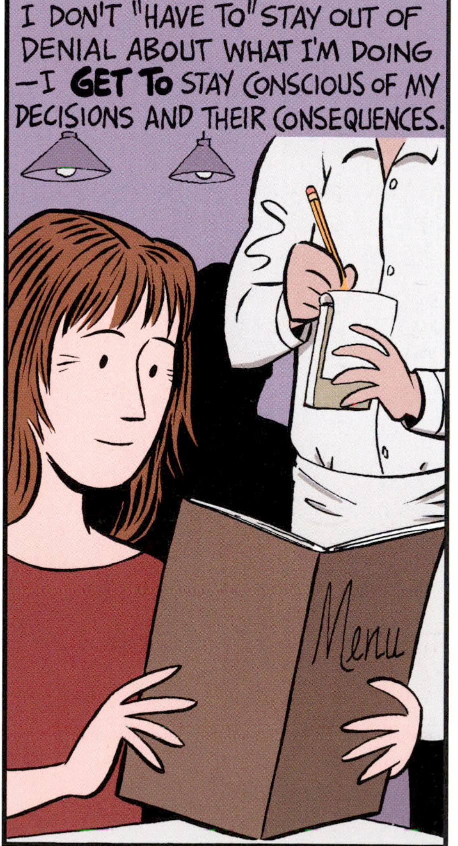
I DON'T "HAVE TO" STAY OUT OF DENIAL ABOUT WHAT I'M DOING —I GET TO STAY CONSCIOUS OF MY DECISIONS AND THEIR CONSEQUENCES.
Menu

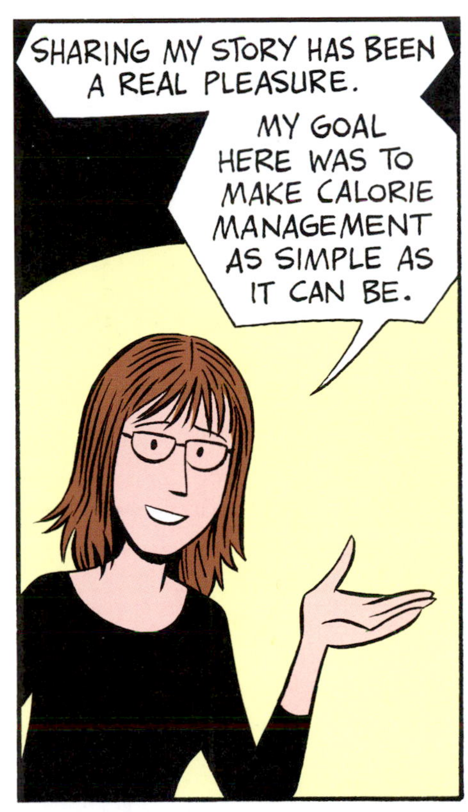
SHARING MY STORY HAS BEEN A REAL PLEASURE.
MY GOAL HERE WAS TO MAKE CALORIE MANAGEMENT AS SIMPLE AS IT CAN BE.

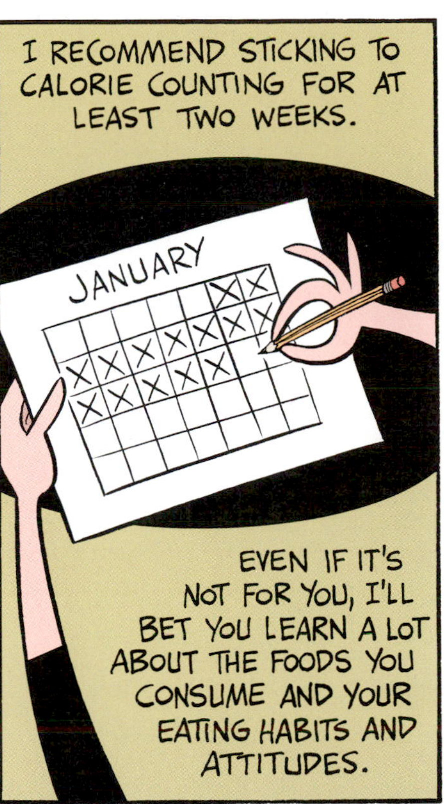
I RECOMMEND STICKING TO CALORIE COUNTING FOR AT LEAST TWO WEEKS.
JANUARY
EVEN IF IT'S NOT FOR YOU, I'LL BET YOU LEARN A LOT ABOUT THE FOODS YOU CONSUME AND YOUR EATING HABITS AND ATTITUDES.

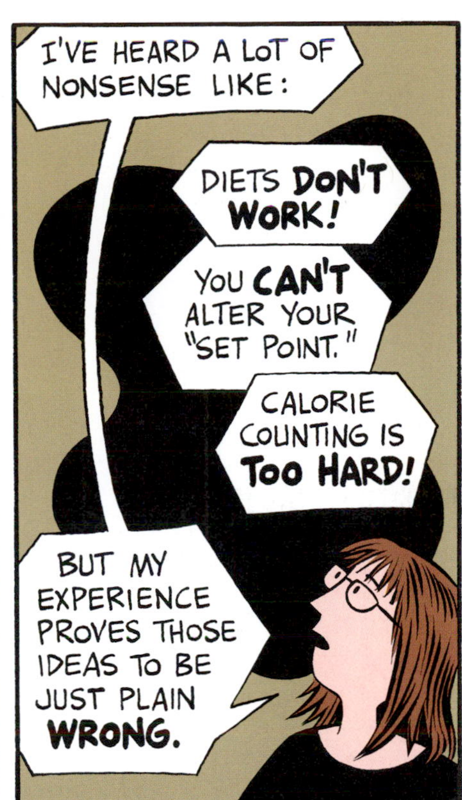
I'VE HEARD A LOT OF NONSENSE LIKE:
DIETS **DON'T WORK!**
YOU **CAN'T** ALTER YOUR "SET POINT."
CALORIE COUNTING IS **TOO HARD!**
BUT MY EXPERIENCE PROVES THOSE IDEAS TO BE JUST PLAIN **WRONG.**

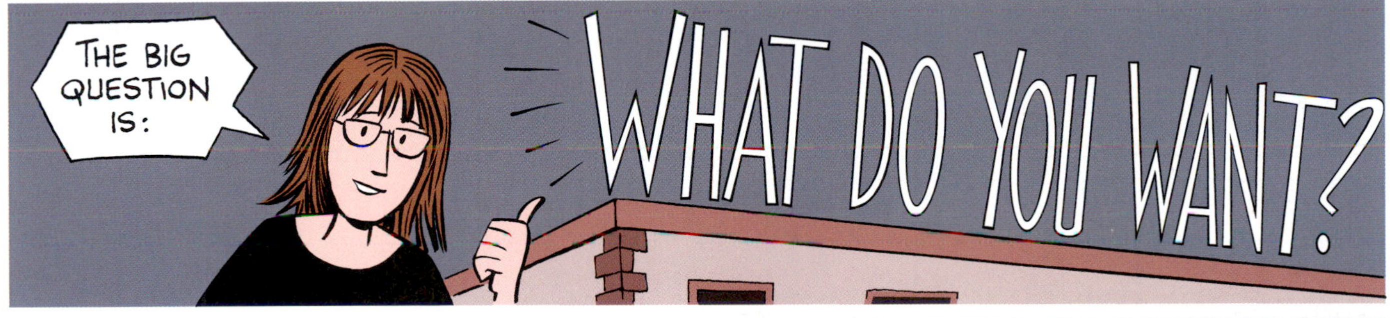
THE BIG QUESTION IS:
WHAT DO YOU WANT?

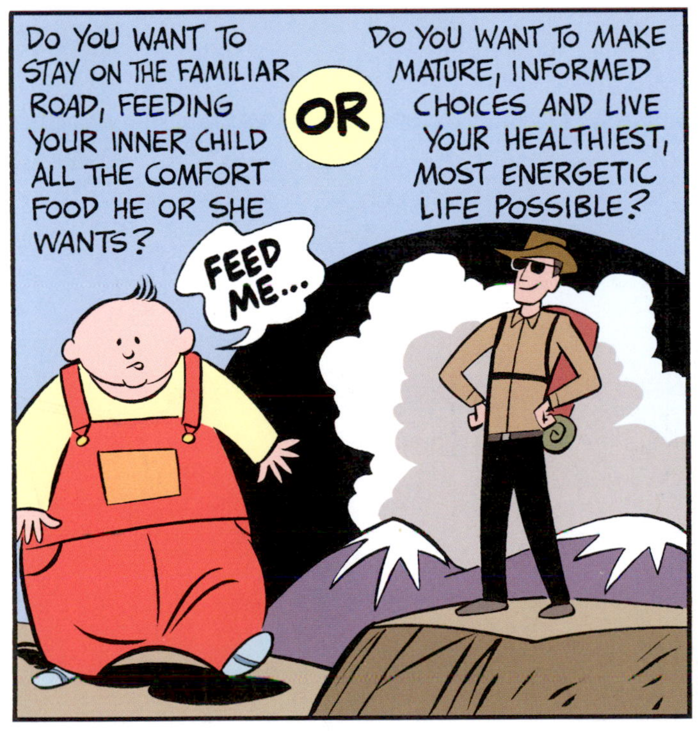
DO YOU WANT TO STAY ON THE FAMILIAR ROAD, FEEDING YOUR INNER CHILD ALL THE COMFORT FOOD HE OR SHE WANTS?
OR
DO YOU WANT TO MAKE MATURE, INFORMED CHOICES AND LIVE YOUR HEALTHIEST, MOST ENERGETIC LIFE POSSIBLE?
FEED ME...

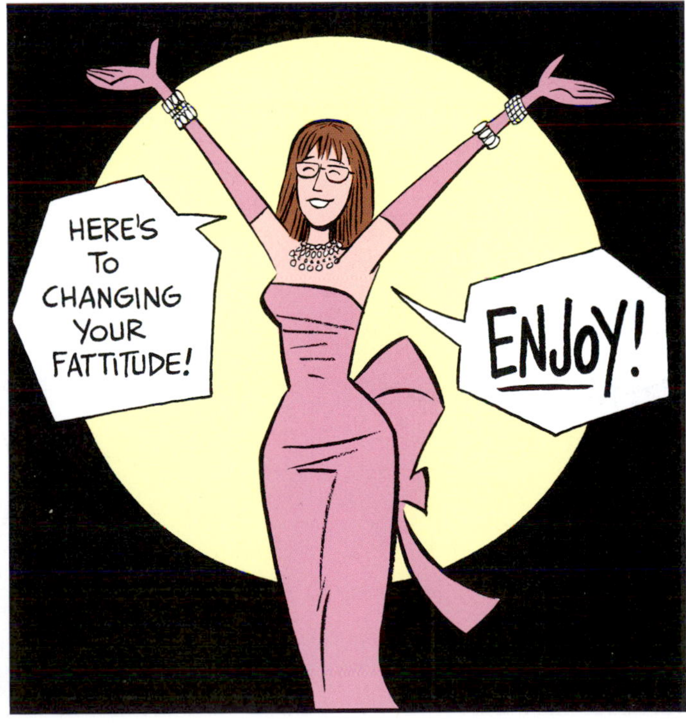
HERE'S TO CHANGING YOUR FATTITUDE!
ENJOY!

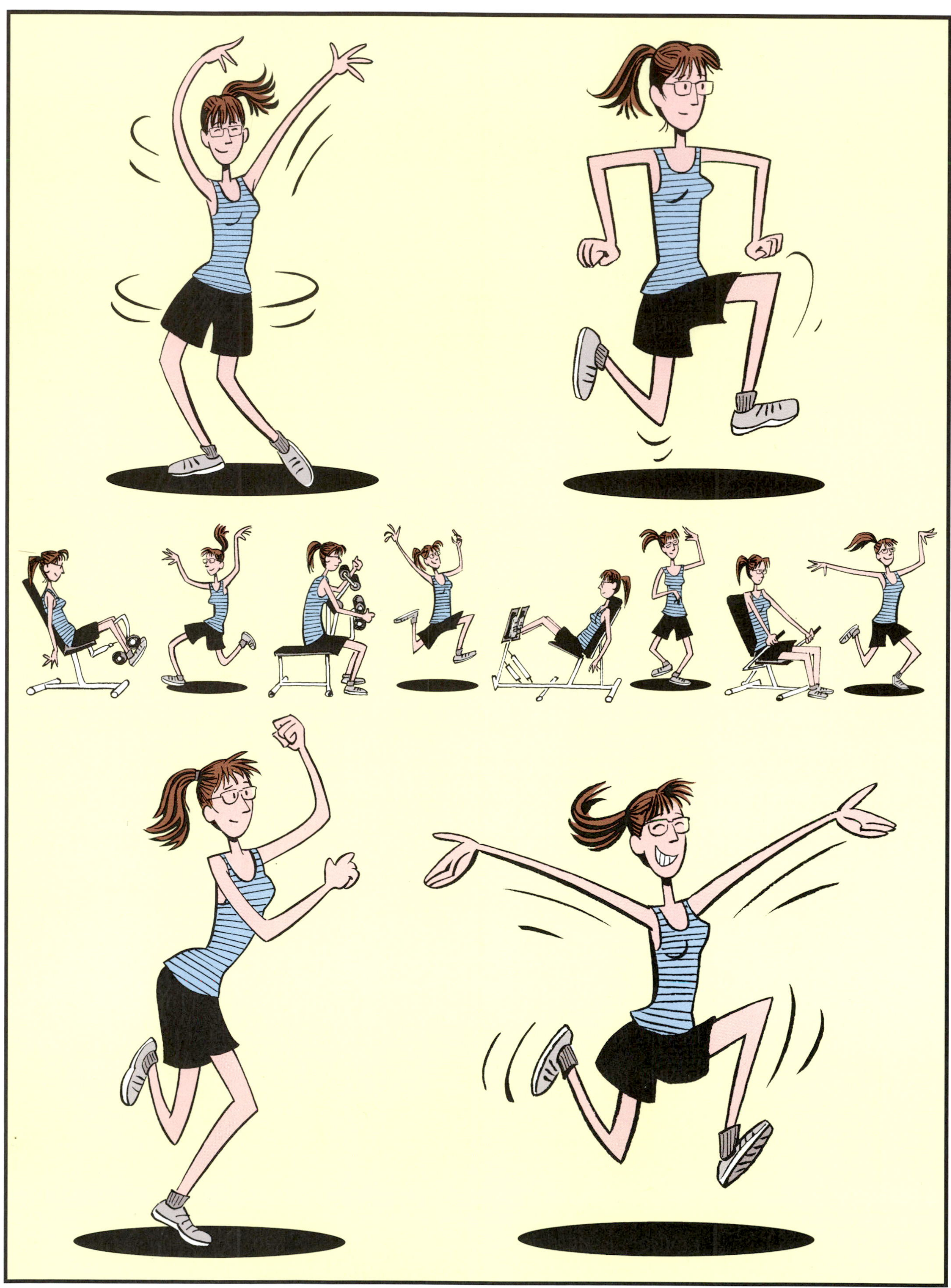

# Calorie Charts

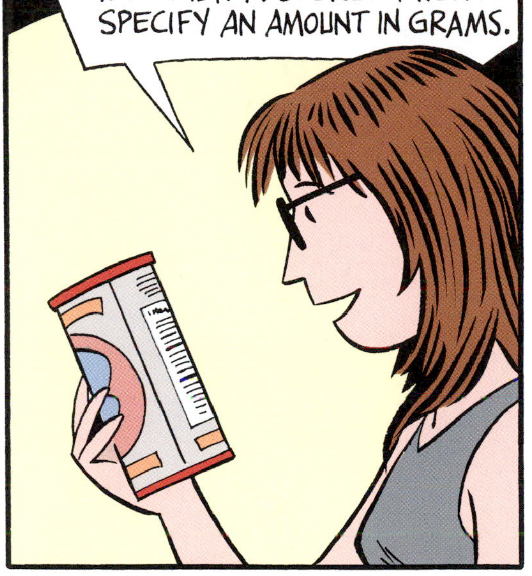
WHILE TRACKING DOWN CALORIE AMOUNTS FOR VARIOUS FOODS, I'VE LOOKED AT A LOT OF LISTS, LABELS, AND CHARTS.
SOMETIMES THE SERVING AMOUNT IS EASY TO GET—"½ GRAPEFRUIT," FOR EXAMPLE—BUT TOO OFTEN A SOURCE MIGHT SPECIFY AN AMOUNT IN GRAMS.

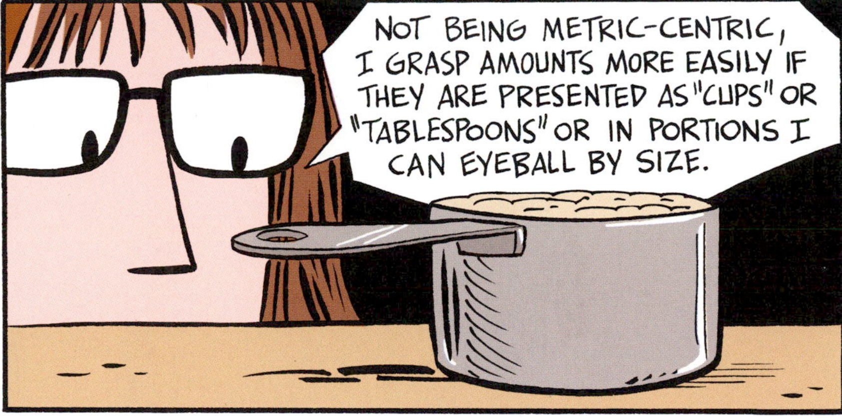
NOT BEING METRIC-CENTRIC, I GRASP AMOUNTS MORE EASILY IF THEY ARE PRESENTED AS "CUPS" OR "TABLESPOONS" OR IN PORTIONS I CAN EYEBALL BY SIZE.

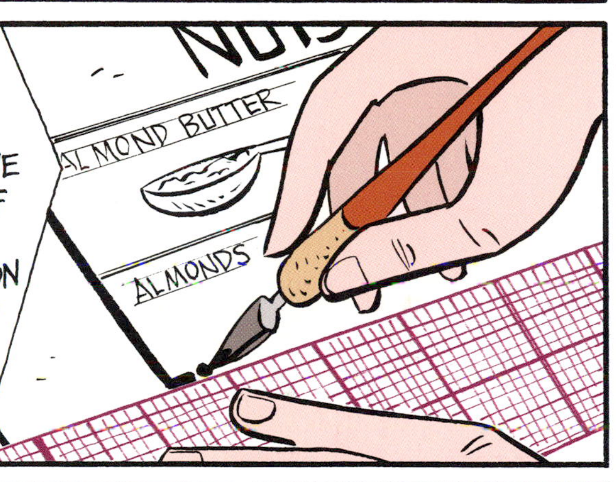
THE FOLLOWING LIST IS BY NO MEANS COMPREHENSIVE. IT IS DESIGNED TO GIVE A GENERAL IDEA OF THE CALORIE AMOUNTS OF COMMON WHOLE FOODS AND TO HELP THE BEGINNER GET STARTED.
ALMOND BUTTER
ALMONDS

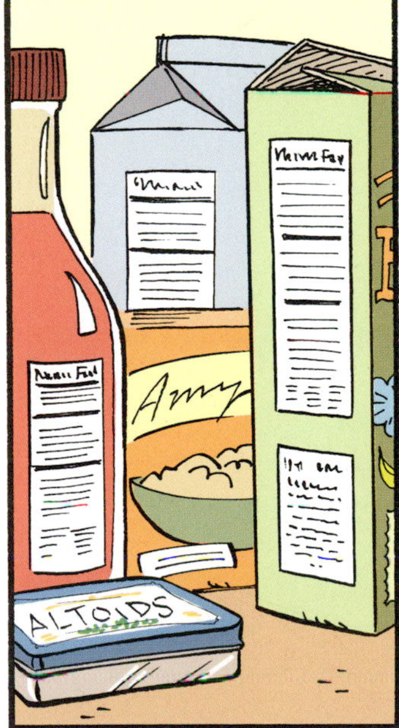
MOST FOODS THAT COME PACKAGED WITH A NUTRITION LABEL—BREADS, CHIPS, CANNED OR FROZEN VEGETABLES, AND SO ON—HAVE NOT BEEN LISTED.
Amy
ALTOIDS

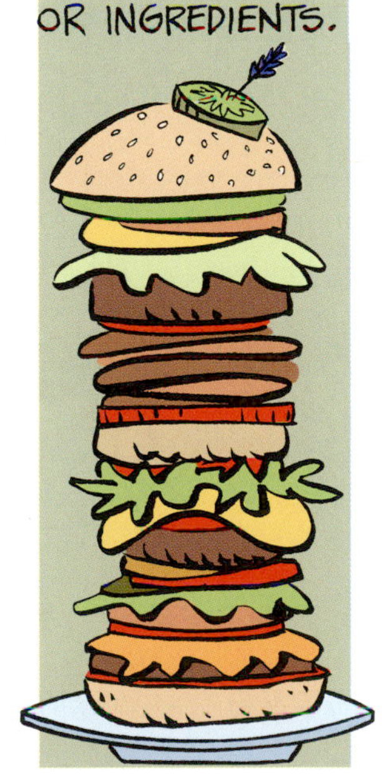
OTHER FOODS I LEFT OUT INCLUDE PREPARED DISHES SUCH AS POTATO SALAD OR PIE, SINCE CALORIE AMOUNTS PER SERVING DEPEND ON THE RECIPES OR INGREDIENTS.

ONLY THE APPROXIMATE CALORIC CONTENT OF FOODS (MOST ARE ROUNDED UP OR DOWN TO THE NEAREST 5) IS LISTED, AND PORTION AMOUNTS HAVE BEEN SIMPLIFIED AS MUCH AS POSSIBLE.
287 CALORIES FOR 368 GRAMS OR .68 OF A LARGE SERVING...

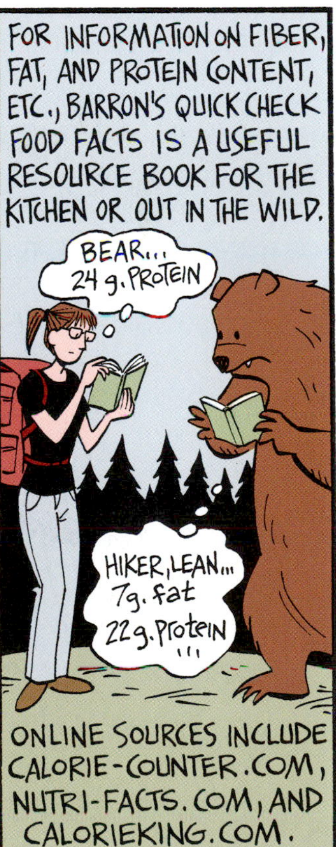
FOR INFORMATION ON FIBER, FAT, AND PROTEIN CONTENT, ETC., BARRON'S QUICK CHECK FOOD FACTS IS A USEFUL RESOURCE BOOK FOR THE KITCHEN OR OUT IN THE WILD.
BEAR... 24 g. PROTEIN
HIKER, LEAN... 7g. fat 22g. Protein ...
ONLINE SOURCES INCLUDE CALORIE-COUNTER.COM, NUTRI-FACTS.COM, AND CALORIEKING.COM.

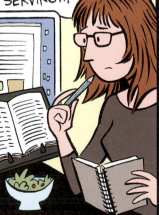

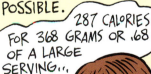

# Vegetables

| | | |
|---|---|---|
| ARTICHOKE | 1 GLOBE | 60 |
| ARUGULA, RAW | 1 LEAF | 1 |
| ASPARAGUS | ½ CUP | 20 |
| BEAN SPROUTS | ¾ CUP | 25 |
| BEANS, STRING/SNAP, COOKED | ½ CUP | 20 |
| BEANS, STRING/SNAP, RAW | ¾ CUP | 25 |
| BEETS, DICED, COOKED | ⅓ CUP | 25 |
| BROCCOLI PIECES, COOKED | ½ CUP | 20 |
| BROCCOLI, RAW | 1 CUP | 25 |
| BRUSSELS SPROUTS, BOILED | ½ CUP | 30 |
| CABBAGE, BOILED | 1 CUP | 30 |
| CABBAGE, RAW | 1 CUP | 20 |
| CABBAGE, RED, RAW | 1 CUP | 20 |
| CARROT JUICE | ½ CUP | 40 |
| CARROT, RAW, GRATED | ½ CUP | 50 |
| CARROT, RAW, WHOLE | 1 MEDIUM | 35 |
| CAULIFLOWER, COOKED | 1 CUP | 30 |
| CAULIFLOWER, RAW | 1 CUP | 25 |
| CELERY | 2 STALKS | 15 |
| CHARD, SWISS, COOKED | 1 CUP | 35 |
| CHIVES, RAW | 1 tsp. | 0 |
| CILANTRO, RAW | 1 tsp. | 0 |
| COLLARD GREENS, COOKED | ½ CUP | 25 |
| COLLARD GREENS, RAW | 2 CUPS | 20 |
| CORN, COOKED | 1 EAR | 45 |
| CORN, COOKED | 1 CUP | 130 |
| CUCUMBER, PEELED & SLICED | ½ CUP | 7 |
| CUCUMBER, WHOLE | 8 INCH | 40 |
| DANDELION GREENS, RAW | 1 CUP | 25 |
| EGGPLANT, COOKED, SLICES | 1 CUP | 30 |
| ENDIVE, RAW | ½ CUP | 4 |
| FENNEL BULB, RAW, SLICED | 1 CUP | 25 |
| GARLIC, RAW | 1 CLOVE | 5 |
| GINGER ROOT, RAW | 1 tsp. | 1 |
| KALE, COOKED | 1 CUP | 40 |
| KOHLRABI SLICES, RAW | 1 CUP | 35 |
| LEEKS, CHOPPED, COOKED | ½ CUP | 15 |
| LETTUCE, ICEBERG, CHOPPED | 2 CUPS | 15 |
| LETTUCE, ROMAINE, CHOPPED | 2 CUPS | 20 |
| LETTUCE, BUTTERHEAD, CHOPPED | 2 CUPS | 15 |
| MUSHROOMS, COOKED | ½ CUP | 25 |
| MUSHROOMS, PORTABELLA, RAW | 1 MEDIUM | 20 |
| MUSHROOMS, RAW | ½ CUP | 10 |
| MUSHROOMS, SHIITAKE, COOKED | 4 'SHROOMS | 40 |
| MUSHROOMS, SHIITAKE, DRIED | 1 'SHROOM | 12 |
| MUSTARD GREENS, COOKED | 1 CUP | 25 |
| MUSTARD GREENS, RAW | 1 CUP | 20 |
| OKRA SLICES, COOKED | ½ CUP | 25 |

# Vegetables

| | | |
|---|---|---|
| ONION, COOKED | 1 T. | 7 |
| ONION, RAW | ½ CUP | 30 |
| ONION, SPRING/GREEN, CHOPPED | ¼ CUP | 8 |
| PARSNIP, COOKED | ½ CUP | 65 |
| PEAS (EDIBLE POD)/SNOW, COOKED | ⅓ CUP | 20 |
| PEAS (EDIBLE POD)/SNOW, RAW | 1 CUP | 70 |
| PEPPER, ANCHO, DRIED | 1 PEPPER | 50 |
| PEPPER, HOT CHILI, GREEN, RAW | 1 PEPPER | 20 |
| PEPPER, HOT CHILI, DRIED | 1 PEPPER | 3 |
| PEPPER, JALAPEÑO, RAW | 1 PEPPER | 4 |
| PEPPER, POBLANO (PASILLA), RAW | 1 PEPPER | 20 |
| PEPPER, SERRANO, RAW | 1 PEPPER | 2 |
| PEPPER, SWEET BELL, COOKED | 1 T. | 3 |
| PEPPER, SWEET BELL, GREEN, RAW | 1 CUP | 25 |
| PEPPER, SWEET BELL, RED, RAW | 1 CUP | 40 |
| PEPPER, SWEET BELL, YELLOW, RAW | 1 CUP | 45 |
| POTATO, BAKED, NO SKIN | ½ CUP | 60 |
| POTATO, BAKED, WITH SKIN | 2½" x 5" SPUD | 220 |
| POTATO, BAKED, SKIN | 1 SKIN | 115 |
| POTATO, BOILED, NO SKIN | ½ CUP | 70 |
| PUMPKIN, FRESH, COOKED | ½ CUP | 25 |
| RADISH, RED, RAW | 1 LARGE | 2 |
| RUTABAGA, COOKED | ½ CUP | 35 |
| RUTABAGA, RAW | ½ CUP | 25 |
| SHALLOTS, RAW | 1 T. | 7 |
| SOYBEANS, COOKED | 1 CUP | 255 |
| SPINACH, COOKED | 1 CUP | 40 |
| SPINACH, RAW | 1 CUP | 7 |
| SQUASH, SUMMER, COOKED | 1 CUP | 35 |
| SQUASH, SUMMER, RAW | 1 CUP | 25 |
| SQUASH, SUMMER, ZUCCHINI, COOKED | ½ CUP | 20 |
| SQUASH, SUMMER, ZUCCHINI, RAW | 1 CUP | 15 |
| SQUASH, WINTER, ACORN, BAKED | 1 CUP | 115 |
| SQUASH, WINTER, ACORN, BOILED | 1 CUP | 85 |
| SQUASH, WINTER, ACORN, RAW | 1 CUP | 55 |
| SQUASH, WINTER, BUTTERNUT, BAKED | 1 CUP | 80 |
| SQUASH, WINTER, BUTTERNUT, RAW | 1 CUP | 65 |
| SQUASH, WINTER, SPAGHETTI, BOILED | 1 CUP | 40 |
| SQUASH, WINTER, SPAGHETTI, RAW | 1 CUP | 30 |
| SWEET POTATO, BAKED WITH SKIN | 1 LARGE | 185 |
| TOMATILLO, RAW | 1 MEDIUM | 10 |
| TOMATO, GREEN, RAW | 1 CUP | 45 |
| TOMATO, RED, BOILED | 1 CUP | 65 |
| TOMATO, RED, RAW | 1 MEDIUM | 20 |
| TOMATO, RED, STEWED | 1 CUP | 70 |
| TOMATO, RED, RAW, CHERRY | 1 CUP | 30 |
| TOMATO, DRIED | 1 PIECE | 5 |
| TURNIP GREENS, COOKED | 1 CUP | 30 |
| YAM, RAW, CUBED | 1 CUP | 180 |
| YAMBEAN (JICAMA) RAW | 1 CUP | 45 |
| YARDLONG BEAN, COOKED | 1 POD | 7 |

# Fruit

| | | |
|---|---|---|
| APPLE, GRANNY SMITH | 1 MEDIUM | 80 |
| APPLE, GALA | 1 MEDIUM | 75 |
| APPLE, GOLDEN DELICIOUS | 1 MEDIUM | 50 |
| APPLE, RED DELICIOUS | 1 MEDIUM | 90 |
| APRICOT | 1 MEDIUM | 20 |
| APRICOT, DRIED | 1/4 CUP | 80 |
| AVOCADO | 1 MEDIUM | 280 |
| AVOCADO, CUBED | 1 CUP | 240 |
| BANANA | 1 MEDIUM | 100 |
| BLACKBERRIES, RAW | 1 CUP | 75 |
| BLUEBERRIES | 1 CUP | 80 |
| BOYSENBERRIES | 1 CUP | 70 |
| CHERRIES, RAW | 10 CHERRIES | 40 |
| CRABAPPLES, RAW | 1 CUP | 85 |
| CRANBERRIES, DRIED | 1/3 CUP | 120 |
| CRANBERRIES, RAW | 1 CUP | 45 |
| CRANBERRY SAUCE, SWEETENED | 1 T. | 30 |
| CURRANTS, ZANTE, DRIED | 1/4 CUP | 100 |
| DATES, DOMESTIC, DRIED | 1 DATE | 25 |
| DATES, MEDJOOL | 1 DATE | 50 |
| ELDERBERRIES, RAW | 1 CUP | 110 |
| FIG, DRIED, UNCOOKED | 1 FIG | 50 |
| FIG, RAW | 1 MEDIUM | 40 |
| GOOSEBERRIES, RAW | 1 CUP | 65 |
| GRAPEFRUIT | 1/2 LARGE | 55 |
| GRAPEFRUIT, WHITE | 1/2 LARGE | 40 |
| GRAPES, RED OR GREEN | 1 CUP | 110 |
| GUAVA, RAW | 1 FRUIT | 45 |
| KIWI, NO SKIN | 1 FRUIT | 55 |
| KUMQUAT | 1 FRUIT | 12 |
| LEMON | 1 FRUIT | 15 |
| LIME | 1 FRUIT | 20 |
| LITCHI, DRIED | 1 FRUIT | 5 |
| LOGANBERRIES, THAWED | 1 CUP | 80 |
| LOQUAT | 1 LARGE | 10 |
| MANGO | 1/2 CUP | 55 |
| MELON, CANTALOUPE | 1 CUP | 55 |
| MELON, CASABA | 1 CUP | 45 |
| MELON, HONEYDEW | 1 CUP | 60 |
| MULBERRIES | 9 BERRIES | 5 |
| NECTARINE | 1 MEDIUM | 70 |
| OLIVES, BLACK | 1 OLIVE | 6 |
| OLIVES, KALAMATA | 3 OLIVES | 45 |
| ORANGE, NAVEL | 1 MEDIUM | 65 |
| ORANGE, VALENCIA | 1 MEDIUM | 60 |
| PAPAYA | 1 CUP | 55 |
| PASSION FRUIT | 1 FRUIT | 20 |
| PEACH | 1 LARGE | 70 |
| PEAR, ASIAN | 1 MEDIUM | 50 |
| PEAR, BOSC | 1 LARGE | 150 |
| PERSIMMON, JAPANESE | 1 FRUIT | 120 |
| PINEAPPLE | 1 CUP | 75 |
| PLANTAIN, COOKED | 1 CUP | 180 |
| PLUM | 1 FRUIT | 35 |
| POMEGRANATE | 1 FRUIT | 105 |
| RASPBERRIES | 1 CUP | 60 |
| RHUBARB | 1 STALK | 10 |
| STRAWBERRIES | 1 CUP | 45 |
| TANGERINE | 1 LARGE | 45 |
| WATERMELON | 1 CUP | 50 |

## Juices

| | | |
|---|---|---|
| APPLE JUICE | 1/2 CUP | 60 |
| GRAPE JUICE | 1/2 CUP | 80 |
| GRAPEFRUIT JUICE | 1/2 CUP | 50 |
| LEMON OR LIME JUICE | 1 OZ. | 8 |
| ORANGE JUICE | 1/2 CUP | 55 |
| TANGERINE JUICE | 1/2 CUP | 50 |

# Legumes

PER 1-CUP SERVING

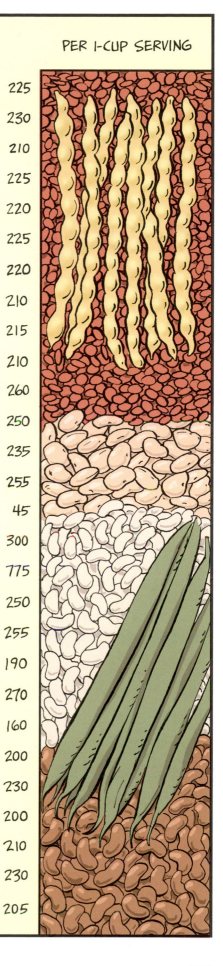

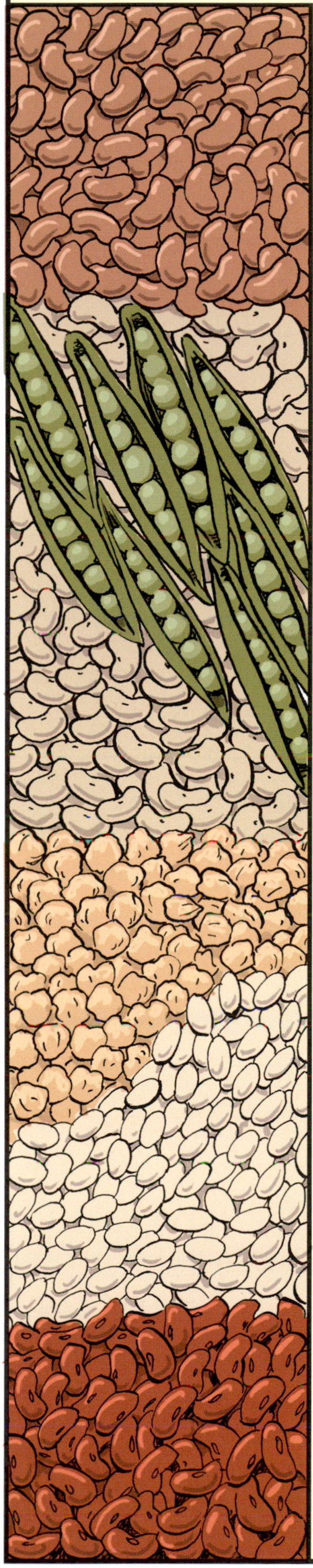

| | |
|---|---|
| BEANS, BLACK, BOILED | 225 |
| BEANS, FRENCH, COOKED | 230 |
| BEANS, GREAT NORTHERN, BOILED | 210 |
| BEANS, KIDNEY, BOILED | 225 |
| BEANS, KIDNEY, CALIF. RED, BOILED | 220 |
| BEANS, KIDNEY, RED, BOILED | 225 |
| BEANS, KIDNEY, ROYAL RED, BOILED | 220 |
| BEANS, LIMA, IMMATURE SEEDS, BOILED | 210 |
| BEANS, LIMA, MATURE SEEDS, BOILED | 215 |
| BEANS, MUNG, MATURE SEEDS, BOILED | 210 |
| BEANS, NAVY, BOILED | 260 |
| BEANS, PINK, BOILED | 250 |
| BEANS, PINTO, BOILED | 235 |
| BEANS, SMALL WHITE, BOILED | 255 |
| BEANS, SNAP, GREEN, BOILED | 45 |
| BEANS, SOY, MATURE SEEDS, BOILED | 300 |
| BEANS, SOY, MATURE SEEDS, DRY ROASTED | 775 |
| BEANS, WHITE, MATURE SEEDS, BOILED | 250 |
| BEANS, YELLOW, MATURE SEEDS, BOILED | 255 |
| BROADBEANS (FAVA), BOILED | 190 |
| CHICKPEAS (GARBANZO), BOILED | 270 |
| COWPEAS (BLACK-EYE BEANS), IMMATURE | 160 |
| COWPEAS, MATURE SEEDS, BOILED | 200 |
| LENTILS, MATURE SEEDS, BOILED | 230 |
| LUPINS, MATURE SEEDS, BOILED | 200 |
| MOTHBEANS, MATURE SEEDS, BOILED | 210 |
| PEAS, SPLIT, MATURE, BOILED | 230 |
| PIGEON PEAS, MATURE SEEDS, BOILED | 205 |

# Peanuts, Nuts, & Seeds

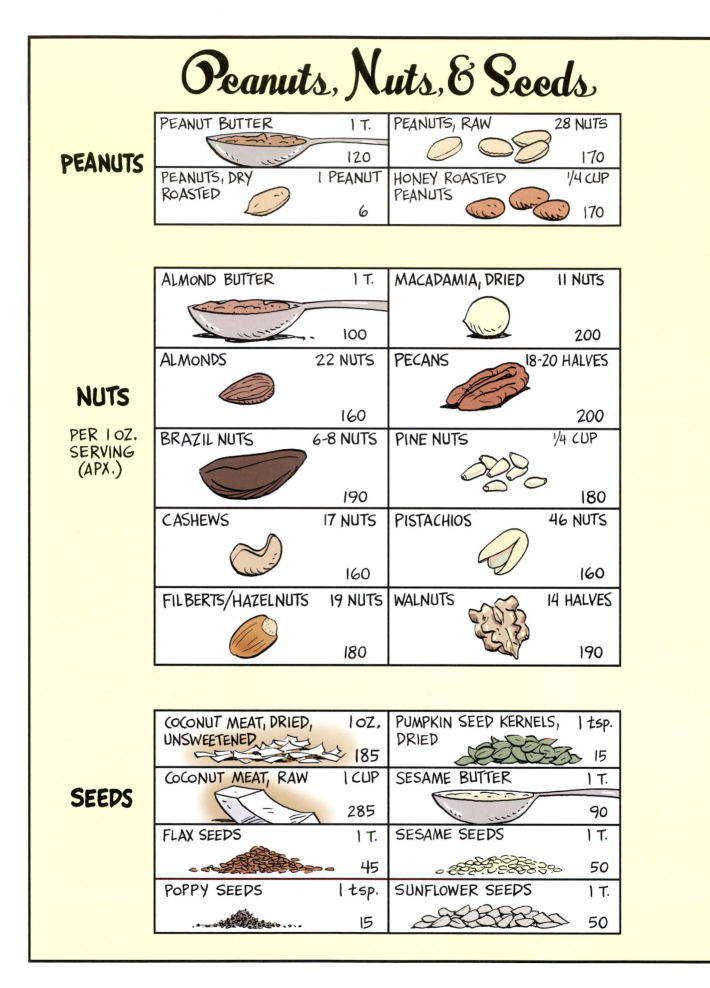

**PEANUTS**

| Item | Serving | Calories |
|---|---|---|
| PEANUT BUTTER | 1 T. | 120 |
| PEANUTS, RAW | 28 NUTS | 170 |
| PEANUTS, DRY ROASTED | 1 PEANUT | 6 |
| HONEY ROASTED PEANUTS | 1/4 CUP | 170 |

**NUTS**

PER 1 OZ. SERVING (APX.)

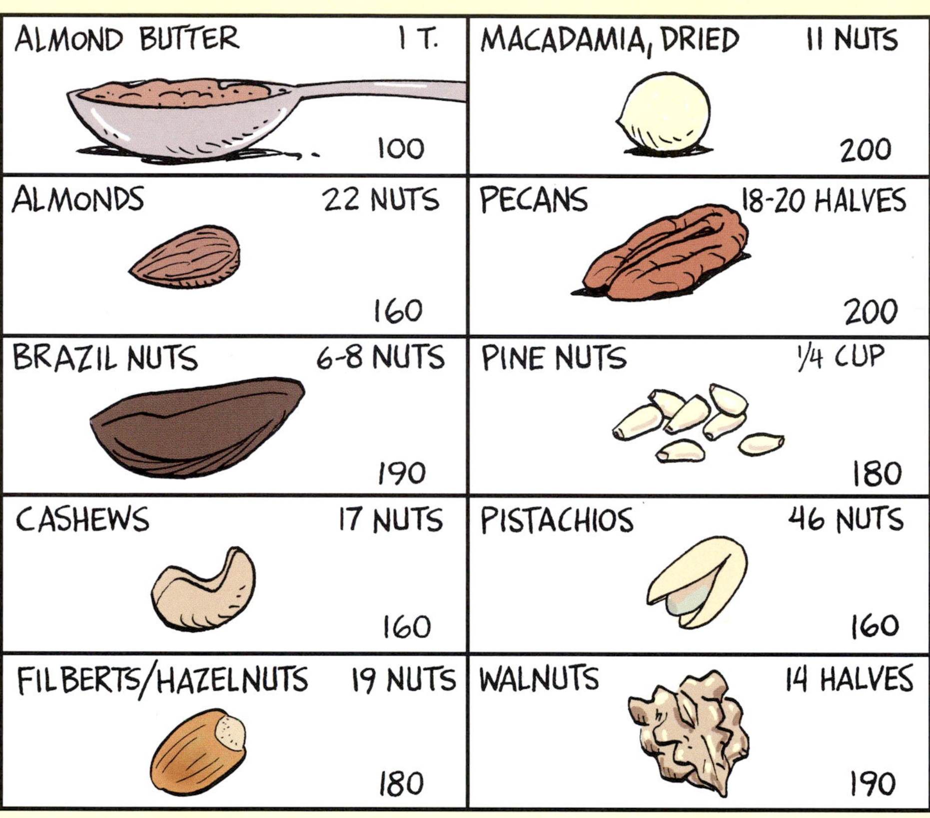

| Item | Serving | Calories |
|---|---|---|
| ALMOND BUTTER | 1 T. | 100 |
| MACADAMIA, DRIED | 11 NUTS | 200 |
| ALMONDS | 22 NUTS | 160 |
| PECANS | 18-20 HALVES | 200 |
| BRAZIL NUTS | 6-8 NUTS | 190 |
| PINE NUTS | 1/4 CUP | 180 |
| CASHEWS | 17 NUTS | 160 |
| PISTACHIOS | 46 NUTS | 160 |
| FILBERTS/HAZELNUTS | 19 NUTS | 180 |
| WALNUTS | 14 HALVES | 190 |

**SEEDS**

| Item | Serving | Calories |
|---|---|---|
| COCONUT MEAT, DRIED, UNSWEETENED | 1 OZ. | 185 |
| PUMPKIN SEED KERNELS, DRIED | 1 tsp. | 15 |
| COCONUT MEAT, RAW | 1 CUP | 285 |
| SESAME BUTTER | 1 T. | 90 |
| FLAX SEEDS | 1 T. | 45 |
| SESAME SEEDS | 1 T. | 50 |
| POPPY SEEDS | 1 tsp. | 15 |
| SUNFLOWER SEEDS | 1 T. | 50 |

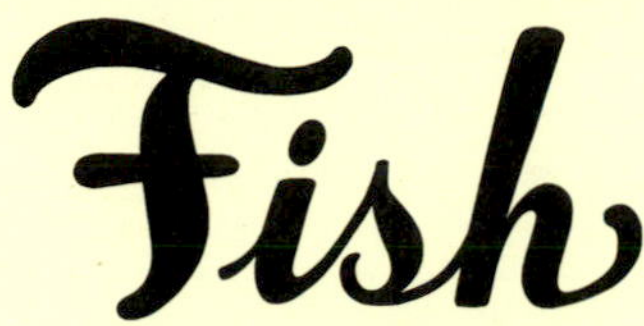

# Fish

3-OZ. PORTIONS UNLESS OTHERWISE NOTED

| | | |
|---|---|---|
| ANCHOVY | 1 FISH | 8 |
| BASS, COOKED W/ DRY HEAT | | 105 |
| BLUEFISH | | 135 |
| CARP | | 140 |
| CATFISH, FARMED, COOKED W/ DRY HEAT | | 130 |
| CATFISH, WILD, COOKED W/ DRY HEAT | | 90 |
| CAVIAR, BLACK AND RED | 1 T. | 40 |
| COD, ATLANTIC, COOKED W/ DRY HEAT | | 90 |
| DOLPHINFISH (MAHI MAHI), BROILED | | 90 |
| DRUM, FRESHWATER | | 130 |
| EEL | | 150 |
| FLATFISH (FLOUNDER OR SOLE) | | 100 |
| GROUPER | | 100 |
| HADDOCK | | 95 |
| HALIBUT, ATLANTIC OR PACIFIC | | 120 |
| HALIBUT, GREENLAND | | 205 |
| HERRING, ATLANTIC | | 175 |
| HERRING, PACIFIC | | 215 |
| MACKEREL, ATLANTIC | | 225 |
| MACKEREL, KING | | 115 |
| MACKEREL, SPANISH | | 135 |
| MONKFISH | | 85 |
| MULLET, STRIPED | | 130 |
| PERCH | | 100 |
| PIKE, NORTHERN OR WALLEYE | | 100 |
| POLLOCK | | 100 |
| POMPANO | | 180 |
| POUT | | 90 |
| ROCKFISH | | 105 |
| ROE | | 170 |
| ROUGHY | | 75 |
| SABLEFISH | | 215 |
| SALMON, ATLANTIC, FARMED | | 175 |
| SALMON, ATLANTIC, WILD | | 155 |
| SALMON, CHINOOK | | 200 |
| SALMON, CHINOOK, SMOKED | | 105 |
| SALMON, COHO, FARMED, COOKED W/ DRY HEAT | | 150 |
| SALMON, COHO, WILD, COOKED W/ DRY HEAT | | 120 |
| SALMON, COHO, WILD, COOKED W/ MOIST HEAT | | 155 |
| SALMON, PINK | | 130 |
| SALMON, SOCKEYE | | 185 |
| SARDINE, PACKED IN WATER | | 110 |
| SEA BASS | | 105 |
| SEA TROUT | | 115 |
| SHAD | | 215 |
| SHEEPSHEAD | | 110 |
| SMELT, RAINBOW | | 105 |
| SNAPPER | | 110 |
| STURGEON | | 120 |
| SUCKER, WHITE | | 100 |
| SWORDFISH | | 130 |
| TILAPIA | | 110 |
| TILEFISH | | 125 |
| TROUT, RAINBOW, WILD | | 130 |
| TUNA, BLUEFIN, FRESH | | 155 |
| TUNA, YELLOWTAIL, FRESH | | 120 |
| TURBOT | | 105 |
| WHITEFISH | | 145 |
| WOLFFISH | | 105 |
| YELLOWTAIL | | 160 |

# Shellfish

| | | |
|---|---|---|
| ABALONE, FRIED | 3 OZ. | 160 |
| ABALONE, RAW | 3 OZ. | 90 |
| CLAM, MOIST | 3 OZ. | 125 |
| CRAB, ALASKA KING | 3 OZ. | 80 |
| CRAB, DUNGENESS | 3 OZ. | 95 |
| CRAYFISH | 3 OZ. | 75 |
| LOBSTER | 3 OZ. | 85 |
| MUSSEL, BLUE, MOIST | 3 OZ. | 145 |
| OCTOPUS | 3 OZ. | 140 |
| OYSTER, EASTERN, FARMED, DRY | 6 MEDIUM | 50 |
| OYSTER, EASTERN, WILD, DRY | 6 MEDIUM | 40 |
| OYSTER, EASTERN, WILD, MOIST | 6 MEDIUM | 60 |
| OYSTER, PACIFIC, MOIST | 1 MEDIUM | 40 |
| OYSTER, PACIFIC, DRY | 1 MEDIUM | 40 |
| SCALLOPS, RAW | 3 OZ. | 90 |
| SCALLOPS, BROILED | 3 OZ. | 150 |
| SHRIMP | 3 OZ. | 85 |
| SPINY LOBSTER | 3 OZ. | 120 |
| SQUID, RAW | 1 OZ. | 25 |
| WHELK | 3 OZ. | 235 |

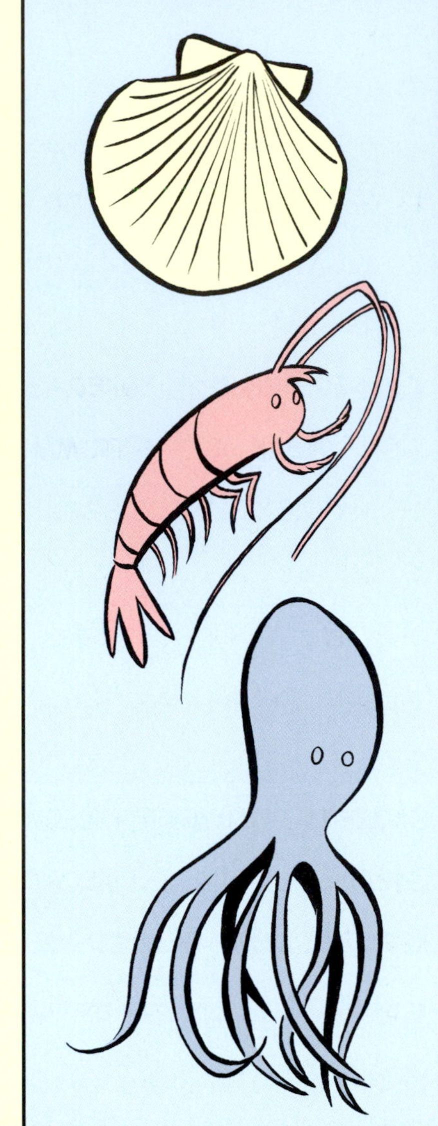

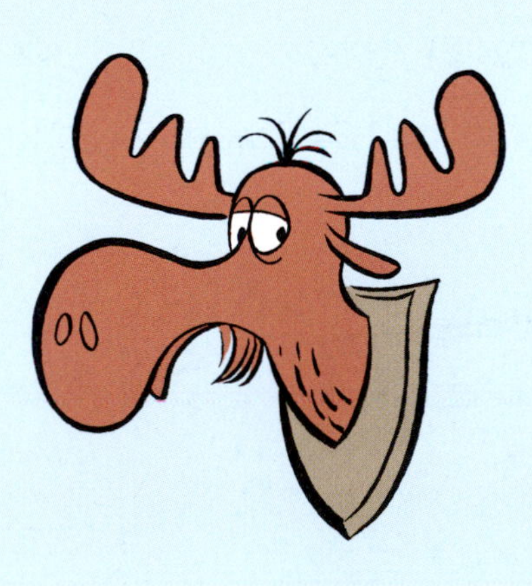

3-OZ. PORTIONS

# Game Meats

| | |
|---|---|
| BEAR, ROASTED | 135 |
| BISON, ROASTED | 120 |
| ELK, ROASTED | 125 |
| MOOSE, ROASTED | 115 |
| RABBIT, ROASTED | 170 |
| RABBIT, WILD, STEWED | 150 |
| VENISON CHOP, ROASTED | 135 |
| VENISON CHOP, STEWED | 145 |

# Beef

3-OZ. PORTIONS

| | |
|---|---|
| BLADE ROAST, BRAISED, TRIMMED | 225 |
| BOTTOM ROUND, CHOICE, BRAISED | 185 |
| CHUCK ARM POT ROAST, TRIMMED | 185 |
| CLUB STEAK, BROILED, TRIMMED | 175 |
| CORNED BRISKET, COOKED, TRIMMED | 215 |
| CUBE STEAK, FRIED, TRIMMED | 195 |
| FLANK STEAK, CHOICE, BROILED, TRIMMED | 175 |
| GROUND, EXTRA-LEAN, BAKED MEDIUM | 210 |
| GROUND, EXTRA-LEAN, BAKED WELL | 235 |
| GROUND, EXTRA-LEAN, BROILED MEDIUM | 220 |
| GROUND, EXTRA-LEAN, BROILED WELL | 225 |
| GROUND, EXTRA-LEAN, FRIED WELL | 225 |
| GROUND, LEAN, BAKED MEDIUM | 230 |
| GROUND, LEAN, BROILED WELL | 240 |
| GROUND, LEAN, FRIED WELL | 235 |
| GROUND, REGULAR, BROILED WELL | 250 |
| GROUND, PATTY, BAKED MEDIUM | 245 |
| HEART, SIMMERED | 150 |
| KIDNEY, SIMMERED | 125 |
| LIVER, FRIED | 135 |
| LONDON BROIL, CHOICE, TRIMMED | 175 |
| PORTERHOUSE STEAK, CHOICE, BROILED, TRIMMED | 185 |
| ROUND EYE, CHOICE, ROASTED, TRIMMED | 150 |
| ROUND CHOICE, BROILED | 235 |
| ROUND, POT, ROASTED | 235 |
| ROUND STEAK, ROASTED | 205 |
| RUMP ROAST, SELECT, BRAISED | 220 |
| RUMP ROAST, SELECT, BRAISED, TRIMMED | 165 |
| SHORT RIBS, CHOICE, BRAISED | 400 |
| SHORT RIBS, CHOICE, BRAISED, TRIMMED | 250 |
| SIRLOIN, CHOICE, BROILED | 240 |
| SIRLOIN STEAK, CHOICE, BROILED, TRIMMED | 170 |
| SIRLOIN STRIP STEAK, BROILED, TRIMMED | 175 |
| STEW MEAT, COOKED, TRIMMED | 200 |
| T-BONE STEAK, CHOICE, BROILED | 255 |
| T-BONE STEAK, CHOICE, BROILED, TRIMMED | 175 |
| TENDERLOIN STEAK, BROILED, TRIMMED | 180 |
| TONGUE, SIMMERED | 240 |
| TOP ROUND STEAK, BROILED, TRIMMED | 155 |
| WELLINGTON | 260 |
| WHOLE RIB, CHOICE, BRAISED | 320 |
| WHOLE RIB, CHOICE, ROASTED, TRIMMED | 210 |

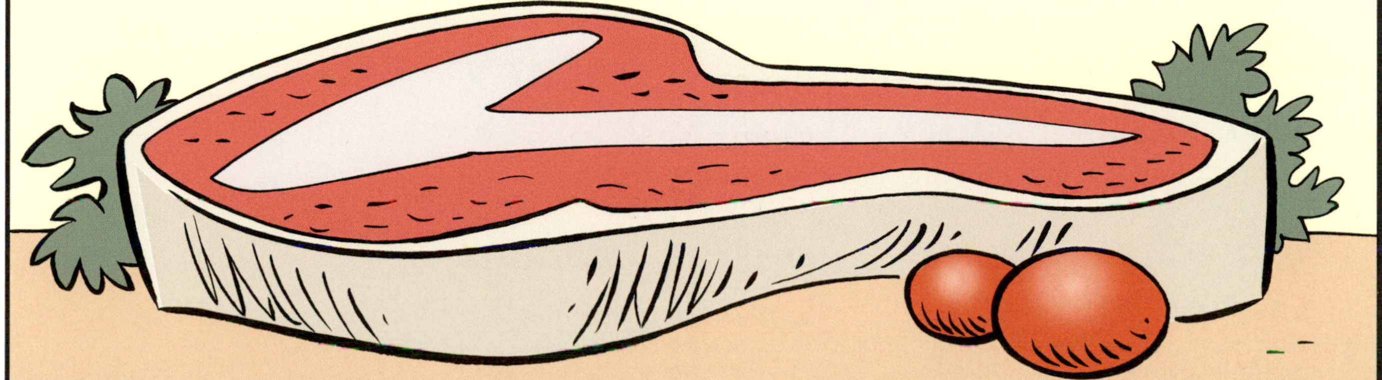

# Pork

3-OZ. PORTIONS

| | |
|---|---|
| BACON, COOKED | 50 |
| BLADE, BRAISED | 275 |
| BLADE, BROILED | 270 |
| BLADE, BROILED, TRIMMED | 200 |
| BLADE CHOP, FRIED | 290 |
| BLADE CHOP, FRIED, TRIMMED | 205 |
| BLADE, ROASTED | 275 |
| BLADE, ROASTED, TRIMMED | 210 |
| BOSTON BLADE, ROASTED | 230 |
| CENTER CHOP, BROILED, TRIMMED | 170 |
| CENTER LOIN CHOP, BRAISED | 210 |
| CENTER LOIN CHOP, FRIED | 235 |
| CENTER LOIN, ROASTED | 200 |
| CENTER RIB, BRAISED | 215 |
| CENTER RIB, CHOP, ROASTED | 115 |
| CENTER RIB, FRIED | 225 |
| CHOP, SMOKED, COOKED | 240 |
| CHOP, SMOKED, COOKED, TRIMMED | 145 |
| FRESH GROUND, COOKED | 255 |
| HAM HOCKS, COOKED | 280 |
| HAM, FRESH, ROASTED, TRIMMED | 180 |
| LEG/FRESH HAM, ROASTED | 230 |
| LEG RUMP, ROASTED, TRIMMED | 175 |
| LOIN, CHOP, BRAISED, TRIMMED | 175 |
| LOIN RIB, RAW, TRIMMED | 125 |
| LOIN, ROASTED | 210 |
| SHOULDER, BRAISED | 280 |
| SIRLOIN, BRAISED | 210 |
| SIRLOIN, BROILED | 220 |
| SPARERIBS, BRAISED | 340 |
| STEAK, BOSTON BLADE, BRAISED | 270 |
| TENDERLOIN, BRAISED | 175 |
| TENDERLOIN, LEAN, BROILED | 160 |
| TOP LOIN, BLADE, FRIED | 220 |
| WHOLE SHOULDER, ROASTED | 250 |

# Lamb

3-OZ. PORTIONS

| | |
|---|---|
| ARM CHOP, BRAISED | 300 |
| ARM CHOP, BRAISED, TRIMMED | 240 |
| BLADE, BRAISED | 295 |
| BLADE, BRAISED, TRIMMED | 245 |
| FORESHANK, BRAISED, TRIMMED | 160 |
| GROUND, BROILED | 240 |
| LEG, ROASTED | 220 |
| LEG, ROASTED, TRIMMED | 160 |
| LOIN, CHOICE, LEAN, ROASTED | 170 |
| LOIN CHOP, BROILED | 270 |
| LOIN CHOP, BROILED, TRIMMED | 185 |
| RIB ROAST, CHOICE | 305 |
| SHOULDER, ROASTED | 235 |
| SHOULDER, ROASTED, TRIMMED | 175 |
| SIRLOIN, LEG, CHOICE, ROASTED | 250 |
| SWEETBREADS, BRAISED | 200 |
| TONGUE, BRAISED | 235 |

# Fine Feathered Friends

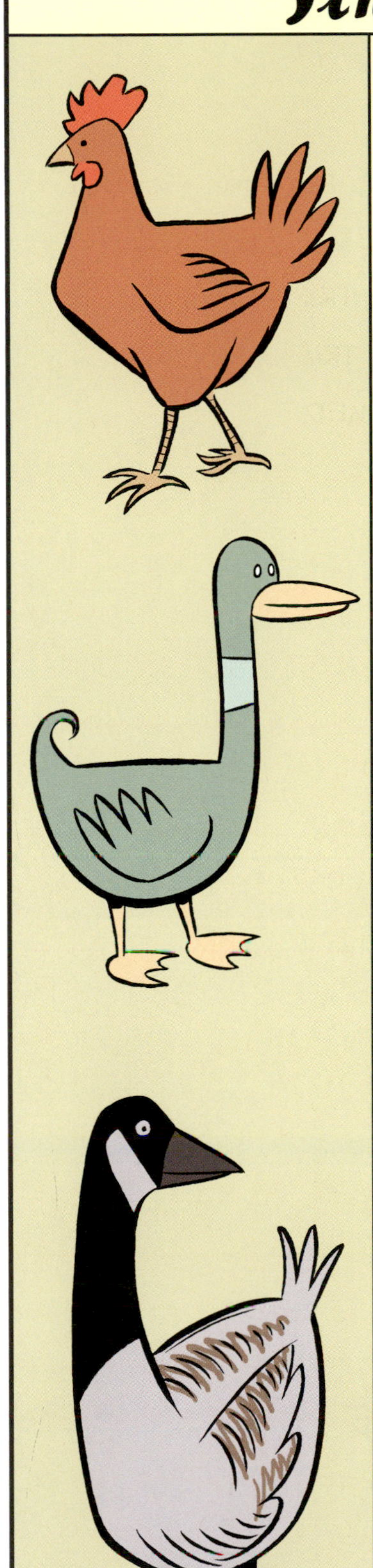

| | |
|---|---|
| CHICKEN BACK, FRIED, NO SKIN | 250 |
| CHICKEN BACK, ROASTED, NO SKIN | 205 |
| CHICKEN BREAST, ROASTED, NO SKIN | 170 |
| CHICKEN, DARK, ROASTED, NO SKIN | 175 |
| CHICKEN, DARK, STEWING, NO SKIN | 220 |
| CHICKEN DRUMSTICK, BATTER-FRIED | 230 |
| CHICKEN LIVERS, SIMMERED | 140 |
| CHICKEN NECK, STEWED | 210 |
| CHICKEN THIGH, FLOUR-FRIED | 225 |
| CHICKEN THIGH, ROASTED | 210 |
| CHICKEN THIGH, ROASTED, NO SKIN | 180 |
| CHICKEN THIGH, STEWED | 200 |
| CHICKEN WING, ROASTED | 250 |
| DUCK, CHINESE, PRESSED | 160 |
| DUCK, ROASTED, NO SKIN | 170 |
| GOOSE, ROASTED | 260 |
| GOOSE, ROASTED, NO SKIN | 200 |
| PHEASANT, ROASTED | 100 |
| TURKEY BACON, 2 SLICES | 70 |
| TURKEY, GROUND PATTY, COOKED | 200 |
| TURKEY HEARTS, SIMMERED | 150 |
| TURKEY, HEN, DARK, ROASTED, NO SKIN | 165 |
| TURKEY, HEN, WHITE, ROASTED, NO SKIN | 140 |
| TURKEY LIVERS, SIMMERED | 150 |
| TURKEY PASTRAMI | 120 |
| TURKEY, ROASTED | 175 |
| TURKEY, WHITE, ROASTED | 170 |
| TURKEY, WHITE, ROASTED, NO SKIN | 120 |

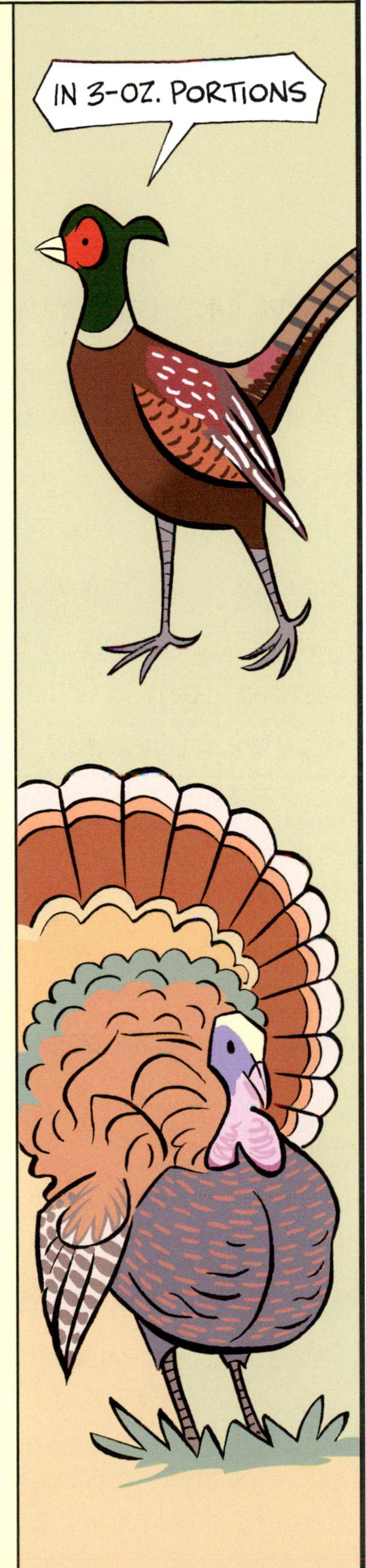

# Dairy and Eggs

## MILK PRODUCTS

| | | |
|---|---|---|
| BUTTER | 1 T. | 100 |
| BUTTER, WHIPPED | 1 T. | 65 |
| CREAM CHEESE | 1 T. | 70 |
| CREAM SUBSTITUTE, POWDERED | 1 T. | 35 |
| CREAM, COFFEE OR TABLE | 1 T. | 30 |
| CREAM, HALF AND HALF | 1 T. | 20 |
| CREAM, SOUR | 1 T. | 25 |
| MILK | 8 OZ. | 160 |
| MILK, 1% LOW-FAT | 8 OZ. | 100 |
| MILK, 2% LOW-FAT | 8 OZ. | 140 |
| MILK, NON-FAT (SKIM) | 8 OZ. | 85 |
| WHIPPED CREAM | 2 T. | 25 |

## CHEESES (1-OZ. PORTIONS)

| | |
|---|---|
| AMERICAN | 95 |
| ASIAGO, AGED | 110 |
| BLUE CHEESE CRUMBLES | 100 |
| CHEDDAR | 115 |
| CHEDDAR, SHARP, YELLOW | 80 |
| CHEDDAR, WHITE | 115 |
| FETA | 75 |
| GOAT, HARD | 125 |
| GOAT, SEMI-SOFT | 105 |
| GOAT, SOFT | 75 |
| GORGONZOLA | 110 |
| MONTEREY JACK | 105 |
| MOZZARELLA | 80 |
| PARMESAN | 110 |
| PROVOLONE | 100 |
| RICOTTA, PART SKIM | 40 |
| ROMANO | 110 |
| ROQUEFORT | 105 |
| SWISS | 105 |

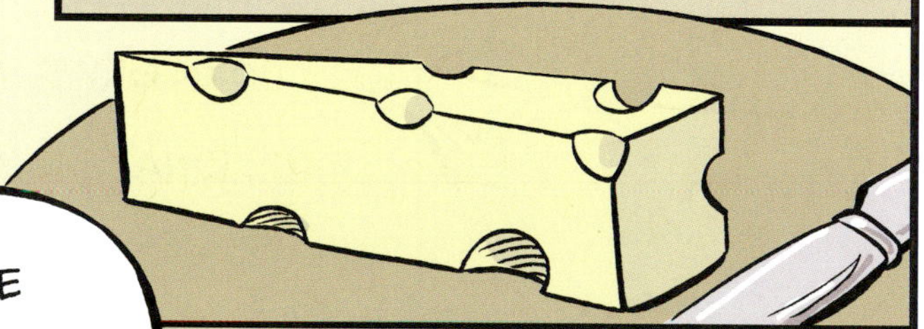

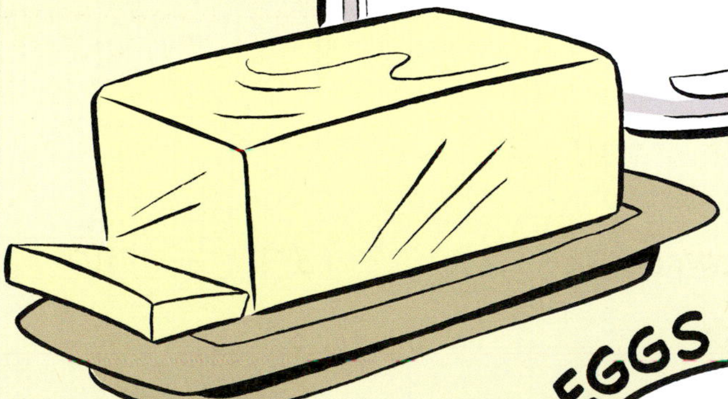

## EGGS

1 LARGE CHICKEN EGG 75

| | |
|---|---|
| CHICKEN EGG WHITES (2) | 35 |
| CHICKEN EGG YOLK | 60 |
| DUCK EGG | 130 |
| GOOSE EGG | 265 |
| QUAIL EGG | 15 |
| TURKEY EGG | 135 |

## Grains

ALL COOKED UNLESS OTHERWISE NOTED

| | | |
|---|---|---|
| BARLEY, PEARLED | 1 CUP | 195 |
| BUCKWHEAT GROATS, ROASTED | 1/4 CUP | 155 |
| BULGUR | 1 CUP | 150 |
| COUSCOUS | 1 CUP | 175 |
| MILLET | 1 CUP | 205 |
| QUINOA | 1 CUP | 220 |
| RICE, BROWN, MEDIUM-GRAIN | 1 CUP | 220 |
| RICE, BROWN, LONG-GRAIN | 1 CUP | 205 |
| RICE, WHITE, MEDIUM-GRAIN | 1 CUP | 240 |
| RICE, WILD | 1 CUP | 165 |
| WHEAT BRAN, TOASTED | 1/4 CUP | 110 |
| WHEAT GERM, RAW | 3 T. | 50 |

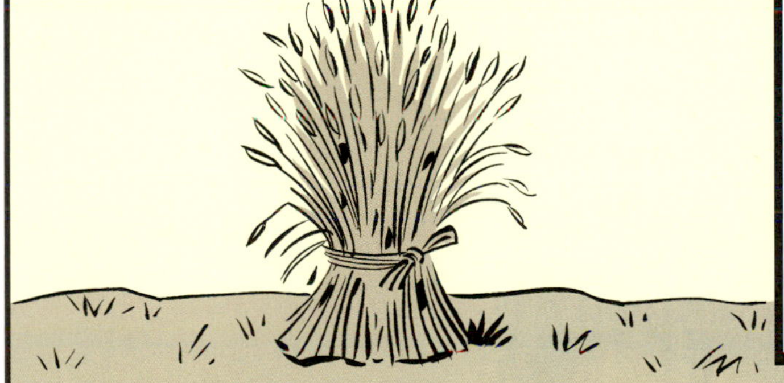

## Pasta

| | | |
|---|---|---|
| MACARONI, SMALL SHELLS | 1 CUP | 180 |
| MACARONI, SPIRAL | 1 CUP | 210 |
| MACARONI, ELBOW | 1 CUP | 220 |
| MACARONI, WHOLE WHEAT | 1 CUP | 175 |
| NOODLES, EGG, ENRICHED | 1 CUP | 220 |
| NOODLES, EGG, SPINACH | 1 CUP | 210 |
| NOODLES, JAPANESE, SOBA | 1 CUP | 115 |
| NOODLES, JAPANESE, SOMEN | 1 CUP | 230 |
| PASTA, CORN | 1 CUP | 175 |
| RICE NOODLES | 1 CUP | 190 |
| SPAGHETTI, ENRICHED | 1 CUP | 220 |
| SPAGHETTI, SPINACH | 1 CUP | 180 |
| SPAGHETTI, WHOLE WHEAT | 1 CUP | 175 |

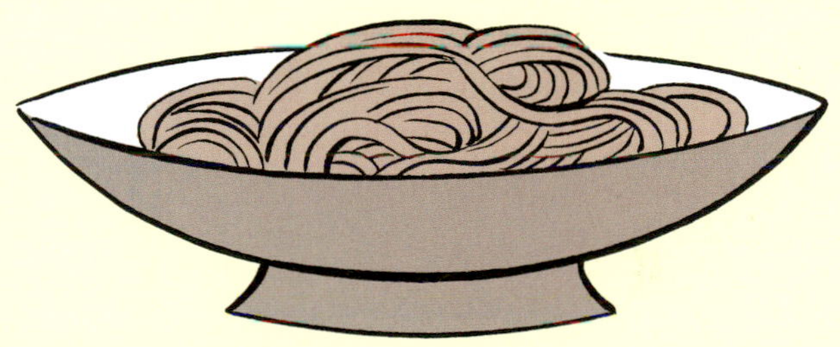

## Hot Cereals

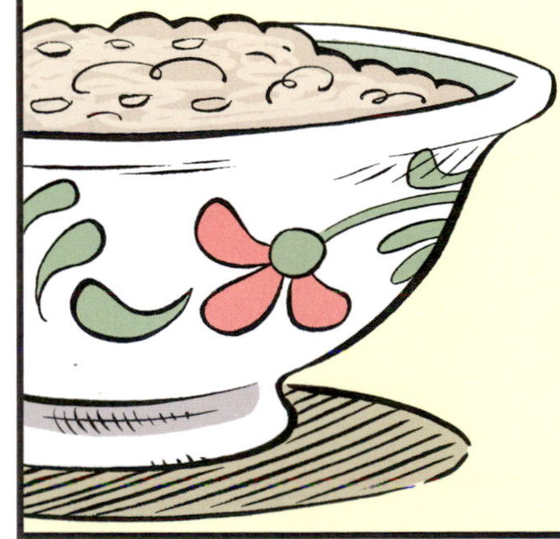

| | | |
|---|---|---|
| CORN GRITS, YELLOW, UNCOOKED | 3 T. | 110 |
| FARINA, UNCOOKED | 3 T. | 115 |
| OAT BRAN, UNCOOKED | 1/2 CUP | 150 |
| OATMEAL, UNCOOKED | 1/2 CUP | 150 |
| WHOLE WHEAT, UNCOOKED | 1/4 CUP | 160 |

# Liquor

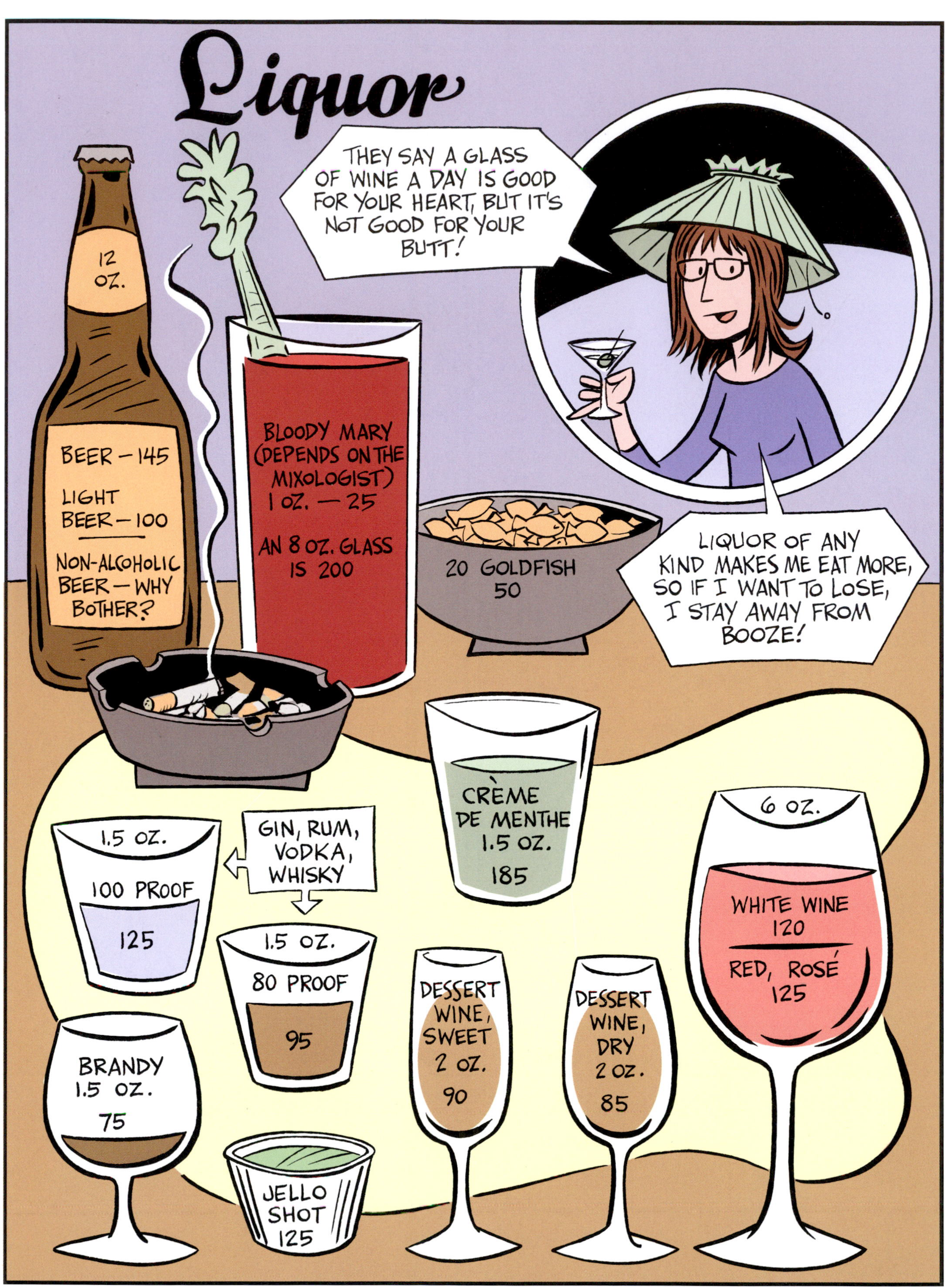
THEY SAY A GLASS OF WINE A DAY IS GOOD FOR YOUR HEART, BUT IT'S NOT GOOD FOR YOUR BUTT!
LIQUOR OF ANY KIND MAKES ME EAT MORE, SO IF I WANT TO LOSE, I STAY AWAY FROM BOOZE!
12 OZ.
BEER – 145
LIGHT BEER – 100
NON-ALCOHOLIC BEER – WHY BOTHER?
BLOODY MARY (DEPENDS ON THE MIXOLOGIST) 1 OZ. — 25
AN 8 OZ. GLASS IS 200
20 GOLDFISH 50
CRÈME DE MENTHE 1.5 OZ. 185
1.5 OZ. 100 PROOF 125
GIN, RUM, VODKA, WHISKY
1.5 OZ. 80 PROOF 95
BRANDY 1.5 OZ. 75
JELLO SHOT 125
DESSERT WINE, SWEET 2 OZ. 90
DESSERT WINE, DRY 2 OZ. 85
6 OZ.
WHITE WINE 120
RED, ROSÉ 125

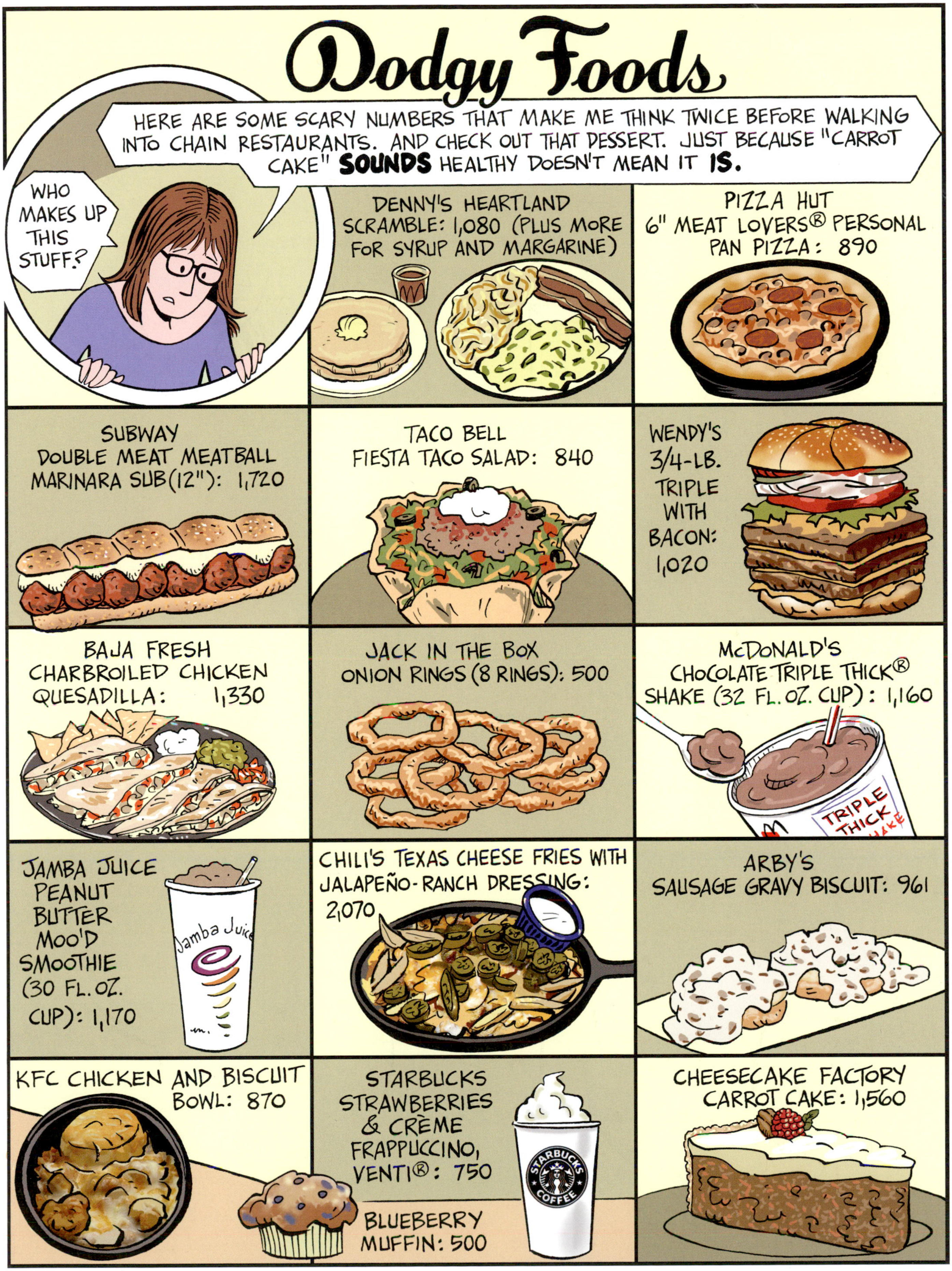

# Dodgy Foods



DENNY'S HEARTLAND SCRAMBLE: 1,080 (PLUS MORE FOR SYRUP AND MARGARINE)

PIZZA HUT 6" MEAT LOVERS® PERSONAL PAN PIZZA: 890

SUBWAY DOUBLE MEAT MEATBALL MARINARA SUB (12"): 1,720

TACO BELL FIESTA TACO SALAD: 840

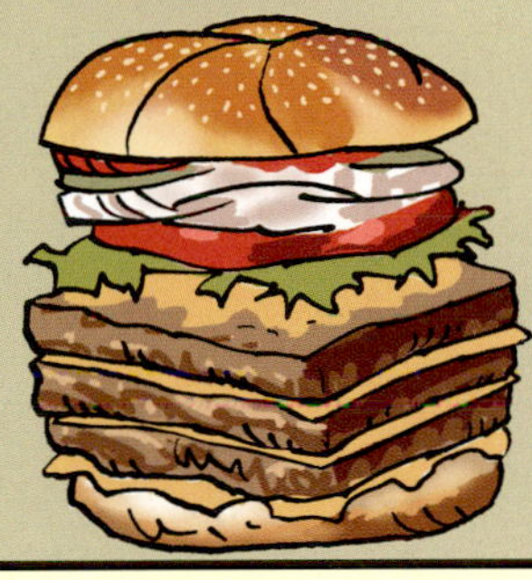

WENDY'S 3/4-LB. TRIPLE WITH BACON: 1,020

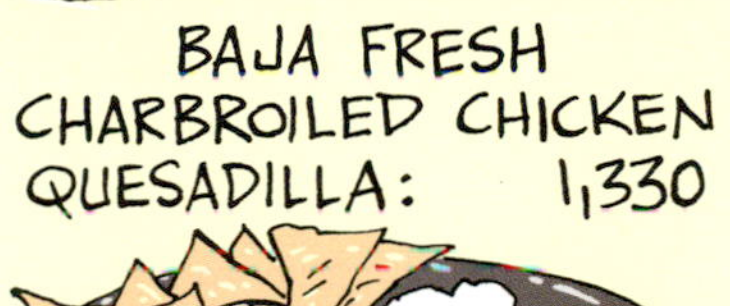

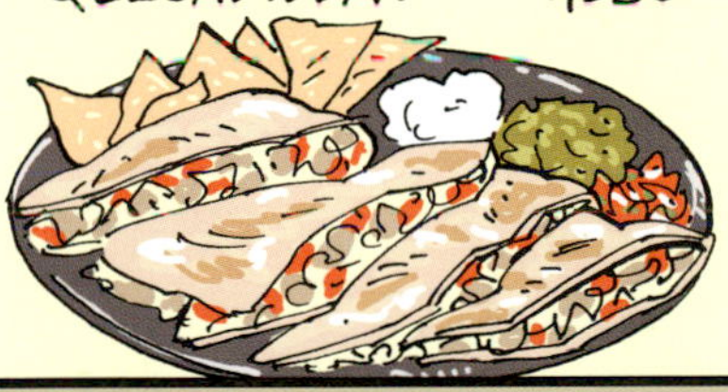

BAJA FRESH CHARBROILED CHICKEN QUESADILLA: 1,330

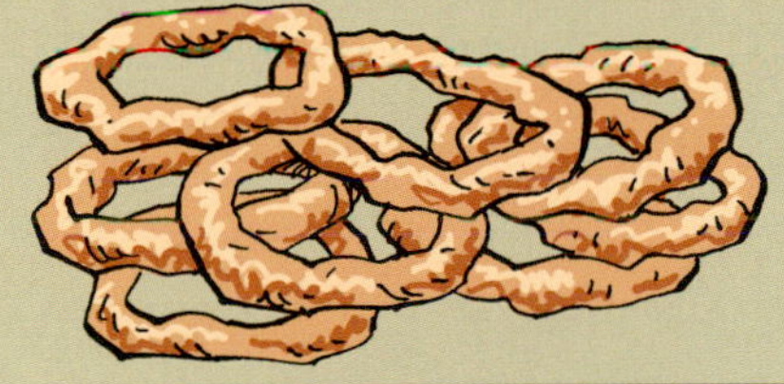

JACK IN THE BOX ONION RINGS (8 RINGS): 500

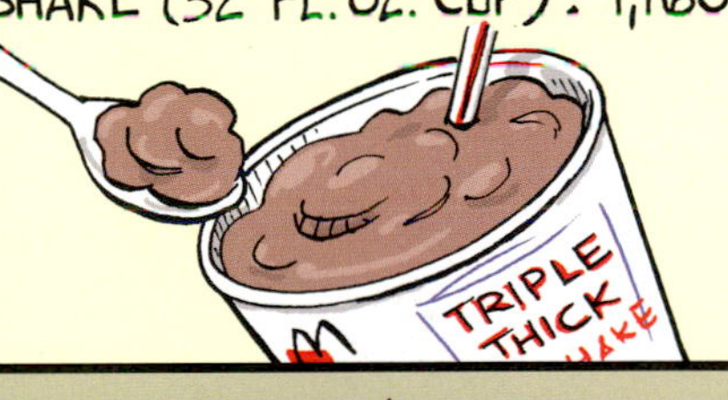


McDONALD'S CHOCOLATE TRIPLE THICK® SHAKE (32 FL. OZ. CUP): 1,160

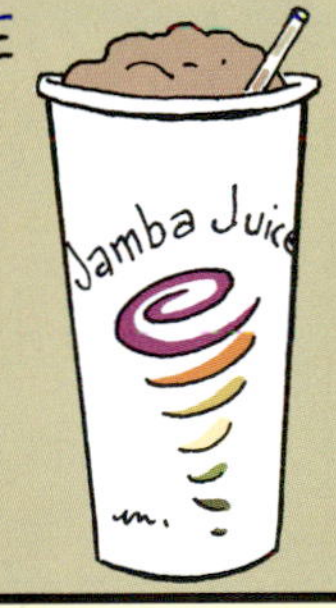


JAMBA JUICE PEANUT BUTTER MOO'D SMOOTHIE (30 FL. OZ. CUP): 1,170

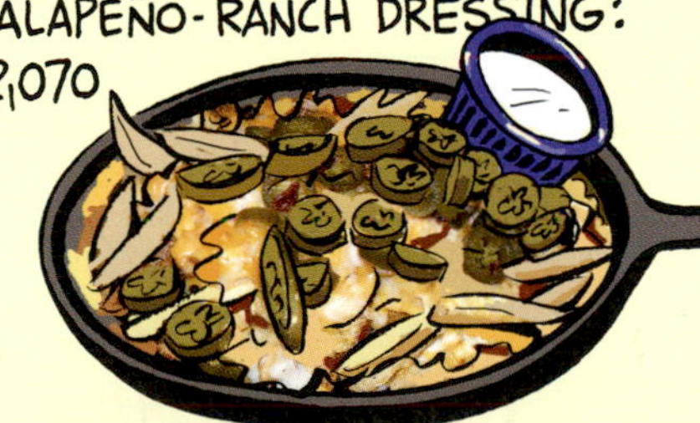

CHILI'S TEXAS CHEESE FRIES WITH JALAPEÑO-RANCH DRESSING: 2,070

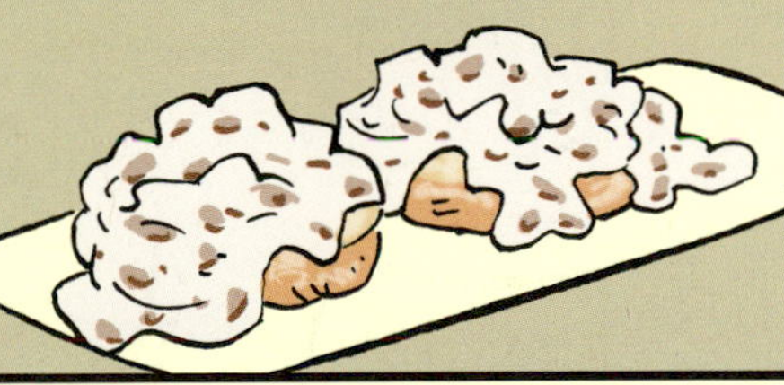

ARBY'S SAUSAGE GRAVY BISCUIT: 961

KFC CHICKEN AND BISCUIT BOWL: 870

BLUEBERRY MUFFIN: 500

STARBUCKS STRAWBERRIES & CRÈME FRAPPUCCINO, VENTI®: 750

CHEESECAKE FACTORY CARROT CAKE: 1,560

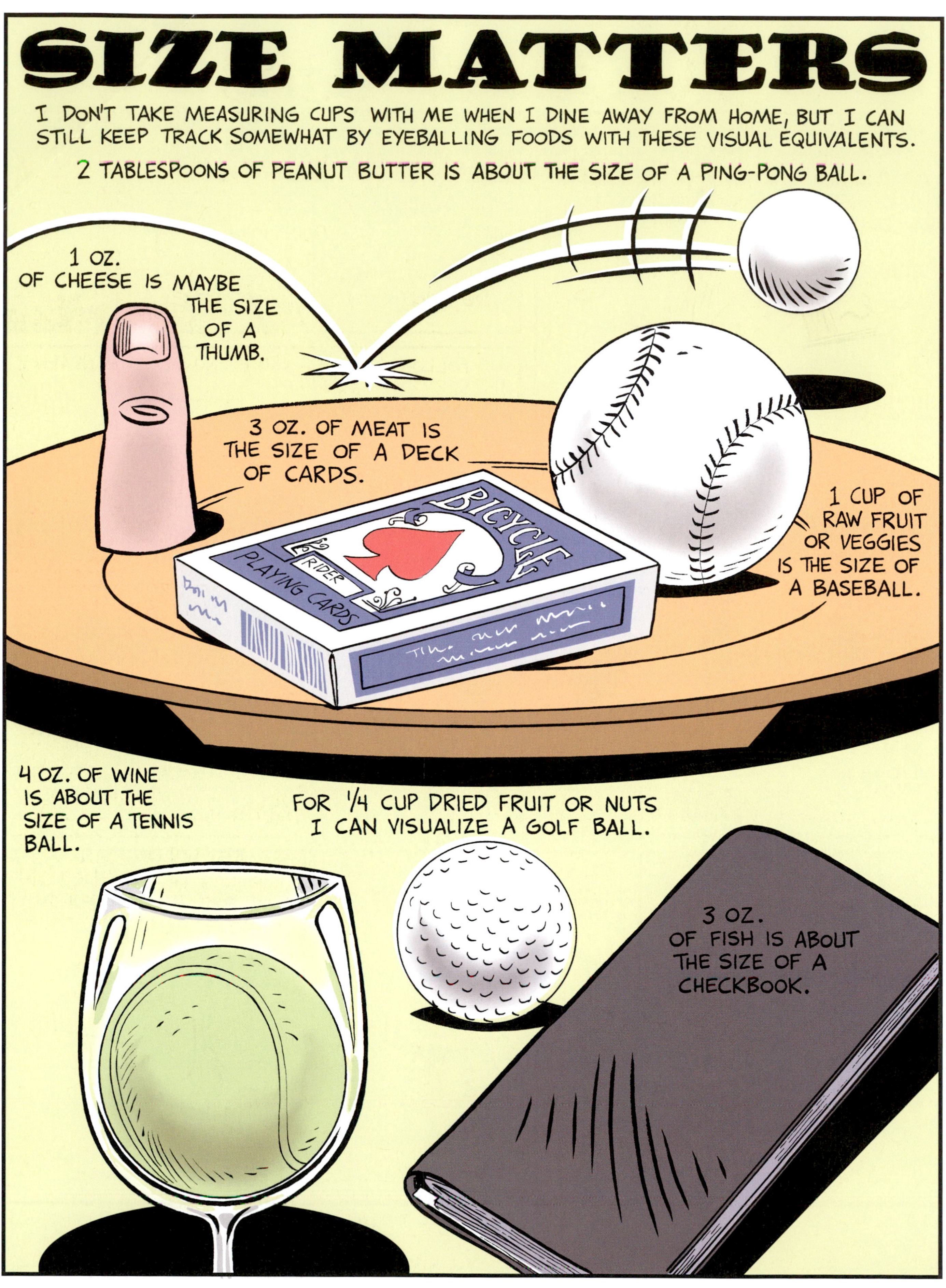
SIZE MATTERS
I DON'T TAKE MEASURING CUPS WITH ME WHEN I DINE AWAY FROM HOME, BUT I CAN STILL KEEP TRACK SOMEWHAT BY EYEBALLING FOODS WITH THESE VISUAL EQUIVALENTS.
2 TABLESPOONS OF PEANUT BUTTER IS ABOUT THE SIZE OF A PING-PONG BALL.
1 OZ. OF CHEESE IS MAYBE THE SIZE OF A THUMB.
3 OZ. OF MEAT IS THE SIZE OF A DECK OF CARDS.
BICYCLE
RIDER
PLAYING CARDS
1 CUP OF RAW FRUIT OR VEGGIES IS THE SIZE OF A BASEBALL.
4 OZ. OF WINE IS ABOUT THE SIZE OF A TENNIS BALL.
FOR 1/4 CUP DRIED FRUIT OR NUTS I CAN VISUALIZE A GOLF BALL.
3 OZ. OF FISH IS ABOUT THE SIZE OF A CHECKBOOK.

# Menu Plans

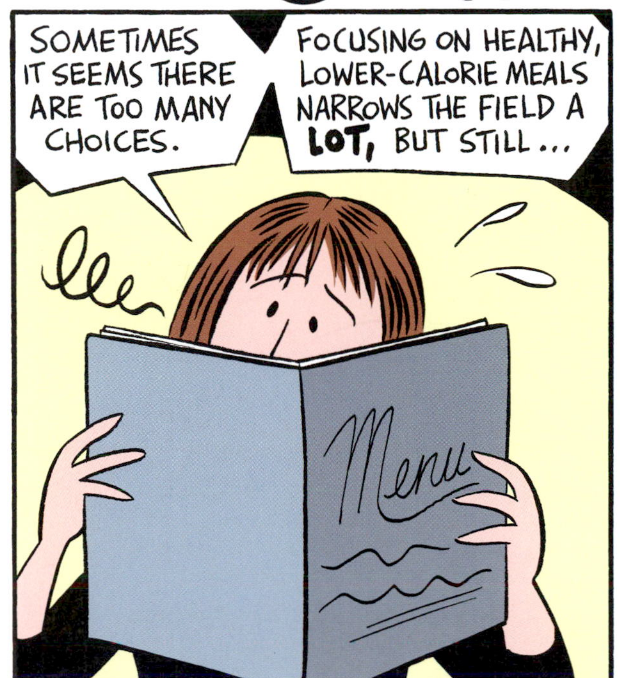

SOMETIMES IT SEEMS THERE ARE TOO MANY CHOICES.
FOCUSING ON HEALTHY, LOWER-CALORIE MEALS NARROWS THE FIELD A **LOT,** BUT STILL ...
Menu

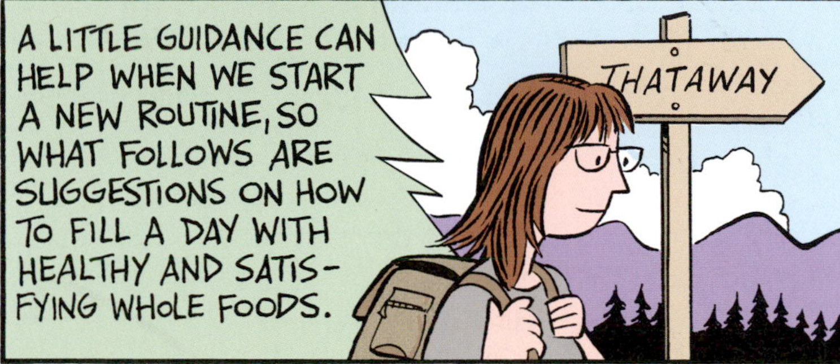

A LITTLE GUIDANCE CAN HELP WHEN WE START A NEW ROUTINE, SO WHAT FOLLOWS ARE SUGGESTIONS ON HOW TO FILL A DAY WITH HEALTHY AND SATISFYING WHOLE FOODS.
THATAWAY

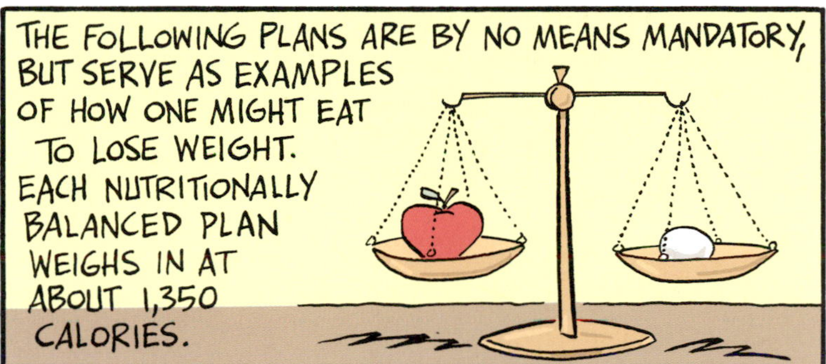

THE FOLLOWING PLANS ARE BY NO MEANS MANDATORY, BUT SERVE AS EXAMPLES OF HOW ONE MIGHT EAT TO LOSE WEIGHT. EACH NUTRITIONALLY BALANCED PLAN WEIGHS IN AT ABOUT 1,350 CALORIES.

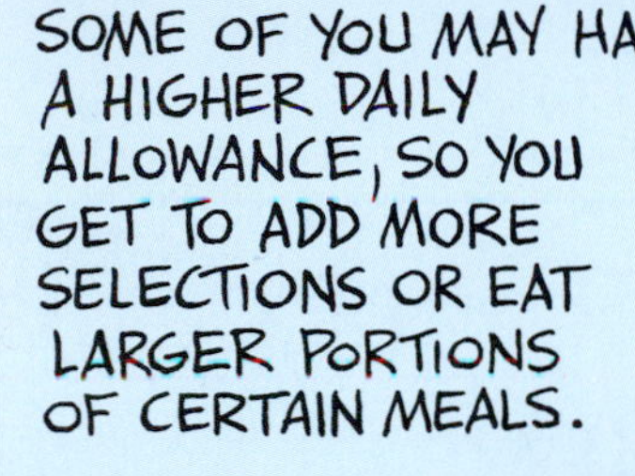

SOME OF YOU MAY HAVE A HIGHER DAILY ALLOWANCE, SO YOU GET TO ADD MORE SELECTIONS OR EAT LARGER PORTIONS OF CERTAIN MEALS.

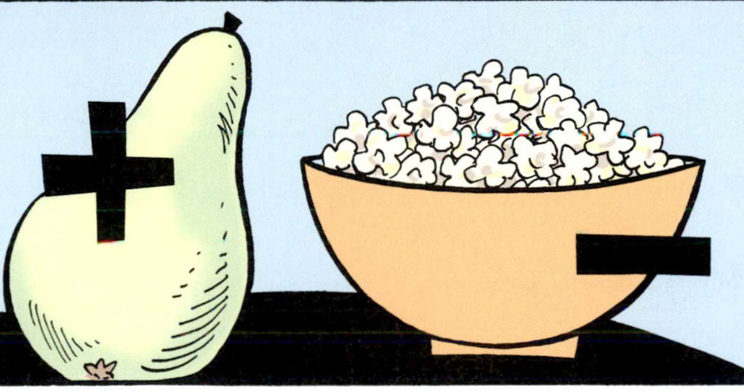

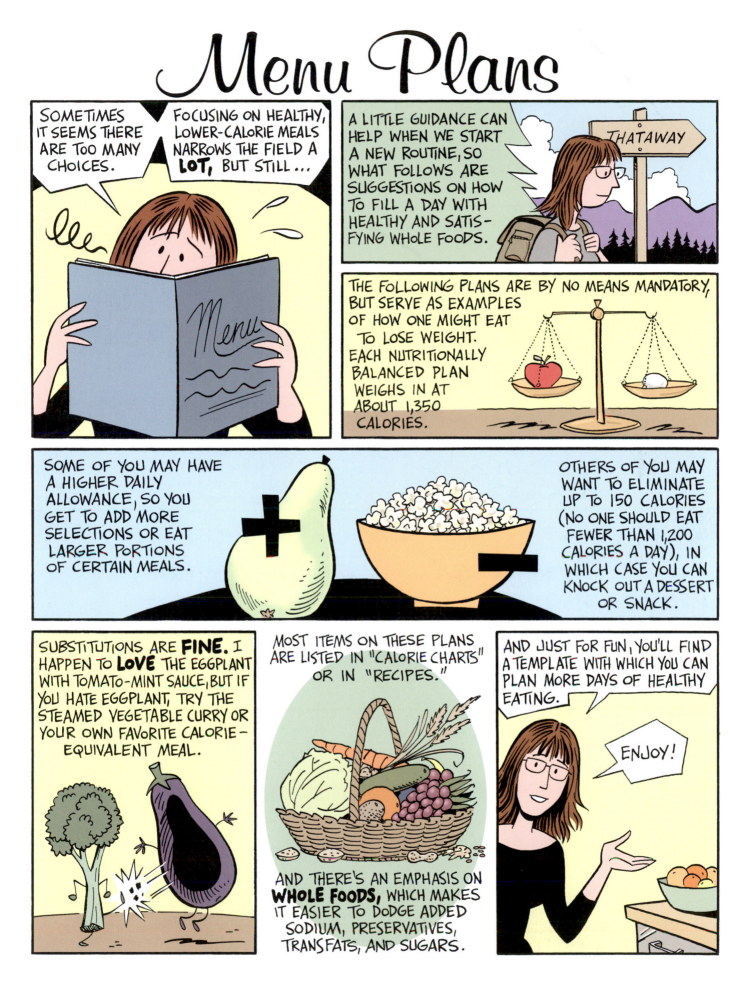

OTHERS OF YOU MAY WANT TO ELIMINATE UP TO 150 CALORIES (NO ONE SHOULD EAT FEWER THAN 1,200 CALORIES A DAY), IN WHICH CASE YOU CAN KNOCK OUT A DESSERT OR SNACK.

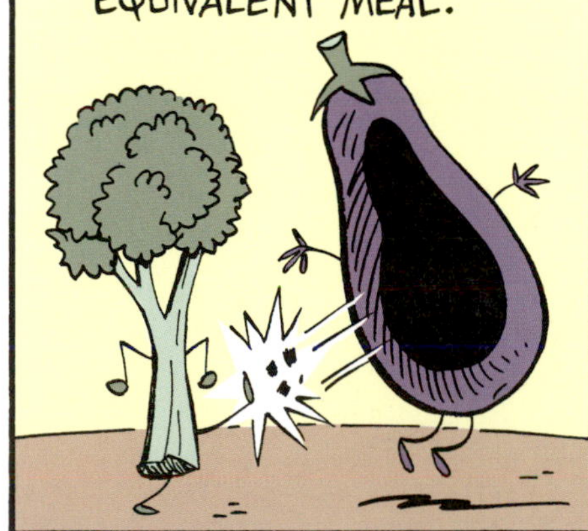

SUBSTITUTIONS ARE **FINE.** I HAPPEN TO **LOVE** THE EGGPLANT WITH TOMATO-MINT SAUCE, BUT IF YOU HATE EGGPLANT, TRY THE STEAMED VEGETABLE CURRY OR YOUR OWN FAVORITE CALORIE-EQUIVALENT MEAL.

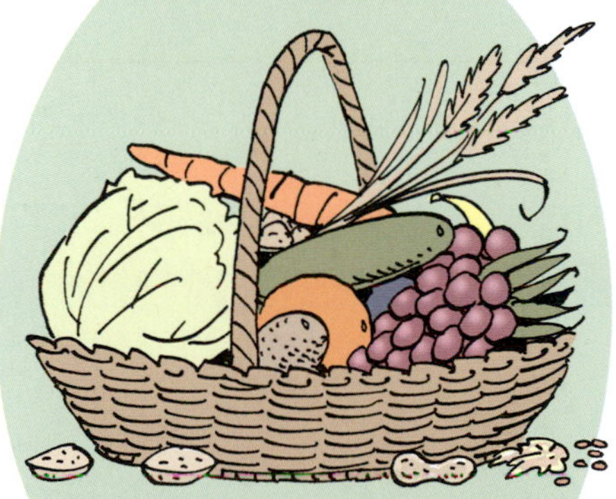

MOST ITEMS ON THESE PLANS ARE LISTED IN "CALORIE CHARTS" OR IN "RECIPES."

AND THERE'S AN EMPHASIS ON **WHOLE FOODS,** WHICH MAKES IT EASIER TO DODGE ADDED SODIUM, PRESERVATIVES, TRANSFATS, AND SUGARS.

AND JUST FOR FUN, YOU'LL FIND A TEMPLATE WITH WHICH YOU CAN PLAN MORE DAYS OF HEALTHY EATING.

ENJOY!

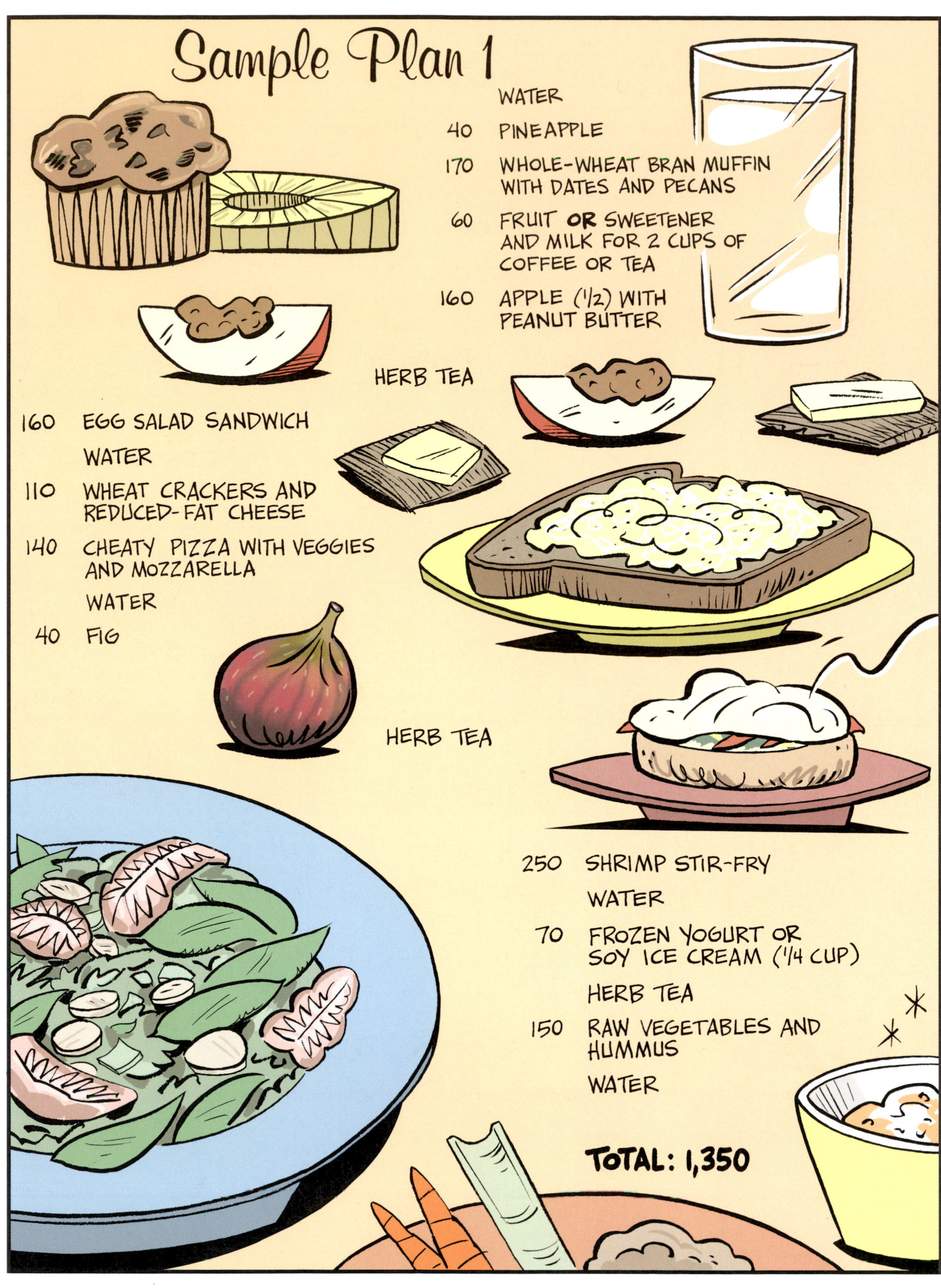
Sample Plan 1
WATER
40 PINEAPPLE
170 WHOLE-WHEAT BRAN MUFFIN WITH DATES AND PECANS
60 FRUIT OR SWEETENER AND MILK FOR 2 CUPS OF COFFEE OR TEA
160 APPLE (1/2) WITH PEANUT BUTTER
HERB TEA
160 EGG SALAD SANDWICH
WATER
110 WHEAT CRACKERS AND REDUCED-FAT CHEESE
140 CHEATY PIZZA WITH VEGGIES AND MOZZARELLA
WATER
40 FIG
HERB TEA
250 SHRIMP STIR-FRY
WATER
70 FROZEN YOGURT OR SOY ICE CREAM (1/4 CUP)
HERB TEA
150 RAW VEGETABLES AND HUMMUS
WATER
TOTAL: 1,350

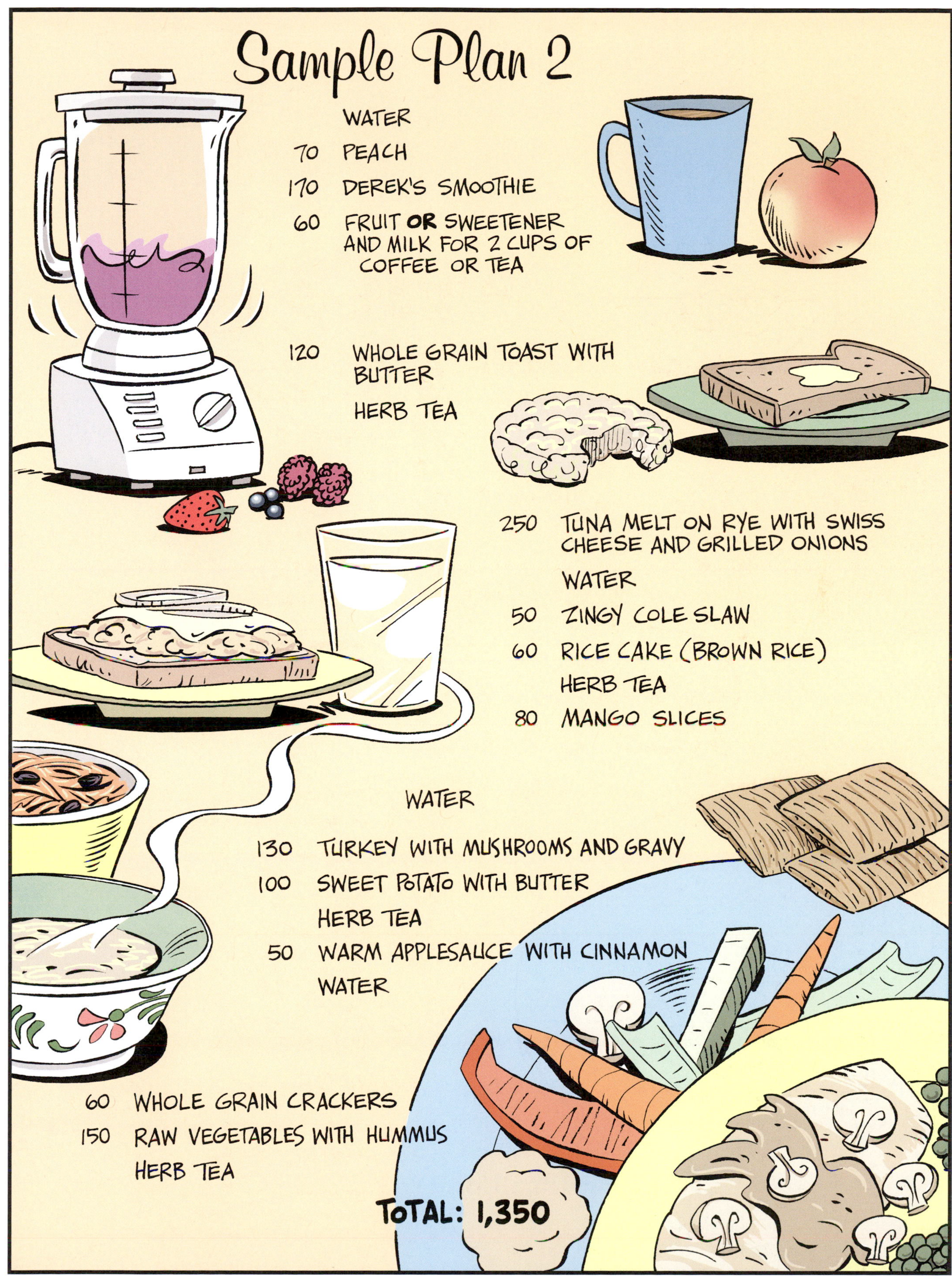
Sample Plan 2
WATER
70 PEACH
170 DEREK'S SMOOTHIE
60 FRUIT OR SWEETENER AND MILK FOR 2 CUPS OF COFFEE OR TEA
120 WHOLE GRAIN TOAST WITH BUTTER
HERB TEA
250 TUNA MELT ON RYE WITH SWISS CHEESE AND GRILLED ONIONS
WATER
50 ZINGY COLE SLAW
60 RICE CAKE (BROWN RICE)
HERB TEA
80 MANGO SLICES
WATER
130 TURKEY WITH MUSHROOMS AND GRAVY
100 SWEET POTATO WITH BUTTER
HERB TEA
50 WARM APPLESAUCE WITH CINNAMON
WATER
60 WHOLE GRAIN CRACKERS
150 RAW VEGETABLES WITH HUMMUS
HERB TEA
TOTAL: 1,350

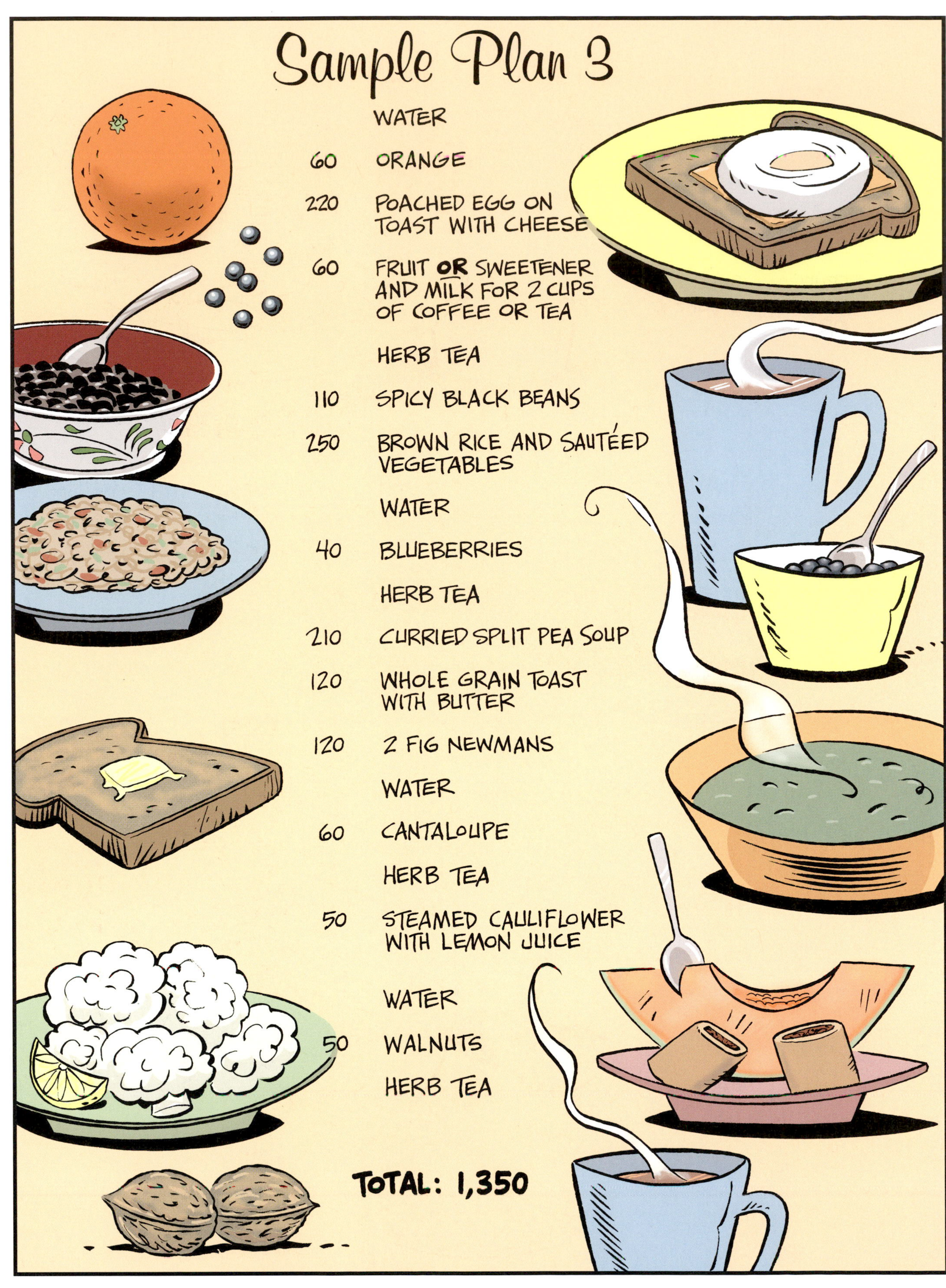
Sample Plan 3
WATER
60 ORANGE
220 POACHED EGG ON TOAST WITH CHEESE
60 FRUIT OR SWEETENER AND MILK FOR 2 CUPS OF COFFEE OR TEA
HERB TEA
110 SPICY BLACK BEANS
250 BROWN RICE AND SAUTÉED VEGETABLES
WATER
40 BLUEBERRIES
HERB TEA
210 CURRIED SPLIT PEA SOUP
120 WHOLE GRAIN TOAST WITH BUTTER
120 2 FIG NEWMANS
WATER
60 CANTALOUPE
HERB TEA
50 STEAMED CAULIFLOWER WITH LEMON JUICE
WATER
50 WALNUTS
HERB TEA
TOTAL: 1,350

# Sample Plan 4

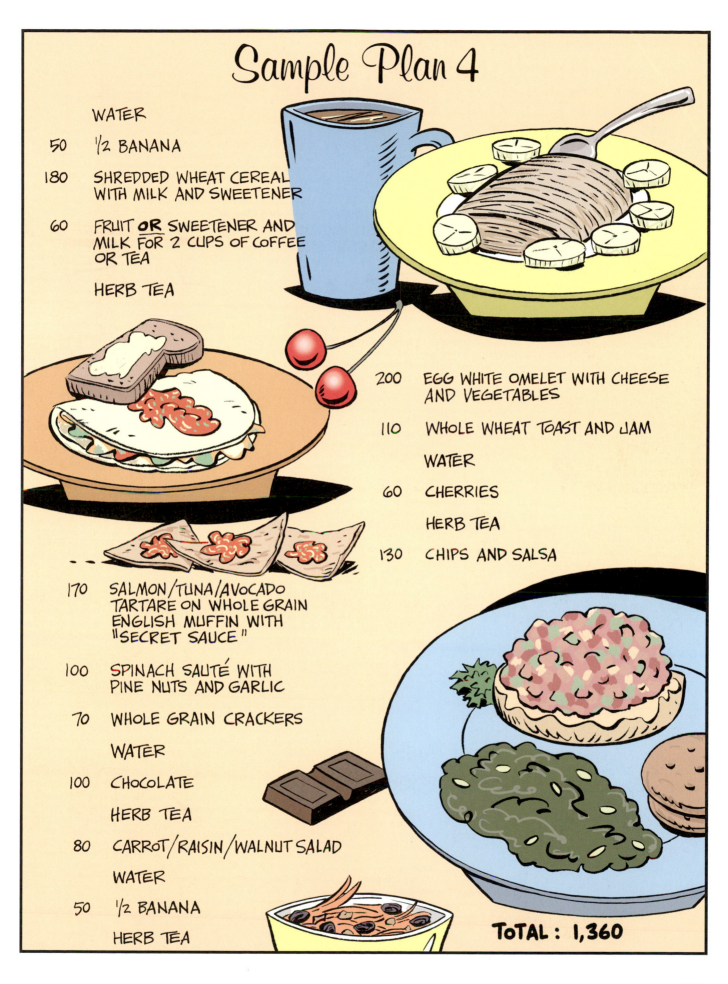

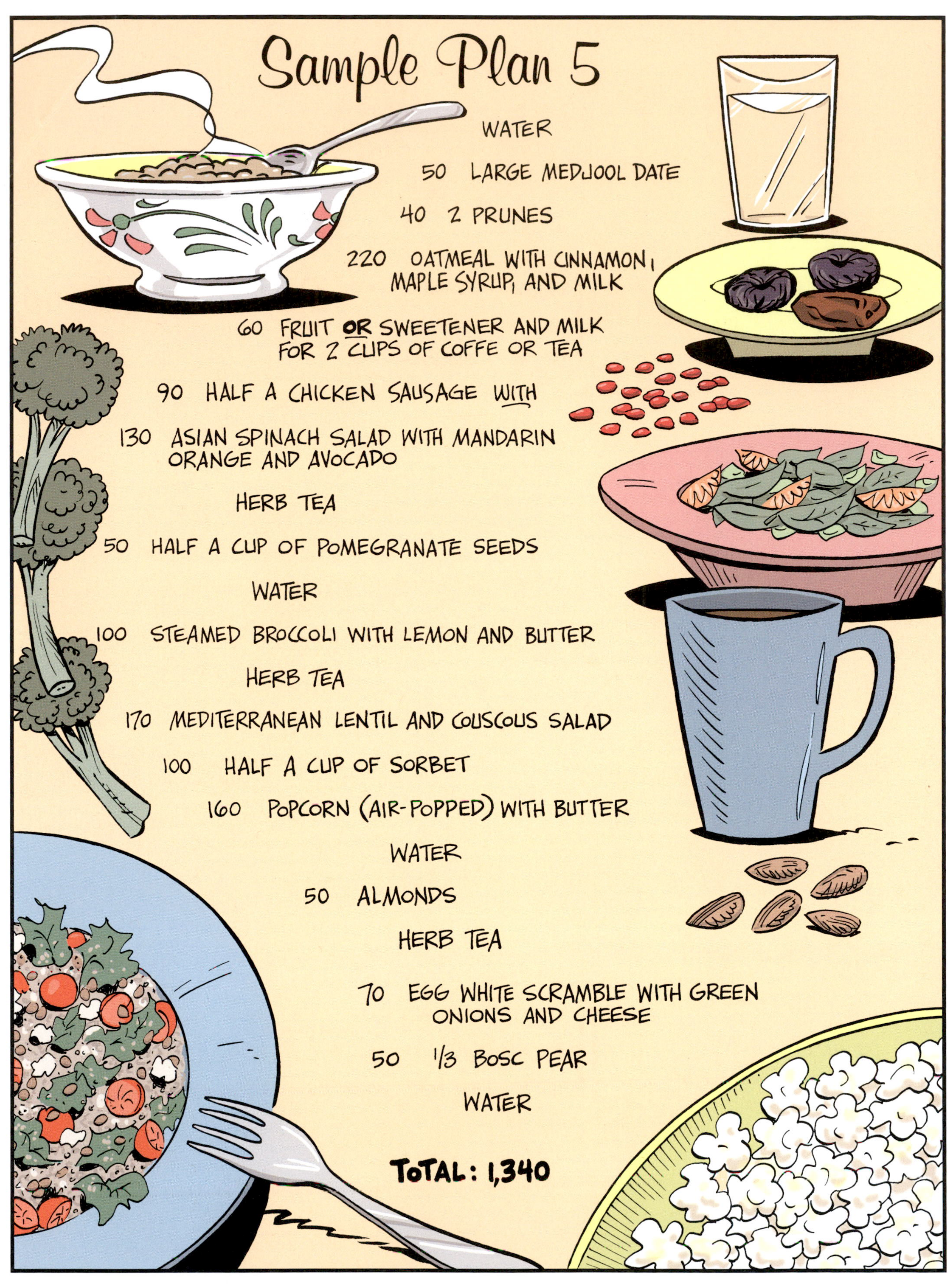
Sample Plan 5
WATER
50 LARGE MEDJOOL DATE
40 2 PRUNES
220 OATMEAL WITH CINNAMON, MAPLE SYRUP, AND MILK
60 FRUIT OR SWEETENER AND MILK FOR 2 CUPS OF COFFE OR TEA
90 HALF A CHICKEN SAUSAGE WITH
130 ASIAN SPINACH SALAD WITH MANDARIN ORANGE AND AVOCADO
HERB TEA
50 HALF A CUP OF POMEGRANATE SEEDS
WATER
100 STEAMED BROCCOLI WITH LEMON AND BUTTER
HERB TEA
170 MEDITERRANEAN LENTIL AND COUSCOUS SALAD
100 HALF A CUP OF SORBET
160 POPCORN (AIR-POPPED) WITH BUTTER
WATER
50 ALMONDS
HERB TEA
70 EGG WHITE SCRAMBLE WITH GREEN ONIONS AND CHEESE
50 1/3 BOSC PEAR
WATER
TOTAL: 1,340

# Menu Template

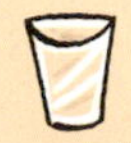
**WATER**—THE FIRST GLASS OF 8 FOR THE DAY!

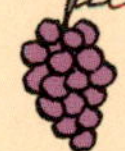
**FRUIT**—SEE "FRUITS" PAGE IN "CALORIE CHARTS" FOR SERVING SIZE INFORMATION

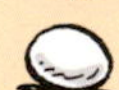
**BREAKFAST**—SEE BREAKFAST RECIPES FOR IDEAS

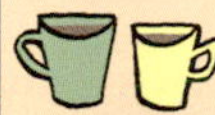
FRUIT **OR** SWEETENER AND MILK FOR 2 CUPS OF COFFEE OR TEA

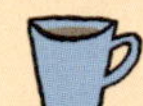
**HERB TEA**—A GREAT WAY TO SNEAK IN WATER WITH FLAVOR

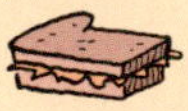
**LUNCH**—SEE "ENTRÉES" RECIPES FOR IDEAS (PAGE 166)

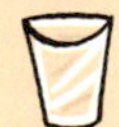
**WATER**—FILLS ONE UP AND KEEPS THINGS RUNNING SMOOTHLY

**FRUIT**—SHOOT FOR ABOUT 3 SERVINGS A DAY

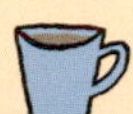
**HERB TEA**—TRY TO AVOID TOO MANY CAFFEINATED BEVERAGES

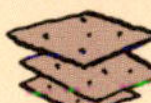
**GRAIN SNACK**—CRACKERS, BROWN RICE CAKES, TOAST—BUT WHOLE GRAIN, PLEASE

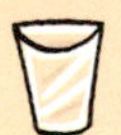
**WATER**—GREAT FOR THE SKIN!

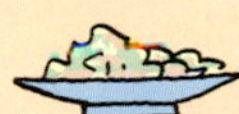
**DINNER**—SEE "ENTRÉES" RECIPES FOR IDEAS

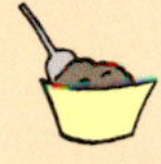
**DESSERT**—MODERATION IS KEY!

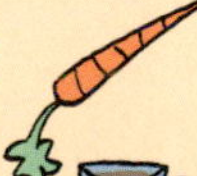
**VEGGIE SNACK**—5 TO 7 SERVINGS A DAY IS GOOD

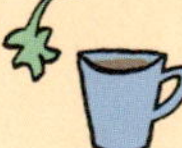
**HERB TEA**—IT'S GOOD TO KEEP A VARIETY OF FLAVORS ON HAND

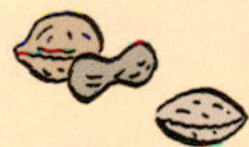
**NUTS OR SEEDS**—GREAT FOR THE HEART, BUT DON'T OVERDO IT!

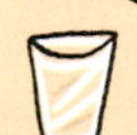
**WATER**—JUST A REMINDER

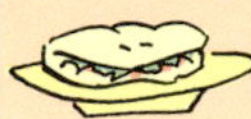
**PROTEIN SNACK**—EGG WHITE OMELETS ARE GOOD... YOGURT...

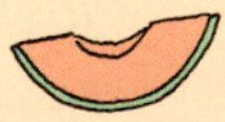
**FRUIT**—SOMETHING "MELLOW" LIKE MELON OR HALF A BANANA

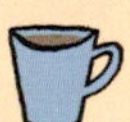
**HERB TEA**—CAMOMILE BEFORE BEDTIME HELPS WITH SLEEP

GAUGING CALORIE TOTALS TO THE TIME OF DAY CAN HELP—I TRY TO BE AT ABOUT 700 BY 7:00 P.M. BUT SEE WHAT WORKS BEST FOR YOU.

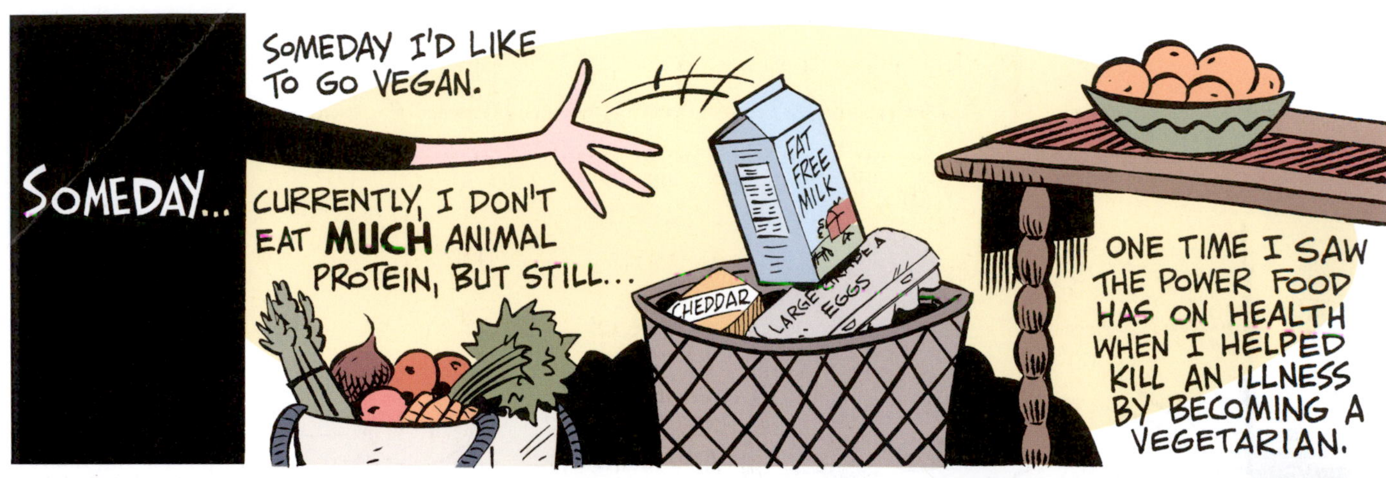
SOMEDAY...
SOMEDAY I'D LIKE TO GO VEGAN.
CURRENTLY, I DON'T EAT MUCH ANIMAL PROTEIN, BUT STILL...
FAT FREE MILK
CHEDDAR
LARGE GRADE A EGGS
ONE TIME I SAW THE POWER FOOD HAS ON HEALTH WHEN I HELPED KILL AN ILLNESS BY BECOMING A VEGETARIAN.

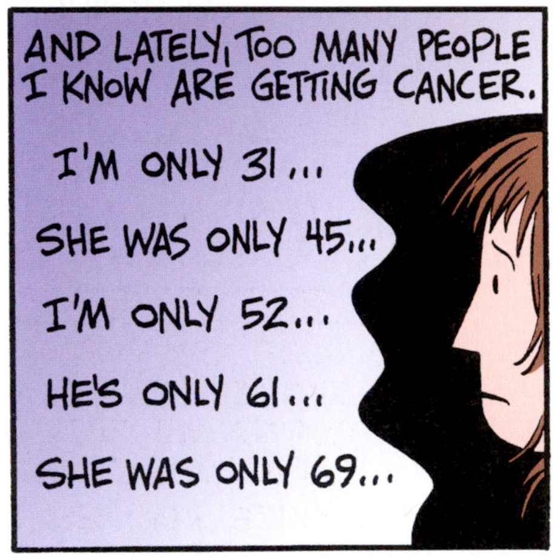
AND LATELY, TOO MANY PEOPLE I KNOW ARE GETTING CANCER.
I'M ONLY 31...
SHE WAS ONLY 45...
I'M ONLY 52...
HE'S ONLY 61...
SHE WAS ONLY 69...

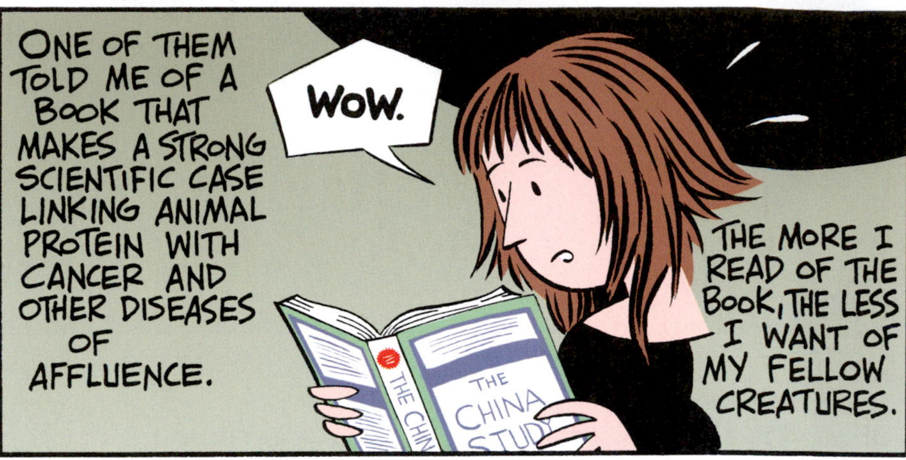
ONE OF THEM TOLD ME OF A BOOK THAT MAKES A STRONG SCIENTIFIC CASE LINKING ANIMAL PROTEIN WITH CANCER AND OTHER DISEASES OF AFFLUENCE.
WOW.
THE CHINA STUDY
THE MORE I READ OF THE BOOK, THE LESS I WANT OF MY FELLOW CREATURES.

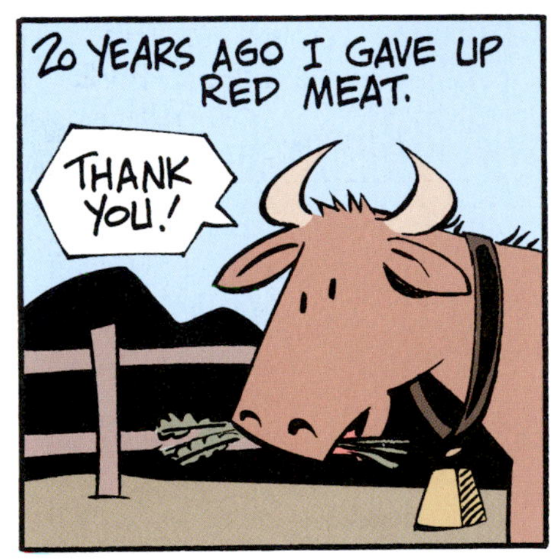
20 YEARS AGO I GAVE UP RED MEAT.
THANK YOU!

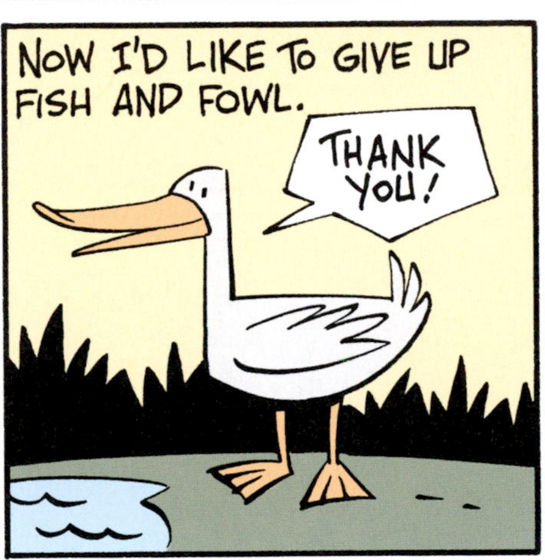
NOW I'D LIKE TO GIVE UP FISH AND FOWL.
THANK YOU!

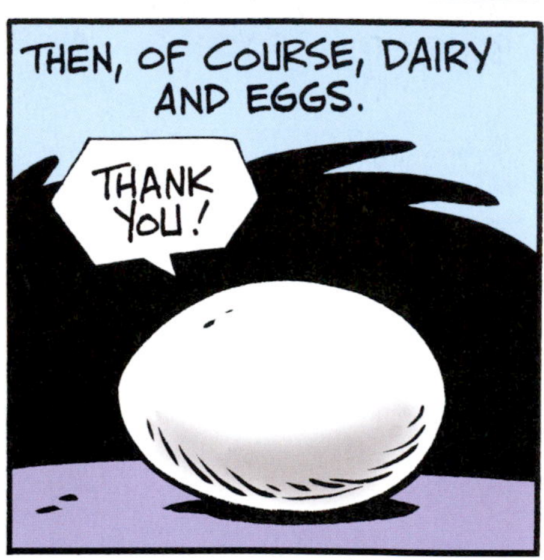
THEN, OF COURSE, DAIRY AND EGGS.
THANK YOU!

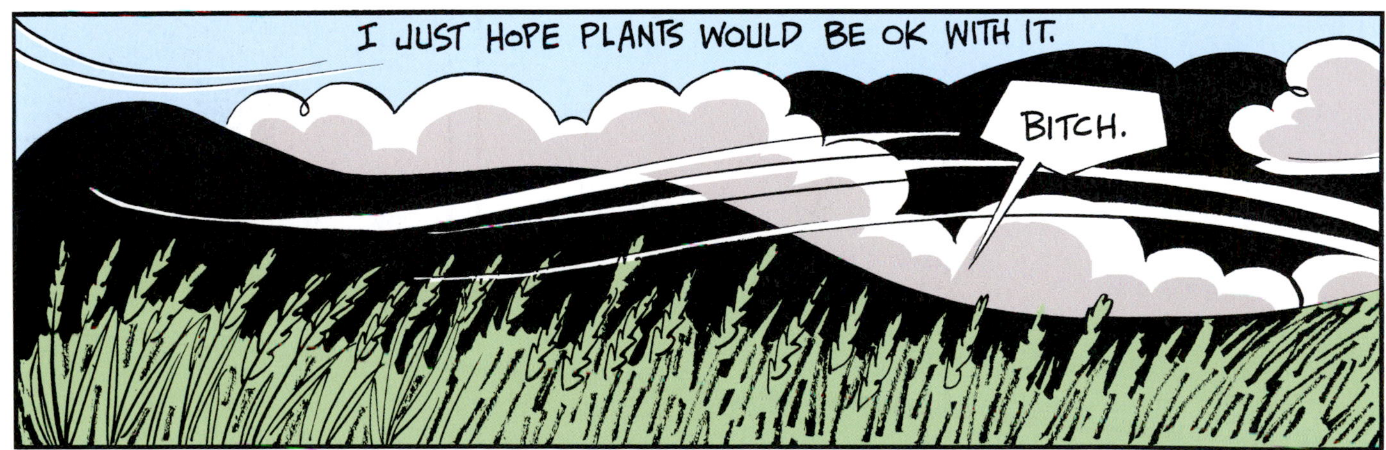
I JUST HOPE PLANTS WOULD BE OK WITH IT.
BITCH.

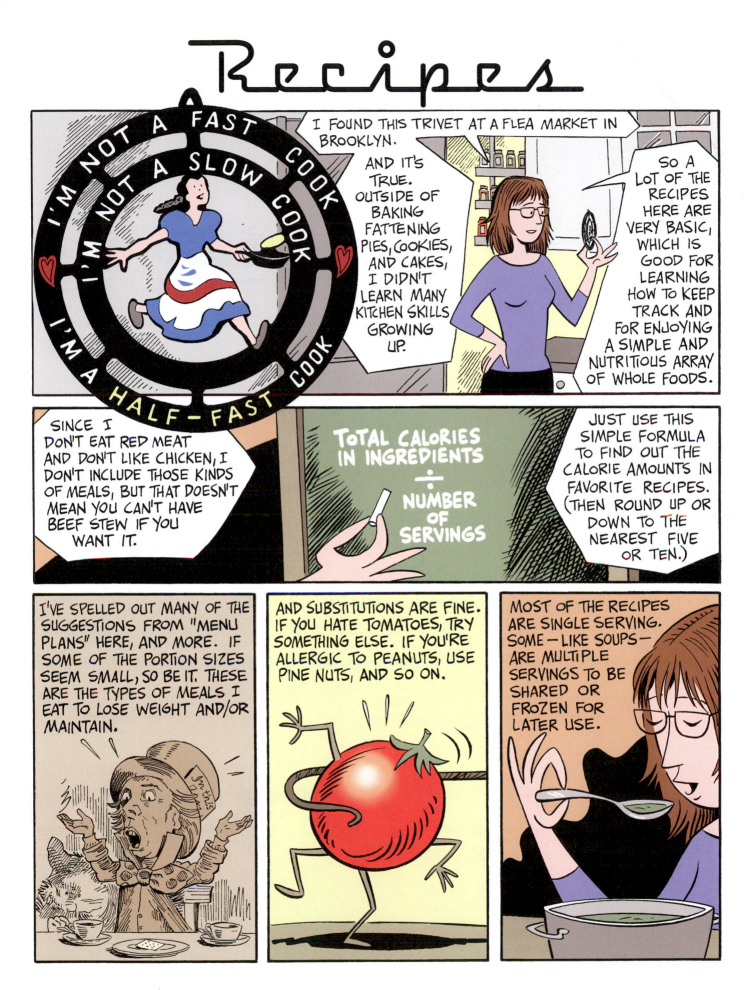

# Recipes

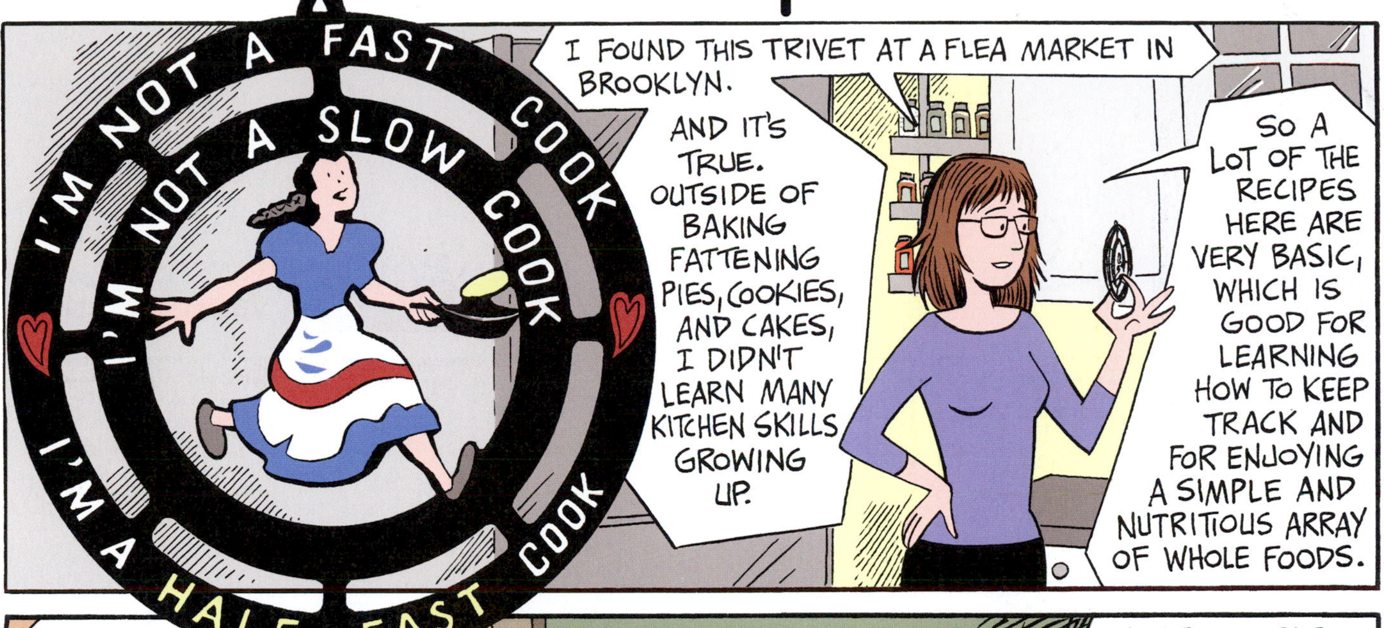

I'M NOT A FAST COOK
I'M NOT A SLOW COOK
I'M A HALF-FAST COOK
I FOUND THIS TRIVET AT A FLEA MARKET IN BROOKLYN.
AND IT'S TRUE. OUTSIDE OF BAKING FATTENING PIES, COOKIES, AND CAKES, I DIDN'T LEARN MANY KITCHEN SKILLS GROWING UP.
SO A LOT OF THE RECIPES HERE ARE VERY BASIC, WHICH IS GOOD FOR LEARNING HOW TO KEEP TRACK AND FOR ENJOYING A SIMPLE AND NUTRITIOUS ARRAY OF WHOLE FOODS.

SINCE I DON'T EAT RED MEAT AND DON'T LIKE CHICKEN, I DON'T INCLUDE THOSE KINDS OF MEALS, BUT THAT DOESN'T MEAN YOU CAN'T HAVE BEEF STEW IF YOU WANT IT.

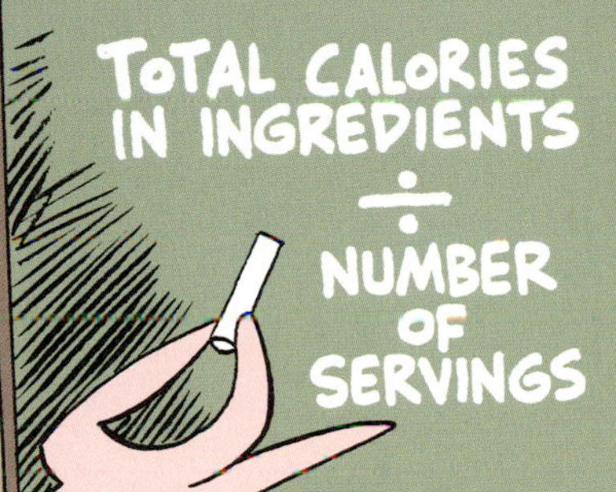


JUST USE THIS SIMPLE FORMULA TO FIND OUT THE CALORIE AMOUNTS IN FAVORITE RECIPES. (THEN ROUND UP OR DOWN TO THE NEAREST FIVE OR TEN.)

I'VE SPELLED OUT MANY OF THE SUGGESTIONS FROM "MENU PLANS" HERE, AND MORE. IF SOME OF THE PORTION SIZES SEEM SMALL, SO BE IT. THESE ARE THE TYPES OF MEALS I EAT TO LOSE WEIGHT AND/OR MAINTAIN.

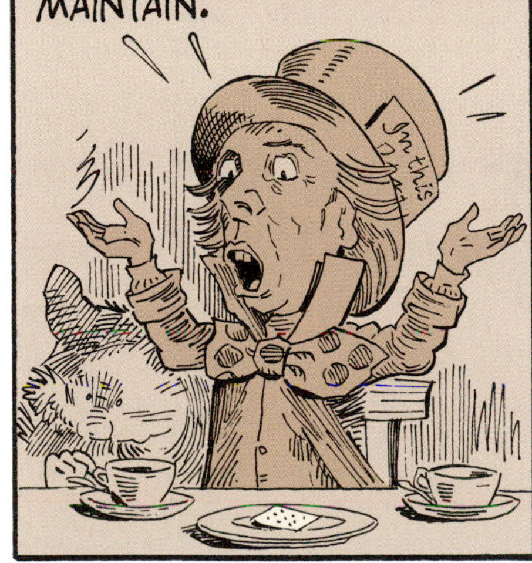

AND SUBSTITUTIONS ARE FINE. IF YOU HATE TOMATOES, TRY SOMETHING ELSE. IF YOU'RE ALLERGIC TO PEANUTS, USE PINE NUTS, AND SO ON.

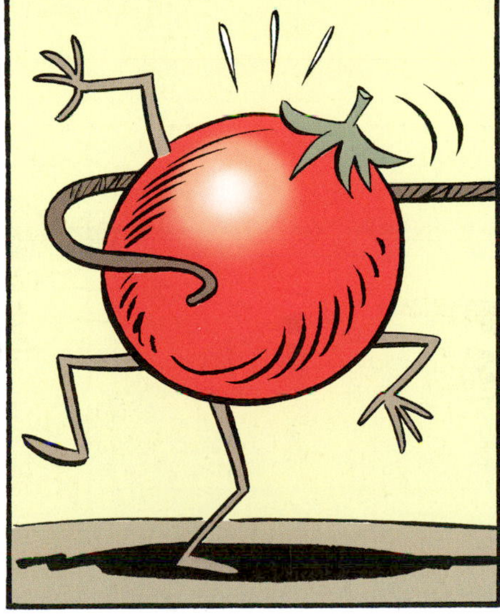

MOST OF THE RECIPES ARE SINGLE SERVING. SOME—LIKE SOUPS—ARE MULTIPLE SERVINGS TO BE SHARED OR FROZEN FOR LATER USE.

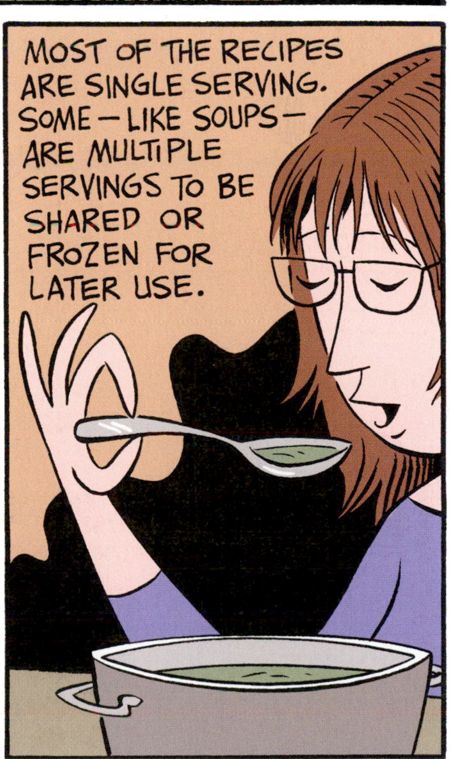

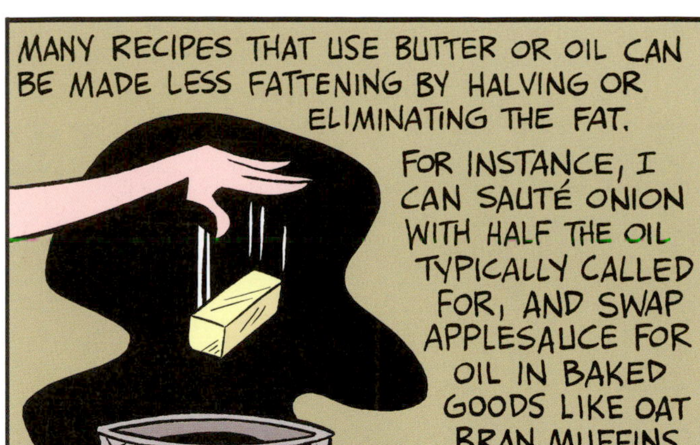
MANY RECIPES THAT USE BUTTER OR OIL CAN BE MADE LESS FATTENING BY HALVING OR ELIMINATING THE FAT.
FOR INSTANCE, I CAN SAUTÉ ONION WITH HALF THE OIL TYPICALLY CALLED FOR, AND SWAP APPLESAUCE FOR OIL IN BAKED GOODS LIKE OAT BRAN MUFFINS.

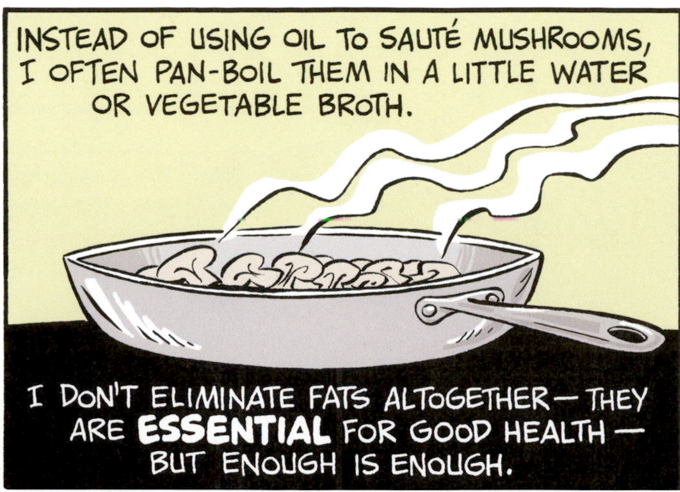
INSTEAD OF USING OIL TO SAUTÉ MUSHROOMS, I OFTEN PAN-BOIL THEM IN A LITTLE WATER OR VEGETABLE BROTH.
I DON'T ELIMINATE FATS ALTOGETHER—THEY ARE ESSENTIAL FOR GOOD HEALTH—BUT ENOUGH IS ENOUGH.

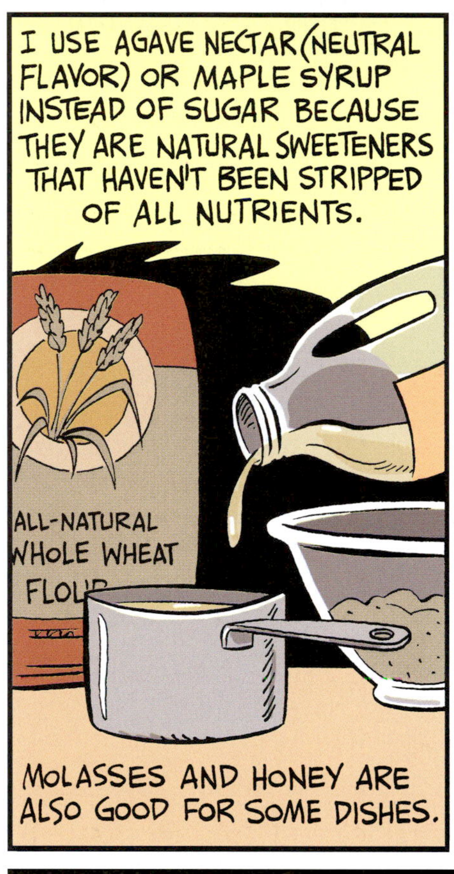
I USE AGAVE NECTAR (NEUTRAL FLAVOR) OR MAPLE SYRUP INSTEAD OF SUGAR BECAUSE THEY ARE NATURAL SWEETENERS THAT HAVEN'T BEEN STRIPPED OF ALL NUTRIENTS.
ALL-NATURAL WHOLE WHEAT
MOLASSES AND HONEY ARE ALSO GOOD FOR SOME DISHES.

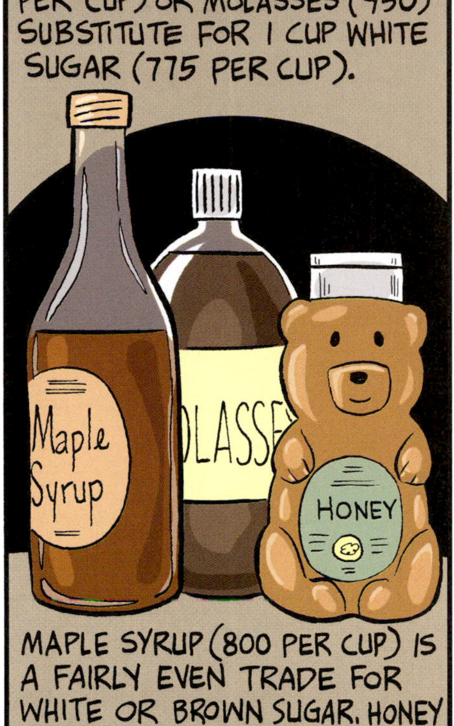
3/4 CUP AGAVE NECTAR (960 PER CUP) OR MOLASSES (950) SUBSTITUTE FOR 1 CUP WHITE SUGAR (775 PER CUP).
Maple Syrup
HONEY
MAPLE SYRUP (800 PER CUP) IS A FAIRLY EVEN TRADE FOR WHITE OR BROWN SUGAR. HONEY COMES IN AT 1,030 PER CUP.

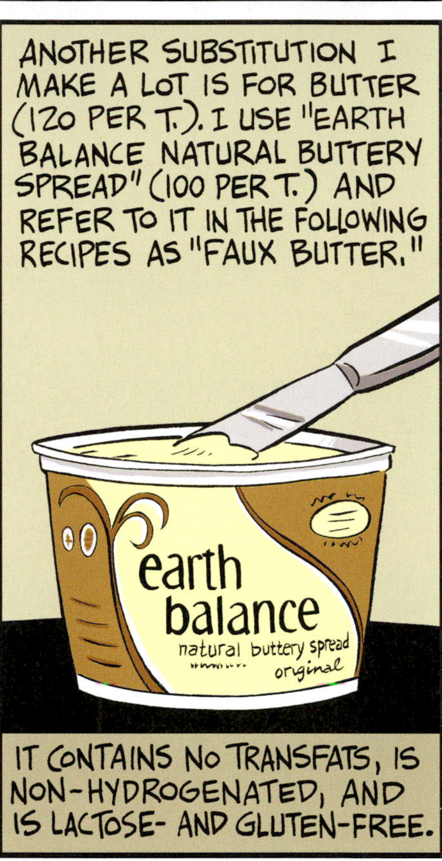
ANOTHER SUBSTITUTION I MAKE A LOT IS FOR BUTTER (120 PER T.). I USE "EARTH BALANCE NATURAL BUTTERY SPREAD" (100 PER T.) AND REFER TO IT IN THE FOLLOWING RECIPES AS "FAUX BUTTER."
earth balance
natural buttery spread
original
IT CONTAINS NO TRANSFATS, IS NON-HYDROGENATED, AND IS LACTOSE- AND GLUTEN-FREE.

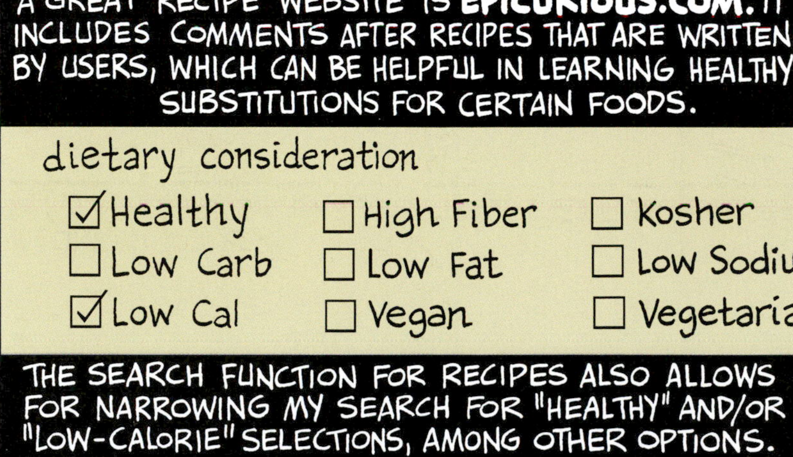
A GREAT RECIPE WEBSITE IS EPICURIOUS.COM. IT INCLUDES COMMENTS AFTER RECIPES THAT ARE WRITTEN BY USERS, WHICH CAN BE HELPFUL IN LEARNING HEALTHY SUBSTITUTIONS FOR CERTAIN FOODS.
dietary consideration
☑ Healthy
☐ High Fiber
☐ Kosher
☐ Low Carb
☐ Low Fat
☐ Low Sodiu
☑ Low Cal
☐ Vegan
☐ Vegetaria
THE SEARCH FUNCTION FOR RECIPES ALSO ALLOWS FOR NARROWING MY SEARCH FOR "HEALTHY" AND/OR "LOW-CALORIE" SELECTIONS, AMONG OTHER OPTIONS.

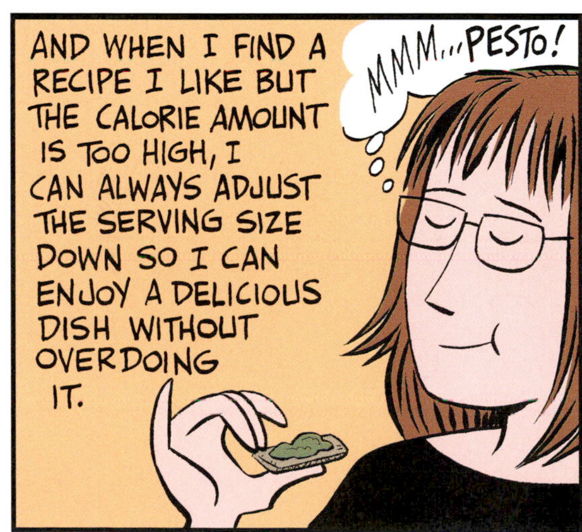
AND WHEN I FIND A RECIPE I LIKE BUT THE CALORIE AMOUNT IS TOO HIGH, I CAN ALWAYS ADJUST THE SERVING SIZE DOWN SO I CAN ENJOY A DELICIOUS DISH WITHOUT OVERDOING IT.
MMM...PESTO!

# Cooking for Rookies

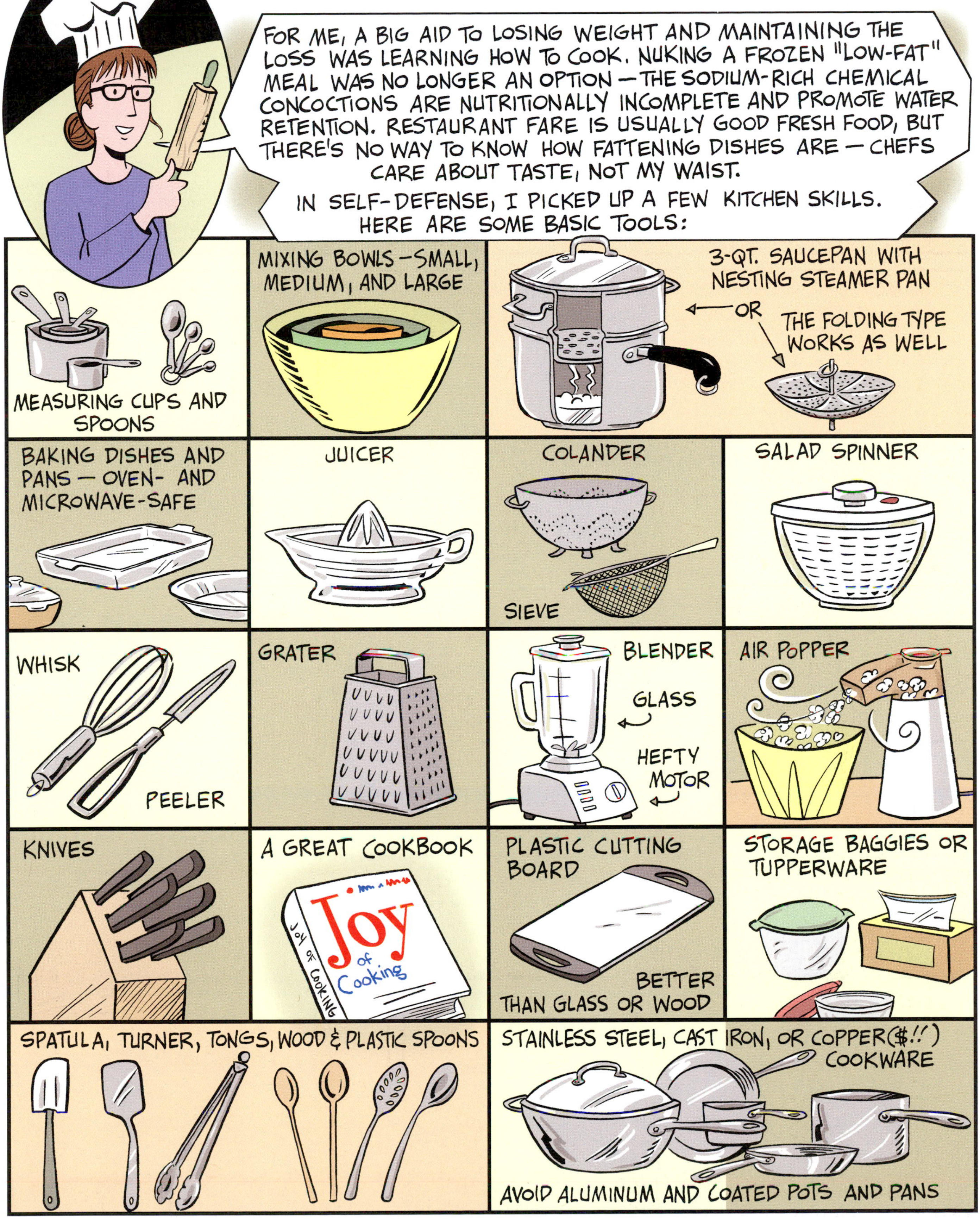

FOR ME, A BIG AID TO LOSING WEIGHT AND MAINTAINING THE LOSS WAS LEARNING HOW TO COOK. NUKING A FROZEN "LOW-FAT" MEAL WAS NO LONGER AN OPTION — THE SODIUM-RICH CHEMICAL CONCOCTIONS ARE NUTRITIONALLY INCOMPLETE AND PROMOTE WATER RETENTION. RESTAURANT FARE IS USUALLY GOOD FRESH FOOD, BUT THERE'S NO WAY TO KNOW HOW FATTENING DISHES ARE — CHEFS CARE ABOUT TASTE, NOT MY WAIST.

IN SELF-DEFENSE, I PICKED UP A FEW KITCHEN SKILLS. HERE ARE SOME BASIC TOOLS:

MEASURING CUPS AND SPOONS

MIXING BOWLS — SMALL, MEDIUM, AND LARGE

3-QT. SAUCEPAN WITH NESTING STEAMER PAN

OR

THE FOLDING TYPE WORKS AS WELL

BAKING DISHES AND PANS — OVEN- AND MICROWAVE-SAFE

JUICER

COLANDER

SIEVE

SALAD SPINNER

WHISK

PEELER

GRATER

BLENDER

GLASS

HEFTY MOTOR

AIR POPPER

KNIVES

A GREAT COOKBOOK

Joy of Cooking

PLASTIC CUTTING BOARD

BETTER THAN GLASS OR WOOD

STORAGE BAGGIES OR TUPPERWARE

SPATULA, TURNER, TONGS, WOOD & PLASTIC SPOONS

STAINLESS STEEL, CAST IRON, OR COPPER ($!!) COOKWARE

AVOID ALUMINUM AND COATED POTS AND PANS

# Breakfasts

I CAN EAT ANY OF THESE MEALS AT ANY TIME OF DAY, BUT SOMEHOW THEY SEEM TO FIT BETTER WITH MORNING.

## EGG MUFFIN WITH VEGGIE SAUSAGE AND CHEESE

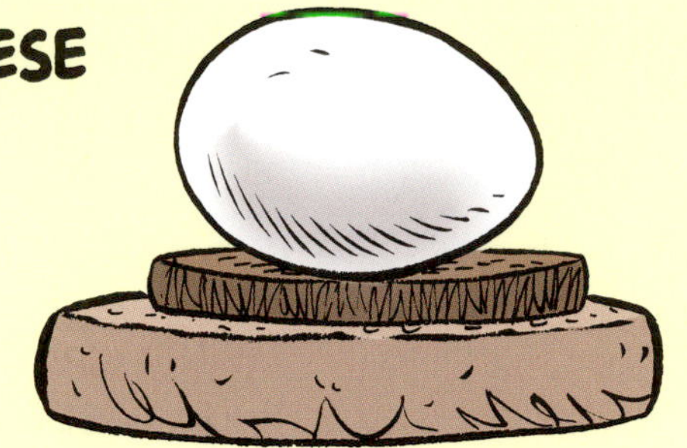

| | |
|---|---|
| 1 EGG, MINUS HALF THE YOLK | 50 |
| 1 VEGGIE SAUSAGE PATTY | 70 |
| ½ WHOLE-WHEAT ENGLISH MUFFIN | 80 |
| ½ OZ. REDUCED-FAT WHITE CHEDDAR | 35 |
| A SHORT BLAST OF SPRAY OIL | 15 |

COOK PATTY IN MICROWAVE OR OVEN, AS PER INSTRUCTIONS ON PACKAGE. WHILE PATTY COOKS, SEPARATE THE YOLK FROM THE EGG WHITE. BREAK THE YOLK AND SCOOP OUT 1½ tsp.; THROW THAT OUT. ADD REMAINING YOLK TO EGG WHITE; ADD A SPLASH OF MILK, SOY MILK, OR WATER; SALT AND PEPPER TO TASTE.
HEAT OMELET PAN OVER MEDIUM HEAT, ADD A SHORT BLAST OF SPRAY OIL, AND SCRAMBLE THAT EGG. LIGHTLY TOAST THE MUFFIN, THEN TOP IT WITH EGG, CHEESE, AND VEGGIE SAUSAGE. BAKE AT 375°F OR BROIL FOR A MINUTE OR UNTIL CHEESE MELTS. A DASH OF HOT SAUCE NEVER HURTS.

TOTAL: 250

## YOGURT AND FRUIT PARFAIT

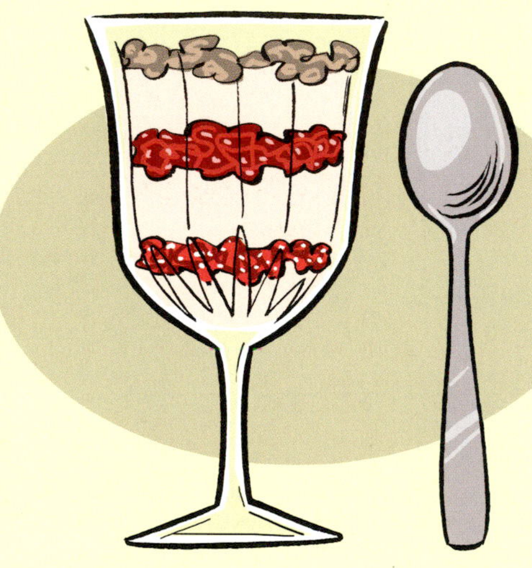

| | |
|---|---|
| ½ CUP PLAIN NON-FAT YOGURT | 60 |
| ½ tsp. AGAVE NECTAR* OR HONEY | 10 |
| 1 SMALL SCOOP STEVIA* | Ø |
| 2 T. POMEGRANATE SEEDS** | 15 |
| 5 CHERRIES, PITTED AND CHOPPED | 20 |
| 2 T. GRANOLA (IF ½ CUP IS 200) | 50 |

TOTAL: 155

* AVAILABLE IN BETTER MARKETS AND HEALTH FOOD STORES.

** AVAILABLE IN SEEDS-ONLY PACKAGES AT MANY MARKETS DURING WINTER MONTHS.

## DEREK'S SMOOTHIE

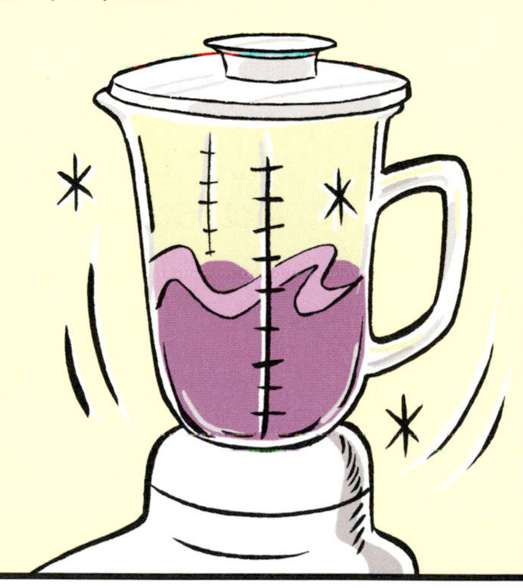

| | |
|---|---|
| ½ BANANA | 50 |
| ¼ CUP ORANGE JUICE | 30 |
| ¼ CUP FAT-FREE VANILLA YOGURT | 45 |
| ¼ CUP BLUEBERRIES, FRESH OR FROZEN | 20 |
| ¼ CUP FROZEN MIXED BERRIES | 20 |

PUREÉ ALL IN BLENDER, THE FROZEN BERRIES ADD A REFRESHING CHILL.

TOTAL: 165

## FRENCH TOAST

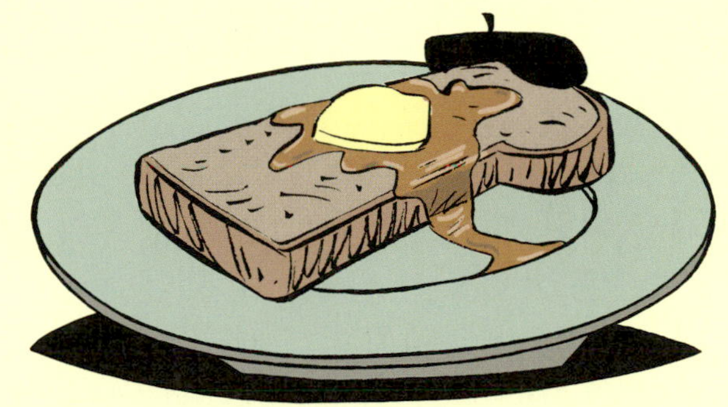

| | |
|---|---|
| 1/2 EGG | 35 |
| 1/2 SLICE WHOLE-GRAIN BREAD | 40 |
| SPLASH OF MILK OR SOY MILK | 5 |
| PINCH OF CINNAMON | Ø |
| 1/2 tsp. BUTTER (GENEROUS) | 20 |
| 1 tsp. MAPLE SYRUP | 15 |
| A SHORT BLAST OF SPRAY OIL | 15 |

WHISK TOGETHER EGG, MILK, AND CINNAMON. SOAK BREAD IN MIX. HEAT SKILLET OVER MEDIUM HEAT AND SPRAY WITH OIL. FRY THE BATTERED BREAD ON BOTH SIDES UNTIL COOKED THROUGH. SERVE WITH BUTTER (OR FAUX BUTTER) AND SYRUP.

TOTAL: 130

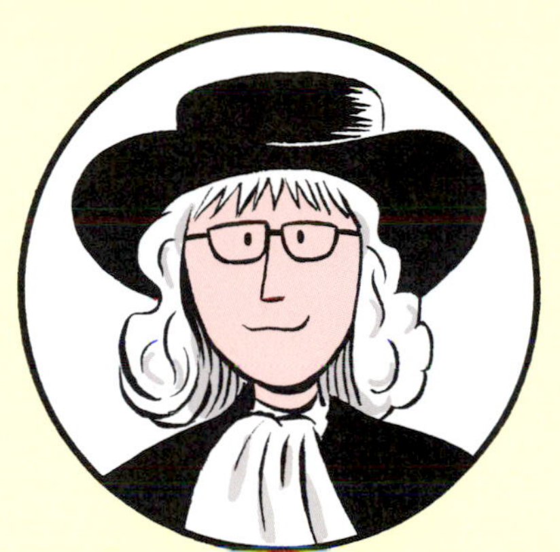

## OATMEAL, FULLY LOADED

| | |
|---|---|
| 2/3 CUP WATER | |
| DASH SALT | |
| 1/3 CUP "OLD-FASHIONED" OATS | 100 |
| 1/4 APPLE, CHOPPED, NO SKIN | 20 |
| 1 T. PECANS, CHOPPED | 50 |
| 1 1/2 tsp. MAPLE SYRUP | 25 |
| 1/4 CUP SOY MILK OR NON-FAT MILK | 25 |
| PINCH OF CINNAMON | Ø |
| 1 SMALL SCOOP STEVIA | Ø |

BOIL WATER IN SMALL SAUCEPAN WITH A PINCH OF SALT. TOSS IN OATS, REDUCE HEAT TO LOW AND SIMMER. ADD APPLE, CINNAMON, AND STEVIA; CONTINUE COOKING UNTIL EXCESS WATER IS GONE. TRANSFER TO BOWL; ADD NUTS, SYRUP, AND MILK.

TOTAL: 220

## MAPLE WALNUT GRANOLA

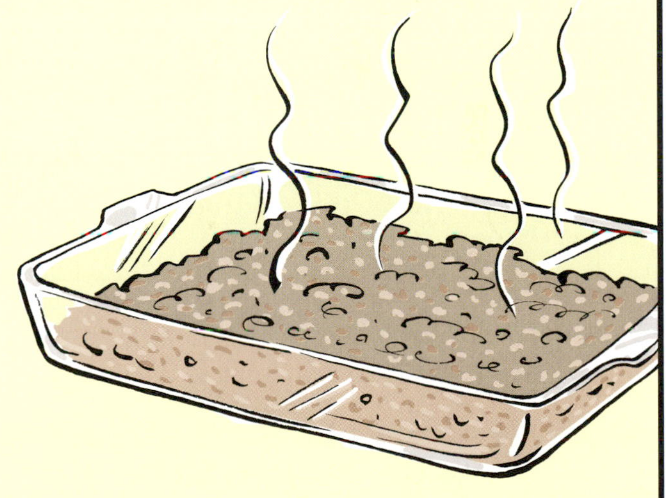

| | |
|---|---|
| 1 1/2 CUP ROLLED OATS | 450 |
| 1/2 CUP WHEAT GERM | 130 |
| 1/4 CUP WALNUTS, CHOPPED | 200 |
| 1/4 CUP RAISINS | 125 |
| 1/4 CUP DRIED CRANBERRIES | 100 |
| 2 T. SESAME SEEDS | 60 |
| 2 T. MAPLE SYRUP | 100 |
| 1 T. MOLASSES | 60 |
| 1/2 tsp. CINNAMON | Ø |

PREHEAT OVEN TO 300°F. STIR ALL INGREDIENTS TOGETHER IN A LARGE MIXING BOWL (ORDER DOES NOT MATTER), THEN TRANSFER TO A 9" X 13" CASSEROLE DISH. BAKE FOR 25 MINUTES, OR UNTIL THE GRANOLA HAS TURNED GOLDEN BROWN. MIX SEVERAL TIMES WITH A SPATULA THROUGHOUT THE BAKING PROCESS.

MAKES 3 CUPS. TOTAL PER 1/2 CUP: 205

## OAT BRAN CEREAL (HOT)

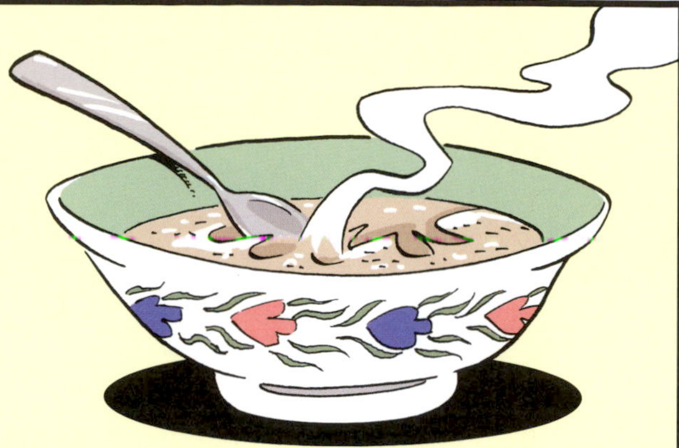

| | |
|---|---|
| 2/3 CUP WATER | |
| 1/3 CUP OAT BRAN | 100 |
| DASH SALT | Ø |
| 1 SMALL SCOOP STEVIA | Ø |
| 1 1/2 tsp. MAPLE SYRUP | 25 |
| 1/4 CUP SOY MILK OR NON-FAT MILK | 25 |

COOK PER INSTRUCTIONS ON BOX. TOTAL: 150

## EGG WITH SPINACH AND MOZZARELLA ON WHOLE-GRAIN TOAST

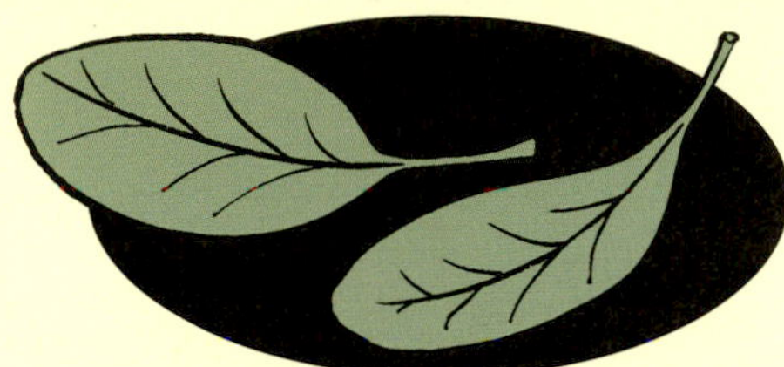

| | |
|---|---|
| 2 1/2 CUPS RAW SPINACH | 20 |
| 1 EGG | 70 |
| 1/2 OZ. MOZZARELLA CHEESE | 35 |
| 1 SLICE WHOLE-GRAIN TOAST | 80 |
| A SHORT BLAST OF SPRAY OIL | 15 |

RINSE SPINACH AND TRIM STEMS. PLACE IN BASKET STEAMER OR STEAMER PAN WITH 1/2" BOILING WATER IN SAUCEPAN; STEAM FOR 7 MINUTES. TURN ON BOILER TO HIGH. HEAT SKILLET OVER MEDIUM HEAT, SPRAY WITH OIL, AND FRY EGG SUNNYSIDE UP OR OVER EASY. SPOON STEAMED SPINACH ONTO TOAST, TOP WITH EGG AND CHEESE. USING OVEN-SAFE PLATE OR PAN, PLACE UNDER BROILER FOR A MINUTE OR UNTIL CHEESE MELTS.

TOTAL: 220

## PEANUT BUTTER NUTTY FRUIT BARS

THESE ARE <u>TOO</u> GOOD—USE SPARINGLY. GREAT FOR TRAVEL, WORK, HIKES—ANY TIME OF DAY.

| | |
|---|---|
| MEDIUM BLAST OF SPRAY OIL | 25 |
| 3 CUPS PUFFED GRAIN CEREAL | 240 |
| 1/4 CUP WALNUTS, CHOPPED | 210 |
| 1/4 CUP PECANS, CHOPPED | 150 |
| 1/4 CUP DATES, CHOPPED | 225 |
| 1/4 CUP DRIED CRANBERRIES | 100 |
| 1/4 CUP RAISINS | 130 |
| 1/3 CUP PEANUT BUTTER | 535 |
| 1/4 CUP HONEY | 240 |
| 1/4 CUP AGAVE NECTAR | 240 |
| 2 T. SESAME SEEDS | 60 |

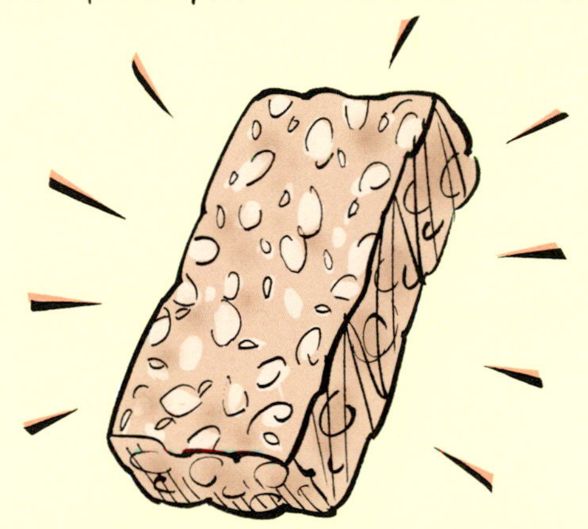

PREHEAT OVEN TO 350°F. SPRAY 9" SQUARE BAKING PAN WITH OIL (<u>NOT</u> OLIVE OIL). MIX CEREAL, NUTS, AND FRUITS IN LARGE BOWL. COMBINE PEANUT BUTTER, HONEY, AND AGAVE NECTAR IN SAUCEPAN. BRING TO BOIL AND CONTINUE COOKING ON FAIRLY HIGH HEAT FOR ABOUT A MINUTE, WHISKING CONSTANTLY, UNTIL MIXTURE BUBBLES VIGOROUSLY AND THICKENS SLIGHTLY. FOLD PEANUT BUTTER GOO INTO CEREAL MIX AND BLEND. SCOOP MIXTURE INTO OILED PAN AND PRESS TO MAKE IT COMPACT. SPRINKLE WITH SESAME SEEDS AND BAKE FOR 10 MINUTES. COOL COMPLETELY, THEN CUT INTO 20 PIECES.

TOTAL: 110 PER PIECE

## POACHED EGG ON TOAST WITH CHEESE

I DON'T HAVE AN EGG POACHER. I LIGHTLY COAT THE INSIDE OF A CUSTARD CUP WITH BUTTERY SPREAD SO THE EGG DOESN'T STICK AND PLACE IT IN THE STEAMER PAN FOR 5 OR 6 MINUTES.

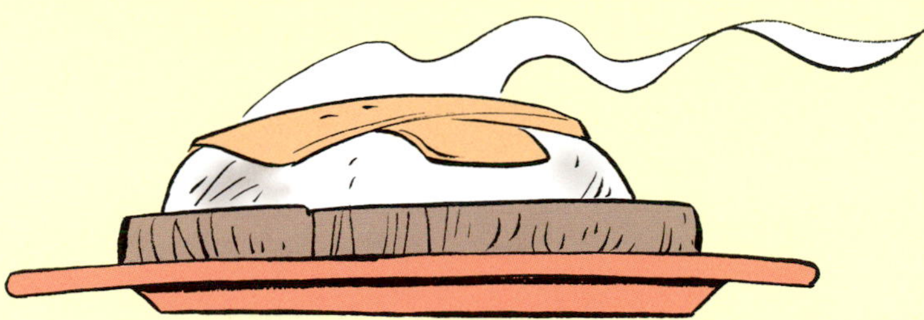

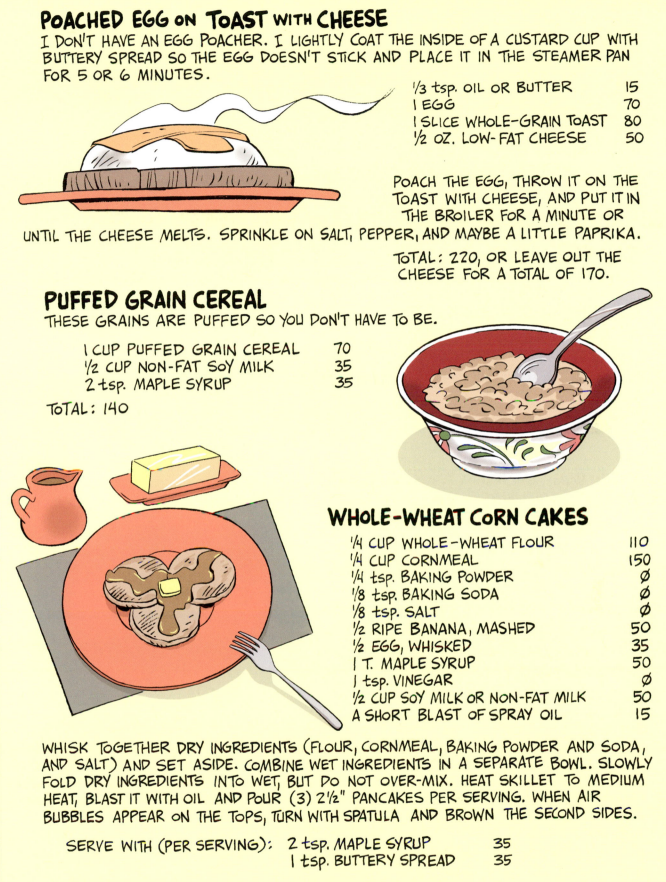

| | |
|---|---|
| 1/3 tsp. OIL OR BUTTER | 15 |
| 1 EGG | 70 |
| 1 SLICE WHOLE-GRAIN TOAST | 80 |
| 1/2 OZ. LOW-FAT CHEESE | 50 |

POACH THE EGG, THROW IT ON THE TOAST WITH CHEESE, AND PUT IT IN THE BROILER FOR A MINUTE OR UNTIL THE CHEESE MELTS. SPRINKLE ON SALT, PEPPER, AND MAYBE A LITTLE PAPRIKA.

TOTAL: 220, OR LEAVE OUT THE CHEESE FOR A TOTAL OF 170.

## PUFFED GRAIN CEREAL

THESE GRAINS ARE PUFFED SO YOU DON'T HAVE TO BE.

| | |
|---|---|
| 1 CUP PUFFED GRAIN CEREAL | 70 |
| 1/2 CUP NON-FAT SOY MILK | 35 |
| 2 tsp. MAPLE SYRUP | 35 |

TOTAL: 140

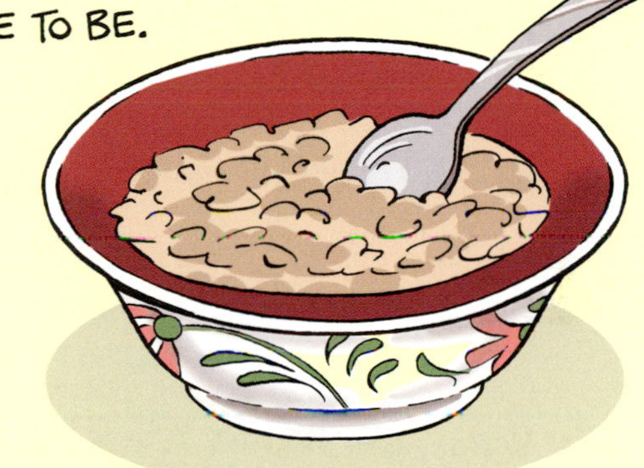

## WHOLE-WHEAT CORN CAKES

| | |
|---|---|
| 1/4 CUP WHOLE-WHEAT FLOUR | 110 |
| 1/4 CUP CORNMEAL | 150 |
| 1/4 tsp. BAKING POWDER | Ø |
| 1/8 tsp. BAKING SODA | Ø |
| 1/8 tsp. SALT | Ø |
| 1/2 RIPE BANANA, MASHED | 50 |
| 1/2 EGG, WHISKED | 35 |
| 1 T. MAPLE SYRUP | 50 |
| 1 tsp. VINEGAR | Ø |
| 1/2 CUP SOY MILK OR NON-FAT MILK | 50 |
| A SHORT BLAST OF SPRAY OIL | 15 |

WHISK TOGETHER DRY INGREDIENTS (FLOUR, CORNMEAL, BAKING POWDER AND SODA, AND SALT) AND SET ASIDE. COMBINE WET INGREDIENTS IN A SEPARATE BOWL. SLOWLY FOLD DRY INGREDIENTS INTO WET, BUT DO NOT OVER-MIX. HEAT SKILLET TO MEDIUM HEAT, BLAST IT WITH OIL AND POUR (3) 2½" PANCAKES PER SERVING. WHEN AIR BUBBLES APPEAR ON THE TOPS, TURN WITH SPATULA AND BROWN THE SECOND SIDES.

| SERVE WITH (PER SERVING): | |
|---|---|
| 2 tsp. MAPLE SYRUP | 35 |
| 1 tsp. BUTTERY SPREAD | 35 |

TOTAL: 200 FOR 3 PANCAKES WITH BUTTER AND SYRUP

## SCRAMBLED EGG WHITES WITH TURKEY BACON

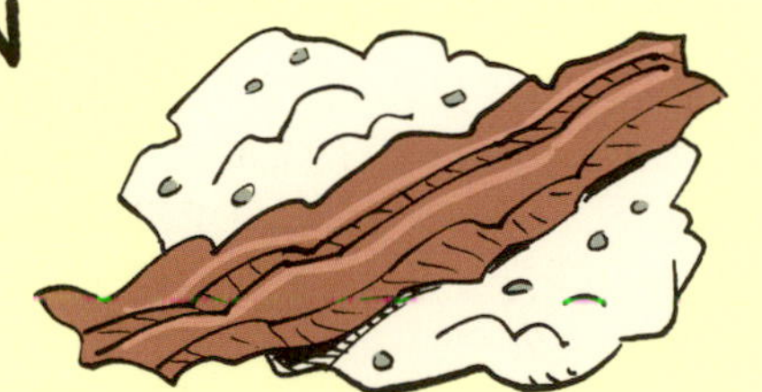

| | |
|---|---|
| 2 EGG WHITES | 30 |
| 1½ tsp. GREEN ONION TOPS, CHOPPED | Ø |
| 1 STRIP TURKEY BACON | 35 |
| A SHORT BLAST OF SPRAY OIL | 15 |

SCRAMBLE THE WHITES IN OILED SKILLET WITH ONION BITS OVER MEDIUM HEAT. NO NEED FOR MORE OIL TO FRY BACON. SALT AND PEPPER TO TASTE.

TOTAL: 80

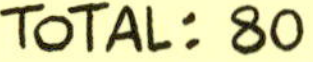

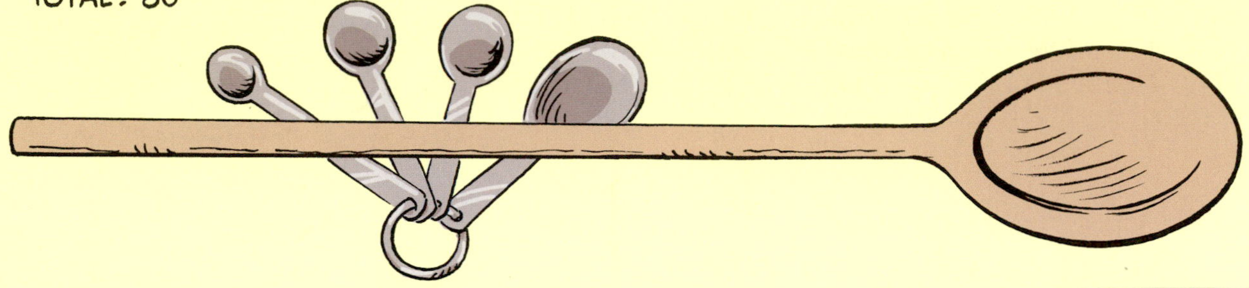

## WHOLE-WHEAT BRAN MUFFINS WITH DATES AND PECANS

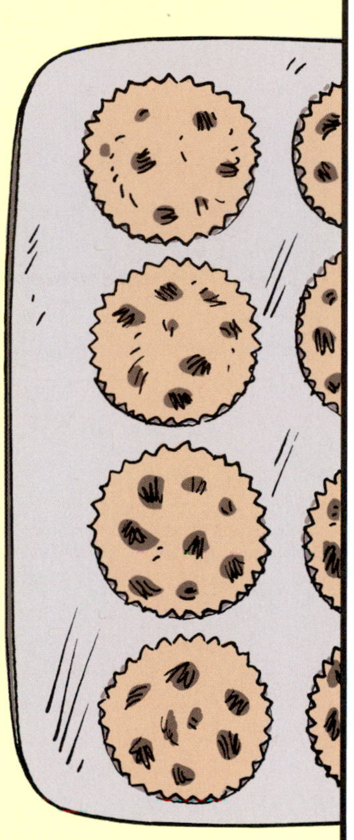

| | |
|---|---|
| A SHORT BLAST OF SPRAY OIL | 15 |
| ½ CUP + 2 T. WHOLE WHEAT FLOUR | 275 |
| 2 T. ALL-PURPOSE (WHITE) FLOUR | 50 |
| ¼ CUP OAT BRAN | 75 |
| 1 tsp. CINNAMON | 5 |
| 1 tsp. BAKING POWDER | 3 |
| ½ tsp. BAKING SODA | Ø |
| ¼ tsp. SALT | Ø |
| ½ CUP (PACKED) MEDJOOL DATES, CHOPPED | 550 |
| ¼ CUP PECANS, CHOPPED | 205 |
| ¼ CUP BROWN SUGAR, PACKED | 180 |
| ¼ CUP UNSWEETENED APPLESAUCE | 25 |
| 1 LARGE EGG | 70 |
| ½ CUP PLAIN NON-FAT YOGURT | 60 |
| 1½ tsp. VANILLA EXTRACT | 20 |
| ¼ tsp. GRATED LEMON PEEL | Ø |

PREHEAT OVEN TO 400°F. FILL 8 MUFFIN CUPS WITH PAPER LINERS THAT YOU HAVE ALREADY BLASTED WITH OIL. COMBINE ALL DRY INGREDIENTS (FLOURS, OAT BRAN, CINNAMON, BAKING POWDER AND SODA, AND SALT) IN A MIXING BOWL, THEN STIR IN DATES AND NUTS. IN ANOTHER BOWL, STIR TOGETHER SUGAR AND APPLESAUCE, THEN WHISK IN ONE AT A TIME THE EGG, YOGURT, VANILLA, AND LEMON PEEL. FOLD THE DRY INGREDIENTS INTO THE WET UNTIL JUST COMBINED. DIVIDE BATTER BETWEEN THE 8 CUPS. BAKE UNTIL GOLDEN BROWN, ABOUT 18 MINUTES, OR UNTIL A TOOTH-PICK INSERTED IN THE CENTER COMES OUT CLEAN.

TOTAL: 190 PER MUFFIN

## PROTEIN PUDDING

| | |
|---|---|
| ½ CUP NON-FAT PLAIN YOGURT | 60 |
| ¼ CUP UNSWEETENED APPLESAUCE | 25 |
| ⅙ APPLE, CHOPPED, NO SKIN | 10 |
| 1 SCOOP SOY PROTEIN POWDER | 65 |
| 2 tsp. AGAVE NECTAR | 40 |
| PINCH CINNAMON | Ø |
| DASH NUTMEG | Ø |

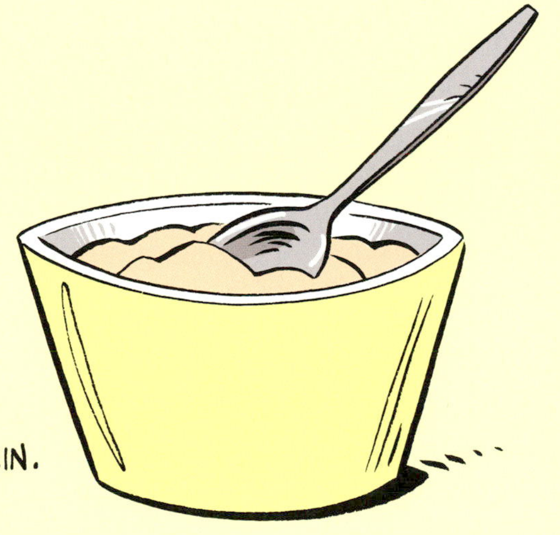

MIX ALL INGREDIENTS TOGETHER, CHILL FOR 20 MINUTES. THIS HIGH-PROTEIN "PUDDING" IS A LITTLE GRAINY FROM THE SOY POWDER, BUT I DON'T CARE—IT SATISFIES MY SWEET TOOTH AND PACKS IN 21g. PROTEIN.

TOTAL: 200

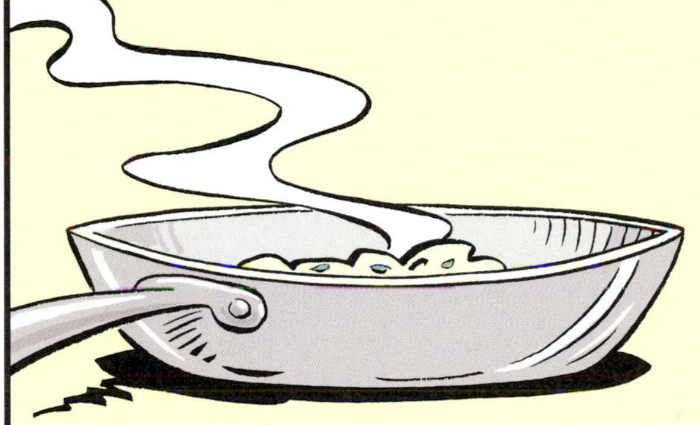

## EGG-WHITE SCRAMBLE

| | |
|---|---|
| 2 EGG WHITES | 35 |
| A SPLASH OF MILK OR SOY MILK | 5 |
| 2 tsp. GREEN ONION, CHOPPED | Ø |
| A SHORT BLAST OF SPRAY OIL | 10 |
| ¼ OZ. REDUCED-FAT CHEDDAR CHEESE | 20 |

WHISK TOGETHER EGG WHITES AND MILK UNTIL FAIRLY FROTHY. HEAT SKILLET OVER MEDIUM HEAT. SPRAY WITH OIL. SAUTÉ ONION FOR 1 MINUTE. ADD EGG WHITES AND COOK UNTIL SOLIDIFIED. TURN DOWN HEAT TO LOW. PLACE CHEESE ON TOP OF SCRAMBLED EGG WHITES, COVER, AND COOK UNTIL CHEESE MELTS, ABOUT 1 MINUTE. SALT AND PEPPER TO TASTE.

TOTAL: 70

## MANGO PROTEIN SMOOTHIE

THIS TASTES SOMEWHAT LIKE THE MANGO "MILKSHAKES" I LIKE AT INDIAN RESTAURANTS. IT'S ULTRA-FILLING, SO I DRINK HALF AND REFRIGERATE THE REST FOR LATER.

| | |
|---|---|
| ¼ CUP PLAIN NON-FAT YOGURT | 30 |
| ¼ CUP SOY MILK | 25 |
| ¼ CUP MANGO NECTAR (CANNED)* | 70 |
| ½ CUP MANGO SORBET | 100 |
| 1 T. SOY PROTEIN POWDER | 20 |
| ½ tsp. AGAVE NECTAR OR HONEY | 10 |

PUT IT ALL IN THE BLENDER AND PULSE UNTIL SMOOTH.

TOTAL: 255

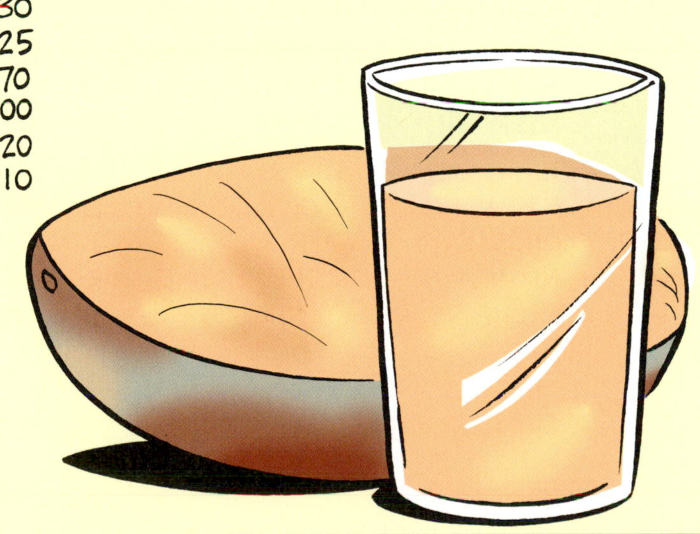

* AVAILABLE IN ETHNIC FOODS SECTIONS IN MANY MARKETS

# Entrées

**WOW**—NOT A SINGLE CHICKEN, PORK, OR BEEF DISH HERE, BUT THAT'S BECAUSE I NO LONGER EAT THEM. MY DIET IS ALWAYS EVOLVING, AND FOR ME THAT MEANS I EAT LESS AND LESS ANIMAL PROTEIN. REASONS WHY INCLUDE LEARNING MORE ABOUT NUTRITION (WE DON'T NEED AS MUCH PROTEIN AS FOOD LOBBYISTS WANT US TO BELIEVE), HEALTH CONSIDERATIONS (MEAT ANIMALS ARE PUMPED FULL OF ANTIBIOTICS AND HORMONES), AND EMPATHY FOR OTHER CREATURES (I'VE STILL GOT A WAY TO GO—I'M WORKING ON IT, FISH AND FOWL).

## SALMON ON MIXED GREENS

| | |
|---|---|
| 3 OZ. SALMON FILLET | 150 |
| 2 CUPS MIXED GREENS | 15 |
| 1 SLICE (ACROSS) RED ONION | 5 |
| 4 ASPARAGUS SPEARS | 20 |
| 4 tsp. HONEY MUSTARD DRESSING | 60 |
| A SHORT BLAST OF SPRAY OIL | 10 |

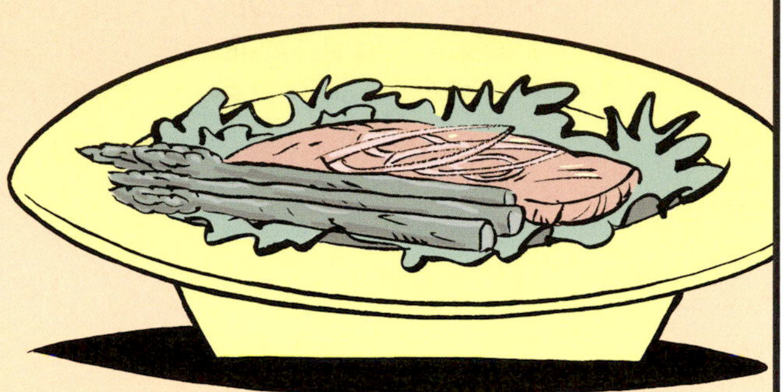

BROIL SALMON FILLET ON HIGH TO DESIRED DONENESS, ABOUT 6 MINUTES, TURNING MIDWAY. HEAT SKILLET OVER MEDIUM HEAT AND SPRAY WITH OIL. LIGHTLY SAUTÉ ONION AND PLACE ON BED OF WASHED AND SPUN-DRY GREENS. STEAM OR PAN-BOIL ASPARAGUS FOR 4 MINUTES AND PLACE ON SALAD BED ALONGSIDE SALMON. DRIZZLE DRESSING ON TOP; SALT AND PEPPER TO TASTE.

TOTAL: 260

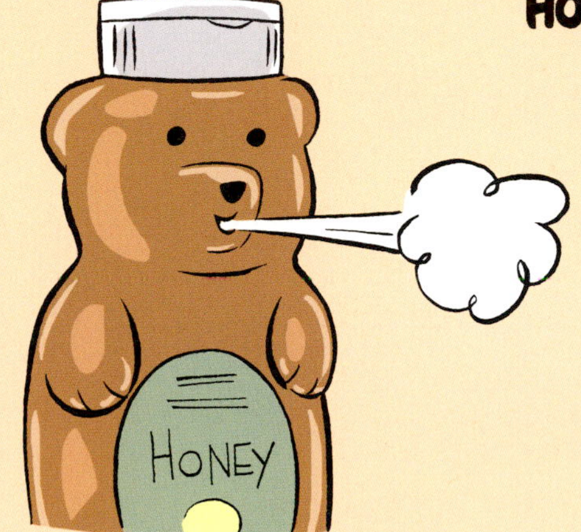


## HONEY MUSTARD DRESSING

| | |
|---|---|
| 3 T. MIRIN* | 105 |
| 1 T. LIGHT MAYONNAISE | 40 |
| 1 T. HONEY MUSTARD | 30 |
| 1/4 tsp. LIME OR LEMON JUICE | Ø |

COMBINE ALL INGREDIENTS AND WHISK TOGETHER IN A SMALL BOWL. MAKES 1/4 CUP (3 SERVINGS) AT 60 CALORIES PER 4 tsp.

*AVAILABLE IN THE ASIAN FOODS SECTIONS OF MANY MARKETS. DOES CONTAIN SOME ALCOHOL.

## TURKEY WITH MUSHROOMS AND GRAVY

| | |
|---|---|
| 1 TURKEY FILLET | 80 |
| 3/4 CUP WHITE MUSHROOMS, CHOPPED | 10 |
| 2 T. CANNED TURKEY GRAVY | 15 |
| A SHORT BLAST OF SPRAY OIL | 15 |

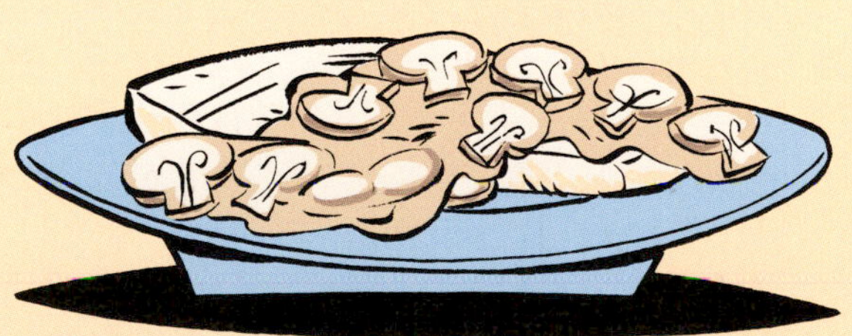

HEAT SKILLET. WHEN HOT, SPRAY WITH OIL AND THROW IN MUSHROOMS. COOK FOR A MINUTE, STIRRING, THEN ADD TURKEY FILLET. TURN HEAT DOWN TO MEDIUM-LOW; COOK UNTIL TURKEY IS DONE THROUGHOUT, SO IT'S NOT PINK WHEN YOU CUT IT OPEN. NUKE GRAVY FOR 25 SECONDS. POUR OVER COOKED TURKEY AND MUSHROOMS; SALT AND PEPPER TO TASTE.

TOTAL: 120

# MEDITERRANEAN COUSCOUS AND LENTIL SALAD

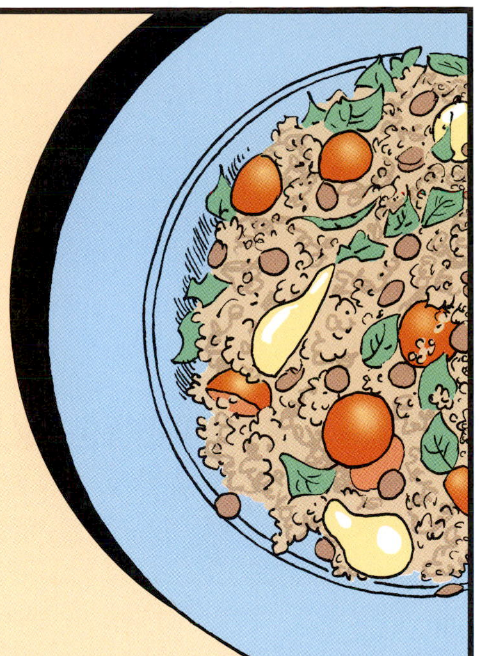

| | |
|---|---|
| ½ CUP LENTILS (UNCOOKED) | 140 |
| 1½ T. WHITE WINE VINEGAR | Ø |
| 1½ T. MIRIN | 60 |
| ¾ CUP WATER | Ø |
| ½ CUP COUSCOUS | 330 |
| ¼ tsp. SALT | Ø |
| 1½ tsp. AND 1 T. EXTRA VIRGIN OLIVE OIL | 180 |
| 1 LARGE GARLIC CLOVE, MINCED AND MASHED TO A PASTE WITH ¼ tsp. SALT | 5 |
| ½ CUP FRESH MINT LEAVES, FINELY CHOPPED | 20 |
| 1 CUP ARUGULA, STEMMED, WASHED, SPUN DRY, AND CHOPPED | 10 |
| 2 CUPS CHERRY TOMATOES, HALVED | 60 |
| ½ CUP REDUCED-FAT FETA, CRUMBLED | 140 |

WASH LENTILS WELL AND SIMMER IN TWO INCHES OF WATER IN A COVERED SAUCE-PAN FOR 15 TO 20 MINUTES, UNTIL THEY ARE TENDER BUT NOT MUSHY. DRAIN THOROUGHLY IN A COLANDER, THEN TRANSFER TO A MIXING BOWL AND STIR TOGETHER WITH 1½ tsp. EACH OF VINEGAR AND MIRIN; SALT AND PEPPER TO TASTE.

IN ANOTHER SAUCEPAN, BRING ¾ CUP OF WATER TO A BOIL. REMOVE PAN FROM HEAT, ADD COUSCOUS, AND COVER FOR 5 MINUTES. WHEN YOU UNCOVER THE PAN, THE COUSCOUS SHOULD HAVE ABSORBED THE WATER. TRANSFER TO A LARGE BOWL, ADD OLIVE OIL, AND FLUFF WITH A FORK.

WHILE THE COUSCOUS AND LENTILS COOL, WHISK TOGETHER GARLIC PASTE, REMAINING VINEGAR, MIRIN, AND OLIVE OIL, AND ADD SALT AND PEPPER TO TASTE.

ADD LENTILS AND DRESSING TO COUSCOUS BOWL AND CHILL FOR AT LEAST 3 HOURS (THIS CAN BE DONE UP TO 24 HOURS IN ADVANCE). JUST BEFORE SERVING, MIX IN MINT, ARUGULA, TOMATOES, AND FETA, AND ADD ADDITIONAL SALT AND PEPPER TO TASTE.

MAKES 6 CUPS. TOTAL PER 1-CUP SERVING: 160

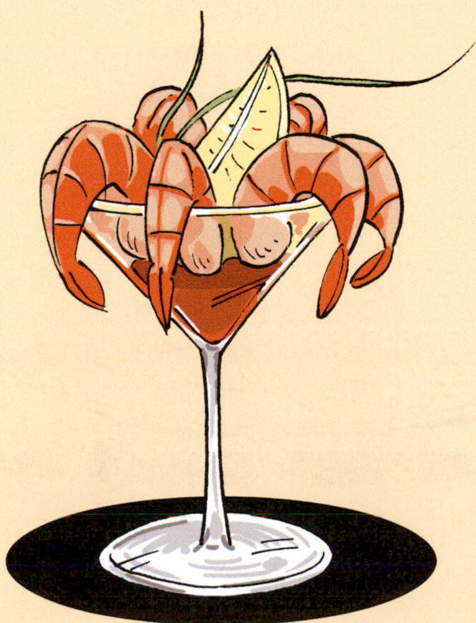

# SPICY SHRIMP COCKTAIL

| | |
|---|---|
| 6 LARGE SHRIMPS, PEELED AND CLEANED | 80 |
| 1 T. TERIYAKI SAUCE | 15 |
| 1 tsp. CHINESE HOT SAUCE* | 5 |
| A SHORT BLAST OF SPRAY OIL | 20 |
| 2 tsp. SHRIMP COCKTAIL SAUCE | 20 |

MIX TOGETHER TERIYAKI SAUCE AND HOT SAUCE; MARINATE SHRIMPS IN IT FOR 20 MINUTES. HEAT PAN, SPRAY WITH OIL, COOK SHRIMPS OVER MEDIUM HEAT UNTIL PINK. SERVE WITH COCKTAIL SAUCE.

TOTAL: 140

* AVAILABLE IN ASIAN FOODS SECTION OF MANY MARKETS

## TILAPIA, ITALIAN STYLE

A CHARMING ITALIAN MAN TOLD ME THIS RECIPE (MORE OR LESS) WHILE I WAITED AT THE FISH COUNTER. VERY NICE.

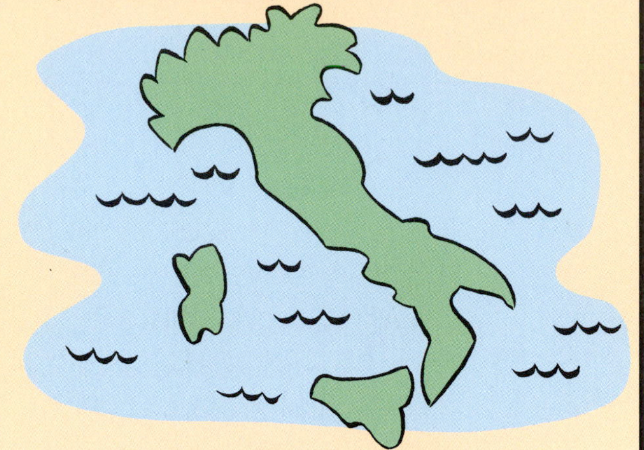

| | |
|---|---|
| 3-OZ. TILAPIA FILLET | 110 |
| ½ SHALLOT, CHOPPED | 5 |
| 1 GARLIC CLOVE, MINCED | 5 |
| 1 tsp. OLIVE OIL | 40 |
| ½ CUP CHERRY TOMATOES, HALVED | 15 |
| ½ tsp. FRESH THYME, SNIPPED (OR ¼ tsp. DRIED THYME) | Ø |
| 2 T. ITALIAN BREAD CRUMBS | 55 |
| 1 tsp. CAPERS | Ø |

PREHEAT OVEN TO 375°F. RINSE FISH; PAT DRY WITH PAPER TOWEL. IN A SMALL BOWL MIX OIL, SHALLOT, GARLIC, AND THYME. DIP FILLET INTO MIXTURE TO COAT BOTH SIDES. PLACE FISH ON BAKING PAN, ADD TOMATOES, AND BAKE FOR 5 MINUTES. REMOVE FROM OVEN AND CHANGE OVEN SETTING FROM BAKE TO BROIL (HIGH). SPRINKLE BREAD CRUMBS AND CAPERS ON FISH AND PLACE UNDER BROILER FOR 5 MINUTES. SALT AND PEPPER TO TASTE.

TOTAL: 230

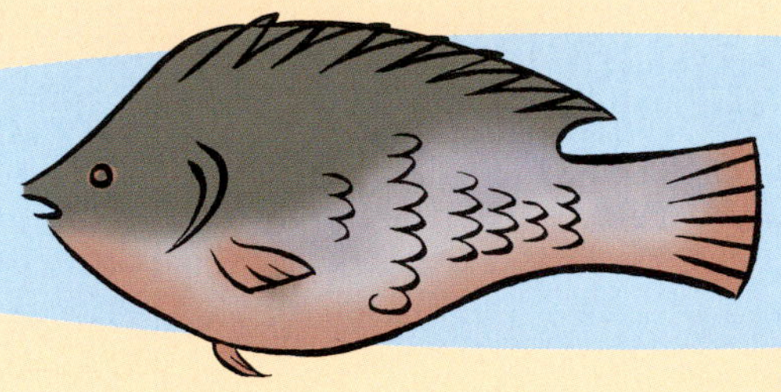

## SHELLS WITH CAULIFLOWER

AN ITALIAN WOMAN COOKED THIS SIMPLE AND SATISFYING DISH FOR A FRIEND, WHO MADE IT FOR ME. I DON'T USUALLY INDULGE IN WHITE FLOUR PASTAS, BUT THE SUBTLE FLAVORS GO WELL WITH THE YELLOW SHELLS.

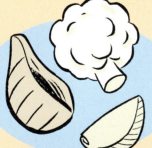

| | |
|---|---|
| ½ CUP (UNCOOKED) ENRICHED PASTA SHELLS | 150 |
| 1 CUP CAULIFLOWER FLORETS | 25 |
| ¼ tsp. SALT | Ø |
| 1 tsp. OLIVE OIL | 40 |
| 1 LARGE GARLIC CLOVE, CHOPPED INTO ⅛" BITS | 5 |
| 2 T. REGGIANO-PARMESAN CHEESE, SHREDDED | 45 |

HEAT 4 CUPS OF WATER WITH SALT IN A 3-QUART SAUCEPAN. RINSE CAULIFLOWER AND BREAK IT INTO VERY SMALL FLORETS. WHEN THE WATER BOILS, THROW IN THE PASTA AND GARLIC AND BOIL, STIRRING OCCASIONALLY, FOR 4 MINUTES. ADD THE CAULIFLOWER AND CONTINUE TO BOIL FOR 4 MORE MINUTES. WHEN DONE, DRAIN. HEAT 1 tsp. OLIVE OIL IN PAN OVER MEDIUM HEAT. TRANSFER SHELLS AND CAULIFLOWER BACK INTO PAN; STIR TO LIGHTLY COAT MIXTURE IN OIL. TRANSFER TO BOWL. SALT AND PEPPER TO TASTE; TOP WITH CHEESE.

TOTAL: 265

# EGGPLANT WITH TOMATO-MINT SAUCE AND GOAT CHEESE

THIS SIMPLE DISH IS PURE HEAVEN!

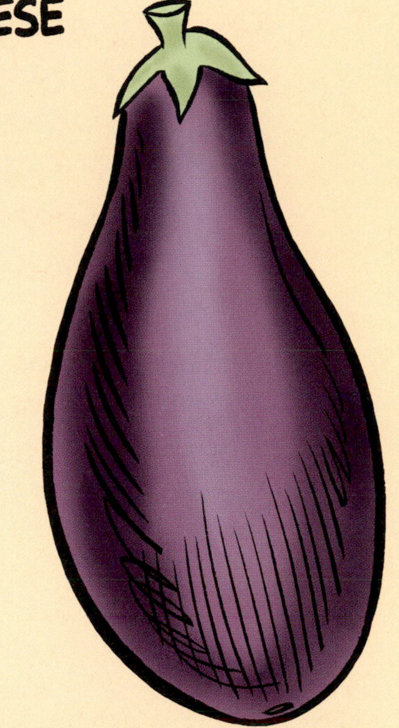

| | |
|---|---|
| A SHORT BLAST OF SPRAY OIL | 15 |
| 1-POUND EGGPLANT, TRIMMED, CUT INTO 1/2"-THICK DISKS | 120 |
| A SECOND SHORT BLAST OF OIL | 15 |
| 1/4 CUP WHITE ONION, CHOPPED | 10 |
| 1 1/4 tsp. OLIVE OIL | 50 |
| 1 GARLIC CLOVE, MINCED | 5 |
| 14.5-OZ. CAN OF ITALIAN-STYLE TOMATOES | 80 |
| 1 1/2 T. FRESH MINT, CHOPPED | Ø |
| 1/4 tsp. DRIED OREGANO | Ø |
| 1/4 CUP CRUMBLED SOFT GOAT CHEESE | 160 |
| 4 FRESH BASIL LEAVES, THINLY SLICED | Ø |

PREPARE EGGPLANT BY LIGHTLY SALTING EACH PIECE AND LETTING THE SALT SOAK IN FOR 10 MINUTES. THIS TAKES AWAY A LOT OF THE NATURAL BITTER TASTE.

PREHEAT OVEN TO 500°F. BLAST A LARGE BAKING SHEET WITH A SHORT SPRAY OF OIL, ARRANGE THE EGGPLANT, AND THEN BLAST AGAIN. ADD SALT AND PEPPER, BAKE FOR 10 MINUTES, THEN TURN DISKS OVER AND BAKE FOR ANOTHER 10 MINUTES. REMOVE BAKING SHEET FROM OVEN AND REDUCE TEMPERATURE TO 350°F.

MEANWHILE, SAUTÉ ONION IN OLIVE OIL ON MEDIUM HEAT FOR ABOUT 5 MINUTES. ONIONS SHOULD BE TRANSLUCENT AND TENDER BUT NOT YET BROWNED. ADD GARLIC AND STIR FOR ANOTHER MINUTE, THEN ADD TOMATOES (WITH JUICES), MINT, AND OREGANO AND SIMMER UNTIL SAUCE THICKENS, ABOUT 20 MINUTES.

WHEN THE SAUCE IS DONE, POUR HALF INTO A BAKING OR CASSEROLE DISH. ARRANGE THE EGGPLANT ON TOP OF THE SAUCE (IT'S GOOD IF THEY OVERLAP) AND THEN ADD THE REST OF THE SAUCE. LAYER THE CHEESE ON TOP AND BAKE FOR 20 MINUTES, UNTIL THE CHEESE IS BUBBLY AND THE CASSEROLE IS HEATED THROUGH. GARNISH WITH BASIL.

MAKES 2 SERVINGS. TOTAL PER SERVING: 230

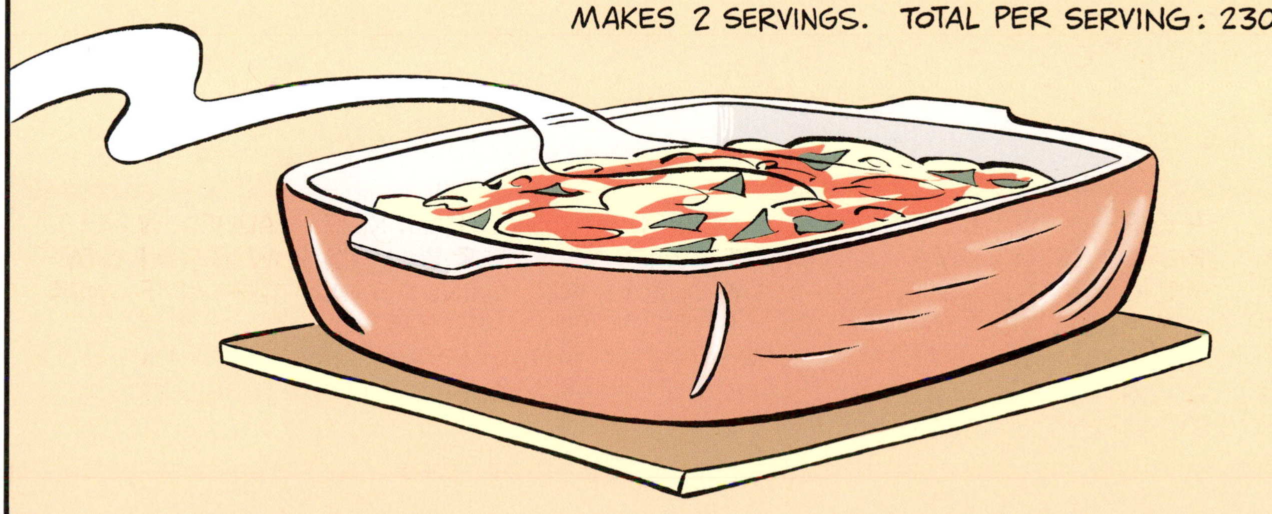

## BROWN RICE WITH SAUTÉED VEGETABLES

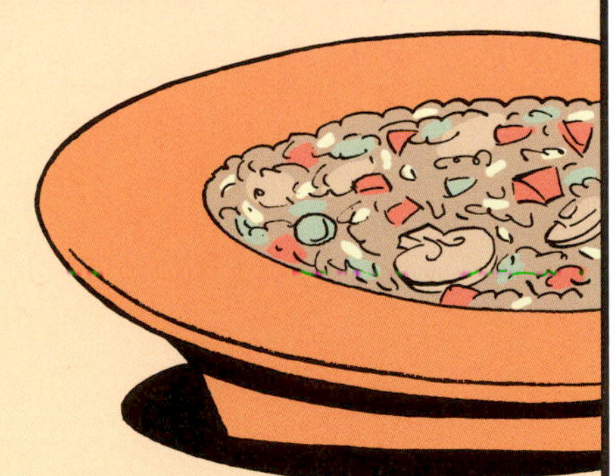

| | |
|---|---|
| 3/4 CUP BROWN RICE, COOKED | 165 |
| 2 T. ONION, CHOPPED | 5 |
| 1/4 CUP SWEET RED PEPPER, CHOPPED | 10 |
| 1/4 CUP ZUCCHINI, CHOPPED | 15 |
| 1/3 CUP MUSHROOMS, SLICED | 5 |
| A SHORT BLAST OF SPRAY OIL | 15 |

HEAT SKILLET OVER MEDIUM HEAT; SPRAY IT WITH OIL. SAUTÉ VEGGIES FOR A FEW MINUTES, STIRRING, THEN ADD RICE. COOK UNTIL RICE IS HEATED. SALT AND PEPPER TO TASTE.

TOTAL: 215

## SCALLOPS PROVENÇALE

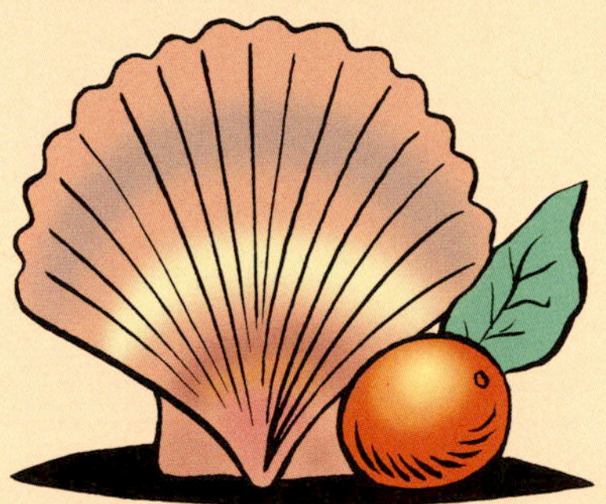

| | |
|---|---|
| 4 OZ. LARGE SEA SCALLOPS, PATTED DRY | 100 |
| 2 tsp. OLIVE OIL | 80 |
| 1 GARLIC CLOVE, SLICED THIN | 5 |
| 1 TOMATO, DICED | 10 |
| 1/8 tsp. DRIED THYME, CRUMBLED | Ø |
| 3 T. FRESH BASIL LEAVES, SHREDDED | Ø |

HEAT OLIVE OIL IN A SKILLET OVER HIGH HEAT AND SEAR SCALLOPS FOR 1 TO 2 MINUTES ON EACH SIDE, UNTIL JUST BROWNED. SET SCALLOPS ASIDE AND COVER TO KEEP WARM. ADD REMAINING OLIVE OIL TO SKILLET AND SAUTÉ THE GARLIC OVER MEDIUM HEAT UNTIL BROWNED. ADD THE TOMATO, THYME, AND HALF OF THE BASIL AND SIMMER, STIRRING CONSTANTLY, FOR ANOTHER MINUTE. SEASON THE SAUCE WITH SALT AND PEPPER, THEN POUR OVER AND AROUND THE SCALLOPS, GARNISHING WITH THE REMAINING BASIL.

TOTAL: 195

SERVE ON PASTA OR ARUGULA.

## CHEATY PIZZA WITH BROCCOLI

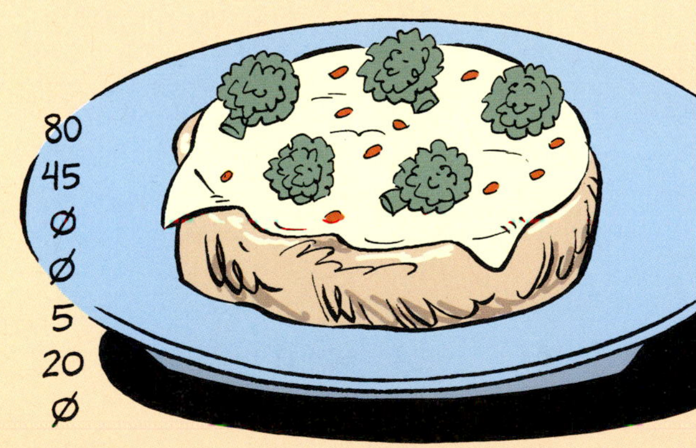

| | |
|---|---|
| 1/2 WHOLE-WHEAT ENGLISH MUFFIN | 80 |
| 1/2 OZ. MOZZARELLA CHEESE | 45 |
| 2 T. BROCCOLI FLORETS | Ø |
| 1/2 tsp. RED ONION, FINELY CHOPPED | Ø |
| 1/2 GARLIC CLOVE, FINELY MINCED | 5 |
| 1/2 tsp. OLIVE OIL | 20 |
| PINCH OF RED PEPPER FLAKES | Ø |

STEAM BROCCOLI FOR 5 MINUTES AND SET ASIDE. TURN BROILER ON HIGH. LIGHTLY TOAST THE MUFFIN HALF, THEN TOP WITH CHEESE, GARLIC, ONION, AND BROCCOLI. SPRINKLE WITH OLIVE OIL AND PUT UNDER BROILER FOR A MINUTE OR UNTIL CHEESE MELTS. SCATTER RED PEPPER FLAKES ON TOP.

TOTAL: 150

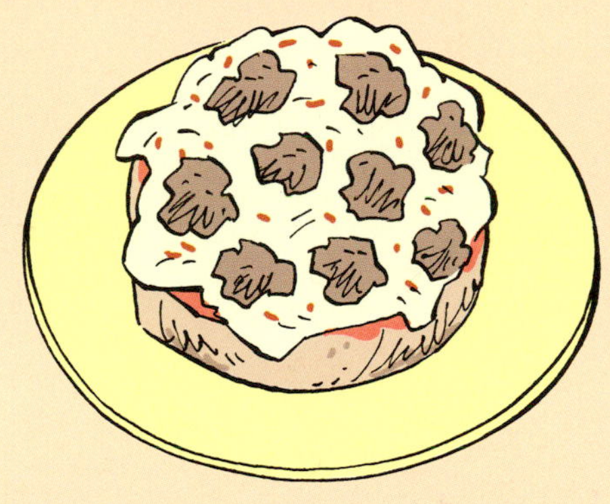

## CHEATY PIZZA WITH VEGGIE SAUSAGE

| | |
|---|---|
| 1/2 WHOLE-WHEAT ENGLISH MUFFIN | 80 |
| 1/2 OZ. MOZZARELLA CHEESE | 35 |
| 1 T. TOMATO PASTE WITH A FEW DROPS OF AGAVE NECTAR | 10 |
| 1/2 VEGGIE PATTY | 35 |

PREHEAT BROILER. LIGHTLY TOAST MUFFIN HALF. NUKE VEGGIE PATTY FOR 30 SECONDS AND SET ASIDE. MIX TOMATO PASTE WITH AGAVE NECTAR (OR HONEY) AND SPREAD ON MUFFIN; TOP WITH CHEESE AND CRUMBLED VEGGIE PATTY. BROIL FOR 1 MINUTE OR UNTIL CHEESE MELTS. SEASON WITH ITALIAN SEASONING AND OR HOT RED PEPPER FLAKES.

TOTAL: 160

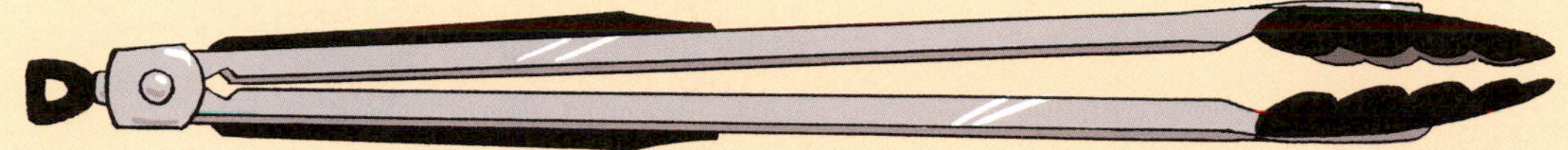

## STIR-FRY WITH TOFU

| | |
|---|---|
| 1 SERVING OF FIRM TOFU | 70 |
| 1 T. PEANUT SAUCE* | 30 |
| 2 tsp. TERIYAKI SAUCE | 10 |
| 1 BABY BOK CHOY | 10 |
| 3 ASPARAGUS STALKS | 15 |
| 1/3 CAN BAMBOO SHOOTS | 20 |
| 3 SHIITAKE MUSHROOMS, HALVED | 30 |
| 1 GARLIC CLOVE | 5 |
| 2 tsp. SOY SAUCE | 10 |
| 5 PEANUTS, CHOPPED | 30 |
| A MEDIUM BLAST OF SPRAY OIL | 20 |

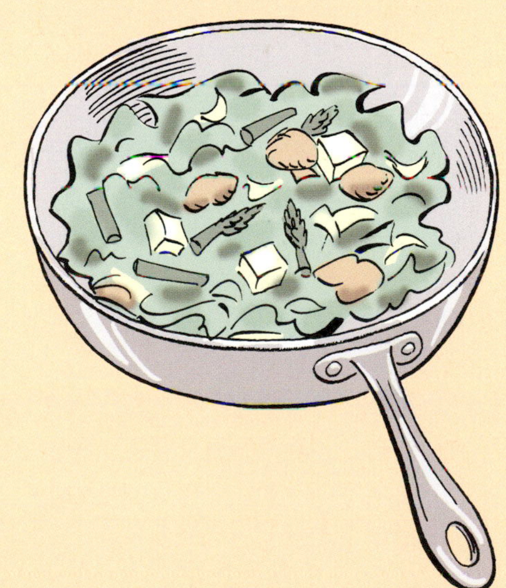

MINCE GARLIC AND SET ASIDE. CUT TOFU INTO CUBES. MIX PEANUT AND TERIYAKI SAUCES IN A BOWL AND ADD TOFU; TOSS TO COVER CUBES IN SAUCE. HEAT WOK OR SKILLET; SPRAY IT WITH OIL. THROW IN THE WHITE BASE OF THE BOK CHOY, CHOPPED, BUT RESERVE THE GREENS TO ADD LATER. STIR IN MUSHROOMS, ASPARAGUS PIECES, AND BAMBOO SHOOTS. AFTER A COUPLE OF MINUTES, ADD THE TOFU WITH SAUCE, GARLIC, AND BOK CHOY GREENS. STIR, AND COOK FOR A MINUTE LONGER. TRANSFER TO SHALLOW DISH OR PLATE. POUR ON 2 tsp. SOY SAUCE AND SPRINKLE WITH PEANUTS.

TOTAL: 250

* AVAILABLE IN ASIAN FOODS SECTION OF MANY MARKETS.

## CURRIED SPLIT PEA SOUP

MY FRIEND DEREK DOESN'T LIKE SPLIT PEA SOUP, BUT ONE TASTE OF THIS CURRIED VERSION AND HE KEPT COMING BACK FOR MORE. SERVE WITH BROWN RICE OR COUSCOUS FOR A COMPLETE PROTEIN COMBO.

| | |
|---|---|
| 1½ tsp. OLIVE OIL | 60 |
| ½ WHITE ONION, CHOPPED | 35 |
| 2 SMALL GARLIC CLOVES, MINCED | 10 |
| 1 T. FRESH GINGER, FINELY MINCED | 10 |
| 1 tsp. CURRY POWDER | Ø |
| ½ tsp. GROUND CUMIN | Ø |
| ⅛ tsp. GROUND CARDAMOM | Ø |
| ⅛ tsp. GROUND CORIANDER | Ø |
| PINCH CINNAMON | Ø |
| 1 tsp. SALT | Ø |
| 4 CUPS WATER | Ø |
| ½ POUND DRIED SPLIT PEAS (ABOUT 1¼ CUP) | 715 |
| ½ CARROT, GRATED | 15 |

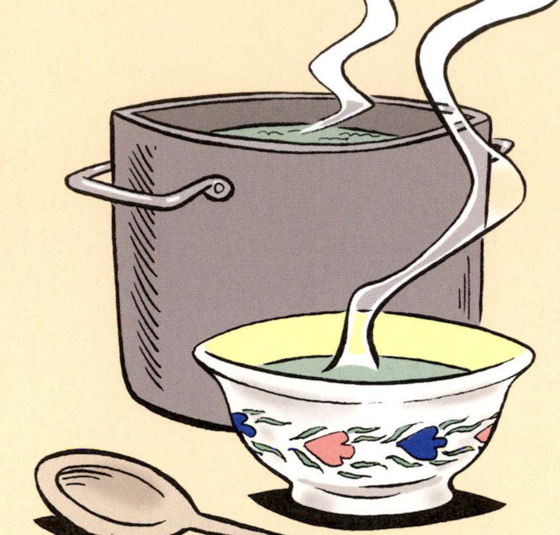

IN A LARGE STOCK POT OVER MEDIUM HEAT, SAUTÉ ONION FOR 5 MINUTES, UNTIL TRANSLUCENT BUT NOT YET BROWNED. ADD GARLIC, GINGER, SPICES, AND SALT AND CONTINUE TO COOK FOR 2 MORE MINUTES.

ADD WATER AND SPLIT PEAS. STIR THOROUGHLY, COVER, AND BRING TO A BOIL. THEN TURN DOWN HEAT TO MEDIUM AND SIMMER—LID SLIGHTLY ASKEW SO STEAM CAN ESCAPE—FOR AN HOUR OR UNTIL PEAS ARE TENDER BUT NOT MUSHY. GARNISH WITH GRATED CARROT.

MAKES 4 SERVINGS OF 1 CUP EACH. TOTAL PER SERVING: 210

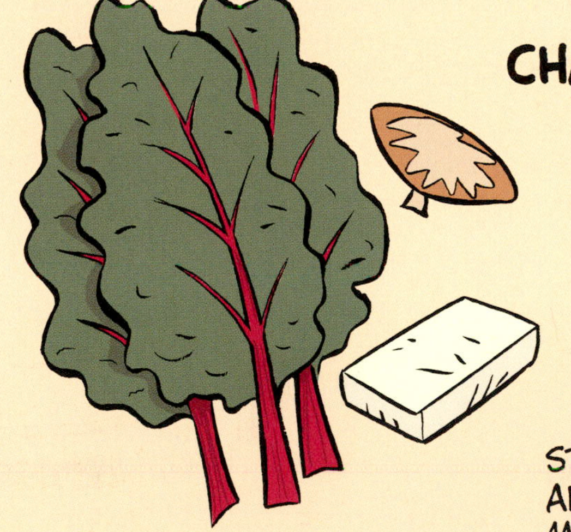

## CHARD, MUSHROOMS, AND TOFU IN SPICY SAUCE

| | |
|---|---|
| 3 LARGE SWISS CHARD LEAVES, TORN | 20 |
| 3 SHIITAKE MUSHROOMS | 10 |
| ⅕ BLOCK OF FIRM TOFU, CHUNKED | 70 |
| ½ GARLIC CLOVE, MINCED | Ø |
| 1 T. TERIYAKI SAUCE | 15 |
| 1 T. SWEET/HOT STIR-FRY SAUCE* | 35 |

STEAM CHARD WITH MUSHROOMS FOR 6 MINUTES. ADD TOFU AND GARLIC; STEAM FOR 2 MORE MINUTES. MIX SAUCES IN SMALL BOWL AND NUKE FOR 25 SECONDS.

WHEN COOKED, DRAIN EXCESS WATER FROM CHARD LEAVES IN COLANDER AND TRANSFER ALL TO BOWL. DRIZZLE WITH WARM SAUCE MIXTURE.

TOTAL: 150

*AVAILABLE IN ASIAN FOODS SECTION OF MANY MARKETS.

## SPINACH SALAD WITH TURKEY BACON AND SPICY ORANGE DRESSING

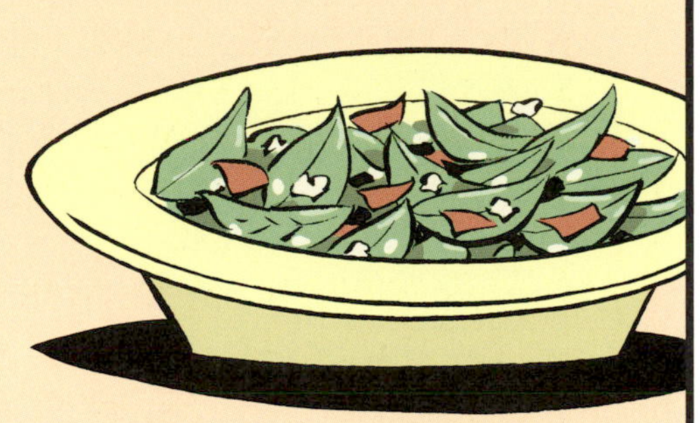

| | |
|---|---|
| 2 ½ CUPS SPINACH LEAVES | 25 |
| 2 T. LOW-FAT FETA | 35 |
| 2 SLICES RED ONION, FINELY SLICED | Ø |
| 1 T. PINE NUTS, LIGHTLY TOASTED | 50 |
| 1 SLICE TURKEY BACON, COOKED AND CRUMBLED | 35 |
| 2 T. SPICY ORANGE DRESSING (SEE BELOW) | 20 |
| A SHORT BLAST OF SPRAY OIL | 15 |

RINSE AND TRIM SPINACH, SPIN DRY OR PAT DRY WITH PAPER TOWELS, AND PLACE ON PLATE. ADD ONION SLICES AND FETA. HEAT PAN, SPRAY WITH OIL. LIGHTLY SAUTÉ BACON AND PINE NUTS; ADD TO SALAD. DRIZZLE WITH DRESSING, AND PEPPER TO TASTE.

TOTAL: 180

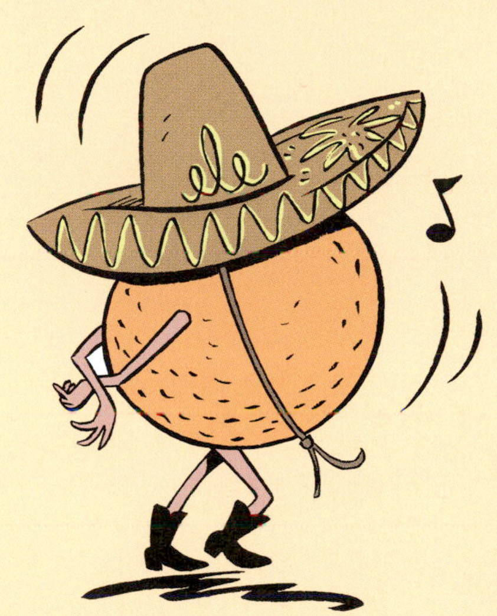


## SPICY ORANGE VINAIGRETTE

| | |
|---|---|
| ½ CUP ORANGE JUICE | 55 |
| ½ tsp. AGAVE NECTAR OR HONEY | 10 |
| 1 SCOOP STEVIA | Ø |
| 1 tsp. SESAME OIL | 40 |
| 1 ½ tsp. SOY SAUCE | 10 |
| 1 T. MIRIN | 35 |
| 2 T. WATER | Ø |
| DASH CAYENNE PEPPER | Ø |
| ½ SHALLOT, CHOPPED | Ø |
| 1 tsp. FRESH GINGER, GRATED | Ø |

WHISK TOGETHER ALL IN A SMALL BOWL. THIS DRESSING KEEPS WELL IN THE FRIDGE. MAKES 2/3 CUP.
TOTAL PER TABLESPOON: 15

## SHRIMP LINGUINI WITH WHOLE-WHEAT PASTA

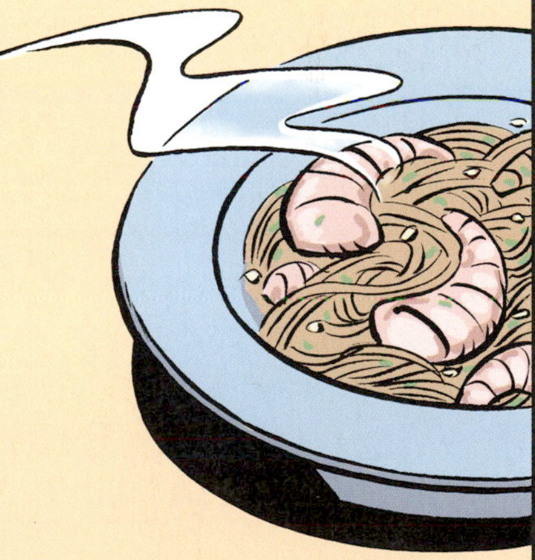

| | |
|---|---|
| 6 SHRIMPS, PEELED AND CLEANED | 80 |
| 2 T. SHALLOT, CHOPPED | 15 |
| 1 tsp. OLIVE OIL | 40 |
| 2 SMALL GARLIC CLOVES, MINCED | 10 |
| ½ tsp. LIME JUICE | Ø |
| 1 T. ITALIAN PARSLEY, CHOPPED | Ø |
| A MEDIUM BLAST OF SPRAY OIL | 20 |
| ½ CUP WHOLE-WHEAT LINGUINI, COOKED (ABOUT A FINGER-WIDTH IN DIAMETER, DRY) | 100 |

MIX OIL, SHALLOTS, GARLIC, PARSLEY, AND LIME JUICE IN BOWL. MIX IN SHRIMP. COOK LINGUINI PER INSTRUCTIONS ON BOX. (TAKE CARE NOT TO UNDER- OR OVERCOOK THE PASTA!) HEAT SKILLET ON MEDIUM HEAT. A FEW MINUTES BEFORE LINGUINI IS DONE, POUR SHRIMP MIXTURE INTO SKILLET AND SAUTÉ UNTIL SHRIMPS ARE PINK ALL AROUND. DRAIN LINGUINI AND TRANSFER TO BOWL; TOP WITH SHRIMP MIXTURE. SALT AND PEPPER TO TASTE.

TOTAL: 265

## EGG-WHITE OMELET WITH CHEESE AND VEGGIES

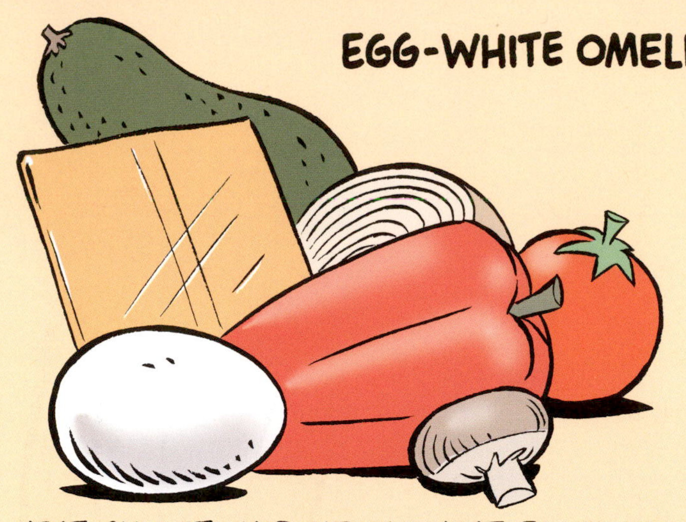

| | |
|---|---|
| 6 T. EGG WHITES | 50 |
| 1 T. SOY MILK | 10 |
| ½ SLICE SOY "CHEDDAR" CHEESE | 30 |
| ¼ CUP SWEET RED PEPPER, CHOPPED | 10 |
| ½ CUP MUSHROOMS, SLICED | 10 |
| ¼ CUP ONION, CHOPPED | 10 |
| 2 T. SALSA | 10 |
| ¼-INCH SLICE AVOCADO | 20 |
| 2 SHORT BLASTS OF SPRAY OIL | 30 |

HEAT SKILLET OVER MEDIUM HEAT, BLAST IT WITH SPRAY OIL, AND SAUTÉ THE PEPPER, MUSHROOMS, AND ONION FOR 5 MINUTES. SET ASIDE. WHISK EGG WHITES WITH MILK. HEAT OMELET PAN, SPRAY WITH OIL, AND COOK THE EGG MIXTURE. FLIP IT, ADD THE CHEESE AND VEGGIES, THEN FOLD IT IN HALF. HEAT BOTH SIDES; TOP WITH AVOCADO AND SALSA. SALT AND PEPPER TO TASTE.

TOTAL: 180

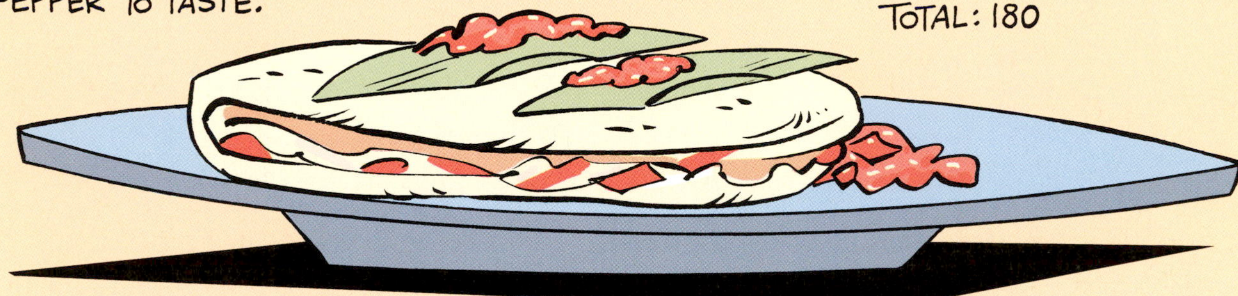

## STIR-FRY WITH SHRIMP

| | |
|---|---|
| 5 RAW SHRIMPS | 70 |
| 1 tsp. TERIYAKI SAUCE | 5 |
| 1 tsp. CHINESE HOT SAUCE | 5 |
| 1 T. SWEET & SOUR SAUCE* | 45 |
| 1 BABY BOK CHOY, CHOPPED | 10 |
| ⅓ CAN WATER CHESTNUTS, SLICED* | 25 |
| ½ CUP SNOW PEAS | 20 |
| 3 SHIITAKE MUSHROOMS, HALVED | 30 |
| 1 GARLIC CLOVE, MINCED | 5 |
| 2 tsp. SOY SAUCE | 10 |
| A SHORT BLAST OF SPRAY OIL | 15 |

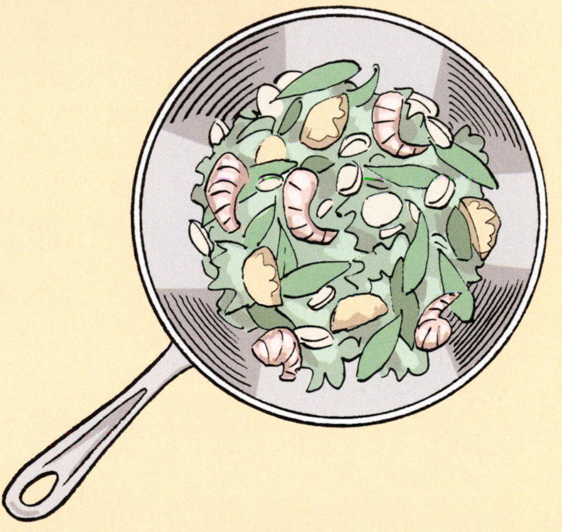

MINCE GARLIC CLOVE AND SET IT ASIDE. MIX CHINESE SAUCES AND MARINATE SHRIMPS IN THE COMBO. HEAT LARGE SKILLET OR WOK OVER HIGH HEAT; SPRAY WITH OIL. THROW IN BASE PART OF BOK CHOY (CHOPPED); RESERVE GREENS FOR LATER. STIR IN MUSHROOMS, SNOW PEAS, AND WATER CHESTNUTS. COOK FOR A COUPLE OF MINUTES UNTIL MUSHROOMS ARE TENDER AND GIVING OFF WATER, THEN TOSS IN SHRIMPS WITH SAUCE, GARLIC, AND BOK CHOY GREENS. TURN THE SHRIMPS SO THEY COOK EVENLY. WHEN THE SHRIMPS ARE DONE (PINK AND WHITE OVER ALL) AND THE GREENS SOFT, TRANSFER TO BOWL AND SPRINKLE ON SOY SAUCE.

TOTAL: 240

* AVAILABLE IN ASIAN FOODS SECTION OF MANY MARKETS

# STUFFED POBLANO PEPPERS

**HOT!** THIS IS MY VERSION OF MY FAVORITE RESTAURANT RELLENOS, MINUS A LOT OF CHEESE...

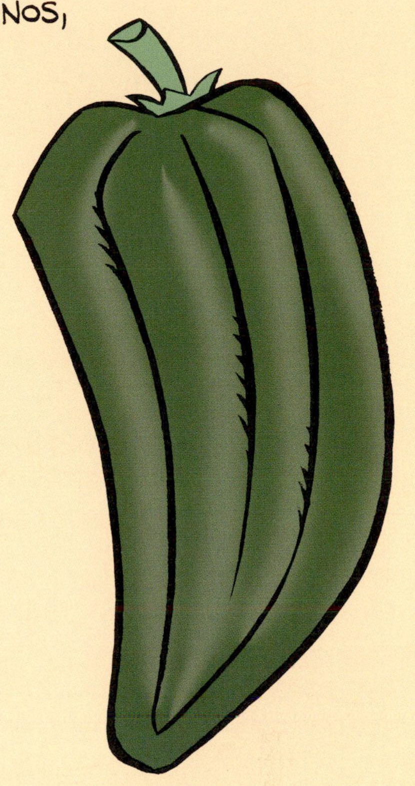

| | |
|---|---|
| 2 LARGE POBLANO PEPPERS* | 40 |
| 2 tsp. OLIVE OIL | 80 |
| 1 CUP ONIONS, CHOPPED | 20 |
| 1 CUP ZUCCHINI, CHOPPED | 20 |
| ½ CUP SWEET RED PEPPER, CHOPPED | 20 |
| ½ CUP BLACK BEANS (COOKED), CLEANED AND RINSED (CANNED IS FINE) | 110 |
| 8 LARGE BLACK OLIVES, CHOPPED | 50 |
| 2 T. CORN KERNELS | 15 |
| PINCH CAYENNE PEPPER | Ø |
| 2 OZ. REDUCED-FAT WHITE CHEDDAR CHEESE, GRATED | 140 |
| 2 T. TOMATO SALSA | 10 |
| 2 T. REDUCED-FAT SOUR CREAM | 30 |
| 4 CORN TORTILLAS | 240 |
| A SHORT BLAST OF SPRAY OIL | 15 |

PREHEAT BROILER TO HIGH. ARRANGE WHOLE PEPPERS ON BAKING SHEET. BROIL UNTIL SLIGHTLY CHARRED ON ALL SIDES, TURNING OCCASIONALLY, ABOUT 10 MINUTES. CUT A LENGTHWISE SLIT IN EACH PEPPER; CAREFULLY REMOVE SEEDS AND PEEL OFF CRUSTY OUTER SKIN.

MEANWHILE, HEAT OIL IN LARGE SKILLET OVER MEDIUM-LOW HEAT. ADD ONIONS AND ZUCCHINI; SAUTÉ UNTIL GOLDEN, ABOUT 20 MINUTES. SEASON WITH SALT AND PEPPER. PREHEAT OVEN TO 350°F. MIX BEANS, OLIVES, CORN, CAYENNE, CHEESE, AND VEGGIES IN BOWL. SPOON MIXTURE INTO PEPPERS. PLACE PEPPERS SEAM SIDE DOWN ON LIGHTLY SPRAY-OILED BAKING DISH. COVER WITH FOIL.

BAKE PEPPERS 20-25 MINUTES. CUT EACH PEPPER IN HALF AND PLACE ON A WARM FLOUR TORTILLA. TOP WITH SALSA AND 1½ tsp. REDUCED-FAT SOUR CREAM.

MAKES 4 SERVINGS — FREEZE EXTRA. TOTAL PER SERVING: 200

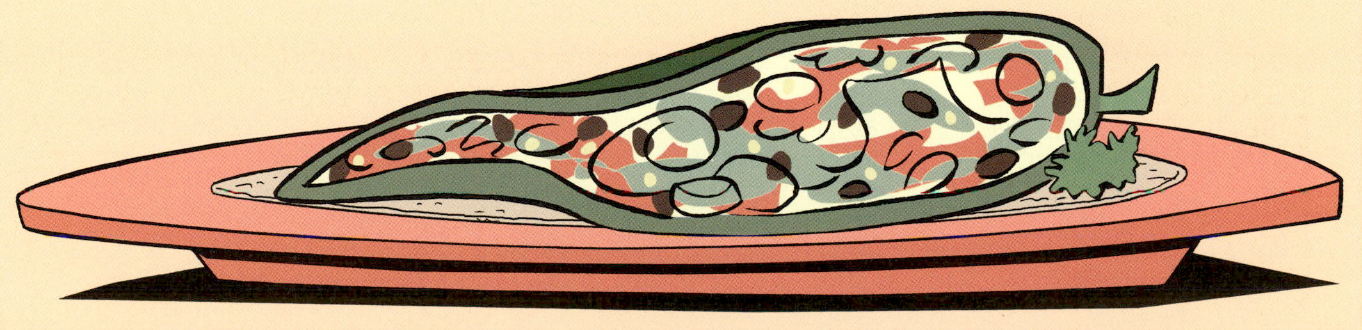

* A MILDLY SPICY CHILE PEPPER AVAILABLE IN MANY MARKETS.

## SALMON/TUNA/AVOCADO TARTARE ON WHOLE-WHEAT ENGLISH MUFFIN

| | |
|---|---|
| 4 tsp. HONEY MUSTARD | 40 |
| 4 tsp. LIGHT MAYONNAISE (40 CAL. PER T.) | 53 |
| 2 OZ. RAW SALMON, SUSHI GRADE, CHOPPED | 80 |
| 2 OZ. RAW TUNA, SUSHI GRADE, CHOPPED | 60 |
| ⅓ CUP AVOCADO, CHOPPED | 80 |
| 1 T. RED ONION, FINELY CHOPPED | 3 |
| 1½ tsp. FRESH DILL, CHOPPED | Ø |
| 1½ tsp. LIME JUICE | 6 |
| 1½ tsp. SHALLOT, MINCED | 4 |
| ½ tsp. OLIVE OIL | 20 |
| ⅛ tsp. GROUND SEA SALT | Ø |
| ⅛ tsp. GROUND BLACK PEPPER | Ø |
| 2 WHOLE-WHEAT ENGLISH MUFFINS, HALVED | 320 |

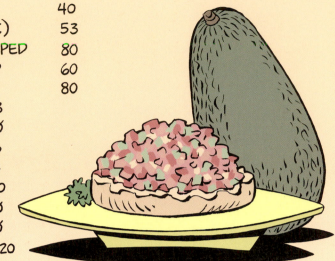

MIX MUSTARD AND MAYO IN SMALL BOWL. SEASON TO TASTE WITH SALT AND PEPPER. COVER AND REFRIGERATE.

MIX ONION, HERBS, OIL, AND SPICES IN MEDIUM BOWL. FOLD IN CHOPPED SALMON, TUNA, AND AVOCADO. COVER AND CHILL FOR AT LEAST 30 MINUTES; KEEP REFRIGERATED. LIGHTLY TOAST ENGLISH MUFFIN HALF; SPREAD 2 tsp. MUSTARD MIXTURE ON ONE SIDE. TOP WITH ¼ CUP TARTARE.

MAKES 4 SERVINGS AT 170 CALORIES EACH.

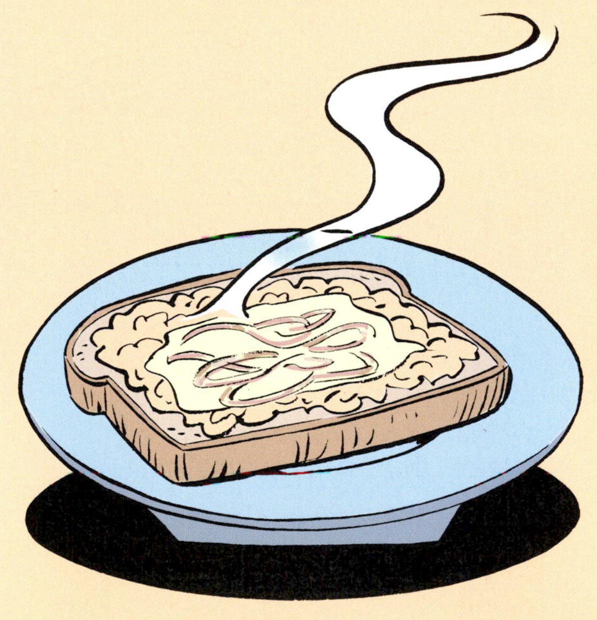

## TUNA MELT

| | |
|---|---|
| ⅓ CAN WHITE TUNA (PACKED IN WATER) | 50 |
| 4 tsp. LOW-FAT MAYONNAISE (15 CAL. PER T.) | 20 |
| ½ tsp. FAUX BUTTER | 15 |
| ⅛" SLICE RED ONION (ABOUT 1½ T.) | Ø |
| A TINY BLAST OF SPRAY OIL | 5 |
| 1 SLICE RYE BREAD | 80 |
| ½ OZ. REDUCED-FAT BABY SWISS CHEESE | 50 |

DRAIN WATER FROM TUNA CAN. (MY CATS **LOVE** "TUNA JUICE.") MIX TUNA WITH MAYO AND SET ASIDE. HEAT SKILLET OVER MEDIUM HEAT. SPREAD BUTTER ON ONE SIDE OF BREAD. FRY UNBUTTERED SIDE FOR 1 MINUTE; TURN OVER AND FRY BUTTERED SIDE. SET ASIDE WHEN DONE. SPRAY A TINY BLAST OF OIL INTO SKILLET—JUST ENOUGH FOR A THIN DISK OF ONION. SAUTÉ OVER MEDIUM HEAT. TURN BROILER ON TO HIGH. SPREAD TUNA ON GRILLED BREAD (I PREFER THE BUTTERED SIDE DOWN); TOP WITH CHEESE AND ONIONS. TRANSFER TO OVEN-SAFE PAN AND PLACE UNDER BROILER FOR 2 MINUTES OR UNTIL CHEESE IS MELTED.

TOTAL: 240

## EGG SALAD SANDWICH

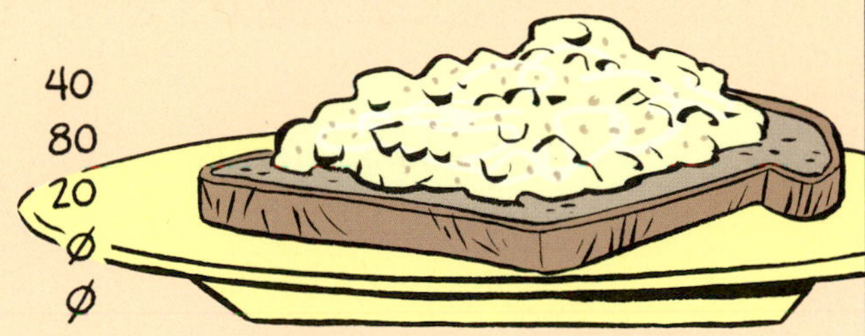

| | |
|---|---|
| 1 HARD-BOILED EGG (WITH ONLY ½ THE YOLK) | 40 |
| 1 SLICE WHOLE-GRAIN BREAD OR TOAST | 80 |
| 4 tsp. LOW-FAT MAYONNAISE | 20 |
| 1 tsp. ONION, FINELY CHOPPED | Ø |
| A DAB OF SPICY MUSTARD | Ø |

SLICE THE PEELED EGG IN HALF. SCOOP OUT HALF OF THE YOLK AND TOSS IT. CHOP THE EGG INTO THE BOWL. MIX IN MAYO, MUSTARD, AND ONION. SPREAD ON TOAST; SALT AND PEPPER TO TASTE.

TOTAL: 140

## ITTY BITTY HOT DOG SANDWICH

I EAT THIS FREQUENTLY BECAUSE IT'S QUICK, SATISFYING, AND THE RIGHT AMOUNT OF CALORIES FOR MY LIGHT LUNCH.

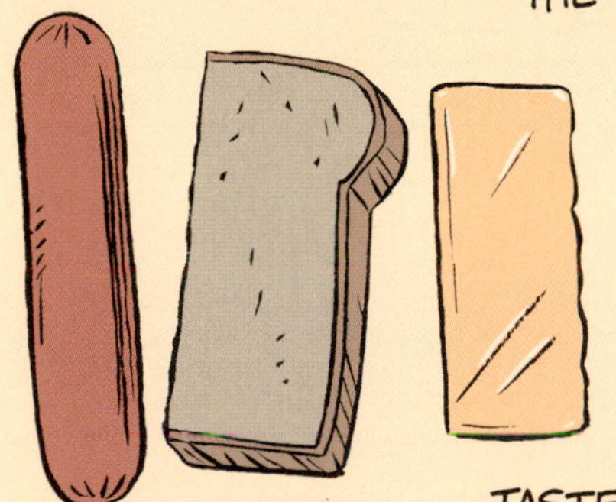

| | |
|---|---|
| 1 VEGGIE DOG (I USE "SMART DOGS") | 45 |
| ½ SLICE SPROUTED-GRAIN BREAD, TOASTED | 40 |
| ½ SLICE SOY "CHEDDAR" CHEESE | 25 |
| 1 T. CATSUP | 10 |
| A DAB OF SPICY MUSTARD | Ø |

SPLIT DOGGIE DOWN CENTER AND BOIL IN ½" WATER FOR A COUPLE OF MINUTES. (SOY PRODUCTS GENERALLY TASTE BETTER COOKED, NOT NUKED.) TOAST THE BREAD, LAY ON THE CHEESE, PLACE DOG HALVES ON CHEESE SO IT MELTS, AND ADD THE CONDIMENTS.

TOTAL: 120

## VEGGIE BURGER ON MINI-PITAS

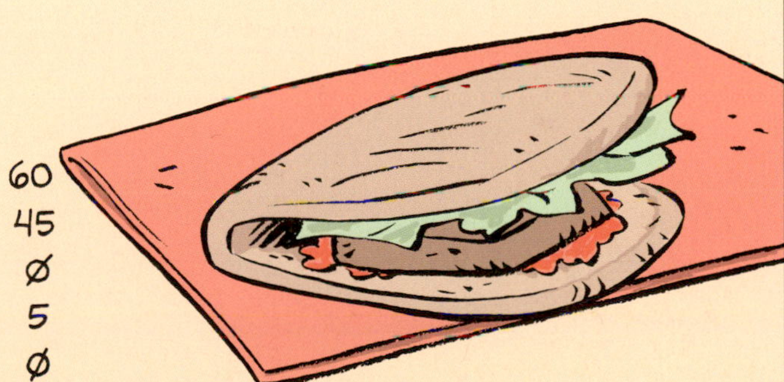

| | |
|---|---|
| ½ VEGGIE BURGER PATTY (I LIKE MORNING STAR FARMS "TOMATO AND BASIL PIZZA BURGER") | 60 |
| 2 WHOLE-WHEAT MINI-PITA POCKETS | 45 |
| 2 tsp. SALSA | Ø |
| MUSTARD, 2 DABS | 5 |
| ROMAINE LETTUCE LEAVES | Ø |

HEAT PATTY AS DIRECTED ON PACKAGE. REFRIGERATE HALF FOR LATER USE; CUT REMAINING HALF IN TWO. TOAST PITAS, SLICE OPEN, SLIDE IN PATTY PARTS, SPOON IN 1 tsp. SALSA PER POCKET ALONG WITH A DAB OF MUSTARD AND LETTUCE.

TOTAL: 110 FOR BOTH MINI-SANDWICHES

## PEANUT BUTTER AND JAM ON TOAST

THIS ISN'T ABOUT **HOW** TO MAKE PB & J, BUT WITH **HOW MUCH** TO MAKE IT.

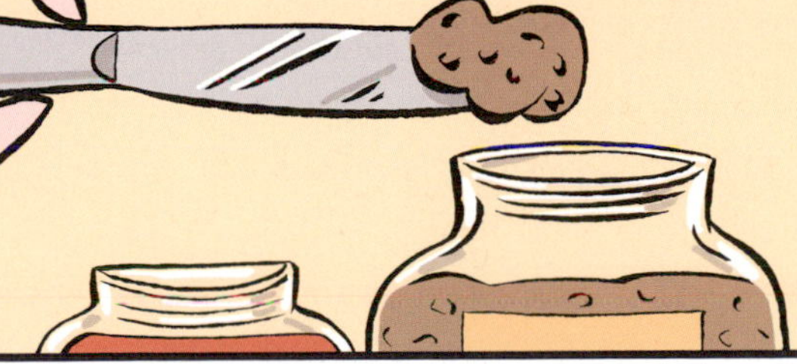

| | |
|---|---|
| 1 SLICE WHOLE-GRAIN TOAST | 80 |
| 2 tsp. PEANUT BUTTER | 80 |
| 1 T. JAM (NO SUGAR ADDED) | 30 |

TOTAL: 190 OR HALVE IT FOR 100

## STEAMED VEGETABLES WITH TOFU AND CURRY SAUCE

THIS DISH WORKS WITH MANY COMBINATIONS OF VEGETABLES—ZUCCHINI, MUSHROOMS, YELLOW SQUASH, AND GREENS LIKE KALE AND SPINACH. I OFTEN PREPARE THE FOLLOWING COMBO WITHOUT TOFU FOR A TOTAL OF 120 CALORIES.

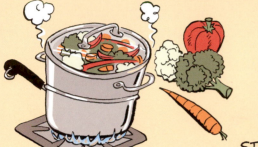

| | |
|---|---|
| 1 CARROT, CHOPPED | 35 |
| 1/2 CUP (GENEROUS) BROCCOLI, CHOPPED | 15 |
| 1/2 CUP (GENEROUS) CAULIFLOWER, CHOPPED | 15 |
| 1/4 OF A SWEET RED PEPPER, CUT INTO STRIPS | 10 |
| 1 SERVING FIRM TOFU, CUBED | 70 |
| 2 T. RED CURRY SAUCE | 40 |

STEAM VEGGIES FOR 6 MINUTES. ADD TOFU AND CONTINUE STEAMING FOR 2 MORE MINUTES. MEANWHILE, NUKE CURRY SAUCE FOR 20 SECONDS. POUR IT OVER STEAMED VEGETABLE MEDLEY. SALT AND PEPPER TO TASTE.

TOTAL: 180

## RED THAI CURRY SAUCE

I USUALLY USE A BOTTLED VERSION THAT COMES TO 40 CALORIES FOR 2 T., BUT IT'S NOT A NATIONAL BRAND SO HERE'S A "LITE" VERSION OF THE REAL DEAL.

HOLLYWOOD HAS A THRIVING THAI COMMUNITY AND SPECIALTY MARKETS, SO I WAS ABLE TO SCORE THE KAFFIR LIME LEAVES WITHOUT TOO MUCH TROUBLE. HOWEVER, IF THESE LEAVES ARE NOT AVAILABLE, USE THE TENDER NEW LEAVES OF LIME, LEMON, OR GRAPEFRUIT. THEY WON'T HAVE THE SAME FRAGRANCE, BUT WORK BETTER THAN DRIED KAFFIR LIME LEAVES. AVOID KUMQUAT LEAVES.

| | |
|---|---|
| 1 14-OZ. CAN UNSWEETENED "LITE" COCONUT MILK* | 315 |
| 12 WHOLE GREEN CARDAMOM PODS, CRUSHED, **OR** HEAPING 1/2 tsp. GROUND CARDAMOM | 4 |
| 3 FRESH KAFFIR LIME LEAVES (3 DOUBLE LEAVES)** | ø |
| 2 GARLIC CLOVES, CHOPPED | 10 |
| 2 T. GOLDEN BROWN SUGAR, PACKED | 105 |
| 1 T. GRATED LEMON PEEL | 3 |
| 1 T. FRESH LIME JUICE | 2 |
| 1 T. THAI RED CURRY PASTE* | 25 |
| 2 tsp. FISH SAUCE (NAM PLA OR NUOC NAM)* | 4 |

BRING ALL INGREDIENTS TO A BOIL IN A SAUCEPAN OVER MEDIUM-HIGH HEAT, WHISKING CONSTANTLY. REDUCE HEAT TO MEDIUM AND SIMMER FOR AN ADDITIONAL MINUTE. REMOVE FROM HEAT, COVER, AND LET SAUCE STAND AT ROOM TEMPERATURE FOR 10 MINUTES. PUSH THROUGH A STRAINER OVER A SMALL BOWL. SEASON TO TASTE WITH SALT AND PEPPER.

SAUCE CAN BE STORED, COVERED, IN THE REFRIGERATOR FOR UP TO TWO DAYS. REWARM BEFORE SERVING. MAKES 1 2/3 CUP SAUCE. TOTAL PER 2-T. SERVING: 35

* AVAILABLE IN THE ETHNIC FOODS SECTION OF MANY SUPERMARKETS OR IN ETHNIC SPECIALTY MARKETS.

** PARTICULAR TO SOUTHEAST ASIAN MARKETS.

# Sides

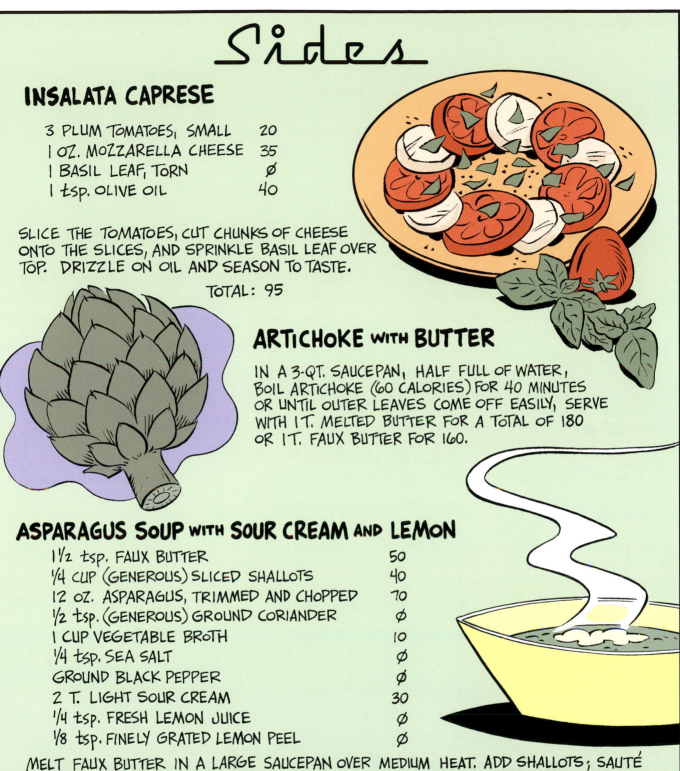

## INSALATA CAPRESE

| | |
|---|---|
| 3 PLUM TOMATOES, SMALL | 20 |
| 1 OZ. MOZZARELLA CHEESE | 35 |
| 1 BASIL LEAF, TORN | ∅ |
| 1 tsp. OLIVE OIL | 40 |

SLICE THE TOMATOES, CUT CHUNKS OF CHEESE ONTO THE SLICES, AND SPRINKLE BASIL LEAF OVER TOP. DRIZZLE ON OIL AND SEASON TO TASTE.

TOTAL: 95

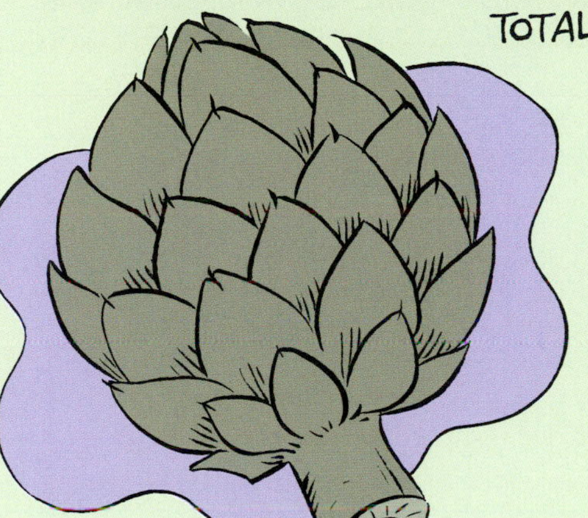

## ARTICHOKE WITH BUTTER

IN A 3-QT. SAUCEPAN, HALF FULL OF WATER, BOIL ARTICHOKE (60 CALORIES) FOR 40 MINUTES OR UNTIL OUTER LEAVES COME OFF EASILY. SERVE WITH 1 T. MELTED BUTTER FOR A TOTAL OF 180 OR 1 T. FAUX BUTTER FOR 160.

## ASPARAGUS SOUP WITH SOUR CREAM AND LEMON

| | |
|---|---|
| 1½ tsp. FAUX BUTTER | 50 |
| ¼ CUP (GENEROUS) SLICED SHALLOTS | 40 |
| 12 OZ. ASPARAGUS, TRIMMED AND CHOPPED | 70 |
| ½ tsp. (GENEROUS) GROUND CORIANDER | ∅ |
| 1 CUP VEGETABLE BROTH | 10 |
| ¼ tsp. SEA SALT | ∅ |
| GROUND BLACK PEPPER | ∅ |
| 2 T. LIGHT SOUR CREAM | 30 |
| ¼ tsp. FRESH LEMON JUICE | ∅ |
| ⅛ tsp. FINELY GRATED LEMON PEEL | ∅ |

MELT FAUX BUTTER IN A LARGE SAUCEPAN OVER MEDIUM HEAT. ADD SHALLOTS; SAUTÉ UNTIL SOFT, ABOUT 5 MINUTES. ADD ASPARAGUS AND CORIANDER AND COOK FOR A MINUTE LONGER, STIRRING CONSTANTLY. ADD VEGETABLE BROTH AND SIMMER FOR 5 MINUTES. LET SOUP COOL A LITTLE, THEN PURÉE IN BLENDER. (YOU WILL PROBABLY NEED TO DIVIDE INTO BATCHES.) POUR BACK INTO SAUCEPAN TO REHEAT, AND SEASON WITH SALT AND PEPPER.

IN A SMALL BOWL, COMBINE SOUR CREAM, LEMON JUICE, AND LEMON PEEL. POUR HALF OF SOUP INTO BOWL AND TOP WITH HALF OF THE SOUR CREAM AND LEMON MIXTURE.

MAKES 2 SERVINGS OF ¾ CUP EACH. TOTAL PER SERVING: 100

## GREEN PEA GUACAMOLE

SOME COOKS LIKE TO MIX GREEN PEAS IN WITH THE AVOCADO TO DILUTE SOME CALORIES. I DON'T USE ENOUGH HERE TO OFFSET THE TOTAL MUCH, BUT NEITHER DO THEY OVERWHELM THE FLAVOR WITH GREEN PEA-NESS. (TAKE CARE NOT TO SAY THAT LAST BIT OUT LOUD.)

| Ingredient | Calories |
|---|---|
| 1 MEDIUM AVOCADO, CHOPPED | 280 |
| 1/2 CUP PEAS, COOKED AND MASHED | 45 |
| 1 SMALL TOMATO, CHOPPED | 10 |
| 2 T. RED ONION, FINELY CHOPPED | 10 |
| 1 1/2 tsp. LIME JUICE | Ø |
| 1/2 GARLIC CLOVE | 5 |
| 3/4 tsp. FRESH JALAPENO PEPPER, CHOPPED | Ø |
| 1/4 tsp. SEA SALT | Ø |
| 1 T. CILANTRO, MINCED | Ø |
| 1/8 tsp. CHILI POWDER | Ø |
| DASH CAYENNE PEPPER | Ø |

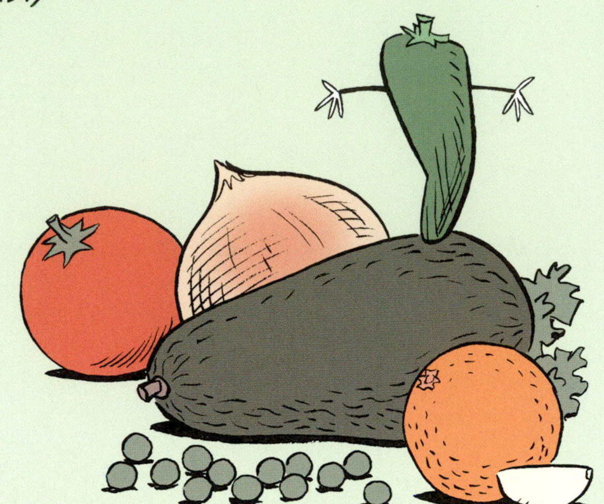

MIX EVERYTHING IN A BOWL, TAKING CARE NOT TO MASH THE AVOCADO TOO MUCH. CHILL FOR AN HOUR BEFORE SERVING. MAKES 1 CUP.

TOTAL PER 1/4-CUP SERVING: 90

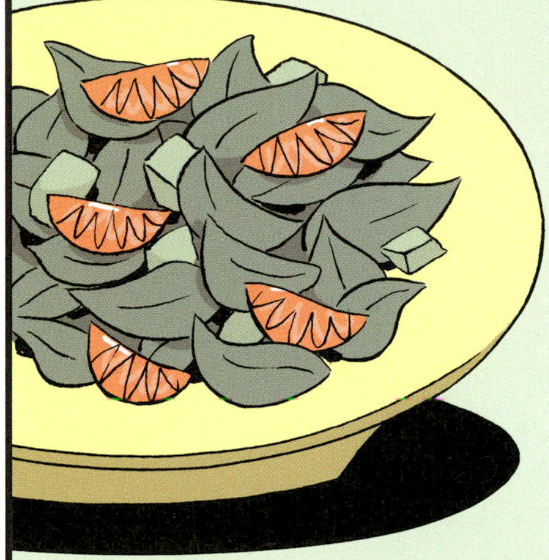

## ASIAN SPINACH SALAD

| Ingredient | Calories |
|---|---|
| 1 1/2 tsp. SHALLOT, FINELY CHOPPED | 5 |
| 1 1/2 tsp. RICE VINEGAR | Ø |
| 1 tsp. MIRIN | 10 |
| 1/2 tsp. VEGETABLE OIL | 20 |
| 1/2 tsp. FRESH GINGER, MINCED | Ø |
| A FEW DROPS OF SESAME OIL | 5 |
| 1 MANDARIN ORANGE | 40 |
| 1 1/2 CUP BABY SPINACH, STEMS TRIMMED | 10 |
| 1/8 AVOCADO (1/4 CUP) | 35 |

WHISK FIRST 6 INGREDIENTS IN LARGE BOWL. SEASON TO TASTE WITH SALT AND PEPPER. SET DRESSING ASIDE. PEEL AND DE-SEED ORANGE AND SEPARATE INTO SECTIONS. CUT AVOCADO INTO THIN SLICES OR CHUNKY BITS. GENTLY TOSS SPINACH, ORANGE, AND AVOCADO TOGETHER. **EXTREMELY** TASTY!

TOTAL: 125

## OYSTERS EXOTICA

COMBINE 1 T. RICE VINEGAR, A SCANT tsp. OF MINCED FRESH GINGER, 1 T. THINLY SLICED GREEN ONION (EQUAL PARTS GREEN AND WHITE), 1/2 tsp. MIRIN, AND 1/8 tsp. GRATED LEMON PEEL IN A SMALL BOWL. LET STAND FOR 15 MINUTES. SERVE SAUCE IN A DIPPING BOWL WITH 3 OYSTERS ON THE HALF SHELL. TOTAL: 130

## CARROT/RAISIN/WALNUT SALAD

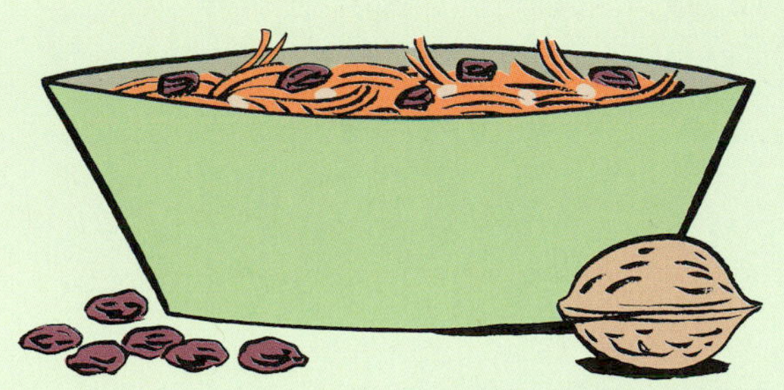

| | |
|---|---|
| 1 CUP CARROT, GRATED | 30 |
| 1 T. WALNUTS, CHOPPED | 50 |
| 2 T. RAISINS | 60 |
| 1 T. ORANGE JUICE | 10 |
| 1/4 CUP PINEAPPLE, FINELY CHOPPED | 20 |
| 2 T. CELERY, FINELY CHOPPED | Ø |
| 1/2 tsp. AGAVE NECTAR | 10 |

MIX INGREDIENTS TOGETHER IN SMALL BOWL AND CHILL.
MAKES 1½ CUP. EACH ½-CUP SERVING TOTALS 60 CALORIES.

## CARROT/BEET/APPLE SALAD

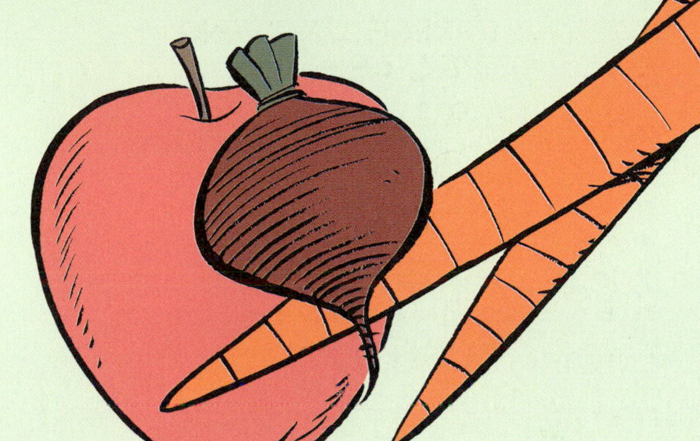

| | |
|---|---|
| 1/2 CUP CARROT, GRATED | 60 |
| 1/2 CUP FRESH BEET, GRATED | 60 |
| 1/2 CUP APPLE, PEELED | 40 |
| 2 tsp. FRESH LEMON JUICE | Ø |
| 1 tsp. SESAME SEEDS | 10 |
| 1/2 tsp. AGAVE NECTAR | 10 |

WASH, PEEL, AND GRATE BEET AND CARROTS; CHOP APPLE. MIX IN LARGE BOWL. MIX IN REMAINING INGREDIENTS. CHILL.

MAKES 2 GENEROUS ½-CUP SERVINGS AT 90 CALORIES EACH.

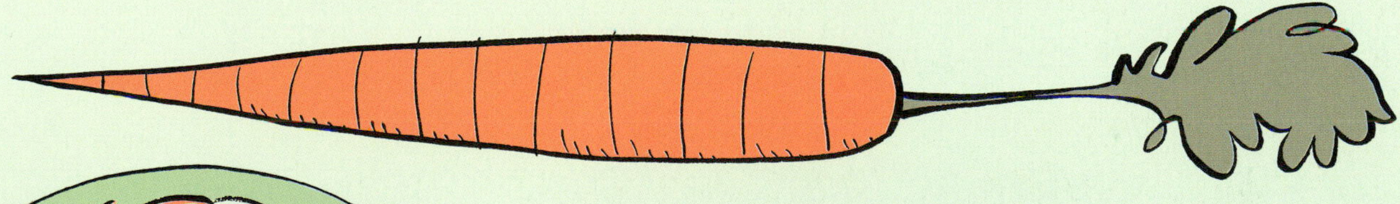

## ZINGY COLESLAW

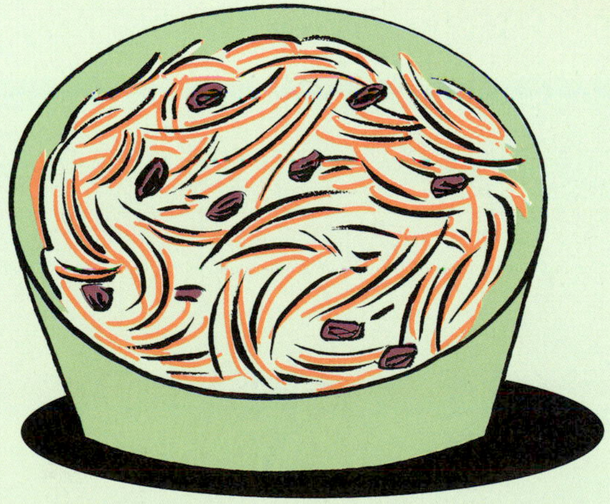

| | |
|---|---|
| 2 1/2 CUP CABBAGE, SHREDDED | 50 |
| 1 MEDIUM CARROT, GRATED | 30 |
| 2 T. RAISINS | 60 |
| 4 tsp. REDUCED-FAT MAYONNAISE | 50 |
| 2 tsp. LEMON JUICE | Ø |
| 4 tsp. ORANGE JUICE | 10 |
| 1 tsp. AGAVE NECTAR OR HONEY | 20 |
| 1 tsp. WHITE WINE VINEGAR | Ø |
| 1/2 tsp. MUSTARD | Ø |

TOSS CABBAGE, CARROT, AND RAISINS TOGETHER IN LARGE BOWL. IN SMALL BOWL, COMBINE MAYONNAISE, JUICES, AGAVE NECTAR, VINEGAR, AND MUSTARD; WHISK UNTIL THOROUGHLY BLENDED. POUR ONTO CABBAGE MIXTURE AND TOSS.

MAKES 2¾ CUPS. TOTAL PER 1-CUP SERVING: 80

## BIELER'S BROTH

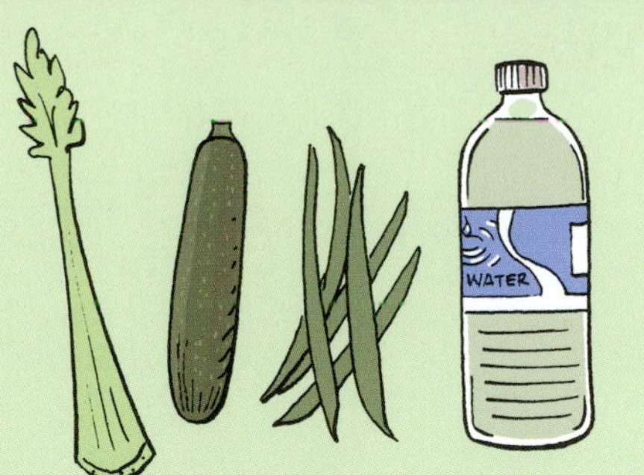


| | |
|---|---|
| 3 CUPS CELERY, CHOPPED | 60 |
| 3 CUPS ZUCCHINI, CHOPPED | 50 |
| 3 CUPS SNAP BEANS, TRIMMED AND CHOPPED | 100 |
| 2 T. SHOYU SAUCE* | 20 |
| SEA SALT | Ø |
| 1 BOTTLE FILTERED WATER (16.9 OZ.) | Ø |

DON'T ASK ME WHY THIS TASTES BETTER WITH BOTTLED WATER – IT JUST DOES. POUR THE WATER INTO THE BOTTOM OF THE STEAMER AND HEAT IT TO BOILING. STEAM CHOPPED VEGGIES FOR 10 MINUTES. WORKING IN BATCHES, USE WATER FROM STEAMER TO PURÉE VEGETABLES IN BLENDER. POUR SOUP BACK INTO SAUCEPAN, WARM IT UP AND ADD SHOYU SAUCE. SEASON TO TASTE WITH SEA SALT.

MAKES 5½ 1-CUP SERVINGS. TOTAL PER SERVING: 40

*SIMILAR TO SOY SAUCE; AVAILABLE IN ASIAN FOODS SECTION OF MANY MARKETS.

## EDAMAME

½ CUP OF COOKED-IN-SHELL SOYBEANS, AVAILABLE IN FRESH OR FROZEN PACKAGES IN MANY MARKETS.

TOTAL: 100

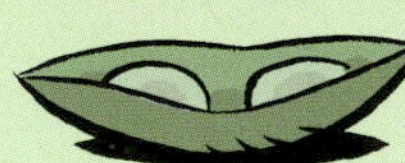

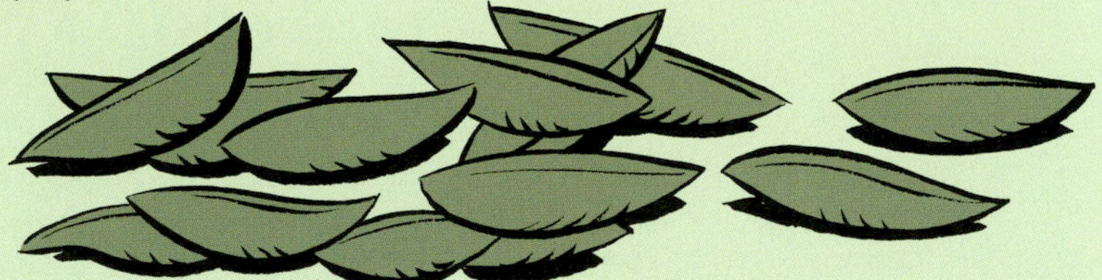

## ROASTED FENNEL WITH OLIVES AND GARLIC

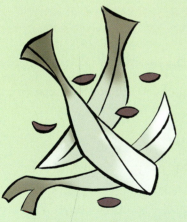

| | |
|---|---|
| A MEDIUM BLAST OF SPRAY OIL | 25 |
| 1 FENNEL BULB | 50 |
| 1½ tsp. OLIVE OIL | 60 |
| 6 KALAMATA OLIVES, PITTED, HALVED | 50 |
| 2 GARLIC CLOVES, MINCED | 10 |
| ¾ tsp. FRESH THYME, CHOPPED | Ø |
| A FEW FLAKES DRIED CRUSHED RED PEPPER | Ø |
| SEA SALT | Ø |
| GROUND BLACK PEPPER | Ø |

PREHEAT OVEN TO 425°F. TRIM AND CUT FENNEL BULB VERTICALLY INTO 8 WEDGES WITH CORE ATTACHED TO EACH WEDGE (SEE ILLUSTRATION). QUICKLY BLAST A LARGE BAKING SHEET WITH OIL. TOSS FENNEL WITH OLIVE OIL, GARLIC, THYME, AND CRUSHED RED PEPPER IN A MIXING BOWL, THEN SPREAD IT OUT EVENLY ON THE BAKING SHEET; SPRINKLE WITH SALT AND PEPPER. ROAST FENNEL FOR 15 MINUTES, TURN, ROAST FOR 10 MORE MINUTES, TURN AGAIN, ROAST FOR 10 MORE MINUTES. THEN ADD THE OLIVES AND RETURN TO THE OVEN FOR A FINAL 8 MINUTES (TOTAL ROASTING SHOULD BE ABOUT 43 MINUTES, AND FENNEL SHOULD BE TENDER AND BROWNING ON THE EDGES). SEASON AGAIN WITH SALT AND PEPPER AND SERVE WARM, OR LET STAND TO ROOM TEMPERATURE.

MAKES ABOUT 2 CUPS (LIGHTLY PACKED). TOTAL FOR 1-CUP SERVING: 100

## HEARTS OF PALM SALAD

| | |
|---|---|
| 2 CUPS BUTTER LETTUCE | 15 |
| 2/3 CUP HEARTS OF PALM | 30 |
| 1 SMALL TOMATO, CHOPPED | 5 |
| 1/8 AVOCADO, CHOPPED | 40 |
| 1 T. SCALLION, CHOPPED | 5 |
| 1 HEAPING tsp. FRESH DILL, CHOPPED | ∅ |
| 1 tsp. OLIVE OIL | 20 |
| 1 tsp. BALSAMIC VINEGAR | ∅ |

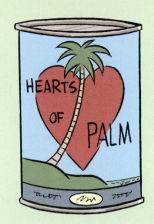

TEAR LETTUCE LEAVES, RINSE, AND SPIN DRY; TRANSFER TO BOWL. RINSE PALM HEARTS AND CUT INTO 1/2" CHUNKS. CHOP AND SHRED THE MIDDLE SECTION OF A SCALLION TO FILL A TABLESPOON. ADD HEARTS, CHOPPED TOMATO, AND SCALLION TO LETTUCE, DRIZZLE ON OIL AND TOSS. ADD DILL, THEN VINEGAR; TOSS AGAIN. SALT AND PEPPER TO TASTE.

TOTAL: 120

## SPINACH WITH OLIVES, RAISINS, AND PINE NUTS

| | |
|---|---|
| A COUPLE OF BLASTS OF SPRAY OIL | 30 |
| 10 OZ. FRESH SPINACH LEAVES, TRIMMED | 100 |
| 1 GARLIC CLOVE | 5 |
| 5 KALAMATA OLIVES, PITTED AND QUARTERED | 42 |
| 1 T. RAISINS | 30 |
| 1 T. PINE NUTS, RAW | 50 |
| 1 tsp. BALSAMIC VINEGAR | ∅ |

HEAT SKILLET OVER MEDIUM HEAT. SPRAY WITH A SHORT BLAST OF SPRAY OIL AND SAUTÉ SPINACH FOR 3 MINUTES; SET ASIDE. HEAT SKILLET OVER MEDIUM HEAT AND SPRAY AGAIN WITH OIL. ADD CHOPPED GARLIC, OLIVES, RAISINS, AND PINE NUTS AND SAUTÉ FOR 3 MINUTES. ADD SPINACH AND TOSS UNTIL HEATED THROUGH. ADD VINEGAR AND TOSS. SALT AND PEPPER TO TASTE.

MAKES 2 SERVINGS. TOTAL PER SERVING: 130

## STUFFED MUSHROOMS

| | |
|---|---|
| 4 LARGE WHITE MUSHROOMS | 10 |
| 2 SHORT BLASTS OF SPRAY OIL | 30 |
| 2 T. WHOLE-GRAIN BREAD, CRUMBLED | 30 |
| 1 tsp. FAUX BUTTER | 35 |
| 1/2 SHALLOT, FINELY CHOPPED | 7 |
| 1/2 GARLIC CLOVE, FINELY CHOPPED | 3 |
| 1 1/2 T. REDUCED-FAT FETA, CRUMBLED | 30 |
| 4 SMALL SPRIGS PARSLEY | ∅ |

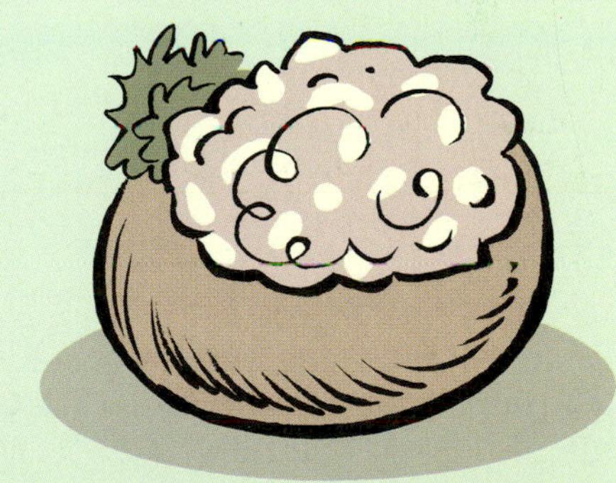

PREHEAT OVEN TO 425°F. SPRAY OIL INTO BAKING DISH. REMOVE STEMS FROM MUSHROOMS AND DISCARD. HEAT SKILLET OVER MEDIUM HEAT, SPRAY WITH OIL, AND SAUTÉ SHALLOT FOR A FEW MINUTES, THEN ADD GARLIC AND CONTINUE COOKING FOR 2 MINUTES MORE. CRUMBLE IN BREAD AND SAUTÉ 2 MINUTES MORE. LET MIXTURE COOL A BIT, THEN MIX WITH FETA. STUFF EACH MUSHROOM CAP, PRESSING GENTLY. TRANSFER TO BAKING DISH AND BAKE ABOUT 12-15 MINUTES. GARNISH WITH PARSLEY AND SERVE WARM.

TOTAL: 35 CALORIES PER STUFFED MUSHROOM

## SWEET POTATO STRIPS

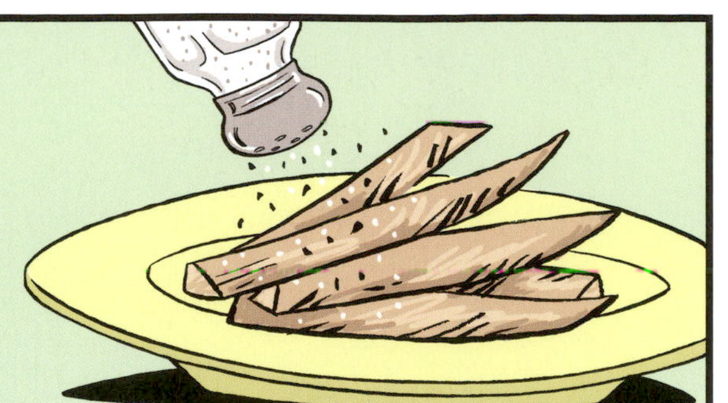

| | |
|---|---|
| 8 OZ. SWEET POTATO WITH SKIN, CLEANED | 190 |
| A BLAST OF SPRAY OIL | 20 |
| 1 tsp. VEGETABLE OIL | 40 |
| ½ tsp. GROUND CUMIN | Ø |
| ½ tsp. GROUND CORIANDER | Ø |
| 2 DASHES FRESH GROUND BLACK PEPPER | Ø |

PREHEAT OVEN TO 425°F. SPRAY OIL ON BAKING SHEET. TOSS POTATO STRIPS AND OIL IN LARGE BOWL; EVENLY COAT. ADD SPICES; TOSS. TRANSFER TO BAKING SHEET, SPRINKLE WITH PEPPER, AND BAKE 15 MINUTES. TURN OVER STRIPS, DUST WITH SECOND DASH OF PEPPER, AND CONTINUE BAKING FOR 10-15 MINUTES. SALT TO TASTE.

MAKES 1 CUP. TOTAL PER ½-CUP SERVING: 130

## BAKED YAM WITH BUTTER

THE YAM CAN BE USED LIKE A SWEET POTATO, BUT IS AN UNRELATED TYPE OF TUBER HIGH IN VITAMIN C, POTASSIUM, FIBER, MANGANESE, AND VITAMIN $B_6$. THEY GENERALLY HAVE A LOWER GLYCEMIC INDEX THAN POTATOES, AND THEREFORE GIVE BETTER PROTECTION AGAINST HEART DISEASE AND DIABETES.

BAKE AT 375°F FOR 40 MINUTES, OR UNTIL EASILY CUT THROUGH.

| | |
|---|---|
| ½ CUP YAM, BAKED | 80 |
| 1 SCANT tsp. FAUX BUTTER | 30 |

TOTAL: 110

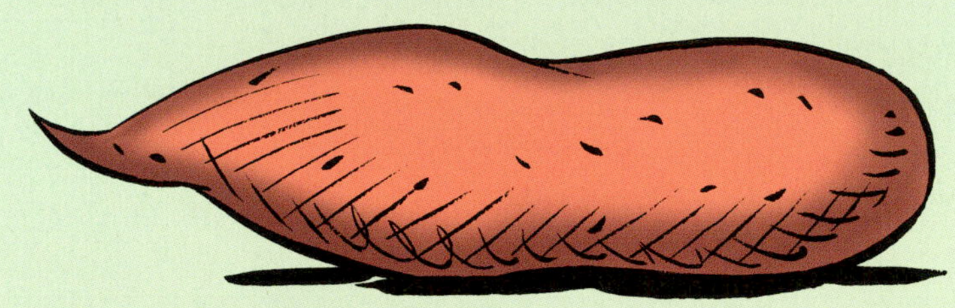

## KALE WITH GARLIC AND CRANBERRIES

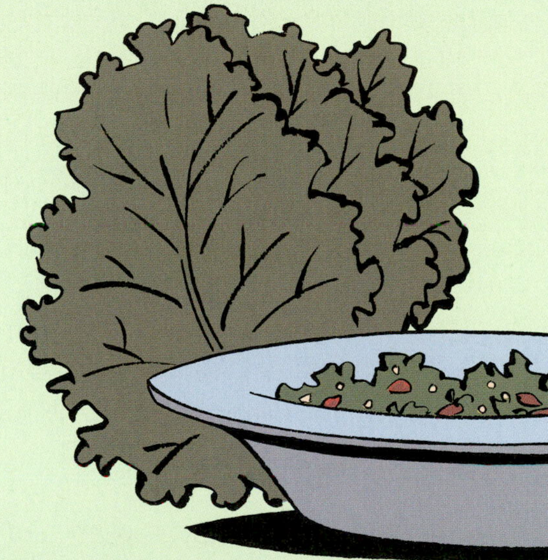

TENDER AND DELICIOUS!

| | |
|---|---|
| ½ POUND KALE, TRIMMED AND TORN | 35 |
| 1 GARLIC CLOVE, MINCED | 5 |
| 1 tsp. OLIVE OIL | 40 |
| 2 T. DRIED CRANBERRIES | 50 |
| ½ tsp. SEA SALT | Ø |
| PINCH GROUND BLACK PEPPER | Ø |

BRING A LARGE POT OF SALTED WATER (1 tsp. SALT) TO A BOIL AND ADD THE KALE. COOK, UNCOVERED, FOR 6 MINUTES. MEANWHILE, PREPARE AN ICE BATH IN A LARGE MIXING BOWL. REMOVE KALE FROM BOILING WATER, DRAIN IN A COLANDER, THEN IMMEDIATELY TRANSFER TO THE ICE BATH TO STOP THE COOKING PROCESS. WHEN KALE IS COOL, DRAIN AGAIN BUT DO NOT SQUEEZE. SAUTÉ GARLIC IN OLIVE OIL IN SAME POT OVER MEDIUM HEAT, STIRRING CONSTANTLY, FOR ABOUT 30 SECONDS. RETURN KALE TO THE POT AND ADD CRANBERRIES, SALT, AND PEPPER. TOSS FREQUENTLY WITH TONGS AND COOK FOR ANOTHER 4 TO 6 MINUTES, UNTIL KALE IS HEATED THROUGH.

MAKES 2 SERVINGS. TOTAL PER SERVING: 70

## ROASTED GREEN BEANS WITH ALMONDS

¼ POUND GREEN BEANS 30
2 PEARL ONIONS, PEELED AND QUARTERED 5
½ tsp. FRESH THYME Ø
½ tsp. OLIVE OIL (SCANT) 15
½ tsp. (SCANT) FRESH LEMON JUICE Ø
PINCH (GENEROUS) LEMON PEEL, GRATED Ø
4 ROASTED ALMONDS 40

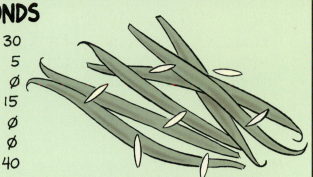

PREHEAT OVEN TO 450°F AND START THE STEAMER BOILING. PLACE BEANS AND ONIONS IN STEAMER FOR 4 MINUTES. WHEN DONE, PLACE ON BAKING DISH AND SPRINKLE WITH OIL AND THYME. SEASON WITH SEA SALT AND PEPPER; TOSS. ROAST FOR 8 MINUTES. TRANSFER VEGETABLES TO BOWL. ADD LEMON JUICE, PEEL, AND HALF OF THE CHOPPED ALMONDS. TOSS TO COAT; SPRINKLE WITH REMAINING ALMONDS.

TOTAL: 90

## CORN ON THE COB

PULL OFF ONLY THE THICK OUTER HUSK—NO NEED TO REMOVE THE SILKS FIRST. ONE AT A TIME, DROP THE EARS (45 CALORIES EACH) INTO A LARGE POT OF BOILING WATER FOR 30 SECONDS TO 1 MINUTE. REMOVE WITH TONGS, STRIP OFF HUSKS, AND TRANSFER TO PLATTER. TASTES GREAT WITH SALT AND GROUND BLACK PEPPER, ½ tsp. BUTTER PER EAR (20 CALORIES), A DASH OF CHILI POWDER, AND A SQUEEZE OF LIME JUICE. TOTAL PER 1-EAR SERVING: 65

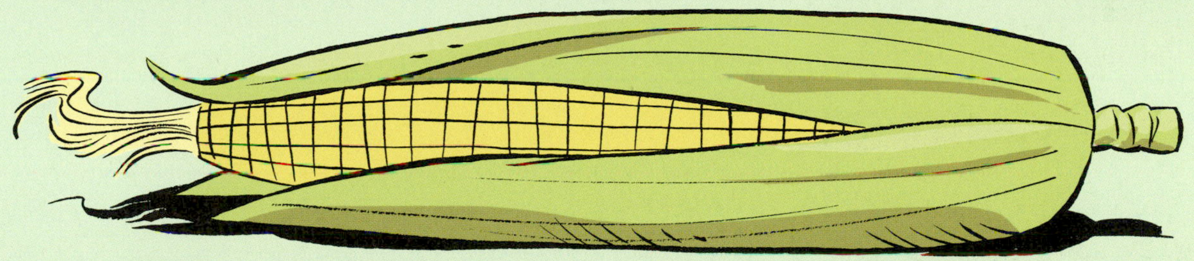

## ROASTED BRUSSELS SPROUTS WITH GARLIC

I'D ONLY HAD BRUSSELS SPROUTS ONCE IN MY LIFE—BOILED TO DEATH, OF COURSE—BEFORE I TRIED THEM THIS WAY. ROASTING WITH GARLIC BRINGS OUT A KIND OF NUTTY FLAVOR. THEY EVEN TASTE GREAT AS LEFTOVERS, COLD FROM THE FRIDGE.

1 POUND BRUSSELS SPROUTS, WASHED, TRIMMED, AND HALVED 210
1 T. VEGETABLE OIL 120
4 GARLIC CLOVES, MINCED 20
¼ tsp. SEA SALT Ø

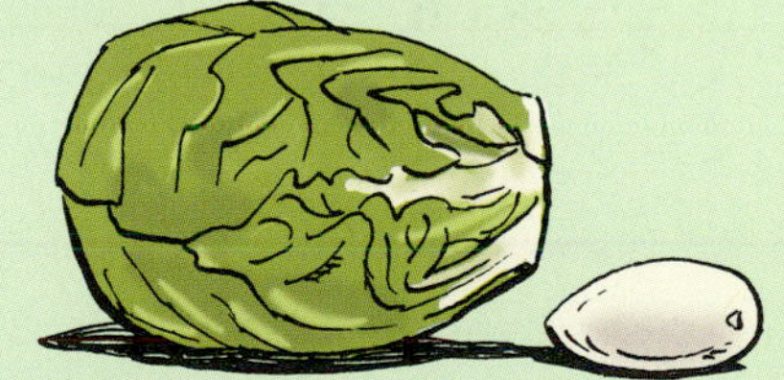

PREHEAT OVEN TO 400°F. MINCE GARLIC AND SET ASIDE.* TOSS SPROUTS WITH OIL IN LARGE BOWL. SPREAD EVENLY ON RIMMED BAKING SHEET AND ROAST FOR 10 MINUTES. REMOVE FROM OVEN AND SPRINKLE WITH GARLIC AND SALT. RETURN SPROUTS TO OVEN FOR 5 MINUTES. WHEN DONE, TRANSFER SPROUTS TO SERVING DISH AND SPRINKLE WITH ROASTED GARLIC REMAINING ON BAKING SHEET. MAKES 3 CUPS.

TOTAL PER ½-CUP SERVING: 60

* AFTER MINCING OR PRESSING RAW GARLIC, LET IT "BREATHE" FOR 15 MINUTES. THIS ALLOWS ENZYMES TO COMBINE FOR GREATER NUTRITIONAL PUNCH.

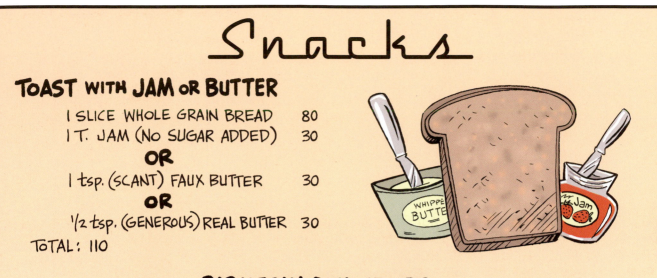

# Snacks

## TOAST WITH JAM OR BUTTER

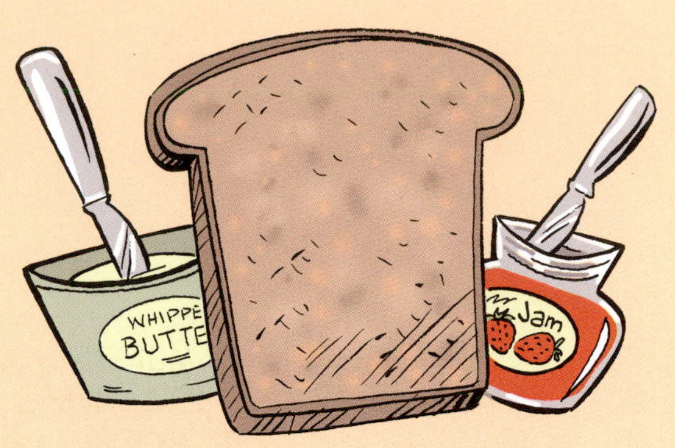


| | |
|---|---|
| 1 SLICE WHOLE GRAIN BREAD | 80 |
| 1 T. JAM (NO SUGAR ADDED) | 30 |
| **OR** | |
| 1 tsp. (SCANT) FAUX BUTTER | 30 |
| **OR** | |
| 1/2 tsp. (GENEROUS) REAL BUTTER | 30 |

TOTAL: 110

## PARMESAN PITA CRISPS

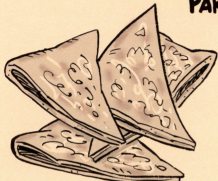

PREHEAT BROILER ON HIGH. SPRINKLE 1 T. GRATED PARMESAN CHEESE (60) OVER HALF OF A LARGE WHOLE WHEAT PITA BREAD (80 CALORIES IF THE WHOLE PITA IS 160). DUST WITH A GENEROUS PINCH OF DRIED OREGANO, PLACE ON OVEN-SAFE PAN, AND BROIL FOR 2 MINUTES OR UNTIL THE CHEESE BROWNS. CUT INTO WEDGES.

TOTAL: 140

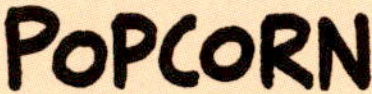

## POPCORN

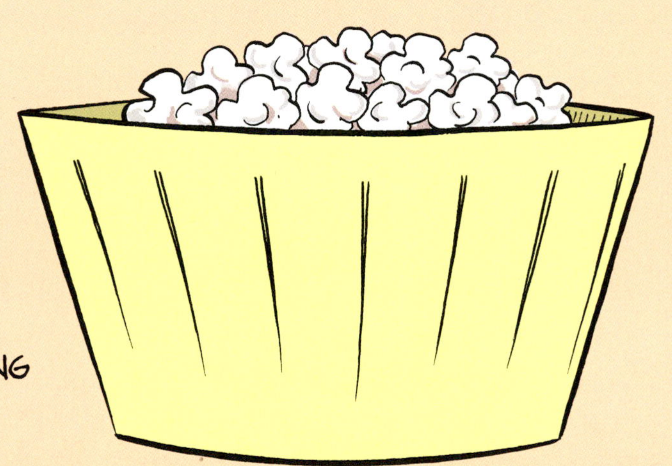

| | |
|---|---|
| 2 T. POPCORN KERNELS (MAKES 4 CUPS) | 120 |
| 2 tsp. FAUX BUTTER | 66 |
| GARLIC SALT OR REGULAR | Ø |

I USE AN AIR-POPPER SO I CAN AFFORD TO DRIZZLE ON A LITTLE BUTTER.

IT'S BEST TO STEER CLEAR OF MICROWAVE POPCORN — THE GASES PRODUCED BY NUKING CHEMICAL INGREDIENTS HAVE MADE MANY CONSUMERS ILL.

TOTAL: 190

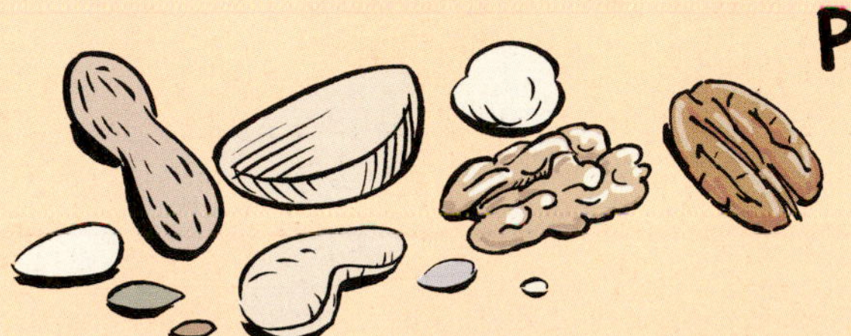

## PEANUTS, NUTS, AND SEEDS

SEE "CALORIE CHARTS" FOR TYPES AND TOTALS. NUTS AND SEEDS ARE A GREAT SOURCE OF PROTEIN AND BENEFIT HEART HEALTH. HOWEVER, I TRY TO LIMIT MY INTAKE TO A MODERATE 50-60 CALORIES A DAY.

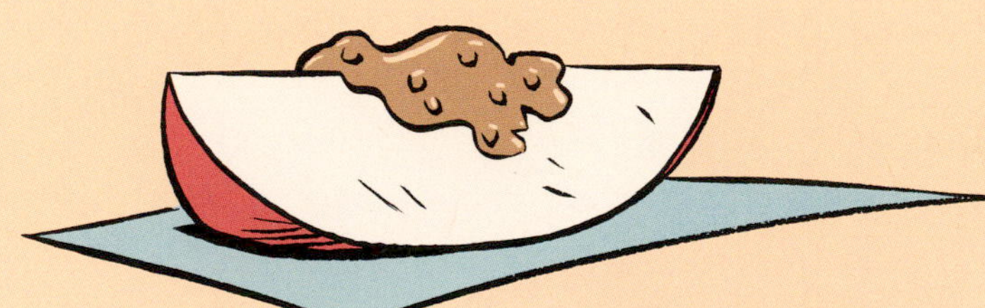

## APPLE WITH PEANUT BUTTER

| | |
|---|---|
| ½ APPLE | 40 |
| 1 T. PEANUT BUTTER | 120 |

TOTAL: 160

## ENGLISH MUFFIN WITH TURKEY BACON AND CHEESE

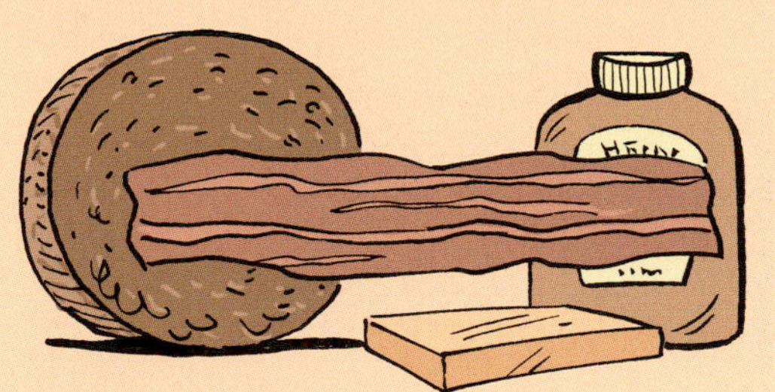

| | |
|---|---|
| ½ WHOLE-WHEAT ENGLISH MUFFIN | 80 |
| ½ OZ. REDUCED-FAT CHEDDAR CHEESE | 35 |
| 1 SLICE TURKEY BACON | 35 |
| 1 tsp. HONEY MUSTARD | 10 |

FRY BACON IN SKILLET OVER MEDIUM HEAT—NO OIL. LIGHTLY TOAST MUFFIN HALF. TOP WITH CHEESE AND BACON AND PLACE UNDER BROILER FOR 1 MINUTE OR UNTIL CHEESE MELTS. SMEAR WITH HONEY MUSTARD.

TOTAL: 160

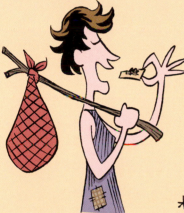

## OLIVE TAPENADE

THE POOR GAL'S CAVIAR—TASTES GREAT ON CRACKERS OR AS A GARNISH ON OMELETS OR SALADS.

| | |
|---|---|
| ½ CUP KALAMATA OLIVES, FINELY MINCED | 430 |
| 1 tsp. OLIVE OIL | 40 |
| 1½ tsp. LEMON JUICE | Ø |
| 1½ tsp. NUTRITIONAL YEAST* | 10 |
| 1 tsp. CAPERS | Ø |
| 1 GARLIC CLOVE, FINELY MINCED | 5 |

MAKES ½ CUP. TOTAL PER 1-tsp. SERVING: 20

*AVAILABLE IN BETTER MARKETS AND HEALTH FOOD STORES

## LEMONADE

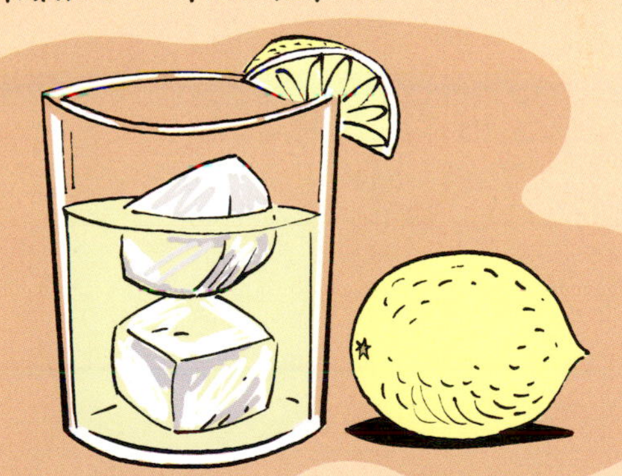

| | |
|---|---|
| 2 Tbsp. LEMON JUICE | 10 |
| 1 tsp. AGAVE NECTAR | 20 |
| SMALL SCOOP STEVIA | Ø |
| ⅔ CUP WATER | Ø |

MIX AND CHILL. TOTAL: 30

## GRILLED CHEESE SANDWICH, HALF

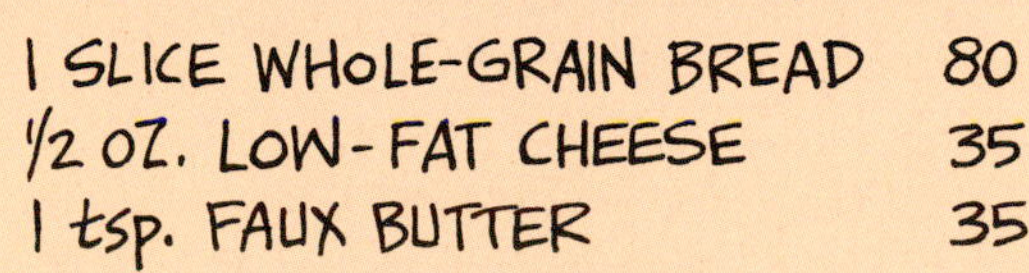

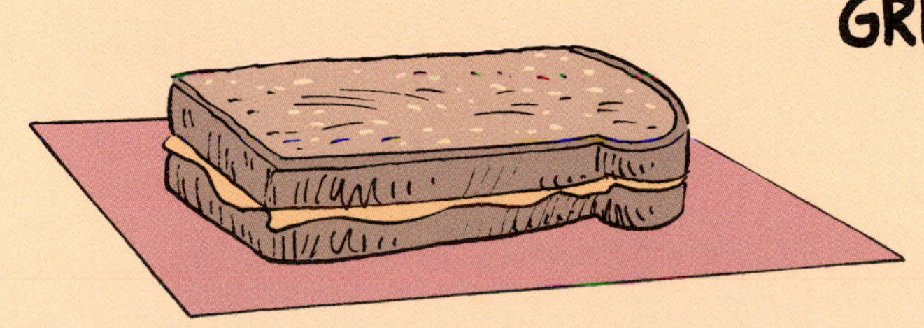

| | |
|---|---|
| 1 SLICE WHOLE-GRAIN BREAD | 80 |
| ½ OZ. LOW-FAT CHEESE | 35 |
| 1 tsp. FAUX BUTTER | 35 |

TOTAL: 150

## RAW VEGGIES WITH HUMMUS

| | |
|---|---|
| 1 CARROT | 35 |
| 4 STALKS CELERY | 30 |
| 3 WHITE MUSHROOMS | 5 |
| 1/4 SWEET RED PEPPER | 10 |
| 1/2 MEDIUM ZUCCHINI | 10 |
| 2 T. HUMMUS | 60 |

CUT UP, DIP, CHEW, REPEAT.

TOTAL: 150

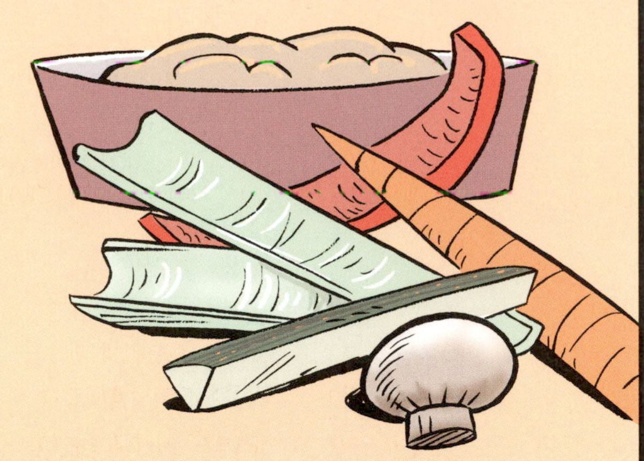

## RICE CAKE WITH EGG-WHITE SALAD

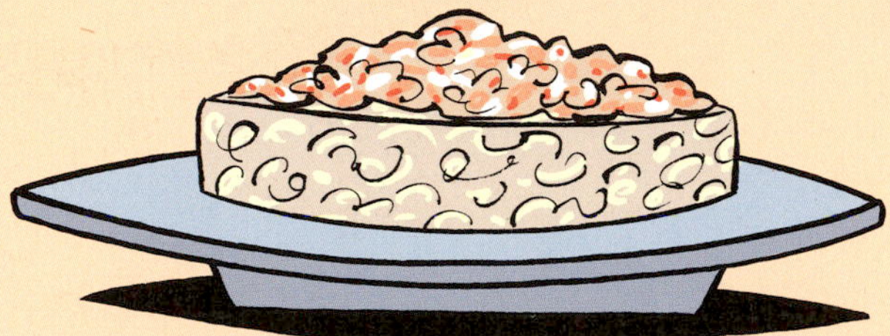

I USE TRADER JOE'S "SPICY RANCHERO EGG-WHITE SALAD" FOR THIS QUICK SNACK WITH CRUNCH AND PROTEIN.

| | |
|---|---|
| 1/4 CONTAINER (1 1/2 OZ.) EGG-WHITE SALAD | 25 |
| 1 RICE CAKE | 35 |

TOTAL: 60

## FRUITS

APPLE, BANANA, CHERRIES, DATES—SEE "FRUITS" PAGE IN "CALORIE CHARTS" FOR COLORFUL AND TASTY SNACKS.

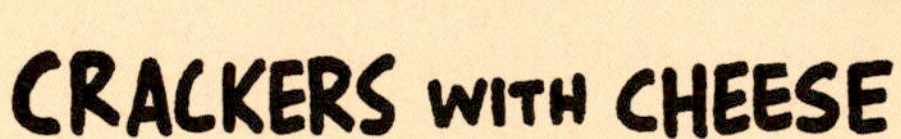

## SMOKED HERRING ON CRACKERS

| | |
|---|---|
| 2 RYE CRACKERS | 60 |
| 1 OZ. SMOKED HERRING | 60 |

TOTAL: 120

## CRACKERS WITH CHEESE

| | |
|---|---|
| 2 RYE CRACKERS | 60 |
| 1/2 OZ. LOW-FAT SWISS | 50 |

TOTAL: 110

| | |
|---|---|
| 2 MULTI-GRAIN CRACKERS | 70 |
| 1/2 OZ. REDUCED-FAT CHEDDAR | 35 |

TOTAL: 105

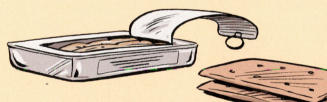

| | |
|---|---|
| 4 REDUCED-FAT WOVEN WHEAT CRACKERS* | 60 |
| 1/2 OZ. GOAT CHEESE | 40 |

TOTAL: 100

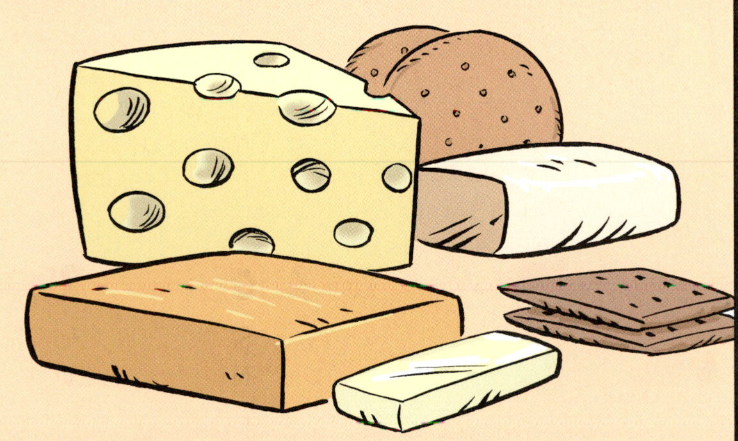

* LOOK FOR "WHOLE WHEAT" LISTED AS THE MAIN INGREDIENT— "WHEAT FLOUR" IS PLAIN OLD OVERPROCESSED WHITE FLOUR.

# Desserts

I LIKE SWEET THINGS. IDEALLY, I SHOULD KNOCK THEM OUT ENTIRELY, BUT THAT'S NO FUN AND IT WOULD MAKE IT HARDER FOR ME TO STICK TO MY GUNS. SO I LEAVE ROOM FOR DESSERT EVERY NIGHT, BUT I KEEP IT LIGHT. HERE ARE A FEW SUGGESTIONS:

## CINNAMON/APPLE TREAT

| | |
|---|---|
| 1/2 APPLE, PEELED, CORED, AND CHOPPED | 40 |
| 1/2 tsp. LEMON JUICE | Ø |
| DASH OF GROUND CINNAMON | Ø |

SPRINKLE CHOPPED APPLE WITH LEMON JUICE AND CINNAMON.

TOTAL: 40 (OR IT CAN VARY PER TYPE OF APPLE.)

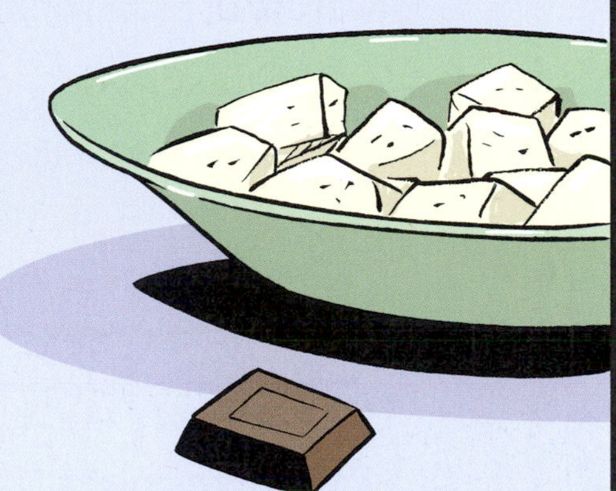

## SORBET AND FRUIT

MANY SORBETS COME IN AT ABOUT 100 PER 1/2-CUP SERVING. TOP WITH A HANDFUL OF RASPBERRIES, STRAWBERRIES, OR OTHER COMPATIBLE FRUIT.

TOTAL: 120

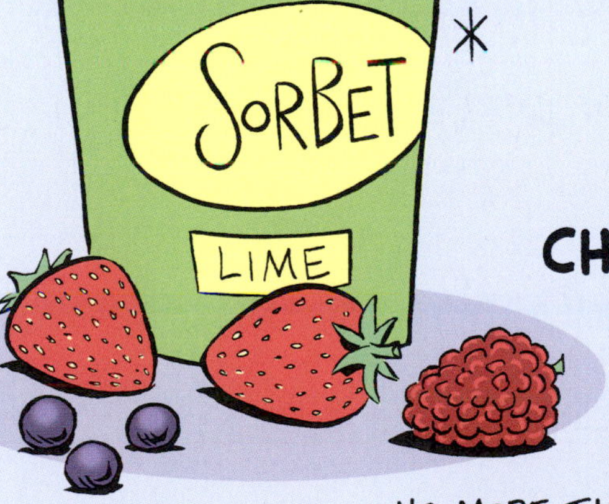


*

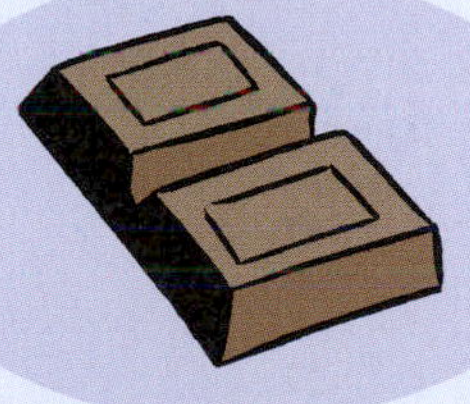

## CHOCOLATE

CHOCOLATE COMES IN ALL KINDS OF PACKAGES, SO FIND ONE YOU LIKE THAT CAN BE BROKEN INTO EASILY MEASURED PIECES. BUT NO MORE THAN 100 CALORIES PER DESSERT, PLEASE—SUGAR IS ADDICTING!

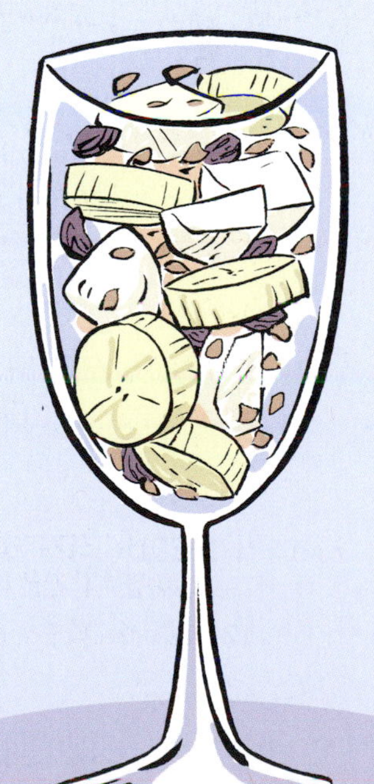

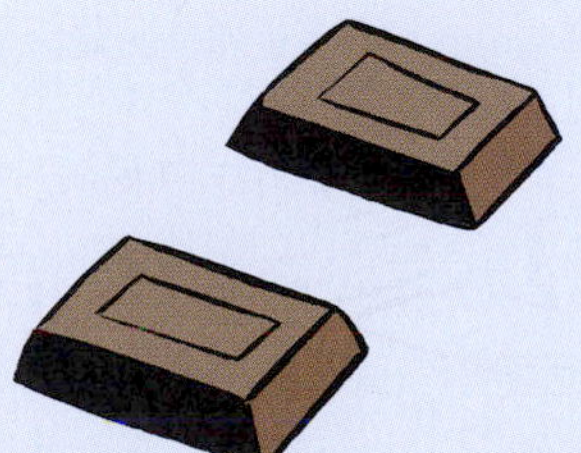

## GRANOLA ON FRUIT

| | |
|---|---|
| 1/3 BOSC PEAR, CHOPPED | 50 |
| 1/2 BANANA, SLICED | 50 |
| 2 T. GRANOLA | 50 |

TOTAL: 150

## CHEWY ALMOND MERINGUES

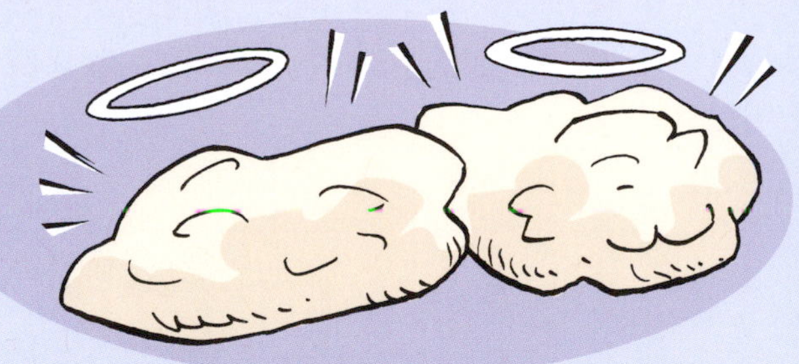

| | |
|---|---|
| 2 LARGE EGG WHITES | 35 |
| 3/4 CUP POWDERED SUGAR | 350 |
| 3/4 CUP BLANCHED SLIVERED ALMONDS | 635 |
| 1 1/2 T. FRESH LEMON JUICE | 10 |
| 1/4 tsp. CINNAMON | Ø |
| 2 (SEPARATE) BLASTS OF SPRAY OIL | 30 |

PREHEAT OVEN TO 300°F. LINE A COUPLE OF BAKING SHEETS WITH PARCHMENT PAPER AND SPRAY THE PAPER WITH OIL, LIGHTLY. (TRUST ME, THESE COOKIES WILL STICK LIKE GLUE TO A REGULAR OILED BAKING SHEET.) IN A LARGE BOWL, BEAT EGG WHITES UNTIL THEY FORM STIFF PEAKS, THEN GENTLY FOLD IN REMAINING INGREDIENTS. AT THIS POINT THE MERINGUE WILL LOSE STIFFNESS AND DEFLATE A BIT. DROP MERINGUE BY MOUNDED TABLESPOONFULS ONTO OILED SHEETS, ABOUT 1 1/2" APART, TO MAKE 16-18 COOKIES. BAKE 25 MINUTES, OR UNTIL COOKIE EDGES ARE GOLDEN. LET COOL COMPLETELY. LIFTING THE PARCHMENT, CAREFULLY "PEEL" COOKIES OFF PAPER AND ONTO TRAY. (CAN BE MADE A DAY IN ADVANCE — STORE IN AIRTIGHT CONTAINER.)

TOTAL PER COOKIE: 60

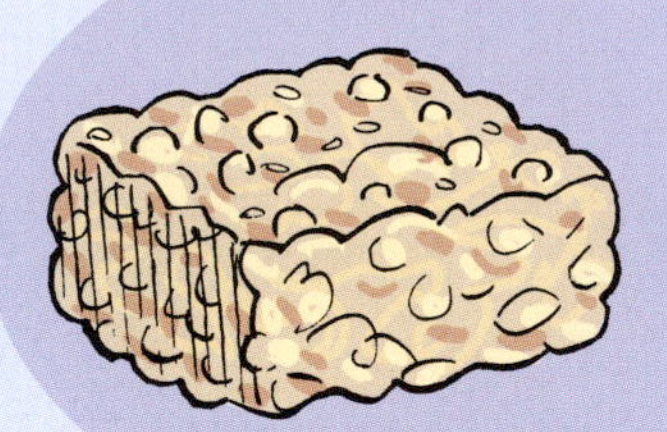

## PEANUT BUTTER NUTTY FRUIT BARS

(SEE "BREAKFASTS" FOR RECIPE.)

1/2 BAR IS PLENTY FOR A DESSERT — GOTTA WATCH THOSE SUGARS SO CLOSE TO BEDTIME.

TOTAL: 60

## PEANUT BUTTER OATMEAL COOKIES

| | |
|---|---|
| 1/2 CUP WHOLE WHEAT FLOUR | 220 |
| 1/2 CUP WHITE FLOUR | 220 |
| 1 1/3 CUP ROLLED OATS | 400 |
| 1 tsp. BAKING POWDER | Ø |
| 1/2 tsp. SALT | Ø |
| 3/8 CUP (1/4 CUP+2T.) CANOLA OIL | 720 |
| 3/8 CUP PEANUT BUTTER | 720 |
| 3/8 CUP AGAVE NECTAR OR HONEY | 360 |
| 1/2 CUP MAPLE SYRUP | 400 |
| 2 T. SOY MILK | 13 |
| 1 tsp. VANILLA EXTRACT | 12 |
| A SHORT BLAST OF SPRAY OIL | 15 |

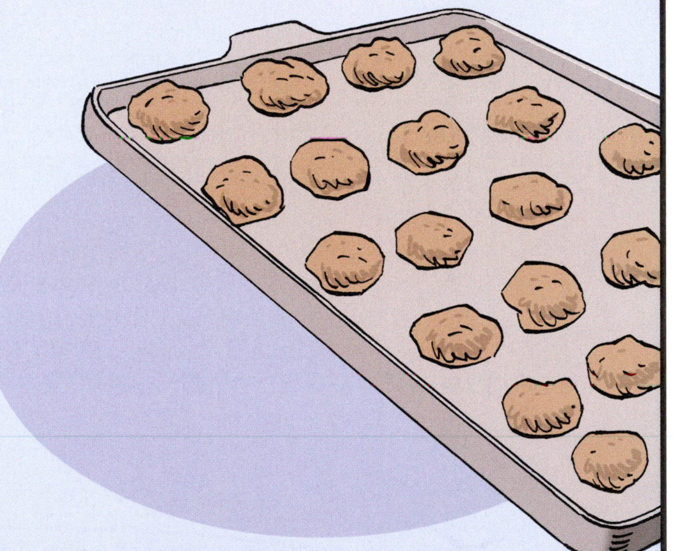

PREHEAT OVEN TO 350°F. USE A SHORT BLAST OF OIL TO GREASE A BAKING SHEET. MIX DRY INGREDIENTS TOGETHER IN LARGE BOWL; MIX WET INGREDIENTS IN ANOTHER BOWL. ADD WET MIXTURE TO DRY AND STIR UNTIL BLENDED EVENLY. SPOON DOLLOPS (ABOUT 1 1/2 T.) ONTO BAKING SHEET TO MAKE 30-32 COOKIES. BAKE FOR 10 MINUTES. COOL ON RACK.

TOTAL PER COOKIE: 100

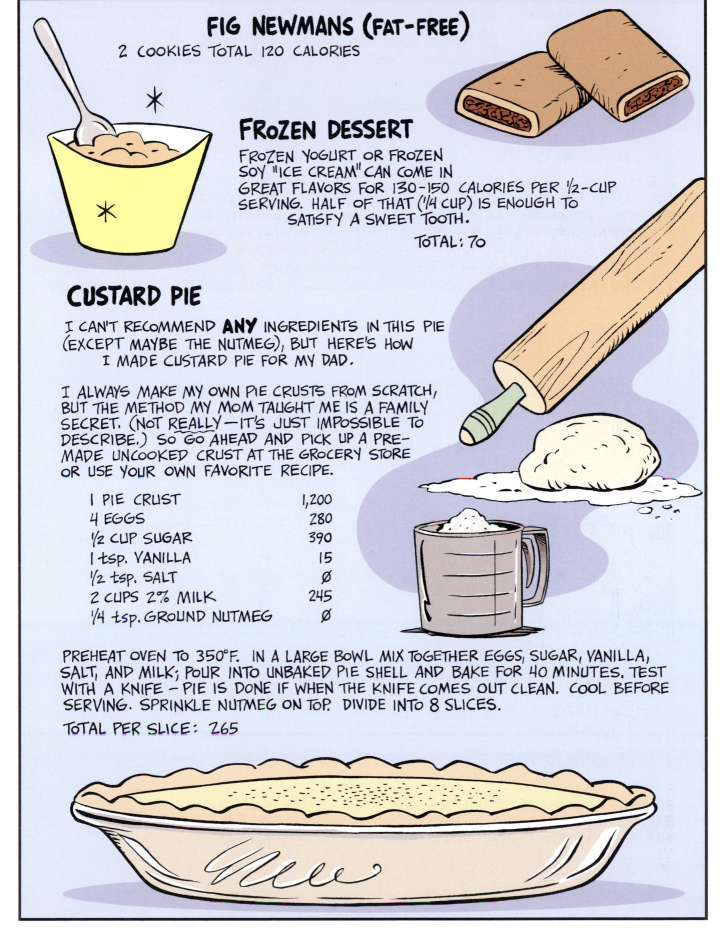

## FIG NEWMANS (FAT-FREE)

2 COOKIES TOTAL 120 CALORIES

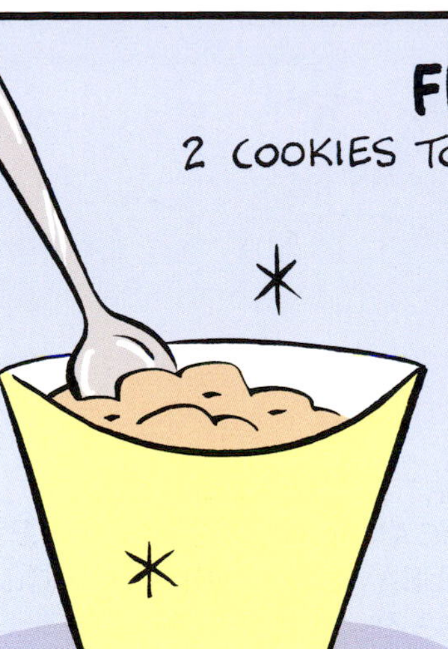

## FROZEN DESSERT

FROZEN YOGURT OR FROZEN SOY "ICE CREAM" CAN COME IN GREAT FLAVORS FOR 130-150 CALORIES PER 1/2-CUP SERVING. HALF OF THAT (1/4 CUP) IS ENOUGH TO SATISFY A SWEET TOOTH.

TOTAL: 70

## CUSTARD PIE

I CAN'T RECOMMEND **ANY** INGREDIENTS IN THIS PIE (EXCEPT MAYBE THE NUTMEG), BUT HERE'S HOW I MADE CUSTARD PIE FOR MY DAD.

I ALWAYS MAKE MY OWN PIE CRUSTS FROM SCRATCH, BUT THE METHOD MY MOM TAUGHT ME IS A FAMILY SECRET. (NOT REALLY—IT'S JUST IMPOSSIBLE TO DESCRIBE.) SO GO AHEAD AND PICK UP A PRE-MADE UNCOOKED CRUST AT THE GROCERY STORE OR USE YOUR OWN FAVORITE RECIPE.

| | |
|---|---|
| 1 PIE CRUST | 1,200 |
| 4 EGGS | 280 |
| 1/2 CUP SUGAR | 390 |
| 1 tsp. VANILLA | 15 |
| 1/2 tsp. SALT | Ø |
| 2 CUPS 2% MILK | 245 |
| 1/4 tsp. GROUND NUTMEG | Ø |

PREHEAT OVEN TO 350°F. IN A LARGE BOWL MIX TOGETHER EGGS, SUGAR, VANILLA, SALT, AND MILK; POUR INTO UNBAKED PIE SHELL AND BAKE FOR 40 MINUTES. TEST WITH A KNIFE – PIE IS DONE IF WHEN THE KNIFE COMES OUT CLEAN. COOL BEFORE SERVING. SPRINKLE NUTMEG ON TOP. DIVIDE INTO 8 SLICES.

TOTAL PER SLICE: 265

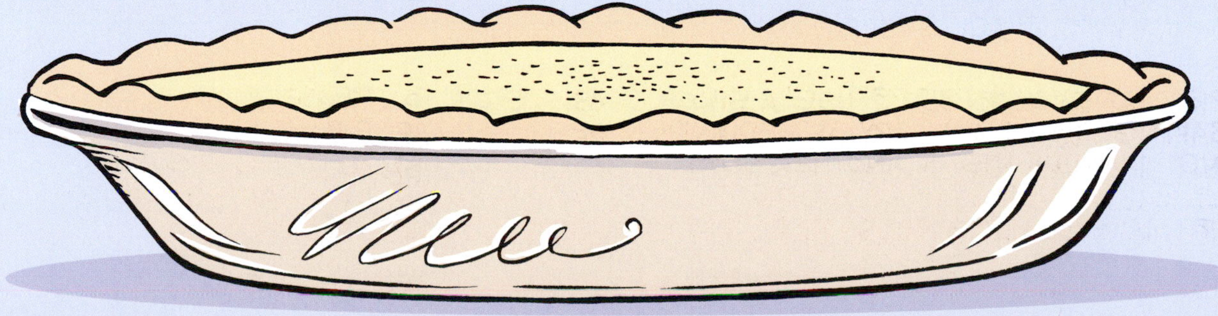

# Checklist

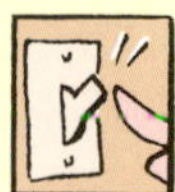

**MAKE A DECISION** TO CHANGE. WE'RE READY WHEN WE'RE READY, BUT WE MAY BE ABLE TO PREPARE OURSELVES FOR CHANGE BY REFLECTING ON HOW OLD BEHAVIORS NO LONGER WORK FOR US.

**WRITE** ABOUT WHY YOU WANT TO CHANGE AND WHAT THE BENEFITS MIGHT BE. WHAT ARE YOUR GOALS? ARE THEY REASONABLE AND ATTAINABLE? DO YOU WANT CHANGE SINCERELY ENOUGH TO DO THE FOOTWORK AND LEARN ABOUT YOURSELF AND NUTRITION?

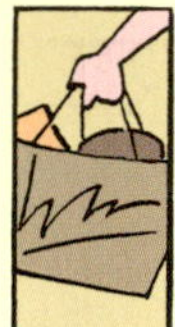

**BUY SOME TOOLS:** AN ACCURATE SCALE, A CALORIE GUIDE, GOOD WORKOUT SHOES, AND MEASURING CUPS ARE MUST-HAVES. OPTIONAL ITEMS INCLUDE A GYM MEMBERSHIP AND/OR TRAINING SESSIONS, WORKOUT CLOTHING, HOME EXERCISE EQUIPMENT, A KITCHEN SCALE (I ONLY RECENTLY BOUGHT ONE, AND I USE IT A LOT), A POCKET CALCULATOR, AND A BOOK OR TWO ON NUTRITION.

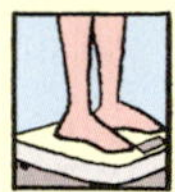

**WEIGH IN** TO FIND OUT WHERE YOU STAND, AND PLEDGE TO DO SO REGULARLY IN ORDER TO STAY OUT OF DENIAL. SUCCESSFUL LOSERS MAKE A HABIT OF KEEPING TRACK.

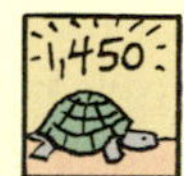


**DEFINE YOUR NUMBERS** BY LOOKING UP HOW MANY CALORIES A DAY WILL HELP YOU REACH YOUR IDEAL WEIGHT. REMEMBER THAT SLOW AND STEADY WEIGHT LOSS TENDS TO STICK BETTER.

**ASK FOR HELP** FROM FRIENDS, FAMILY, OR CO-WORKERS. OR KEEP YOUR DECISION TO CHANGE TO YOURSELF IF EXPERIENCE SHOWS THAT CERTAIN PEOPLE MAY NOT SUPPORT YOUR GOALS.

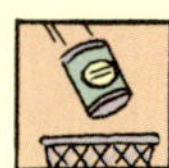

**THROW OUT** UNHEALTHY FOOD FROM YOUR PANTRY AND FRIDGE.

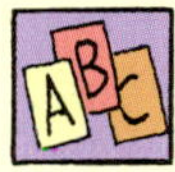


**DESIGN MEAL PLANS** FOR AT LEAST THE FIRST FEW DAYS—THIS WILL MAKE SHOPPING EASIER. ALSO, THERE'S COMFORT IN STRUCTURE WHEN TRYING SOMETHING NEW.

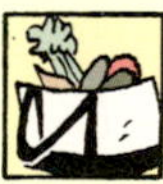

**STOCK UP** ON FRESH WHOLE FOODS. TRY NEW VEGETABLES OR GRAINS. THE MORE HEALTHFULLY YOU EAT, THE MORE YOUR BODY WILL CRAVE WHOLE FOODS.

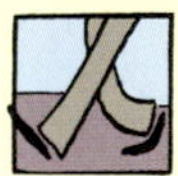

**START AN EXERCISE ROUTINE.** AT A MINIMUM, WALK FOR 20 MINUTES A DAY.

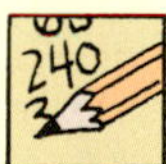


**KEEP TRACK OF CALORIES** THROUGHOUT THE DAY.

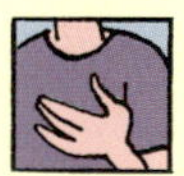

**STAY IN REALITY** BY BEING HONEST WITH YOURSELF.

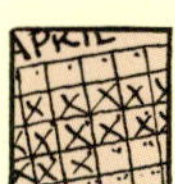

**STICK WITH THE PROGRAM FOR TWO WEEKS.** IF YOU LOSE RESOLVE, YOU'LL LEARN SOMETHING ABOUT FOOD AND YOUR EATING HABITS. YOU'LL ALSO KNOW WHAT TO DO WHEN YOU ARE TRULY READY TO MAKE A LIFELONG CHANGE.

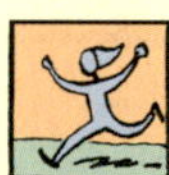

**ENJOY** YOUR LIFE, YOUR FRIENDS AND FAMILY, YOUR WORK AND PLAY, AND ALL THAT WHOLESOME FOOD!

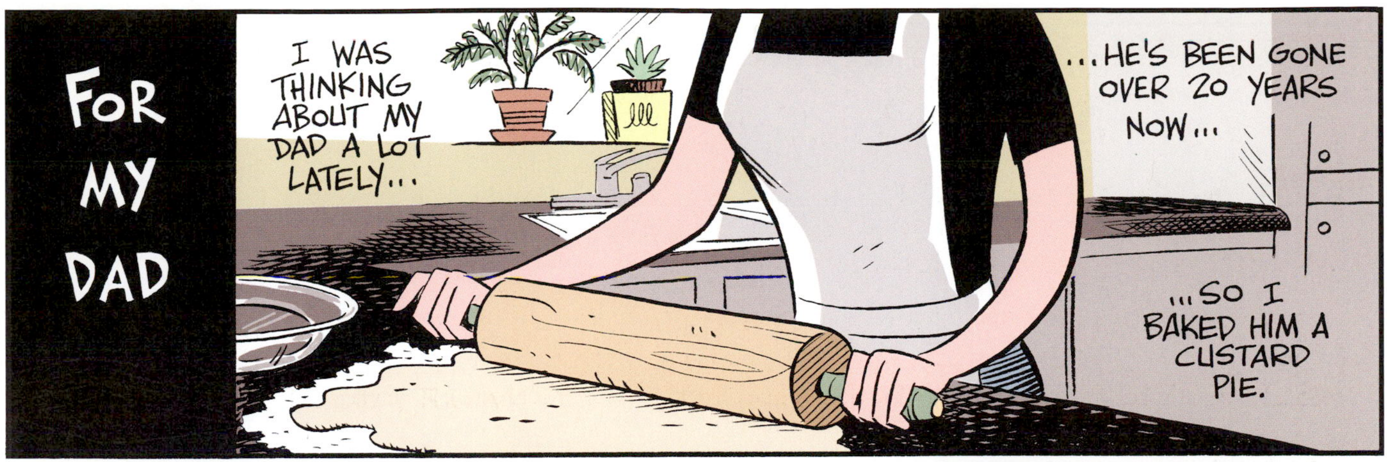
FOR MY DAD
I WAS THINKING ABOUT MY DAD A LOT LATELY...
...HE'S BEEN GONE OVER 20 YEARS NOW...
...SO I BAKED HIM A CUSTARD PIE.

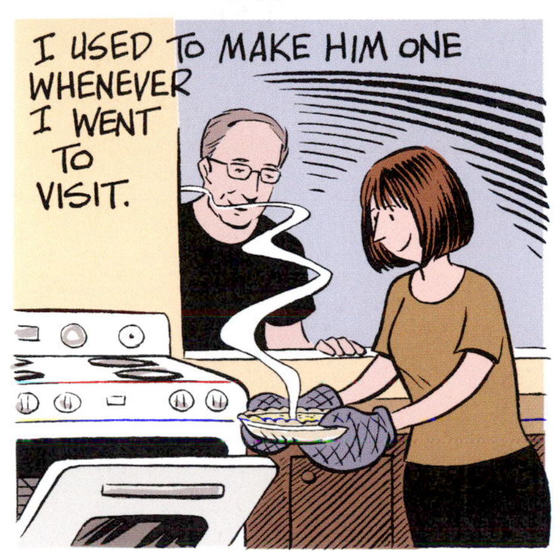
I USED TO MAKE HIM ONE WHENEVER I WENT TO VISIT.

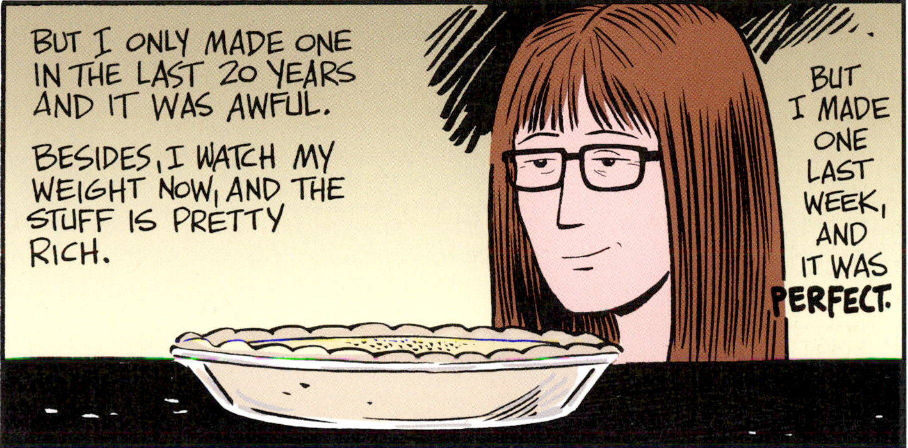
BUT I ONLY MADE ONE IN THE LAST 20 YEARS AND IT WAS AWFUL.
BESIDES, I WATCH MY WEIGHT NOW, AND THE STUFF IS PRETTY RICH.
BUT I MADE ONE LAST WEEK, AND IT WAS PERFECT.

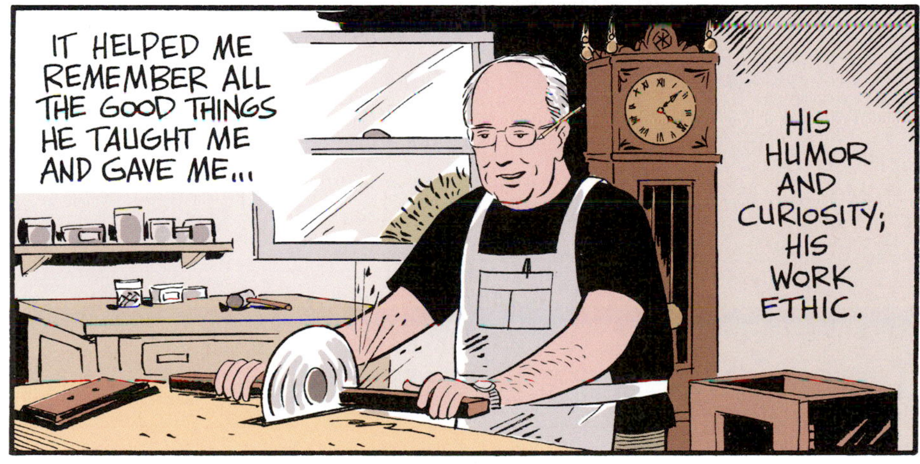
IT HELPED ME REMEMBER ALL THE GOOD THINGS HE TAUGHT ME AND GAVE ME...
HIS HUMOR AND CURIOSITY; HIS WORK ETHIC.

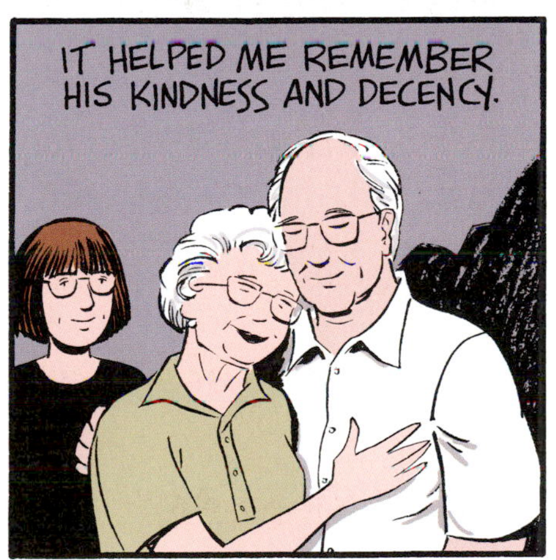
IT HELPED ME REMEMBER HIS KINDNESS AND DECENCY.

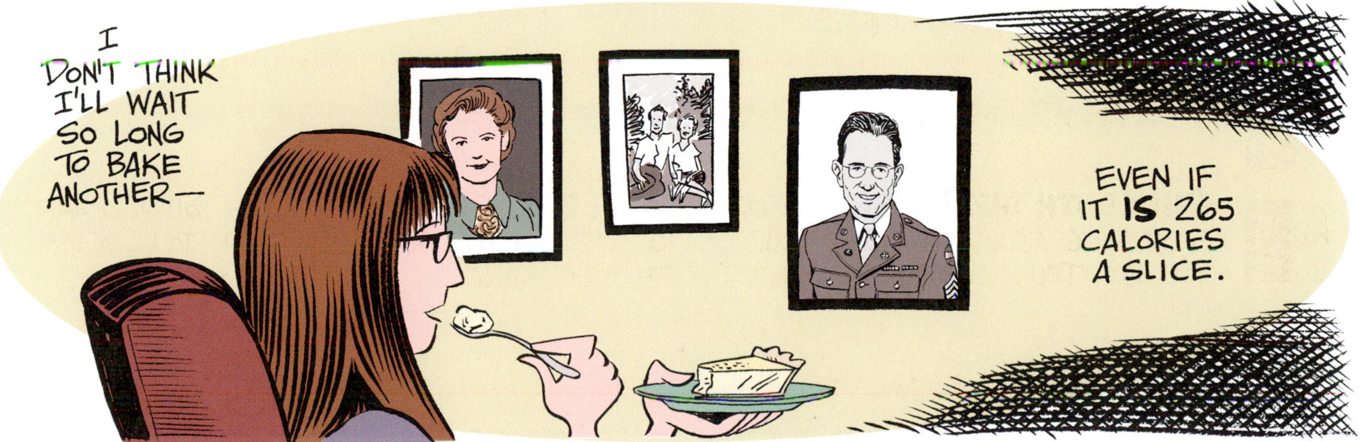
I DON'T THINK I'LL WAIT SO LONG TO BAKE ANOTHER—
EVEN IF IT IS 265 CALORIES A SLICE.

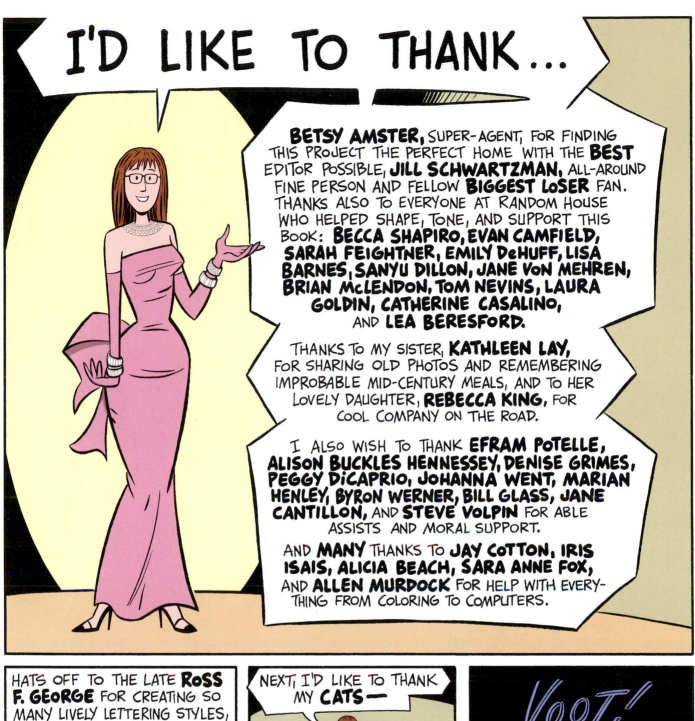

# I'D LIKE TO THANK...

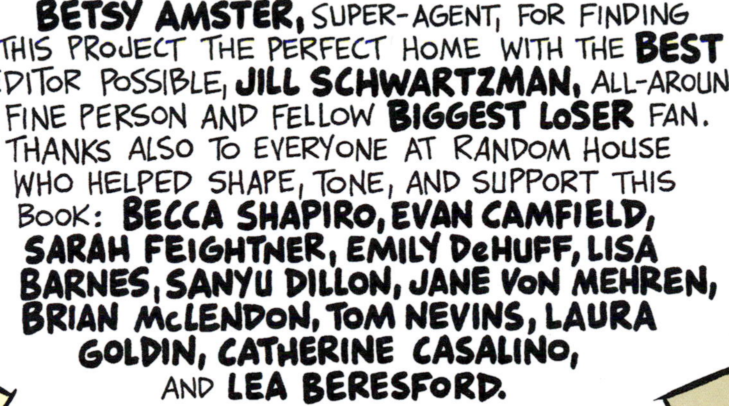

**BETSY AMSTER,** SUPER-AGENT, FOR FINDING THIS PROJECT THE PERFECT HOME WITH THE **BEST** EDITOR POSSIBLE, **JILL SCHWARTZMAN,** ALL-AROUND FINE PERSON AND FELLOW **BIGGEST LOSER** FAN. THANKS ALSO TO EVERYONE AT RANDOM HOUSE WHO HELPED SHAPE, TONE, AND SUPPORT THIS BOOK: **BECCA SHAPIRO, EVAN CAMFIELD, SARAH FEIGHTNER, EMILY DeHUFF, LISA BARNES, SANYU DILLON, JANE VON MEHREN, BRIAN McLENDON, TOM NEVINS, LAURA GOLDIN, CATHERINE CASALINO,** AND **LEA BERESFORD.**

THANKS TO MY SISTER, **KATHLEEN LAY,** FOR SHARING OLD PHOTOS AND REMEMBERING IMPROBABLE MID-CENTURY MEALS, AND TO HER LOVELY DAUGHTER, **REBECCA KING,** FOR COOL COMPANY ON THE ROAD.

I ALSO WISH TO THANK **EFRAM POTELLE, ALISON BUCKLES HENNESSEY, DENISE GRIMES, PEGGY DiCAPRIO, JOHANNA WENT, MARIAN HENLEY, BYRON WERNER, BILL GLASS, JANE CANTILLON,** AND **STEVE VOLPIN** FOR ABLE ASSISTS AND MORAL SUPPORT.

AND **MANY** THANKS TO **JAY COTTON, IRIS ISAIS, ALICIA BEACH, SARA ANNE FOX,** AND **ALLEN MURDOCK** FOR HELP WITH EVERYTHING FROM COLORING TO COMPUTERS.

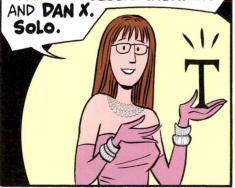

HATS OFF TO THE LATE **ROSS F. GEORGE** FOR CREATING SO MANY LIVELY LETTERING STYLES, AS WELL AS TO CURRENT TYPOGRAPHERS **LESLIE CABARGA** AND **DAN X. SOLO.**

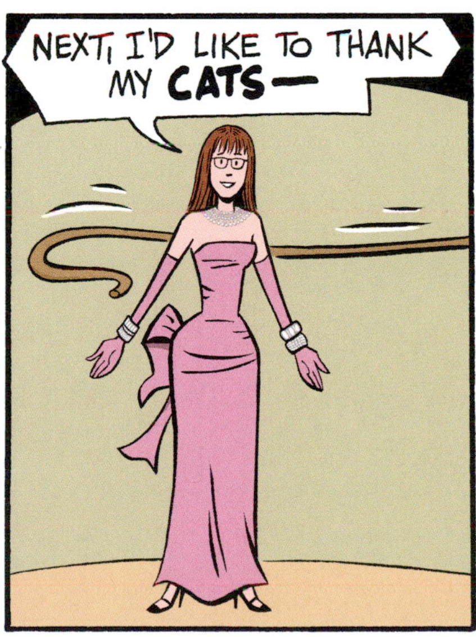
NEXT, I'D LIKE TO THANK MY CATS—

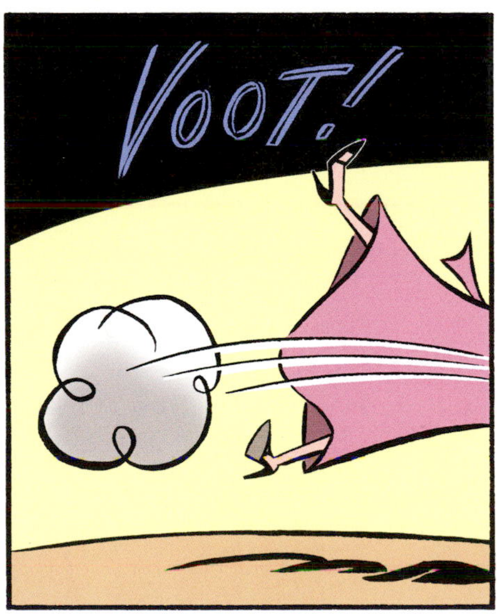
VOOT!

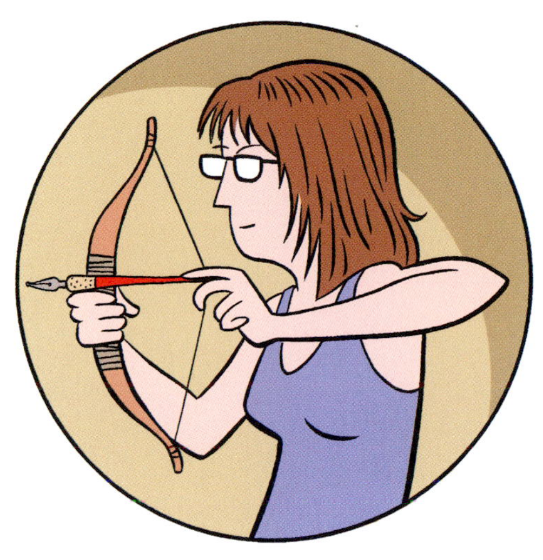

FOR 30-ODD YEARS **CAROL LAY** HAS BEEN DRAWING AND WRITING FOR BOOKS, FILMS, PERIODICALS, ANIMATION, AND—HER FIRST LOVE—COMICS. SHE CURRENTLY LIVES IN LOS ANGELES.
WWW.CAROLLAY.COM